A Guide to
Physical Examination
and History Taking

A Guide to
Physical

With a chapter on the
pediatric examination by

Robert A. Hoekelman, M.D.

Professor and Chairman, Department of Pediatrics
University of Rochester School of Medicine and Dentistry

Professor of Nursing
University of Rochester School of Nursing
Rochester, New York

and
a chapter on the **pregnant woman** by

Joyce E. (Beebe) Thompson, C.N.M.,

Dr.P.H., F.A.A.N.

Professor and Director
Graduate Program in Nurse-Midwifery
University of Pennsylvania School of Nursing
Philadelphia, Pennsylvania

Illustrations by
Susan Shapiro Brenman, M.S.
Medical Illustrator

Robert Wabnitz and Staff
University of Rochester School of Medicine

Examination
and History Taking
Fifth Edition

Barbara Bates, M.D.

Lecturer in Medicine, Department of Medicine
University of Pennsylvania School of Medicine

Lecturer in Nursing
University of Pennsylvania School of Nursing
Philadelphia, Pennsylvania

J.B. Lippincott Company   Philadelphia

Acquisitions Editor: Donna L. Hilton, R.N., B.S.N.
Coordinating Editorial Assistant: Barbara Nelson Cullen
Project Editor: Dina Kamilatos
Manuscript Editor: Mary Norris
Indexer: Katherine Pitcoff
Art Director: Ellen C. Dawson
Design Coordinator: Kathy Kelley-Luedtke
Production Manager: Caren Erlichman
Production Coordinator: Pamela Milcos
Compositor: Tapsco, Incorporated
Printer/Binder: R. R. Donnelley & Sons Company
Color Insert Printer: Southeastern Color Graphics, Inc.

5th Edition

6

Library of Congress Cataloging-in-Publication Data

Bates, Barbara
    A guide to physical examination and history taking/
Barbara Bates: with a chapter on the pediatric examination
by Robert A. Hoekelman and chapter on the pregnant
woman by Joyce E. Thompson: illustrations by Susan
Shapiro Brenman, Robert Wabnitz and staff, University of
Rochester School of Medicine.—5th ed.
        p.   cm.
    Includes bibliographical references.
    Includes index.
    ISBN 0-397-54781-1
    1. Physical diagnosis.   2. Medical history taking.
3. Children—Medical examinations.
I. Hoekelman, Robert A.   II. Thompson, Joyce
Beebe.   III. Title.
    [DNLM: 1. Physical Examination.   WB 205 B329g]
RC76.B37   1990
616.07'54—dc20
DNLM/DLC
for Library of Congress   90-13517
                                                CIP

Any procedure or practice described in this book should be applied by the health-care
practitioner under appropriate supervision in accordance with professional standards
of care used with regard to the unique circumstances that apply in each practice
situation. Care has been taken to confirm the accuracy of information presented and to
describe generally accepted practices. However, the authors, editors, and publisher
cannot accept any responsibility for errors or omissions or for any consequences from
application of the information in this book and make no warranty, express or implied,
with respect to the contents of the book.

Every effort has been made to ensure drug selections and dosages are in accordance
with current recommendations and practice. Because of ongoing research, changes in
government regulations and the constant flow of information on drug therapy,
reactions and interactions, the reader is cautioned to check the package insert for each
drug for indications, dosages, warnings and precautions, particularly if the drug is new
or infrequently used.

*To our readers and colleagues, whose
questions and suggestions have contributed so
much to the book and with whom we have
enjoyed an interprofessional dialogue*

Acknowledgments

Many people have contributed to this book and we are pleased to thank them publicly. For their knowledge, suggestions, and advice, we are grateful to Edward C. Atwater, M.D., Michael J. Barrett, M.D., Frank P. Brooks, M.D., Sc.D., Michael M. Cohen, M.D., Alicia M. Connill, M.D., Lois K. Evans, D.N.Sc., F.A.A.N., David M. Kozart, M.D., Margaret L. Lancefield, M.D, Ph.D., Sal Mangione, M.D., and Cathy Stevenson, M.S.N., R.N. Shelley Schuler, M.D., reviewed Chapter 6, "The Skin," and selected, titled, and labeled most of its new photographs.

It remains a pleasure to work with a team of people who care about the quality of their work. Susan Shapiro Brenman, M.S., medical illustrator, has again created the new art. Art Siegel, director of the Biomedical Communications Facility, School of Medicine, University of Pennsylvania, has taken all but one of the new photographs. Mary Norris, manuscript editor, again improved the style and organization of the text.

For Chapter 19, Sydney Sutherland provided editorial assistance and Tamera Davies prepared the manuscript.

Contents

List of Color Plates and Tables

Color Plates

Tables

Chapter 2
An Approach to Symptoms

Color tabs identify tables at the end of respective chapters

2

3

6

7

8

9

10

11

12

13

14

15

16

17

18

19

Introduction

A Guide to Physical Examination and History Taking is designed for students in health care who are learning to talk with patients, to examine them, and to understand and assess their problems. The first three chapters deal with interviewing and the health history, common and important symptoms, and the assessment of mental status. Then, in chapters devoted to body regions or body systems, the book reviews the relevant anatomy and physiology, describes the sequence and techniques of physical examination, and helps the student to identify selected abnormalities. Two final chapters deal with clinical thinking and organizing the patient's record.

We assume that the learners have had basic courses in human anatomy and physiology. The anatomical and physiological sections in this book are designed to help students apply their knowledge to interpreting symptoms, examining the human body, and understanding physical signs.

Throughout the book we have tried to emphasize common or important problems, rather than the infrequent or esoteric. Occasionally a physical sign has been included despite its rarity because it enjoys a solid niche in classic physical diagnosis, or because recognizing the abnormality is especially important for the health or even the life of the patient.

We assume that students will learn their examination skills by practicing first on other adults. Most of the anatomy and physiology, some of the techniques, and many of the abnormalities are common to both adults and children. Dr. Hoekelman's chapter on the examination of infants and children describes variations that occur in the younger age groups together with signs or conditions that are unique to them.

THE FIFTH EDITION

In the fifth edition, we welcome a new contributor, Joyce E. (Beebe) Thompson, C.N.M., Dr.P.H., F.A.A.N., author of a new chapter on "The Pregnant Woman." Like other chapters on the physical examination, this one includes anatomy, physiology, techniques, and common abnormalities; it also deals with some of the relevant history. Dr. Thompson focuses chiefly on early pregnancy and the information important to a provider of primary care.

Another major change is the addition of color illustrations in two chapters where color has the most relevance: the skin and the peripheral vascular system. Illustrations have been improved or added in other chapters also, especially in Chapter 10, "The Breasts and Axillae," Chapter 11, "The Abdomen," Chapter 13, "Female Genitalia," and Chapter 15, "The Anus, Rectum, and Prostate."

Chapters on mental status, the thorax and lungs, the cardiovascular system, the peripheral vascular system, and the nervous system have been substantially revised or reorganized. Throughout the book, we have tried to update the text and further clarify difficult topics. Judicious pruning and consolidation have helped to keep the book from growing too much.

Despite these changes, we have retained our basic format. Students may study or review the anatomy and physiology sections according to their individual needs. From the sections on techniques and with faculty guidance, they can learn how to do an examination and then review the methods as necessary after practice. Abnormalities described or illustrated in the right-hand column of the sections on techniques help the student to compare abnormal findings with the normal. Tables that follow these sections help the learner to compare and contrast common abnormalities. These tables also serve as subsequent references.

SUGGESTIONS FOR USING THE BOOK

Although a health history and a physical examination have somewhat similar goals in patient care, students often learn them separately, even from different faculty members. Nevertheless, interconnections should be made between them. We suggest that, as students learn successive parts of the physical examination, they also read the relevant sections in Chapter 2, "An Approach to Symptoms." In a few areas, the history and the examination do not quite match. Symptoms described under "The Chest" pertain to the chapters on both the thorax and lungs and the cardiovascular system. The symptoms of the urinary tract, moreover, relate unavoidably to chapters on the abdomen, the anus, rectum, and prostate, and both male and female genitalia.

As students proceed through the body systems and regions, they should refer periodically to Chapter 4, "Physical Examination: Approach and Overview," and to Chapter 21, "The Patient's Record." They can thereby place their newly learned techniques in the sequence of both doing a comprehensive examination and describing it. A review of Chapter 20, "Clinical Thinking: From Data to Plan," will help them to select and analyze the data that they are learning to collect.

Skimming the tables of abnormalities serves to familiarize students with what they should be looking for and why they are asking certain questions. They should not, however, try to memorize the details that are presented there. The best time to learn about abnormalities and diseases is when a patient (real or described) appears with a problem. The student should then try to analyze the problem with this book and pursue the subject as necessary in other relevant clinical texts.

RELATED LEARNING MATERIAL

A Pocket Guide to Physical Examination and History Taking by Barbara Bates and Robert A. Hoekelman is an abbreviated version of this text, designed for portability, review, and convenience. This pocket guide does not stand alone; reference to the text and illustrations of *A Guide to Physical Examination and History Taking* is required for a more comprehensive study and understanding of these subjects.

EQUIPMENT

Equipment necessary for a physical examination includes the following:

An ophthalmoscope and an otoscope (The latter should have appropriate specula for the ears and ideally a short, wide [9 mm] nasal speculum, with magnification, for the nose. See note on page 189.)
A flashlight
Tongue depressors
A ruler and flexible tape measure, preferably marked in centimeters
A thermometer
A watch with a second hand
A sphygmomanometer
A stethoscope with the following characteristics:
- Ear tips that fit snugly and painlessly. To get this fit, choose ear tips of the proper size, align the ear pieces with the angle of your ear canals, and adjust the spring of the connecting metal band to a comfortable tightness.
- Thick-walled tubing as short as feasible to maximize the transmission of sound: about 30 cm (12 inches) if possible and no longer than 38 cm (15 inches)
- A bell and a diaphragm with a good changeover mechanism

Gloves ⎤
Lubricant ⎦ For vaginal and rectal examination

Vaginal specula and equipment for cytological and perhaps bacterio-
   logical study
A reflex hammer
Tuning forks, ideally one of 128 Hz and one of 512 Hz
Safety pins
Cotton
Two test tubes (needed only for selected neurologic examinations)
Paper and pen or pencil

Chapter 1
Interviewing and the Health History

Barbara Bates and Robert A. Hoekelman

The purposes of this chapter are (1) to introduce the concepts of disease and illness, (2) to describe the structure, purposes, and content of the health history, (3) to review the principles and methods of interviewing, and (4) to suggest some ways to talk with patients of different ages and to deal with special situations and problems.

DISEASE AND ILLNESS

"EVERY MAN is
   . . . like all other men,
   . . . like some other men,
   . . . like no other man."*

Symptoms identified by taking a history provide some of the most important items of information used in the process of diagnosing a *disease* —the label that designates the medical understanding of a biologic or psychologic abnormality. Patients recognize and report symptoms, and clinicians translate them into technical terms, group them, analyze them, and make tentative hypotheses about the bodily structures and processes most likely involved in causing them. Symptoms guide the focus and extent of the physical examination and laboratory investigation. Ultimately, the clinician uses data from all these sources to determine the patient's disease or other disorder and to initiate appropriate treatment.

When patients describe the symptoms for which they are seeking professional attention, they are also reporting the story of an *illness* as they

* Kluckhohn C, Murray HA: Personality in Nature, Society, and Culture, p 35. New York, Alfred A. Knopf, 1948.

have lived and remembered it. To some extent, symptoms are a universal human experience. Virtually every person may feel pain, weakness, nausea, or shortness of breath. The meaning of symptoms to that person, however, varies with many factors such as age, socioeconomic status, religion, and ethnic background. Groups of people tend to share a set of meanings common to their culture. For some groups, pain may be the will of God or divine punishment. For others, it is a natural part of life to be borne with little complaint, and for still others it is a sensation for which the proper pill or procedure should give prompt relief. Even within homogeneous groups of people, however, a symptom or an illness often has unique personal meanings that affect an individual's self-image, aspirations, and social relationships. The symptoms themselves, the cultural meanings attributed to them, and the unique personal meanings all contribute to your understanding of patients, and your skills in taking a history should become sufficiently flexible and sensitive to encompass them all.

In addition to enabling you to learn about a person's illness and to gather data with which to diagnose disease, talking with a patient has a third function: it helps that person to feel that he or she is understood, and it thereby helps to establish a therapeutic relationship. A style of questioning narrowly shaped for the sole purpose of diagnosing disease ignores much of what patients have experienced and many of their concerns and questions. It therefore often prevents the development of a trusting relationship, inhibits the patient's willingness to confide further in the practitioner, and diminishes the chances of helping the patient. Even with technically competent health care, patients may leave the hospital or office dissatisfied. "She didn't seem to understand what I was trying to tell her." "He said the pain wasn't cancer, but I knew that already from the mammogram. What does my pain mean? Will it get worse? Will it ever go away?" "All they seem to care about is my wheezing. What about me?"

Talking with a patient about the experience of being ill, on the other hand, can have great value even when nothing can be done about the disease. In the example that follows, research protocol made the patient ineligible for treatment of her long-standing and severe arthritis.

She had never talked about what the symptoms meant to her. She had never said: "This means that I can't go to the bathroom by myself, put my clothes on, even get out of bed without calling for help."

When we finished [the physical assessment] I said something like: "Rheumatoid arthritis really has not been nice to you." She burst into tears, and her daughter did also, and I sat there, very close to losing it myself.

She said: "You know, no one has ever talked about it as a personal thing before, no one's ever talked to me as if this were a thing that mattered, a personal event.

That was the significant thing about the encounter. I didn't really have much else to offer. . . . Something really significant had happened between us, something that she valued and would carry away with her.*

Understanding of illness can come from several sources, the most important of which are the patients themselves. Answers to questions in the "Present Illness" (p. 5) and the "Psychosocial History" (p. 7) are especially relevant. By listening carefully to the patient and by trying to put yourself into the situation described, you can sometimes imagine what it might be like to have a paralyzed leg or chronic diarrhea, for example, or to be raising two children, one of them sick, on a minimum wage. You can then inquire about how the person deals with certain activities or situations that would probably be difficult. Both clinical experience and reading should broaden your knowledge of groups of people different from those you already know, and you can gradually expand your more general insights.

Generalizations based on ethnic group, sex, race, class, and other variables are sometimes useful in making tentative hypotheses about a person's life and experience of illness. To some extent, rich people differ from poor people, men from women, blacks from whites, immigrants from the native-born, the old from the young, the fat from the thin, heavy drinkers from abstainers, and college graduates from those who left school after the tenth grade. The skillful use of such generalizations may lead to questions that give you important knowledge about a patient's illness, treatments, personal problems, strengths, burdens, and options. Moreover, the prevalence of certain diseases varies with most of these factors. Generalizations, however, easily lead to stereotypes that preclude the very understanding that you are seeking. Within each group there are subgroups, within each subgroup there are diverse individuals. Generalizations should be used as carefully selected and provisional hypotheses, not as assumptions or conclusions.

THE STRUCTURE AND PURPOSES OF A HEALTH HISTORY

The traditional health history has several parts, each with a specific purpose. Together they give structure to your data collection and to your final record, but they do not dictate the exact sequence of the interview. Certain introductory materials in the health history typically precede the account of the patient's story. The *date* is always important, and in rapidly changing circumstances the time should be added. *Identifying data,* such as age, sex, race or ethnic origin, birthplace, and occupation, serve not only to establish who the patient is but also to give you some tentative suggestions as to what kind of person you are talking to and

* Hastings C: The lived experience of the illness: Making contact with the patient. In Benner P, Wrubel J: The Primacy of Caring: Stress and Coping in Health and Illness, p 11. Menlo Park, CA, Addison-Wesley, 1989.

even what the likely problems might be. When patients do not initiate their own visits, the *source of referral* becomes important. It indicates that a written report may be necessary, and it helps you to understand the patient's possible motivations. Persons seen at the request of school authorities or an insurance company may have different goals than those who come on their own initiative. The *source of the history*, whether it be the patient, family, friends, police, a letter of referral, or the past medical record, also deserves comment. It helps you to assess the value and possible biases of the information. Under some circumstances it is also helpful to comment on the probable *reliability* of the source of your data. Reliability varies with knowledge, memory, trust, and motivation, among other factors, and is a judgment made at the end of the interaction, not at the beginning.

The main part of the history starts with the patient's *chief complaints*. These are the one or more symptoms or other concerns for which the patient is seeking care or advice. The *present illness* amplifies the chief complaints and gives a full, clear, chronological account of how each of the symptoms developed and what events were related to them. It also includes how the patient thinks and feels about the illness, what concerns have led to seeking attention, and how the illness has affected the patient's life and functions. The *past history* explores prior illnesses, injuries, and medical interventions, while the *current health status* focuses on the present state of health and on environmental conditions, personal habits, and health-related measures that may impinge on it.

The *family history* helps you to assess the patient's risks of developing certain diseases and may also suggest what the patient might be worrying about. Further, a pattern of familial illness may emerge that will prove useful in the care of related persons. The *psychosocial history* sometimes suggests some contributory factors in the patient's illness and helps you to evaluate the patient's sources of support, likely reactions to illness, coping mechanisms, strengths, and concerns. It helps you in getting to know your patient as a person. In the *review of systems* you ask about common symptoms in each major body system and thus try to identify problems that the patient has not mentioned.

THE CONTENT OF A COMPREHENSIVE HISTORY

The items in a comprehensive history necessarily vary with the patient's age, sex, and illness, with the clinician's specialty and available time, and with the goals of the visit. Under many circumstances the clinician's efforts are targeted on a specific complaint, such as a sore throat or burning on urination. A limited approach, tailored to the problem, is then indicated. In other circumstances, however, a comprehensive history is needed. By learning and understanding all the items in such a history you can use them to the best advantage, either all together or in clusters, depending on the situation. Two patterns of such a comprehensive history are detailed in the next few pages: one for adults, the other for children. Technical terms for symptoms appear in these histories. Definitions of these terms, together with ways to ask about the symptoms, are included in Chapter 2.

COMPREHENSIVE HISTORY: ADULT PATIENT

DATE OF HISTORY

IDENTIFYING DATA, including age, sex, race, place of birth, marital status, occupation, and religion

SOURCE OF REFERRAL, if any, and the purpose of it

SOURCE OF HISTORY, such as the patient, a relative, a friend, the patient's medical record, or a referral letter

RELIABILITY, if relevant

CHIEF COMPLAINTS, when possible in the patient's own words. "My stomach hurts and I feel awful." Sometimes patients have no overt complaints; ascertain their goals instead. "I have come for my regular checkup" or "I've been admitted for a thorough evaluation of my heart."

PRESENT ILLNESS. This is a clear, chronological narrative account of the problems for which the patient is seeking care. It should include the onset of the problem, the setting in which it developed, its manifestations, and any past treatments. The principal symptoms should be described in terms of (1) location, (2) quality, (3) quantity or severity, (4) timing (*i.e.*, onset, duration, and frequency), (5) the setting in which they occur, (6) factors that have aggravated or relieved them, and (7) associated manifestations. Relevant data from the patient's chart, such as laboratory reports, also belong in the present illness, as do significant negatives (*i.e.*, the absence of certain symptoms that will aid in differential diagnosis).

A present illness should also include patients' responses to their own symptoms and incapacities. What does the patient think has caused the problem? What are the underlying worries that have led to seeking professional attention? ("I think I may have appendicitis.") And why is that a worry? ("My Uncle Charlie died of a ruptured appendix.") Further, what effects has the illness had on the patient's life? This question is especially important in understanding a patient with chronic illness. "What can't you do now that you could do before? How has the backache, shortness of breath, or whatever, affected your ability to work? . . . your life at home? . . . your social activities? . . . your role as a parent? . . . your role as a husband, or wife? . . . the way you feel about yourself as a man, or a woman?"

PAST HISTORY

General State of Health as the patient perceives it

Childhood Illnesses, such as measles, rubella, mumps, whooping cough, chicken pox, rheumatic fever, scarlet fever, polio

Adult Illnesses

Psychiatric Illnesses

Accidents and Injuries

Operations

Hospitalizations not already described

CURRENT HEALTH STATUS. Although some of the variables grouped under this heading have past as well as current components, they all have potential impact on current health and possible health-related interventions.

Allergies

Immunizations, such as tetanus, pertussis, diphtheria, polio, measles, rubella, mumps, influenza, hepatitis B, *Hemophilus influenzae,* type b, and pneumococcal vaccine

Screening Tests appropriate to the patient's age, such as hematocrits, urinalyses, tuberculin tests, Pap smears, mammograms, stools for occult blood, and cholesterol tests, together with the results and the dates they were last performed

Environmental Hazards, including those in the home, school, and workplace

Use of Safety Measures, such as seat belts and other methods related to specific hazards

Exercise and Leisure Activities

Sleep Patterns, including times that the person goes to bed and awakens, daytime naps, and any difficulties in falling asleep or staying asleep

Diet, including all the dietary intake for a recent 24-hour period, and any dietary restrictions or supplements. Be specific in your questions. "Take yesterday, for example. Starting from when you woke up, what did you eat or drink first? . . . then what? . . . and then?" Ask specifically about coffee, tea, cola drinks, and other caffeine-containing beverages.

Current Medications, including home remedies, nonprescription drugs, vitamin/mineral supplements, and medicines borrowed from family or friends. When a patient seems likely to be taking one or more medications, survey one 24-hour period in detail. "Let's look at yesterday. Starting from when you woke up, what was the first medicine you took? How much? How often in the day did you take it? What are you taking it for? What other medicines . . . ?"

Tobacco, including the type (smoked, *e.g.,* cigarettes, or smokeless, *e.g.,* chewing tobacco or snuff), amount, and duration of use, *e.g.,* cigarettes, a pack a day for 12 years

Alcohol, Drugs, and Related Substances. See pp. 20–21 for suggested methods of inquiry.

FAMILY HISTORY

The age and health, or age and cause of death, of each immediate family member (*i.e.,* parents, siblings, spouse, and children). Data on grandparents or grandchildren may also be useful.

The occurrence within the family of any of the following conditions: diabetes, tuberculosis, heart disease, high blood pressure, stroke, kidney disease, cancer, arthritis, anemia, headaches, epilepsy, mental illness, alcoholism, drug addiction, and symptoms like those of the patient.

PSYCHOSOCIAL HISTORY. This is an outline or narrative description that captures the important and relevant information about the patient as a person:

Home Situation and Significant Others. "Who lives at home with you? Tell me a little about them . . . and about your friends." "Who helps you when you are sick, or need assistance?"

Daily Life, from the time of arising to bedtime. "What is a typical day like? What do you do first? . . . Next?"

Important Experiences, including upbringing, schooling, military service, job history, financial situation, marriage, recreation, retirement

Religious Beliefs relevant to perceptions of health, illness, and treatment

The Patient's Outlook on the present and on the future

REVIEW OF SYSTEMS

General. Usual weight, recent weight change, any clothes that fit tighter or looser than before. Weakness, fatigue, fever

Skin. Rashes, lumps, sores, itching, dryness, color change, changes in hair or nails

Head. Headache, head injury

Eyes. Vision, glasses or contact lenses, last eye examination, pain, redness, excessive tearing, double vision, blurred vision, spots or specks, glaucoma, cataracts

Ears. Hearing, tinnitus, vertigo, earaches, infection, discharge. If hearing is decreased, use of hearing aids

Nose and Sinuses. Frequent colds; nasal stuffiness, discharge, or itching; hay fever, nosebleeds, sinus trouble

Mouth and Throat. Condition of teeth and gums, bleeding gums, dentures, if any, and how they fit, last dental examination, sore tongue, dry mouth, frequent sore throats, hoarseness

Neck. Lumps, "swollen glands," goiter, pain or stiffness in the neck

Breasts. Lumps, pain or discomfort, nipple discharge, self-examination

Respiratory. Cough, sputum (color, quantity), hemoptysis, wheezing, asthma, bronchitis, emphysema, pneumonia, tuberculosis, pleurisy; last chest x-ray film

Cardiac. Heart trouble, high blood pressure, rheumatic fever, heart murmurs; chest pain or discomfort, palpitations; dyspnea, orthopnea, paroxysmal nocturnal dyspnea, edema; past electrocardiogram or other heart tests

Gastrointestinal. Trouble swallowing, heartburn, appetite, nausea, vomiting, regurgitation, vomiting of blood, indigestion. Frequency of bowel movements, color and size of stools, change in bowel habits, rectal bleeding or black tarry stools, hemorrhoids, constipation, diarrhea. Abdominal pain, food intolerance, excessive belching or passing of gas. Jaundice, liver or gallbladder trouble, hepatitis

Urinary. Frequency of urination, polyuria, nocturia, burning or pain on urination, hematuria, urgency, reduced caliber or force of the urinary stream, hesitancy, dribbling, incontinence; urinary infections, stones

Genital

Male. Hernias, discharge from or sores on the penis, testicular pain or masses, history of sexually transmitted diseases and their treatments. Sexual preference, interest, function, satisfaction, and problems

Female. Age at menarche; regularity, frequency, and duration of periods; amount of bleeding, bleeding between periods or after intercourse, last menstrual period; dysmenorrhea, premenstrual tension; age at menopause, menopausal symptoms, postmenopausal bleeding. If the patient was born before 1971, exposure to DES (diethylstilbestrol) from maternal use during pregnancy. Discharge, itching, sores, lumps, sexually transmitted diseases and their treatments. Number of pregnancies, number of deliveries, number of abortions (spontaneous and induced); complications of pregnancy; birth control methods. Sexual preference, interest, function, satisfaction; any problems, including dyspareunia

Peripheral Vascular. Intermittent claudication, leg cramps, varicose veins, past clots in the veins

Musculoskeletal. Muscle or joint pains, stiffness, arthritis, gout, backache. If present, describe location and symptoms (*e.g.*, swelling, redness, pain, tenderness, stiffness, weakness, limitation of motion or activity).

Neurologic. Fainting, blackouts, seizures, weakness, paralysis, numbness or loss of sensation, tingling or "pins and needles," tremors or other involuntary movements

Hematologic. Anemia, easy bruising or bleeding, past transfusions and any reactions to them

Endocrine. Thyroid trouble, heat or cold intolerance, excessive sweating; diabetes, excessive thirst or hunger, polyuria

Psychiatric. Nervousness, tension, mood including depression; memory

COMPREHENSIVE HISTORY: CHILD PATIENT

In addition to the obvious age-related differences between histories of children and those of adults, there are present and past historical data specifically pertinent to the assessment of infants, children, and adolescents. These relate particularly to the patient's chronological age and stage of development. The child's history, then, follows the same outline as the adult's history, with certain additions that are presented here.

IDENTIFYING DATA. Date and place of birth. Nickname, particularly for those between 2 and 10 years of age. First names of parents (and last name of each, if different), their occupations, and where they may be reached during work hours

CHIEF COMPLAINTS. Make clear whether these are concerns of the patient, the parent(s), or both. In some instances a third party, such as a schoolteacher, may have expressed concerns about the child.

PRESENT ILLNESS. Should include how all members of the family respond to the patient's symptoms, what they think about them, and whether the patient achieves any secondary gains from the illness

PAST HISTORY

Birth History. Particularly important during the first 2 years of life and for neurologic and developmental problems. Hospital records should be reviewed if preliminary information from the parent(s) indicates significant difficulties before, during, or after delivery.

Prenatal. Maternal health before and during pregnancy, including nutrition and specific illnesses related to or complicated by pregnancy; doses and duration of all drugs taken during pregnancy; weight gain; vaginal bleeding; duration of pregnancy; parental attitudes concerning the pregnancy and parenthood in general and this child in particular

Natal. Nature of labor and delivery, including degree of difficulty, analgesia used, and complications encountered; birth order if a multiple birth; birth weight

Neonatal. Onset of respirations; resuscitation efforts; Apgar scores (see pp. 567–568) and estimation of gestational age. Specific problems with feeding, respiratory distress, cyanosis, jaundice, anemia, convulsions, congenital anomalies, or infection. Mother's health postpartum; separation of mother and infant and reasons for it; mother's initial reaction to her baby and the nature of bonding. Patterns of crying and sleeping, and of urination and defecation

Feeding History. Particularly important during the first 2 years of life and in dealing with problems of under- and overnutrition

Infancy. Breast feeding—frequency and duration of feeds, use of complementary or supplementary artificial feedings, difficulties encountered, timing and method of weaning. *Artificial feeding*—type, concentration, amount, and frequency of feeds, difficulties (regurgitation, colic, diarrhea) encountered, timing and method of weaning. *Vitamin and iron supplements*—type, amount given, frequency, and duration. *Solid foods*—types and amounts of baby foods given, when introduced, infant's response, introduction of table foods, self-feeding, parental and infant responses to feeding process

Childhood. Eating habits—likes and dislikes, specific types and amounts of food eaten, parental attitudes toward eating in general and toward this child's under- or overeating, parental response to feeding problems (if present). A *diet diary* kept over a 7- to 14-day period may be required for an accurate assessment of food intake in childhood feeding problems.

Growth and Developmental History. Particularly important during infancy and childhood and in dealing with problems of delayed physical growth, psychomotor and intellectual retardation, and behavioral disturbances

Physical Growth. Actual (or approximate) weight and height at birth and at 1, 2, 5, and 10 years; history of any slow or rapid gains or losses; tooth eruption and loss pattern

Developmental Milestones. Ages at which patient held up head while in a prone position, rolled over from front to back and back to front, sat with support and alone, stood with support and alone, walked with support and alone, said first word, combinations of words, and sentences, tied own shoes, dressed without help

Social Development. Sleep—amount and patterns during day and at night, bedtime routines, type of bed and its location; nightmares, terrors, and somnambulation. *Toileting*—methods of training used, when bladder and bowel control attained, occurrence of accidents or of enuresis or encopresis, parental attitudes, terms used within the family for urination and defecation (important to know when a young child is admitted to the hospital). *Speech*—hesitation, stuttering, baby talk, lisping, estimate of number of words in vocabulary. *Habits*—bed rocking, head banging, tics, thumb sucking, nailbiting, pica, ritualistic behavior. *Discipline*—parental assessment of child's temperament and response to discipline; methods used, success or failure, negativism, temper tantrums, withdrawal, aggressive behavior. *Schooling*—experience with day care, nursery school, and kindergarten; age and adjustment upon entry; current parental and child satisfaction; academic achievement; school's concerns. *Sexuality*—relations with members of opposite sex; inquisitiveness regarding conception, pregnancy, and girl–boy differences; parental responses to child's questions and the sex education they have offered regarding masturbation, menstruation, nocturnal emissions, development of secondary sexual characteristics, and sexual urges; dating patterns. *Personality*—degree of independence; relationship with parents, siblings, and peers; group and independent activities and interests, congeniality, special friends (real or imaginary); major assets and skills; self-image

Childhood Illnesses. In addition to specific illnesses experienced, mention of any recent exposures to childhood illnesses should be made here.

Operations
Accidents and Injuries } The reactions of the child and parents to these
Hospitalizations events should be ascertained.

CURRENT HEALTH STATUS

Allergies. Particular attention should be given to the allergies that are more prevalent during infancy and childhood—eczema, urticaria, perennial allergic rhinitis, and insect hypersensitivity.

Immunizations. Specific dates of administration of each vaccine should be recorded so that an ongoing booster program can be maintained throughout childhood and adolescence. Any untoward reactions to specific vaccines should also be recorded.

Screening Procedures. The dates and results of any screening tests performed should be recorded. These include, for all children, vision, hearing, and tuberculin tests, urinalyses, hematocrits, tests for phenylketonuria, galactosemia, and other genetic–metabolic disorders, and, for certain high-risk populations, sickle cell, blood lead, cholesterol, $alpha_1$-antitrypsin deficiency, and other tests that may be indicated.

FAMILY HISTORY. The education attained, job history, emotional health, and family background of each parent or parent substitute. The family socioeconomic circumstances, including income, type of dwelling, and neighborhood in which the family lives. Parental work schedules; family cohesiveness and interdependence; support available from relatives, friends, and neighbors; the ethnic and cultural milieu in which the family lives. Parental expectations, and attitudes toward the patient in relation to siblings. (All or portions of this information may be recorded in the present illness section, if pertinent to it, or under psychosocial history.) Consanguinity of the parents should be ascertained (by inquiring if they are "related by blood").

Once you know what kind of information to gather, you should lay that knowledge aside temporarily lest it come between you and the patient. At least at the start of the interview, and often at other times, you should be guided primarily by what the patient says and does rather than by a printed form or a rigid format.

SETTING THE STAGE FOR THE INTERVIEW

REVIEWING THE CHART. Before seeing the patient, quickly review the chart. Note the identifying data. Age, sex, race, marital status, address, occupation, and religion give you important glimpses into the patient's likely life experiences and may even guide your diagnostic hypotheses. If the patient has been referred from elsewhere, you should know both the source and the goals of the referral. Reviewing the medical chart may also give you invaluable information about past diagnoses and treatments, although it should not prevent you from developing new approaches or ideas.

THE ENVIRONMENT. Although you may have to talk with the patient under difficult circumstances—for example, in a four-bed room or in the corridor of a busy emergency department—a proper environment will improve communication. Your relationship may have begun with the patient's first telephone call to the clinic or office. If the response projected courtesy, interest, and a desire to be helpful, if the patient could be seen reasonably promptly, and if you are punctual for the appointment, the stage has been set for a trusting relationship.

The early stages in the patient–clinician communication, including the proper use of names and titles, are the critical determinants of patients' "reflexive self-concept" (what they think you think of them). If this is high, patients are more likely to be satisfied and more likely to cooperate with your diagnostic and therapeutic recommendations. If it is low, what you say or do later in the visit may have little impact on gaining their trust and cooperation.

The environment itself tells the patient something about your interest. Is the setting quiet? Does it afford privacy? Are you free of interruptions? There should be places where both you and the patient can sit down in clear view of each other, preferably at eye level. Leaning against the far wall, inching toward the door, or shifting around uncomfortably from foot to foot discourages the patient's attempts at communication. So do arrangements that indicate inequality of power or even disrespect, such as greeting and interviewing a woman while she is lying supine, positioned for a pelvic examination.

Your distance from the patient should probably be several feet, not so close as to be uncomfortably intimate nor too distant for easy conversation. Patients may be able to talk with you more easily when sitting next to your desk than when peering over it as if over a barrier. When patients prefer greater social distance they are telling you something about themselves, psychologically or perhaps culturally. Lighting also makes a difference. Beware of sitting between patients and a bright light or window. Although your view may be fine, the patient must squint uncomfortably toward your silhouette. You unwittingly conduct an interrogation, not a helping interview.

Finally, your personal appearance may also affect the ease with which you establish a relationship. Cleanliness, neatness, conservative dress, a white coat, and a name tag are usually desirable but casual dress may be preferable in some circumstances, as in dealing with children or young people.

NOTE TAKING. Since no one can remember all the details of a comprehensive history, you need to take notes. Most patients are accustomed to note taking but some may seem uncomfortable with it. If so, explore their concerns and explain your desire to make an accurate record. With practice you may be able to record most of the past history, current health status, family history, and review of systems in final form as you talk with the patient, especially if you have the help of a written questionnaire. Note taking should not divert your attention from the patient, however, nor should a written form prevent you from following a patient's leads. While eliciting the present illness, the psychosocial history, or other complex portions of the patient's account, do not attempt to write your final report. Instead, jot down short phrases, words, and dates that will aid your memory later. When the patient is talking about sensitive or disturbing material it is best not to take notes at all.

APPROACH TO THE PRESENT ILLNESS

GREETING THE PATIENT. You are now ready to make your approach, greet the patient by name, and give your undivided attention. Shake hands if you feel comfortable doing so. Unless you are talking with a child or adolescent or unless you already know the patient well, use the appropriate title—for example, Mr. O'Neill or Ms. Washington. Use of first names or terms of endearment with unfamiliar adults and use of "Granny" for an aged woman or "Mother" for a child's parent tend to depersonalize and demean. Introduce yourself by name. If there is any ambiguity in your role, such as your status as a student, explain your relation to the patient's care.

THE PATIENT'S COMFORT. Be alert to the patient's comfort. In the office or clinic, there should be a suitable place for coats and belongings other than the patient's own lap. In the hospital, inquire how the patient is feeling and whether your visit now is convenient. Watch for indications of discomfort such as poor positioning, evidence of pain or anxiety, or signs of the need to urinate. An improved position in bed or a short delay so that the patient can say goodbye to visitors or make a trip to the bathroom may be the shortest route to a good history.

OPENING QUESTIONS. Now you are ready to find out why the patient is here—the chief complaints, if any, and the present illness. (Occasionally a patient may come for a checkup or may wish to discuss a health-related matter without having either complaint or illness.) Begin your interview with a general question that allows full freedom of response—for example, "What brings you here?" or "What seems to be the trouble?" After the patient answers, inquire again, or even several times, "Anything else?" When the patient has finished, encourage further description by saying "Tell me about it," or, if there seems to be more than one problem, ask about one of them. "Tell me about the headaches" or ". . . about what bothers you most." As the patient answers, pick up the thread of the history and follow wherever it leads.

FOLLOWING THE PATIENT'S LEADS. Not all histories are complicated. Many patients want help with relatively straightforward medical problems. Others, however, have illnesses with complex psychosocial and pathophysiological causes, and may have complicated feelings about themselves, their illnesses, potential treatments, and those who are trying to help them. At the start you cannot tell one kind of patient from another. In order to do so, your interviewing technique must allow patients to recount their own stories spontaneously. If you intervene verbally too soon, if you ask specific questions prematurely, you risk trampling on the very information you are seeking. Your role, however, is not passive. You should listen actively and watch for clues to important symptoms, emotions, events, and relationships. You can then guide the patient into telling you more about these areas. Methods of helping and guiding patients without diverting them from their own accounts include facilitation, reflection, clarification, empathic responses, confrontation, interpretation, and questions that elicit feelings. Your demeanor throughout is also important.

Facilitation. You use facilitation when by posture, actions, or words you encourage the patient to say more but do not specify the topic. Silence itself, when attentive yet relaxed, is facilitative. Leaning forward, making eye contact, saying "Mm-hmm" or "Go on" or "I'm listening," all help the patient to continue.

Reflection. Closely akin to facilitation is reflection, a repetition of the patient's words that encourages the patient to give you more details. Reflection may be useful in eliciting both facts and feelings, as in the following example:

Patient:	The pain got worse and began to spread. (Pause)
Response:	It spread?
Patient:	Yes, it went to my shoulder and down my left arm to the fingers. It was so bad that I thought I was going to die. (Pause)
Response:	You thought you were going to die?
Patient:	Yes. It was just like the pain my father had when he had his heart attack, and I was afraid the same thing was happening to me.

Here a reflective technique has helped you to discover not only the location and severity of the pain, but also its meaning to the patient. There was no risk of biasing the story or interrupting the patient's train of thought.

Clarification. Sometimes the patient's words are ambiguous or the associations are unclear. If you are to understand their meaning you must request clarification, as in "Tell me what you meant by 'a cold'," or "You said you were behaving just like your mother. What did you mean?"

Empathic Responses. As patients talk with you, they may express—with or without words—feelings about which they are embarrassed, ashamed, or otherwise reticent. These feelings may well be crucial to how you understand their illnesses or plan treatment. If you can recognize and respond to them in a way that shows understanding and acceptance, you show empathy for the patients, make them feel more secure, and encourage them to continue. Empathic responses may be as simple as "I understand." Other examples include, "You must have been very upset," or "That must have been very difficult for you." Empathic responses may also be nonverbal—for example, offering a tissue to a crying patient or gently placing your hand on an arm to convey understanding. In using an empathic response, be sure that you are responding correctly to what the patient has already expressed. If you have acknowledged how upset a patient must have been at the death of a parent, when in fact the death relieved the patient from a long-standing financial and emotional burden, you have seriously misunderstood your patient and possibly blocked further communication on the subject.

Confrontation. While an empathic response acknowledges expressed feelings, confrontation points out to patients something about their own words or behaviors. If you observe clues of anger, anxiety, or depression, for example, confrontation may help to bring these feelings out in the open. "Your hands are trembling whenever you talk about that," or "You say you don't care but there are tears in your eyes." Confrontation may also be useful when the patient's story has been inconsistent. "You say you don't know what brings on your stomach pains, yet whenever you've had them you were feeling picked on."

Interpretation. Interpretation goes a step beyond confrontation. Here you make an inference, rather than a simple observation. "Nothing has been right for you today. You seem fed up with the hospital." "You are asking a lot of questions about the x-rays. Are you worried about them?" In interpreting a patient's words or behavior, you take some risk of making the wrong inference and impeding further communication. When used wisely, however, an interpretation can both demonstrate empathy and increase understanding.

Asking About Feelings. Rather than making an inference or reflecting a feeling, you may simply ask patients how they feel, or felt, about something such as symptoms or events. Unless you let them know that you are interested in feelings as well as in facts, they may withhold the feelings and you may miss important insights.

YOUR GENERAL DEMEANOR. Just as you have been observing the patient throughout the early portions of the interview, the patient has been watching you. Consciously or not, you have been sending messages through both your words and your behavior. You should be sensitive to those messages and control them as well as you can. Posture, gestures, eye contact, and words can all express interest, attention, acceptance, and understanding. The skilled interviewer seems calm and unhurried, even when time is limited. Reactions that betray disgust, disapproval, embarrassment, impatience, or boredom block communication, as do behaviors that condescend, stereotype, or make sport of the patient. Although negative reactions such as these are normal and often quite understandable, they should not be expressed. Guard against them not only when talking with the patient but also when discussing the patient with your colleagues or instructors, either at the bedside or in the hall.

Beginning practitioners may have special problems in dealing with their own limited knowledge; all practitioners confront this problem at least occasionally. When you do not know the answer to a patient's direct question, it is usually best to be honest about it and say so but add that you will try to find out the answer. Clearly acknowledging your status as a student may help you out of otherwise awkward situations.

GETTING MORE DATA. Using the nondirective techniques described thus far, you will usually be able to obtain a general idea of the patient's principal problems. You can encourage a chronological account by such questions as "What then?" or "What happened next?" Most of the time, however, you will need further specific information. Fill in the details with more direct questions that ask for specific information not already offered by the patient. If the present illness involves pain, for example, you should determine the following:

Attributes of a Symptom

1. Its location. Where is it? Does it radiate?
2. Its quality. What is it like?
3. Its quantity or severity. How bad is it?
4. Its timing. When did (does) it start? How long does it last? How often does it come?
5. The setting in which it occurs, including environmental factors, personal activities, emotional reactions, or other circumstances that may have contributed to the illness
6. Factors that make it better or worse
7. Associated manifestations

Most other symptoms can be described in the same terms.

As you learn about a patient's symptoms and their attributes, you should start to think analytically about what bodily systems might be involved by an underlying pathologic process. Leg pain, for example, suggests a problem in the peripheral vascular, the musculoskeletal, or the nervous system. Mild aching in the lower leg along with a swollen ankle at the end of the day suggests a venous problem (part of the peripheral vascular system). Pain in the joints suggests a musculoskeletal problem, while a severe pain that shoots down the back of one leg to below the knee suggests that the pain originates in a nerve root. For additional data that will contribute to your analysis, use items from the relevant parts of the review of systems. In the case of the aching leg with a swollen ankle, a history of varicose veins or of clots in the veins strengthens the hypothesis of a venous problem, while their absence diminishes it but does not rule it out entirely. Lack of ankle swelling would make a venous problem even more unlikely. The absence of certain attributes of symptoms or of commonly associated manifestations or of likely causes becomes significant negative information in the history and, together with the positive findings, shapes your diagnostic ideas. This kind of clinical thinking is discussed further in Chapter 20.

DIRECT QUESTIONS. Several principles apply to the use of direct questions. They should *proceed from the general to the specific.* A possible sequence, for example, might be "What was your chest pain like? Where did you feel it? Show me. Did it stay right there or did it travel anywhere? . . . to which fingers?"

Direct questions *should not be leading questions.* If a patient says "yes" to "Did your stools look like tar?" you must wonder if the description is the patient's or yours. A better wording is "What color were your stools?"

When possible, ask questions that *require a graded response* rather than a "yes" or "no" answer. "How many stairs can you climb before stopping for breath?" is better than "Do you get short of breath climbing stairs?"

Sometimes patients seem quite unable to describe their symptoms without help. To minimize bias here, *offer multiple choice answers*. "Is your pain aching, sharp, pressing, burning, shooting, or what?" Almost any direct question can provide at least two possible answers. "Do you bring up any phlegm with your cough, or not?"

Ask one question at a time. "Any tuberculosis, pleurisy, asthma, bronchitis, pneumonia?" may lead to a negative answer out of sheer confusion.

Finally, *use language that is understandable and appropriate* to the patient. Although you might ask a trained health professional about dyspnea, the more customary term is shortness of breath. When talking with an Appalachian coal miner, on the other hand, it may help to use the colloquial phrase "smothering spells." Appropriate words for technical terms are given in Chapter 2.

THE REST OF THE STORY

While the present illness is usually the single most important part of a history, important data are also discovered in subsequent parts of the interview. In most of these later sections, direct questions constitute your major technique. Stay alert, however, for important medical or emotional material, and be prepared to revert to a nondirective style whenever indicated. While taking a family history, for example, you may learn of a parent's death or a child's illness. Here is a good opportunity to find out what it meant to the patient. "How was it for you then?" or "What were your feelings at the time?" The review of systems may also uncover material that requires as full an exploration as the present illness. Keep your technique flexible.

TRANSITIONS. As you move from one part of the history to another, it helps to orient the patient with brief transitional phrases. "Now I'd like to ask some questions about your past health," or "about other parts of your body."

THE REVIEW OF SYSTEMS. The main purpose of the review of systems is to make sure that you have not missed any important symptoms, particularly in areas that you have not already thoroughly explored while discussing the present illness. A fairly general question that introduces each system, or subset of a system, is helpful. It focuses the patient's attention, allows you to move from the general to the more specific in each system, and on occasion may be all you need to ask. For example:

How are your ears and hearing?
How about your lungs and breathing?
Any trouble with your heart?
How is your digestion? How about your bowels?

The detail in which you ask additional questions within each area depends on the patient's age, complaints, and general state of health and the purpose of the visit, among other variables. An older patient, who is at greater risk of heart disease, cancer, and hearing loss, for example, needs more detailed questioning in certain areas than does an apparently healthy 20-year-old.

Some clinicians like to combine the review of systems with the physical examination, asking about the ears, for example, while looking at them. When a patient has few symptoms, this combination can be efficient. When a patient has multiple symptoms, however, the flow of both the history and the examination is disrupted and necessary note taking becomes awkward. If you want to try the combination, it is probably wise to wait until you master the flow of the examination. Then avoid two common errors. Do not ask a patient a question just as you place your stethoscope on the patient's chest. Voice sounds heard through the chest wall are unintelligible, and the situation is frustrating for both you and the patient. And be careful how and when you ask a question. "Have you ever had any heart trouble?" sounds ominous when the examiner has just finished listening to the heart.

TAKING A HISTORY ON SENSITIVE TOPICS. Beginning students always have difficulties in talking with patients about topics that are emotionally laden or culturally sensitive. At first the list of such subjects may be long, including sexual activities, death and dying, the financial concerns of patients, their racial and ethnic experiences, family interactions, domestic violence, psychiatric illnesses, physical deformities, and the functions of the urinary tract and bowel. Most of us will always feel a little uncomfortable in a few of these areas. Many adult patients, however, respond fairly easily to such questions, and you may thereby learn of important factors that have contributed to their illnesses. A woman's evening headaches may be related to sexual problems with her husband, a man's abdominal pain may worsen whenever his employer makes racial slurs, or a person's blood pressure may still be high because the prescriptions were too expensive to renew.

There are several ways of becoming more comfortable in difficult areas: special courses, professional and general reading, and your own life experiences. Use them all. Further, familiarize yourself with some opening questions on sensitive topics, and learn the additional kinds of data you need in order to make the desired assessments. Whenever possible, listen to experienced clinicians as they discuss such subjects with patients, and then try some of the difficult areas yourself. The range of topics that you can explore with comfort will widen progressively, sometimes to your surprise.

Alcohol and Drugs. One difficult area for many clinicians is asking patients about their use of alcohol and illicit drugs. Yet alcohol and drugs are often directly related to a patient's symptoms, and tolerance to and dependence upon a substance may importantly affect future management. It is not your role to pass judgment on the use of these substances, but it is your job (if the patient is willing) to gather the data with which to make a correct assessment and plan treatment. A nonjudgmental demeanor will help patients discuss their practices with you.

Questions about alcohol and other drugs follow naturally after questions about coffee and cigarettes. "How much alcohol do you drink?" is a good opening question that avoids the easy "yes" or "no" response. Listen carefully to the answer and tailor your next questions accordingly. "I haven't had a drink for 15 months" suggests an important decision to stop drinking, while "I just drink socially" is too vague to have meaning. In each case, further exploration is indicated. Specific questions about the duration, frequency, and quantity of drinking may be useful and should be asked. "When did you start to drink? What do you drink? How much do you drink on the average weekday? . . . during the weekend?" Try to learn the size of each drink in ounces, shotglasses, or other clear terms. Each beer, for example, might be 32 ounces, not the 12 ounces you might have assumed.

These questions have limitations, however. They fail to identify a large proportion of people considered alcoholic, and patients often underreport their consumption.

Affirmative answers to several of the following questions suggest a likelihood of alcoholism:

Have you ever thought that you drank too much in general?
Have family members or friends ever criticized your drinking?
Has their criticism annoyed you?
Have you ever felt guilty about your drinking?
Have you ever had a drink in the morning to get rid of a hangover or steady your nerves?

If indicated, inquire further about blackouts (loss of memory for events during drinking), about accidents or injuries while drinking, and about alcohol-related job losses, marital problems, or arrests.

Questions about drugs take a somewhat similar pattern. "How much marijuana do you use? cocaine? heroin? other drugs like these? How about sleeping pills? diet pills? pain-killers?" And further:

How do you feel when you take it?
Have you had any bad reactions? What happened?
Any drug-related accidents, injuries, or arrests? Job or family problems?
Have you ever tried to quit?

Less directly, it may be helpful to ask first about the use of such substances by friends or family members. "A lot of college students are using drugs these days. How about your school? your friends?" After patients have found your response nonjudgmental and concerned, they may feel more comfortable telling you about their own patterns of use.

Physical Violence. Physical abuse—often not mentioned by the victim—should be considered (1) when injuries are unexplained, seem inconsistent with the patient's story, are concealed by the patient, or cause embarrassment; (2) when the patient has delayed getting treatment for trauma; (3) when there is a past history of repeated injuries or "accidents"; and (4) when the patient or a person close to the patient has a history of alcoholism or drug abuse. At times, the behavior of the abuser raises suspicion: he (she) tries to dominate the interview, will not leave the room, or seems unusually anxious or concerned.

Suitable questions relate to what the patient has told you and what you have observed:

> When he comes home drunk like that, does he ever hit (beat, abuse) you, or the children? What does he do? What do you do?
> You mentioned that you and your husband were having lots of arguments. Do they ever lead to physical fighting?
> I notice you have some bruises on your breasts and abdomen. Can you tell me what happened? Did somebody hit you?

By suggesting that the problem is common, you may enable patients to talk about their experiences. "Many women tell me that someone at home is abusing or hurting them. How is it for you?" In cases of suspected child abuse, you might proceed as follows: "Most parents get very upset when their baby cries or their child has been naughty. How do *you* feel when *your* baby cries? What do you do when your baby won't stop crying? What sort of discipline do you use when your child has done something wrong? Are you ever afraid you might hurt your child?"

The Sexual History. Asking questions about sexual functions and practices serves at least four purposes. (1) Many patients have sex-related questions or problems that they would like to discuss with a professional if given the opportunity. Even if they choose not to discuss these questions on the first visit, they may feel freer to do so at a later time if you have introduced the topic. (2) Sexual practices may be directly related to specific symptoms, and they need to be understood for diagnostic, therapeutic, and preventive reasons. (3) Sexual dysfunctions are sometimes the consequence of medications and, if recognized, may be reversible. (4) Sexual practices are obviously related to the risks of unwanted pregnancy and sexually transmitted diseases, including AIDS. Through discussion, prevention may be possible for the patient or for the patient's partners.

Questions about sexual functions or practices may be relevant at more than one point in a person's history. If a patient's chief complaint involves genitourinary symptoms, a sexual history often becomes a necessary part of taking a present illness. Whenever a person has a chronic illness or serious symptoms such as pain or shortness of breath, sexual function may be affected. Asking about it in the context of other effects on the patient's life is a natural sequence of inquiry. Most commonly, a sexual history is taken during the genitourinary portion of the review of systems. This fairly late point in the history has the advantage of having given you time to establish rapport with the patient.

An introductory sentence or two is often helpful in preparing the patient for what is sometimes an embarrassing topic. "Now, to figure out why you have this discharge and what we should do about it, I need to ask you some questions about your sex life." If there have been no apparent sex-related complaints, a somewhat longer introduction may be indicated. "I'd like to ask you some questions about your sexual health and practices. This information helps me (us) to provide better care for you. If you prefer, I won't write down your answers in the chart. May I go ahead?" If the patient does not wish to go on, accept the choice and make clear (if it is true) that you are available to discuss any such matters in the future.

If the patient assents, proceed with the following questions:

1. "Are you sexually active? That is, have you had sex with anyone in the past few months?" If the answer is no, skip to question 7.
2. "Do you have sex with men, women, or both?"
3. "Do you have more than one partner?" or "How many partners have you had in the last two months?"
4. If the patient is a woman or girl of child-bearing age and is sexually active with males, "Are you interested in getting pregnant or are you using some form of contraception, or doing something, to try to prevent pregnancy?"
5. "Do you think your partner(s) is (are) having sex with other people who might be using IV drugs? or who might be exposed to the AIDS virus or other sexual infections?"
6. "Do you take any precautions to avoid infection?"
7. "Do you have any problems or concerns about your sexual function?"

Note that these questions make no assumptions about marital status, sexual preference, or attitudes toward pregnancy or contraception. Listen to each of the patient's responses, and ask additional questions as indicated. For further lines of inquiry, see pp. 57–60.

CLOSING. After you have completed the history, return the initiative briefly to the patient: "Is there anything else we should talk about?" or "Have we omitted anything?" You may want to recapitulate part of the present illness to be sure of a common understanding. Finally, make clear to the patient what to do or what to expect next. "I will step out for a few minutes. Please get completely undressed and put on this gown. I would like to examine you.''

PATIENTS AT DIFFERENT AGES

As people develop, have families, and age, they provide you with special opportunities and require certain adaptations in your interviewing style.

TALKING WITH PARENTS. To obtain histories on infants and children under 5 years of age, you gather all or at least most of your information from a third party, the parent(s) or legal guardian. Pediatric practitioners usually conduct interviews with both the parent and the child present. This is convenient, and it offers an opportunity to observe both parent–child interactions and the child's capacity for self-amusement. These observations may provide a clearer picture of the relationship between parent and child (and between parents if both are present) than can the answers to any number of questions. For the younger child, moreover, this interlude may help to dispel fears of the practitioner or of the visit, and it may allow for a smooth transition from the interview to the examination.

Interviewing a parent with the child present, however, has its disadvantages. The history may be incomplete and less accurate than when you interview the parent(s) alone. When sensitive areas are not fully explored because the child is present, you will need to interview the parent at a later time (often at the end of the visit when the child has left the room) to clarify certain points or to fill in missing data.

The techniques for talking with parents are much the same as those for talking with adult patients, with some special modifications. When parents describe a child's symptoms, they often do so accurately but they also have their own assumptions, perceptions, biases, and needs. For example, parents may assume that their child's chronic cough is due to a series of colds, not to bronchial asthma; they may perceive their child's poor performance in school as the fault of an overbearing teacher rather than as the result of a learning disability; or their bias toward their child as being exceptional may cause them to play down inappropriate social behaviors. Parents need to feel that they are doing a good job. When you ask a mother questions about her child's health you are, in a sense, testing her capabilities as a mother, and you should evaluate her responses in that context. There is a lot at stake for most parents as they try to cope with the problems of their children, so they need health practitioners who are supportive rather than judgmental or critical. Comments like, ''Why didn't you bring him in sooner?'' or ''Why, in heaven's name, did you do that?'' will not improve your rapport with a worried parent whose infant or child is acutely ill.

Refer to the infant or child by name rather than by ''him,'' ''her,'' or ''the baby.'' When the mother's marital status is not immediately clear, you may avoid embarrassment in asking about the father by saying ''Is Jane's father in good health?" rather than "Is your husband in good health?" Address the parents as "Mr. Smith" and "Ms. Smith" rather than by their first names or, heaven forbid, "Mom" or "Dad." First names may be used with permission when you have established a reasonably long-standing relationship. On the other hand, be prepared for the parent who calls you by your first name.

In interviewing parents, open-ended questions are usually more productive than direct questions. In the realm of psychosocial issues and problems, however, you must more often than not use explicit direct questions, since parents rarely introduce these subjects spontaneously even when given the opportunity with open-ended approaches.

Finally, you need to recognize that the chief complaint may not relate at all to the apparent reason the parent has brought the child to see you. The complaint may serve as a "ticket of admission" to care, through which if the circumstances are right the parent may bring up another concern that by itself is not viewed as a "legitimate" reason for seeking care. Try to create an atmosphere that will allow parents to express all their concerns. If necessary, ask questions that will facilitate the process.

Are there any other problems with Johnny that you would like to tell me about?

What did you hope I would be able to do for you when you came today?

Is there anything special you would like me to explain to you about Jody?

Is there anything else bothering you about the other children, your husband (wife), or yourself that you'd like to talk about?

TALKING WITH CHILDREN. Children of 5 years or older are able to add significantly to the history and can describe more accurately than can parents the severity of the symptoms and their own level of concern regarding them. You can sometimes improve the accuracy of your information by interviewing the child without the parent.

Starting with open-ended questions helps to place children at ease and get them to talk about their problems.

Your mother tells me that you get a lot of stomachaches. What can you tell me about them?

Do they worry you?

Does it bother you that they cause you to miss going to school a lot?

What helps to make them go away?

What do you think causes them?

Questions may also be used to obtain a subjective assessment of the child's symptoms:

Show me where you get the pain. Is it like a pin prick, or does it ache?
Does it stay in the same spot, or does it move around?
Does it make you feel like you are going to throw up?

TALKING WITH ADOLESCENTS. Many adults find talking with an adolescent difficult and frustrating because the adolescent often does not answer questions in an "adult" manner and may appear laconic and disdainful. This need not be the case. Adolescents, like most other people, will usually respond positively to anyone who demonstrates a genuine interest in them, not as "cases" but as people. That interest must be established early and then sustained if communication is to be effective. Adolescents tend to open up when the focus of the interview is on themselves and not on their problems. Thus, a good way to begin the interview with adolescents is to chat informally about their friends, school, hobbies, and family.

Adolescents seek health care on their own initiative or at the suggestion or insistence of their parents. They may come alone or with at least one parent. In the latter case, it is best to explain to both parent and adolescent that health care at this stage of one's individual development requires some degree of confidentiality. This requires speaking to the adolescent alone after obtaining past medical and social information from the parent(s). A confidential relationship is not based on "keeping secrets"; it is based on mutual respect. If it becomes necessary for the adolescent's own sake or for the sake of others to share confidential information, it is important to include the adolescent in that process.

Certain techniques of promoting good communication with an adult patient may be threatening to an adolescent. Reflection is a technique that should be avoided with the younger, cognitively immature adolescent, since it requires thinking skills not yet acquired. The use of silence in an attempt to get the patient to talk is rarely successful with adolescents, who usually do not have sufficient self-assurance to respond appropriately to this form of facilitation. Confrontation, rather than "bringing feelings out in the open," may cause an anxious adolescent to retreat into silence. Closely related to this is the technique of asking about feelings. Adolescents often find discussing their feelings with adults very difficult.

These caveats need not deter you from talking with adolescents. Most adolescents will talk with someone they respect and accept when given the opportunity in a friendly, informal atmosphere. You are more likely to succeed as a professional if you "play it straight," act your age, and do not stretch too far in trying to bridge the generation gap.

AGING PATIENTS. At the other end of the life cycle, aging patients also pose special problems and special opportunities. Their hearing and vision may be impaired, their responses may be slow, and they often have chronic illnesses with their associated discomforts and difficulties in getting about. For several reasons, elderly people may not report their symptoms. They may be afraid or embarrassed to do so, they may be trying to avoid medical expenses or the discomforts of diagnosis and treatment, they may think that their symptoms are merely a part of the aging process, or they may have simply forgotten about them. Aging patients also tell their histories more slowly than do younger ones.

Give an elderly person extra time to respond to your questions. Speak slowly and in a lower voice. A comfortable room, free of distractions and noise, is helpful. Do not try to accomplish everything in one visit. Multiple visits may be less fatiguing and more productive.

From middle age on, people become increasingly aware of their personal aging and begin to measure their lives in terms of the years left rather than the years lived. It is normal for older people to reminisce about the past and to reflect upon previous experience, including joys, regrets, and conflicts. Listening to this process of life review can give you important insights into your patients and may help them work through some of their painful feelings.

Try to determine the patients' priorities and goals. Learn how they have handled crises in the past. Because they may pursue similar adaptive patterns in the present situation, this knowledge will help you plan with them. Find out how they perceive themselves and their situation. "Can you tell me how you feel about getting older? What kinds of things do you find most satisfying? What kinds of things worry you? What would you like to change if you could?"

Learning how elderly people (and others with chronic illness) function in their daily lives is essential to your understanding of and care for them. Can they perform the ordinary activities of daily living independently, do they need some help, or are they entirely dependent? Inquire about walking, eating, dressing, grooming, bathing, and toileting. Are there any problems such as incontinence or falls? Inquire too about using a telephone, shopping, preparation of food, housekeeping, house repairs, laundry, transportation, taking medications, and handling financial affairs such as paying the bills. Are there problems with stairs, distance from shops or the bank, and fears for personal safety? Who is available for help?

SPECIAL PROBLEMS

Regardless of patient age, certain behaviors and special situations may particularly vex or perplex the practitioner.

SILENCE. Neophyte interviewers may grow uncomfortable during periods of silence, feeling somehow obligated to keep the conversation going. They need not feel so. Silences have many meanings and many uses. When recounting their present illnesses, patients frequently fall silent for short periods in order to collect their thoughts, remember details, or decide whether or not they trust you enough to report something. An attentive silence on the interviewer's part is usually the best response here, sometimes followed by brief encouragement to continue. During periods of silence be particularly alert to nonverbal signs of distress. Patients may fall silent because they are having difficulty controlling their emotions. If so, these are almost invariably significant feelings that are best expressed. A gentle confrontation may help: "You seem to be having trouble talking about this." Depressed patients or those with organic brain syndrome may have lost their usual spontaneity of expression, give short answers to questions, and fall silent quickly after each one. If you sense one of these problems, shift your inquiry to an exploratory mental status examination (see pp. 102–112).

At times, a patient's silence results from interviewer error or insensitivity. Are you asking too many direct questions in rapid sequence? The patient may simply have yielded the initiative to you and taken the passive role you seem to expect. Have you offended the patient in any way—for example, by signs of disapproval or criticism? Have you failed to recognize an overwhelming symptom such as pain, nausea, dyspnea, or the need to urinate or defecate? If so, you may need to abbreviate the interview considerably or return after the patient has been relieved.

OVERTALKATIVE PATIENTS. The garrulous, rambling patient may be just as difficult as the silent one, and possibly more so. Faced with limited time and the perceived need to "get the whole story," the interviewer may grow impatient, even exasperated. Although there are no perfect solutions for this problem, several techniques are helpful. First, you may need to lower your own goals and accept less than a comprehensive history. It may be unobtainable. Second, give the patient free rein for the first 5 or 10 minutes of the interview. You will then have the chance to observe the patient's pattern of speech. Does the patient seem obsessively detailed or unduly anxious? Is there a flight of ideas or a disorganization of thought processes that suggests a psychotic disorder? Third, try to focus the account on what you judge to be most important. Show interest and ask questions in those areas. Facilitate sparingly. Interrupt if you must, but courteously. A brief summary may help you change the topic while letting the patient know that you have both heard and understood. "As I understand it, your chest pains come frequently, last a long time, and do not necessarily stay in any one place. Now tell me about your breathing." Finally, do not let your impatience show. If you have used up the allotted time or, more likely, gone over it, explain that to the patient and arrange for a second meeting. Setting a time limit for the next appointment may be helpful. "I know we have much more to talk about. Can you come again next week? We will have a full half hour then."

PATIENTS WITH MULTIPLE SYMPTOMS. Some patients seem to have every symptom that you mention. They have an "essentially positive review of systems." Although it is conceivable that such a patient has multiple organic illnesses, serious emotional problems are much more likely. In such cases it will profit little to explore each symptom in detail. Guide the interview into a psychosocial assessment instead.

ANXIOUS PATIENTS. Anxiety is a frequent and natural reaction to sickness, to therapy, and to the health-care system itself. For some patients, anxiety has importantly colored their reactions to life stress and may have contributed to their illnesses. Be sensitive to nonverbal and verbal clues.

For example, anxious patients may sit tensely, fidgeting with their fingers or clothes. They may sigh frequently, lick their dry lips, sweat more than average, or actually tremble. Carotid pulsations may betray a rapid heart rate. Some anxious patients fall silent, unable to speak freely or confide. Others try to cover their feelings with words, busily avoiding their own basic problems. When you sense an underlying anxiety, encourage such patients to talk about their feelings.

REASSURANCE. When you are talking with anxious patients, it is tempting to reassure them: "Don't worry. Everything is going to be all right." This approach is usually counterproductive. Unless you and the patient have had a chance to explore the nature of the anxiety, you may well be giving reassurance about the wrong thing. Moreover, premature reassurance blocks further communication. Since admitting anxiety exposes a weakness, it requires encouragement, not a coverup. The first step to effective reassurance involves identifying and accepting the patient's feelings. This promotes a feeling of security. The final steps come much later in the health-care process, after you have completed the interview, the physical examination, and perhaps some laboratory studies. Then you can interpret for the patient what is happening and deal openly with the real concerns.

ANGER AND HOSTILITY. Patients have reasons to be angry: they are ill, they have suffered loss, they lack their accustomed control over their own lives, they feel relatively powerless in the health-care system. They may direct this anger toward you. It is possible that you have justly earned their hostility. Were you late for your appointment, inconsiderate, insensitive, or angry yourself? If so, recognize the fact and try to make amends. More often, however, patients are displacing their anger onto the clinician as a symbol of all that is wrong. Allow them to get it off their chests. Accept their feelings without getting angry in return. Beware of joining such patients in their hostility toward another part of the clinic or hospital, even when you privately harbor similar feelings. After a patient has calmed down, you may be able to identify specific steps that will help in the future. Rational solutions to emotional problems are not always possible, however, and people need time to resolve their angry feelings.

THE OBSTREPEROUS INEBRIATE. Few patients can disrupt the clinic or emergency room more quickly than acutely intoxicated persons who are angry, belligerent, and uncontrolled. Before interviewing such patients, it is wise to alert the security force of the hospital. As you make your approach greet the patient by name and title, introduce yourself, and offer a handshake. In this situation it is especially important to appear accepting, not challenging. To do this, avoid all but the briefest eye contact and keep your posture relaxed and nonthreatening, your hands loosely open rather than clenched into fists. Do not try to make inebriated patients lower their voices or stop cursing at you or the staff, but listen carefully and try to understand what they are saying. Since some such persons feel trapped in small rooms it is usually best to talk with them in an open area, and you too are likely to feel more comfortable there. In addition, an offer of food or coffee may help to quiet the agitated person and bring some calm to the stormy scene.

CRYING. Like anger, crying is an important clue to emotions. Rarely should it be suppressed. If the patient seems on the verge of tears, gentle confrontation or an empathic response may simply allow crying. Quiet acceptance is then appropriate. Offer a tissue; wait for recovery; perhaps make a facilitating or supportive remark: "It's good to get it out." In that kind of accepting context, most patients will soon compose themselves and will feel better and capable of continuing the discussion.

DEPRESSION. Masquerading as fatigue, weight loss, insomnia, or mysterious aches and pains, depression is one of the most common problems in clinical medicine, and is commonly missed or ignored. Be alert for it, identify it, and explore its manifestations. Be sure you know how bad it is. Just as you would evaluate the severity of angina pectoris, you must evaluate the severity of depression. Both are potentially lethal. You need not fear that asking about suicide will suggest it to the patient. For appropriate questions about depression, see Chapter 3.

SEXUALLY ATTRACTIVE OR SEDUCTIVE PATIENTS. Clinicians of both sexes may occasionally find themselves attracted to their patients. If you become aware of such feelings, accept them as normal human responses but prevent them from affecting your behavior. Keep your relationship with the patient within professional bounds.

Occasionally patients may be frankly seductive or may make sexual advances. Calmly, but firmly, you should make clear that your relationship is professional, not personal. You may also wish to review your own image. Have you been overly warm with the patient? expressed your affection physically? sought his or her emotional support? Has your dress or demeanor been unconsciously seductive? Avoid these problems when you can.

CONFUSING BEHAVIORS OR HISTORIES. At times you may find yourself baffled, frustrated, and confused in your interaction with the patient. The history is vague and difficult to understand, ideas are poorly related to one another, and language is hard to follow. Even though you word your questions carefully, you seem unable to get clear answers. The patient's manner of relating to you may also seem peculiar: distant, aloof, inappropriate, or bizarre. Symptoms may be described in bizarre terms: "My fingernails feel too heavy," or "My stomach knots up like a snake." These characteristics should alert you to possible mental illnesses, such as schizophrenia. With the usual nondirective techniques you may be able to get more information about the unusual qualities of the symptoms. You should also include in your interview an assessment of the patient's mental status, with special attention to mood, thought, and perceptions (see pp. 105–108).

Many psychotic patients are functioning, with varying degrees of success, in the community. Such patients are frequently capable of telling you freely about their diagnoses, their symptoms, their hospitalizations, and their current medications. You should feel comfortable inquiring about these without embarrassment or circumlocution.

Schizophrenia is not the only cause of confusing histories. Some patients have organic disorders of cognitive function such as delirium or dementia. Be particularly alert for delirium when dealing with an acutely ill or intoxicated patient, and for dementia when dealing with an elderly patient. Patients with these problems may be unable to give clear histories. They are vague and inconsistent about symptoms or events and unable to report when and how things happened. They may be inattentive to your questions and hesitant in their answers. Occasionally such patients may confabulate, that is, make up part of their histories in order to fill in the gaps in their memories. When you suspect an organic brain syndrome or disorder, do not spend too much time trying to get a detailed history. You will only tire and frustrate the patient as well as yourself. Switch your inquiry instead to an evaluation of mental status, checking particularly on level of consciousness, orientation, and memory (see pp. 103 and 108–110). You can work the initial questions smoothly into the interview. "When was your last appointment in the clinic? Let's see, then, that was about how long ago?" "Your address now is? . . . and your phone number?" Responses can all be checked against the chart (presuming, of course, that the chart is accurate).

PATIENTS WITH LIMITED INTELLIGENCE. Patients of moderately limited intelligence can usually give adequate histories. You may, in fact, overlook their limitations and thereby make mistakes, such as omitting their dysfunction from a disability evaluation or giving instructions they cannot understand. If you suspect such problems, pay special attention to the patients' schooling. How far did they go in school? Why did they drop out? How were they doing at the time? What kinds of courses are (were) they taking? High school seniors of normal intelligence are not usually taking simple arithmetic. If your patient is, you can make a smooth transition into a mental status examination, including simple calculations, vocabulary, information, and tests of abstract reasoning (see pp. 110–111).

When patients suffer from severe mental retardation, you will have to obtain their history from family or friends. By showing interest in the patients themselves, however, and by engaging them in simple conversation, try to establish a personal relationship. As with children, avoid "talking down" to mentally retarded patients and using affectations of speech or condescending behaviors. If the patient does not perceive these postures, family members or friends will.

ABILITY TO READ. Before giving written instructions, it may be advisable to assess a patient's reading ability. Some people who cannot read because of a language barrier, learning disorder, or poor vision admit it when questioned. Others do not. You can check, as if testing their vision, by asking them to read some words or sentences for you. Illiterate people may try to hide their inability to read. Respond sensitively, and remember that literacy and intelligence are not synonymous.

LANGUAGE BARRIERS. Nothing will more surely convince you that a history is essential than having to do without one. When you cannot communicate with your patient because you speak different languages, take every possible step to find a translator. A few broken words and gestures are no substitute. The ideal translator is a neutral, objective person who is familiar with both languages. When family members or friends try to help, they are more likely to distort meanings and may also present problems in confidentiality to both the patient and the interviewer. Many translators try to speed the process by telescoping a long communication into a few words. Try to make clear at the beginning that you need the translator to translate everything, not to interpret or summarize. Make your questions clear and short. You can also help the translator by outlining the goals for each segment of your history.

When available, written bilingual questionnaires are invaluable, especially for the review of systems. Before using one, however, be sure patients can read in their own language or can get help with the questionnaire.

THE HEARING-IMPAIRED. Communicating with people whose hearing is severely impaired presents many of the problems of communicating with a patient who speaks a different language. Here, again, written questionnaires are a great help. Although very time-consuming, handwritten questions and answers may be the only solution. If the patient knows sign language, make every effort to find a translator who speaks, hears, and can use it. When patients have partial hearing impairment or can read lips, face them directly, in good light. Speak slowly and in a relatively low-pitched voice. Do not let your voice trail off at the ends of sentences, avoid covering your mouth, and use gestures to reinforce your words. If the patient has a "good" ear, arrange the seating to take advantage of it. A person who has a hearing aid should, of course, wear it, and you should check to be sure that it is working. Patients who wear glasses should use them too; visual cues may help them to understand you better. Supplement any oral instructions with writing.

BLIND PATIENTS. When talking with a blind patient, be especially careful to announce yourself and explain who you are and why you are there. Taking the patient's hand may help to establish contact and indicate where you are. If the room is unfamiliar, orient the patient to it and explain what is there and whether anyone else is present. Remember to respond vocally to such patients when they speak, since facilitative postures and gestures will not work. At the same time guard against raising your voice unnecessarily.

FATALLY ILL PATIENTS. In communicating with fatally ill or dying patients, most interviewers face problems within themselves—their own discomforts, anxieties, and desires to avoid the subject or even the patients. With the help of reading and discussion, you will need to work through your own feelings. As in any clinical situation, it is helpful to know what reactions the patient is likely to have. Kübler-Ross has described five stages in a patient's response to impending death: denial and isolation, anger, bargaining, depression or preparatory grief, and acceptance. At each stage, your approach is basically the same. Be alert to the feelings of such patients and to cues that they want to talk about them. Help them to bring out their concerns with nondirective techniques. Make openings for them to ask questions: "I wonder if you have any concerns about the operation? . . . your illness? . . . how it will be when you go home?" Explore these concerns and provide whatever information the patients are asking for. Be wary of inappropriate reassurance. If you can explore and accept the patients' feelings, if you can answer the patients' questions, if you can assure and demonstrate your ability to stay with the patients throughout the illness, reassurance will grow where it really matters—within the patients themselves.

Fatally ill or dying patients rarely want to talk about their illnesses all the time, nor do they wish to confide in everyone they meet. Give such patients opportunities to talk, and listen receptively, but if the patient prefers to keep the conversation on a lighter plane you need not feel like a failure. Remember that illness—even a terminal one—is only one small part of personhood. A smile, a touch, an inquiry after a family member, a comment on the day's ballgame, or even some gentle kidding all recognize and reinforce other parts of the patient's individuality and help to sustain the living person. To communicate appropriately you have to get to know the patient: that is part of the helping process.

TALKING WITH FAMILIES OR FRIENDS. Some patients are totally unable to give their own histories. Others may be unable to describe parts of them, such as their behavior during a convulsion. Under these circumstances you must try to find a third person from whom to get the story. At times, although you may think you have a reasonably comprehensive knowledge of the patient, other sources may offer surprising and important information. A spouse, for example, may report significant family strains, depressive symptoms, or drinking habits that the patient has denied. When you suspect such discrepancies, look for opportunities to get additional information from persons other than the patient.

When you decide to seek information from a third person, it is usually wise to get the patient's approval. Assure such patients that you will keep confidential what they have already told you, or get their permission to share certain information. Data from other persons must also be held in confidence.

The basic principles of interviewing apply to your conversations with relatives or friends. Find a private place to talk. Leaning against opposite sides of a hospital corridor is not conducive to good communication. Introduce yourself, state your purpose, inquire how they are feeling under the circumstances, and recognize and acknowledge their concerns. As you listen to their versions of the history, be alert for clues to the quality of their relationships with the patient. These may color their credibility or give you helpful ideas in planning the patient's care.

Occasionally a relative or friend insists on accompanying the patient during the history or even the physical examination. If you can, ascertain his or her reasons as well as the patient's wishes. When patients are completely unable to give their own histories, help from an informed person is essential. When patients can communicate at all, however, even just by facial expressions or gestures, it is important that they be given the chance to do so with complete confidentiality. It is usually possible to divide the interview into two parts—one with the patient alone and the other with both the patient and the second person. Each part has its own value.

RESPONDING TO PATIENTS' QUESTIONS. Patients' questions may seek simple factual information. More often, however, they express feelings or concerns. Try to elicit these feelings or delve further, lest you offer a misguided answer.

Patient:	What are the effects of this blood pressure medicine?
Response:	There are several effects. Why do you ask?
Patient:	(Pause) Well, I was reading up on it in a friend's book. I read it could make me impotent.

Similar caution is indicated when patients seek advice for personal problems. Should the patient quit a stressful job, for example, or move to Arizona, or have an abortion? Before responding, find out what approaches he or she has considered, what pros and cons there might be to the possible solutions. A chance to talk through the problem with you is usually much more valuable than any answer you could give.

Finally, when the patient is asking for specific information about the diagnosis, progress, or treatment plan, answer when you can but be careful that your responses do not conflict with those provided by others. When you are unsure of the answer, offer to find out if you can. Alternatively, you can suggest that the patient ask Dr. X because Dr. X knows more about the case or is making that decision. Beware, however, of using this approach simply to avoid a difficult issue. If you carry the primary patient responsibility yourself, share your opinions and plans and the patient's prognosis with other members of the health team so that each in turn can communicate with the patient effectively.

Chapter 2
An Approach to Symptoms

While Chapter 1 deals with the general methods of interviewing, this chapter tailors those methods to common or important symptoms. It (1) defines the technical terms for the symptoms, (2) suggests ways of asking about them, and (3) outlines some of their most common mechanisms and causes.

Technical terms, of course, are not intended for use with most patients. As a clinician you must learn, however, to translate the patient's observations into words such as tinnitus, hemoptysis, or nocturia. You can then understand the professional literature and communicate clearly with your colleagues.

Data to gather about symptoms appear here in bold-faced type. Specific questions are suggested, especially in difficult or sensitive areas. When no suggestions are made, identify the seven attributes of the symptom, as described on page 17, and use the general principles of interviewing that you have already learned.

The order used in this chapter resembles the review of systems in a comprehensive history. Interpretive comments on the meaning of certain symptoms appear in the right-hand columns, together with examples of specific abnormalities that may cause them. Tables at the end of the chapter compare various disorders and diseases according to their symptoms. Where assessment of symptoms depends heavily on physical examination, reference is made to later chapters.

Obviously no table exhausts all the possible explanations for symptoms, nor can any table, which is necessarily oversimplified, capture the infinite variety of human perceptions and experience. Real patients seldom match a textbook in every detail.

One of the qualities that is difficult for one person to communicate to another is color. A chart that includes the various colors of sputum, urine, and feces is often helpful in getting an accurate history. You can easily make such a chart by cutting rectangles out of the colored pages of a magazine and taping them to a small card. Colors should range from white to yellowish and light green for sputum; from pale to deep yellow, orange, pink, reddish, and brown for urine; and from gray and light tan to brown and black for feces. The bright and dark red colors of blood should also be included. These colors can be arranged into one scheme from which the patient can select the closest match.

Symptoms and Approaches to Them

GENERAL SYMPTOMS

Changes in *body weight* result from quantitative changes in either the body tissues or the body fluids. *Weight gain* occurs when caloric intake exceeds caloric expenditure over a period of time, and typically appears as increased body fat. Weight gain may also result from an abnormal accumulation of body fluids. When the retention of fluid is relatively mild it may not be visible, but as several pounds of it accumulate it usually appears as edema.

Weight loss is an important symptom that has many causes. Mechanisms include one or more of the following: decreased intake of food for reasons that include anorexia, dysphagia, vomiting, and insufficient supplies of food; defective absorption of nutrients through the gastrointestinal tract; increased metabolic requirements; and loss of nutrients through the urine, feces, or injured skin.

A person may also lose weight when a fluid-retaining state improves or responds to treatment. Moreover, the greater part of the weight lost when a person starts on a low-calorie diet is fluid.

Good opening questions include "How often do you check your weight? Has it changed in the past year? . . . in what manner? Why has it changed, do you think? What would you like to weigh?" If weight change in either direction appears to be a problem, try to ascertain the amount of change, its timing, the setting in which it occurred, and any associated symptoms.

In the *overweight patient*, for example, when did the weight gain begin? Was the patient heavy as an infant or a child? Using milestones appropriate to the patient's age, inquire about the weight at the time of birth, on entrance to kindergarten, on graduation from high school or college, on discharge from the service, at marriage, following each pregnancy, at menopause, and on retirement. What was going on in the patient's life during the periods of weight gain? Has the patient tried to lose weight? How? With what results?

When the problem is *weight loss*, try to determine whether the intake of food has diminished proportionately or whether it has remained normal or even increased.

Symptoms associated with the weight loss often suggest its likely cause. So does a good psychosocial history. Who cooks and shops for the patient? Where and with whom does the patient eat? Are there

Rapid changes in weight (over a few days) suggest changes in body fluids, not tissues.

See Table 15-3, Mechanisms and Patterns of Edema, pp. 455–456.

Causes of weight loss include gastrointestinal diseases; endocrine disorders (diabetes mellitus, hyperthyroidism, adrenal insufficiency); chronic infections; malignancies; chronic cardiac, pulmonary, or renal failure; depression; and anorexia nervosa.

Weight loss with a relatively high food intake suggests diabetes mellitus, hyperthyroidism, or malabsorption. Consider also binge eating (*bulimia*) with clandestine vomiting.

Poverty, old age, social isolation, physical disability, emotional or mental impairment,

any difficulties in getting, storing, preparing, or chewing the food? Does the patient restrict certain foods for medical, religious, or other reasons?

lack of teeth, ill-fitting dentures, alcoholism, and drug abuse increase the likelihood of malnutrition.

Throughout the history, be alert for manifestations of malnutrition. Symptoms here are often subtle and nonspecific: weakness, easy fatigability, cold intolerance, flaky dermatitis, and ankle swelling, among other examples. A good dietary history is mandatory.

Like weight loss, *fatigue* is a relatively nonspecific symptom with many causes. It refers to a sense of weariness or loss of energy that patients describe in various ways. "I've lost my pep. . . . I just feel blah. . . . I'm all in. . . . I can hardly get through the day. . . . By the time I get to the office I feel as though I've done a day's work." Because fatigue is a normal response to hard work, sustained stress, or grief, you must consider the context in which it occurs, but fatigue that is unrelated to such factors needs an explanation.

Fatigue is a common symptom of depression and anxiety states, but consider also infections (such as hepatitis, infectious mononucleosis, and tuberculosis); endocrine disorders (hypothyroidism, adrenal insufficiency, diabetes mellitus, and panhypopituitarism); heart failure; chronic disease of the lungs, kidneys, or liver; electrolyte imbalance; moderate to severe anemia; malignancies; nutritional deficits; medications; and drug withdrawal.

In infants and children, fatigue is not expressed verbally but is manifested by withdrawal from normal activities, irritability, loss of interest in the surroundings, and excessive sleeping.

Use open-ended questions to explore the attributes of the patient's fatigue, and get as clear an idea as possible of what the patient is experiencing. Important clues to the cause of the problem often lie in a good psychosocial history, review of systems, and exploration of sleep patterns.

Weakness is different from fatigue. It denotes a demonstrable loss of muscular power, and will be discussed later with other neurologic symptoms (see p. 64).

Weakness, especially if localized in a neuroanatomic pattern, suggests a disorder of the nervous system or muscles.

Fever refers to an abnormal elevation in body temperature (see p. 136). **Ask about it when the patient has an acute or a chronic illness. Find out whether the patient has measured the temperature with a thermometer. Has the patient felt feverish or unusually hot, noted excessive sweating, or felt chilly and cold? Try to distinguish between subjective *chilliness* and a *shaking chill* in which the body shivers and the teeth chatter.**

Recurrent shaking chills suggest more extreme swings in temperature.

Feelings of coldness, gooseflesh, and shivering accompany a rising temperature, while hot feelings and sweats accompany defervescence. The normal temperature rises during the day and falls during the night. When fever exaggerates this swing, *night sweats* occur. Malaise, headache, and pain in the muscles and joints often accompany fever.

Feelings of heat and sweating also accompany menopause.

Fever has many causes. **Focus your questions on the timing of the illness and its associated symptoms. Become familiar with patterns of infectious diseases to which your patient may have been subject, and** inquire about travel, contacts with sick persons, or other unusual exposures. Inquire about medications. They may cause fever, while aspirin, acetaminophen, corticosteroids, and nonsteroidal anti-inflammatory drugs (NSAIDs) may mask it.

THE SKIN

Start your inquiry about the patient's skin with a few open-ended questions: "Have you noticed any changes in your skin? . . . your hair? . . . your nails? Have you had any rashes? . . . sores? . . . lumps? . . . itching? . . . any moles that have changed in appearance? Where? When?" Further questions are usually best deferred until the physical examination, when you can see what the patient is talking about.

See Chapter 6, The Skin, and pp. 583–585.

Causes of generalized itching without obvious reason include dry skin, aging, pregnancy, uremia, obstructive jaundice, lymphomas and leukemia, drug reactions, and body lice.

THE HEAD

Headache is an extremely common symptom. Although only a very small fraction of people with headaches harbor life-threatening problems as the cause, the symptom requires careful evaluation. Get as full a description as possible. After your usual open-ended approach, ask the patient to show you where the discomfort is. Is it one-sided or bilateral? steady or throbbing? The single most important attribute of headache is its chronological pattern. Are you dealing with a new and acute problem, a chronic and recurring one that has not changed very much in its pattern, or a chronic, recurring one that has recently changed in its characteristics or has become progressively severe? Does the pain recur at the same time every day? Associated symptoms and a family history may also give you important clues.

See Table 2-1, Headaches, pp. 66–69.

Subarachnoid hemorrhage and meningitis cause acute severe headaches. Tension and migraine headaches are the most common kinds of recurring headaches. Changing or progressively severe headaches increase the likelihood of tumor or other demonstrable organic cause.

Inquire specifically about associated nausea and vomiting and about neurologic symptoms. Explore the physical and emotional settings in which the headaches occur.

Nausea and vomiting are common with migraine but also occur with brain tumors.

Ask whether coughing, sneezing, or changing the position of the head affects the headache.

Such maneuvers may increase the pain of brain tumor and acute sinusitis.

THE EYES

"How is your vision?" and "Have you had any trouble with your eyes?" conveniently start your inquiry about ocular problems. If the patient has noted a visual disturbance,

Refractive errors most commonly explain gradual blurring. High blood sugar levels may cause blurring.

● Has it started suddenly or gradually?

Sudden visual loss suggests retinal detachment, vitreous hemorrhage, or occlusion of the central retinal artery.

- **Is it troublesome only with close work or only at distances?**

Difficulty with close work suggests *hyperopia* (farsightedness) or *presbyopia* (aging vision); with distances, *myopia* (nearsightedness).

- **Is the entire visual field blurred or are only parts of it? Is the defect central or peripheral in the visual field, or does it involve only one side of it?**

Slow central loss in nuclear cataract (p. 202), macular degeneration (p. 184); slow peripheral loss in open-angle glaucoma (p. 178); one-sided loss in hemianopsia and quadrantic defects (p. 198).

- **Are there specks in the vision or spots where the patient cannot see (*scotomas*)? If so, do they move around in the visual field when the patient shifts gaze, or are they fixed?**

- **Does the patient wear glasses?**

Moving specks or strands suggest vitreous floaters; fixed defects (scotomas) suggest lesions in the retinas or visual pathways.

Continue with questions about *pain* in or around the eyes, *redness*, and *excessive tearing or watering*.

See Table 7-5, Red Eyes, p. 201.

Ask about double vision (*diplopia*). If diplopia is present, find out whether the images are side-by-side (*horizontal diplopia*) or on top of each other (*vertical diplopia*).

Diplopia indicates a weakness or paralysis of one or more extraocular muscles (pp. 161, 179, 594–599). Horizontal diplopia implicates the 3rd or 6th cranial nerve; vertical diplopia, the 3rd or 4th cranial nerve.

One kind of horizontal diplopia is physiologic. Hold one finger upright about 6 inches in front of your face, a second at arm's length. When you focus on either finger, the image of the other is double. A patient who notices this phenomenon can be reassured.

THE EARS

Opening questions for the ears are "How is your hearing?" and "Have you had any trouble with your ears?" If the patient has noticed a *hearing loss*, does it involve one or both ears? Did it start suddenly or gradually? What are the associated symptoms, if any?

See Table 7-17, Patterns of Hearing Loss, pp. 220–221.

Try to distinguish between two basic types of hearing impairment: *conduction loss*, which results from problems in the external or middle ear, and *sensorineural loss*, which results from problems in the inner ear, the cochlear nerve, or its central connections in the brain. **Two questions may be helpful here. Does the patient have special difficulty understanding people as they talk? What difference does a noisy environment make?**

Persons with sensorineural loss have particular trouble understanding speech, often complaining that others mumble. Noisy environments make it worse. In conduction loss, noisy environments may help.

Symptoms associated with hearing loss, such as earache or vertigo, help you to assess the likely causes. In addition, inquire specifically about medications that might contribute to the impairment and ask about sustained exposure to loud noise.

Medications include aminoglycosides, aspirin, NSAIDs, quinine, furosemide, and others.

Hearing loss or total deafness in infants is usually suspected when the parents note a lack of response to their voices or to environmental sounds. Such concerns deserve thorough investigation. Toddlers with hearing loss often manifest this by a delay in the development of speech.

Tinnitus is a perceived sound that has no external stimulus. It is commonly heard as a musical ringing but may also be heard as a rushing or roaring noise. One or both ears may be involved. Tinnitus may accompany hearing loss of any kind and often remains unexplained. Occasionally, popping sounds originate in the temporomandibular joint or patients become aware of vascular noises from their own necks.

Tinnitus is a common symptom, increasing in frequency with age. When associated with hearing loss and vertigo it suggests Meniere's disease.

Vertigo refers to the false perception that either the patient or the environment is rotating or spinning. These sensations point primarily to a problem in the inner ear, the cochlear nerve, or its central connections in the brain.

See Table 2-2, Vertigo, p. 71.

Vertigo poses a great challenge to the interviewer. **"Are there times when you feel dizzy?" is an appropriate first question,** but patients often have great difficulty describing their sensations. Try to distinguish vertigo from (1) a sense of unsteadiness without the feeling of movement, (2) faintness or an impending loss of consciousness, and (3) a vague lightheadedness. **Get the story without biasing it. You may need a multiple-choice question. Determine whether or not the patient has felt pulled to the ground or off to one side during the dizziness. Does a change in position alter or provoke the dizziness? Ask about nausea and vomiting, which typically accompany vertigo, and about other associated symptoms. Pay special attention to the timing and course of the problem.**

A feeling of being pulled suggests true vertigo.

Further symptoms relevant to the ears include:

● *Discharge* from the ear

Unusually soft wax, debris from inflammation or rash in the ear canal, or discharge through a perforated eardrum secondary to acute or chronic otitis media.

● *Pain* in the ear, or *earache*

Inquire about these in your usual manner.

Pain suggests a problem in the external or middle ear but may also be referred from other structures in the mouth, throat, or neck.

THE NOSE AND SINUSES

Rhinorrhea refers to a nasal discharge and is often associated with *nasal stuffiness*, a sense of obstruction. These symptoms frequently occur together with *sneezing*, watery eyes, and discomfort in the throat. *Itching* may also be felt in the eyes, nose, and throat. **Assess the chronology of the illness. Does it occur for a week or so, especially when common colds and related syndromes are prevalent, or does it occur seasonally when pollens are in the air? Is it associated with specific contacts or environments? What remedies has the patient used? for how long? and how well do they work?**

Causes include viral infections, allergic rhinitis ("hay fever"), and vasomotor rhinitis. Itching favors an allergic cause.

Relation to seasons or environmental contacts suggests allergy.

Excessive use of decongestants can worsen the symptoms.

Inquire about drugs that might cause stuffiness.

Oral contraceptives, reserpine, guanethidine, and alcohol

Are there other symptoms associated with the nasal ones, such as pain and tenderness in the face, local headache, or fever?

These together suggest sinusitis.

Is the patient's nasal stuffiness limited to one side? If so, you may be dealing with a different problem that requires careful physical examination.

Consider a deviated nasal septum, foreign body, or tumor.

Epistaxis means bleeding from the nose. The blood usually originates from the nose itself but may come from a paranasal sinus or the nasopharynx. There is usually no difficulty in getting a history of epistaxis. When the patient is lying down, however, or when the bleeding originates in posterior structures, blood may pass into the throat rather than out the nostrils. You must then differentiate it from coughing or regurgitating blood. **Try to determine the site of the bleeding, its severity, and associated symptoms. Is it a recurrent problem, and has there been easy bruising or bleeding elsewhere in the body?**

Local causes of epistaxis include trauma (especially nose picking), inflammation, drying and crusting of the nasal mucosa, tumors, and foreign bodies.

Bleeding disorders may contribute to epistaxis.

THE MOUTH, THROAT, AND NECK

Bleeding from the gums is a common symptom, most often noted when brushing teeth. **Inquire about local lesions and any tendency to bleed or bruise elsewhere.**

Bleeding gums are most often caused by gingivitis (p. 225).

A *sore tongue* may be caused by local lesions as well as by general conditions.

Aphthous ulcers (p. 224); sore smooth tongue of nutritional deficiency (p. 227)

Sore throat is a frequent complaint, usually developing as part of an acute illness with other upper respiratory symptoms.

See Table 7-23, Abnormalities of the Pharynx (p. 228)

Hoarseness refers to an altered quality of the voice that is often described as husky, rough, or harsh. The pitch may be lower than before. Hoarseness most often results from disease of the larynx, but may also develop

Overuse of the voice (as in cheering) and acute infections are the most likely causes.

when extralaryngeal lesions press on the nerves that supply it. **Inquire about overuse of the voice, allergy, smoking or other inhaled irritants, and any associated symptoms. Distinguish between an acute and a chronic problem.** Hoarseness lasting two or more weeks usually makes visual examination of the larynx advisable.

"**Have you noticed any 'swollen glands' or lumps in your neck?" is a useful question, even though "glands" is not the proper technical term for lymph nodes. Ask about an enlarged thyroid gland or** *goiter* (although symptoms of thyroid dysfunction will be discussed later in the chapter). You may also wish to include *pain or stiffness in the neck* here, but these are discussed with the musculoskeletal system.

Causes of chronic hoarseness include smoking, allergy, voice abuse, hypothyroidism, chronic infections such as tuberculosis, and tumors.

Enlarged, tender lymph nodes commonly accompany pharyngitis. Increased, decreased, or normal thyroid function may accompany a goiter.

THE BREASTS

Questions about a woman's breasts may be included in the history or deferred to the physical examination. **Inquire about** *pain or discomfort,* *lumps,* **and any** *discharge from the nipples.* **Has the patient ever examined her own breasts? How often does she do it?** Approximately 50% of women have palpable lumps or nodularity in their breasts. Premenstrual enlargement and tenderness are common.

Lumps may be physiologic or pathologic. They include cysts, benign tumors, and cancers. See Table 10-2, Differentiation of Common Breast Nodules (p. 337).

THE CHEST

Pain or discomfort in the chest frequently raises concern about heart disease, but it commonly originates in other structures as well.

See Table 2-3, Chest Pain (pp. 72–73).

Chief among the sources of chest pain are:

● The myocardium

Myocardial infarction, angina pectoris

● The aorta

Dissecting aneurysm

● The trachea and large bronchi

Tracheobronchitis

● The parietal pleura

Pleurisy, pericarditis

● The esophagus

Reflux esophagitis, esophageal spasm

● The chest wall, including the musculoskeletal system and the skin

Costochondritis, herpes zoster

● Extrathoracic structures, such as the neck, gallbladder, and stomach

Cervical arthritis, biliary colic

Lung tissue itself has no pain fibers; if lung conditions such as pneumonia or pulmonary infarction cause pain, they usually do so by inflammation of the adjacent parietal pleura. Muscle strain produced by coughing may also be responsible. The pericardium has few pain fibers, and the pain of pericarditis usually arises from inflammation of adjacent parietal pleura. Chest pain commonly accompanies anxiety but its mechanism remains obscure.

Your initial questions should be as broad as possible. "Do you have discomfort or unpleasant feelings in your chest?" As you proceed to the full history, ask the patient to show you exactly where the discomfort is, and watch for any gestures used to describe it. Follow your usual style of questioning. All seven attributes (see p. 20) of this symptom may be helpful in differentiating among the various causes of chest pain.

Palpitations are an unpleasant awareness of the heartbeat. Patients report their sensations in various terms such as skipping, racing, fluttering, pounding, or stopping of the heart. Palpitations may result from an irregular heartbeat, from rapid acceleration or slowing of the heart, or from increased forcefulness of cardiac contraction, but the perception also depends on patients' sensitivities to their own bodily sensations. Palpitations do not necessarily mean heart disease, and the most serious arrhythmias, such as ventricular tachycardia, often do not produce palpitations.

You may ask directly about palpitations, but if the patient does not understand your question, reword it. "Are you sometimes aware of your heartbeat? What is it like?" Ask the patient to show you how it feels by tapping out the rhythm with a hand or finger. Was it fast or slow? regular or irregular? How long did it last? If there was an episode of rapid heart action, did it start and stop suddenly or gradually?

You may wish to teach selected patients how to make serial measurements of their pulse rates in case they have further episodes.

Dyspnea refers to a nonpainful but uncomfortable awareness of breathing that is inappropriate to the circumstances. Only the patient can report dyspnea. An observer may notice abnormally rapid or deep breathing, but these cannot be equated with the subjective sensation. Dyspnea commonly results from cardiac or bronchopulmonary disease but also frequently accompanies anxiety.

Ask if the patient has had any difficulty in breathing. Dyspneic patients may describe shortness of breath, a smothering feeling, inability to get enough air, or difficulty in taking a deep enough breath. **Ask when the symptom occurs, at rest or with exercise, and how much effort produces it.** Because of variations in age, body weight, and physical fitness there is no absolute scale on which to quantify dyspnea, but **try to determine its severity according to the patient's everyday activities.**

Anxiety is the most common cause of chest pain in children. Among organic causes, costochondritis is most common.

A clenched fist over the sternum suggests angina pectoris; a finger pointing to a small area "over my heart" suggests a noncardiac origin; a hand moving up and down from epigastrium to neck suggests heartburn.

Transient skips and flipflops suggest premature contractions; persisting irregularity, atrial fibrillation. A rapid regular beating of sudden onset and cessation suggests paroxysmal tachycardia.

See Tables 9-1 to 9-3 for the differentiation of selected heart rates and rhythms (pp. 304–307). A rapid regular rate of less than 120 per minute is usually sinus tachycardia.

See Table 2-4, Dyspnea, pp. 74–75.

Episodic dyspnea that occurs at rest as well as with exercise suggests anxiety with hyperventilation. Such patients often report that they cannot get a deep enough breath. Deep sighs are frequently observed.

How many steps can the patient climb without pausing for breath? or how many flights of stairs? How about work? carrying the groceries? mopping the floor or making a bed? Has the symptom altered the patient's activities? How? Qualitative descriptions are not often helpful in assessing the nature of dyspnea, but carefully determine the timing, setting, associated symptoms, and factors that aggravate it or relieve it.

Orthopnea is dyspnea that occurs when the patient is lying down and improves upon sitting up. It is classically quantified according to the number of pillows on which the patient sleeps, or the fact that the patient prefers to sleep sitting up. Be sure, however, that the patient uses the extra pillows or sleeps in a sitting position because of dyspnea, not for other reasons.

Orthopnea suggests left ventricular failure or mitral stenosis but may also accompany obstructive lung disease.

Paroxysmal nocturnal dyspnea describes episodes of sudden dyspnea and orthopnea that waken a patient from sleep, usually one or two hours after going to bed. The patient typically sits up, stands up, or goes to a window for air. Wheezing and cough may be associated. The episode usually subsides spontaneously but may recur at about the same time on subsequent nights.

Paroxysmal nocturnal dyspnea suggests left ventricular failure or mitral stenosis and may be mimicked by nocturnal asthmatic attacks.

Wheezes are musical respiratory sounds that may be audible both to the patient and to others.

Wheezing suggests partial airway obstruction.

Edema refers to the accumulation of excessive fluid in the interstitial spaces, and appears as swelling. Although questions about edema are typically included in the chest history, it has many other causes and may signify local problems as well as more general ones. **Focus your questions on the distribution and timing of the swelling, and explore the associated symptoms and the setting in which it occurs. "Have you had any swelling anywhere? Where? . . . anywhere else? When does it occur? Is it worse in the morning or at night? Do your shoes get tight? Do the rings on your fingers get too tight? Are your eyelids puffy or swollen in the morning? Have you had to let your belt out? Have your clothes gotten too tight around your middle?"** Because several liters of extra fluid may accumulate in a person's body before overt edema appears, it is useful to ask the patient who tends to retain fluid to record daily morning weights.

See Table 15-3, Mechanisms and Patterns of Edema, pp. 455–456.

Dependent edema appears in the lowest body parts—the feet and legs except in bedridden persons. Consider peripheral, cardiac, and other causes. Puffy eyelids and tight rings, when associated with edema elsewhere, suggest renal disease or hypoalbuminemia. An enlarged waistline may indicate *ascites* (fluid in the peritoneal cavity) or fat.

Cough is a frequent symptom that varies in significance from the trivial to the ominous. A person may cough voluntarily, but more typically cough is a reflex response to stimuli that irritate receptors in the larynx, trachea, or large bronchi. These stimuli include both external agents such as irritating dusts, foreign bodies, and even extremely hot or cold air, and internal substances such as mucus, pus, and blood. Inflammation of the respiratory mucosa, and pressure or tension on the air passages as from a tumor or enlarged peribronchial lymph node, may also cause coughing.

See Table 2-5, Cough and Hemoptysis, p. 76.

Although cough typically signals a problem in the respiratory tract, the underlying cause may also be cardiovascular.

Cough is an important symptom of left-sided heart failure.

"Do you have a cough?" may be an adequate opening question, but for some patients, especially those who smoke, a morning cough has become so habitual that they fail to mention it. Further questions here are "Do you have to clear your throat in the morning?" and "Do you have a cigarette cough?" Determine the timing of the cough. Is it a new symptom or more chronic? How frequent is it? When does it occur? Is it seasonal? Are there factors that seem to precipitate or aggravate it? Has a chronic cough changed in any way?

Assess the cough qualitatively by whether it is dry or productive of *sputum* **(phlegm). Because some patients, especially women, may swallow their sputum, you may have difficulty here. If possible, however, try to get a description of the volume of the sputum and its color, odor, and consistency. Many patients have difficulty in describing the volume of their sputum. A multiple-choice question may be helpful in eliciting a rough estimate. "How much do you think you cough up in 24 hours: a teaspoon, tablespoon, quarter cup, half cup, cupful, or what?"** If the patient coughs in your presence, offer a tissue and ask the patient to cough any phlegm into it so that you can inspect it. A specimen from deep in the chest is desirable. **Symptoms associated with the cough often lead you to its cause.**

Mucoid sputum is translucent, white, or gray. *Purulent* sputum is yellowish or greenish. *Mucopurulent* sputum has components of both. Large volumes of purulent sputum suggest bronchiectasis or lung abscess.

Hemoptysis refers to the coughing or "spitting up" of blood, which may vary from blood-streaked phlegm to pure blood. **Ask if the patient has ever experienced either of these. Assess the volume of blood produced together with other attributes of the sputum. Focus your further questions on the setting in which the hemoptysis occurred and the associated symptoms.**

See Table 2-5, Cough and Hemoptysis, p. 76. Hemoptysis is a rare and usually terminal event in infants, children, and adolescents, seen most often in older children with cystic fibrosis.

Before labeling this symptom, you should try to determine by history and examination the origin of the bleeding. If the blood or blood-streaked material appears without coughing, it may originate in the mouth or pharynx. If it is vomited rather than coughed, it probably originates in the gastrointestinal tract. Blood from either the nasopharynx or the gastrointestinal tract, however, is occasionally aspirated and then coughed out.

Blood originating in the stomach is usually darker than that from the respiratory tract and may be mixed with food particles.

THE GASTROINTESTINAL TRACT

Dysphagia refers to difficulty in swallowing, the sense that food or liquid is sticking, hesitating, or "won't go down right." The sensation of a lump in the throat or in the retrosternal area, unassociated with swallowing, is not true dysphagia. Dysphagia may result from esophageal disorders or from difficulty in transferring food from the mouth to the esophagus.

For transfer and esophageal dysphagia, see Table 2-6, Dysphagia, p. 77.

Ask the patient to show you where the dysphagia is felt.

Pointing to the chest suggests an esophageal disorder; point-

Timing is helpful in assessing dysphagia. When did it start? Is it intermittent or persistent? Is it progressing, and if so, how quickly?

Determine what precipitates it: relatively solid foods such as meat, softer foods such as ground meat and mashed potatoes, or hot or cold liquids. Has the pattern changed? What are the associated symptoms and medical conditions?

Odynophagia, pain on swallowing, may occur in two forms. A sharp, burning pain suggests mucosal inflammation, while a squeezing, cramping pain suggests a muscular cause. Odynophagia may accompany dysphagia, but either symptom may occur by itself.

Indigestion is a common complaint that generally refers to distress associated with eating, but people use the term for many different symptoms. Find out just what your patient means. Possibilities include:

- *Heartburn,* a sense of burning or warmth that is felt retrosternally and may radiate from the epigastrium to the neck. It usually originates in the esophagus. When severe, however, it may raise the question of heart disease, in both your mind and that of the patient. Some patients with coronary artery disease, moreover, describe their pain as burning, "like indigestion." Pay particular attention to what brings on the discomfort and what relieves it.

- *Excessive gas,* as manifested by frequent belching, abdominal bloating or distention, or *flatus* (the passage of gas by rectum). Inquire about specific foods that seem to produce these symptoms. Start with open-ended questions here, but be sure to discover any relationship to the ingestion of milk or milk products. (A deficiency in intestinal lactase commonly causes gaseousness after the ingestion of milk or milk products.) A normal person passes roughly 600 ml of gas per rectum daily.

- Unpleasant *abdominal fullness after meals* of normal size or *inability to eat a full meal*

- *Abdominal pain*
- *Nausea and vomiting*

ing to the throat may occur in either a transfer or an esophageal disorder.

Dysphagia with only solid foods suggests a mechanical narrowing of the esophagus; dysphagia related to both solids and liquids suggests a disorder of esophageal muscle.

Causes of mucosal inflammation include reflux esophagitis and esophageal infections due to herpesvirus or *Candida.*

Heartburn points to reflux of gastric acid into the esophagus and is often precipitated by a heavy meal, lying down, or bending forward. Ingested alcohol, citrus juices, or aspirin may also cause it. When it is chronic, consider reflux esophagitis. See Table 2-3, Chest Pain, pp. 72–73.

Swallowing air (*aerophagia*) is the normal cause of belching but does not cause bloating or excessive flatus. Consider instead gas-producing foods such as legumes, deficiency in intestinal lactase, and irritable bowel syndrome.

Causes include anticholinergic drugs, obstruction of the gastric outlet, gastric cancer, and gastroparesis (a complication of diabetes mellitus).

In order to approach the problem of *abdominal pain*, you should understand its possible mechanisms and clinical patterns. There are three broad categories.

1. *Visceral pain* originates in the abdominal organs. Hollow structures such as the intestine or biliary tree may become painful when they contract unusually forcefully or when they are distended or stretched. Solid organs such as the liver become painful when their capsules are stretched. Visceral pain is rather poorly localized but is typically, though not necessarily, felt near the midline, at levels that vary according to the structure involved, as illustrated below.

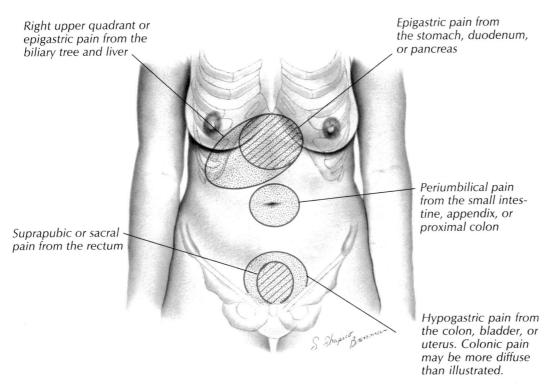

Right upper quadrant or epigastric pain from the biliary tree and liver

Epigastric pain from the stomach, duodenum, or pancreas

Periumbilical pain from the small intestine, appendix, or proximal colon

Suprapubic or sacral pain from the rectum

Hypogastric pain from the colon, bladder, or uterus. Colonic pain may be more diffuse than illustrated.

Renal and ureteral pain are illustrated on p. 53.

Visceral pain varies in quality and may be gnawing, burning, cramping, or aching. When it becomes severe, it may be associated with sweating, pallor, nausea, vomiting, and restlessness.

2. *Parietal pain* originates in the parietal peritoneum and is caused by inflammation. It is a steady, aching pain that is usually more severe than visceral pain and more precisely localized over the involved structure. It is typically aggravated by movement or coughing, and patients with this kind of pain usually prefer to lie still.

Acute appendicitis exemplifies both visceral and parietal pain. Early distention of the inflamed appendix produces periumbilical pain, which is gradually replaced by right lower quadrant pain due to inflammation of the adjacent parietal peritoneum.

3. *Referred* pain is felt in more distant sites that are innervated at approximately the same spinal levels as the disordered structure. Referred pain often develops as the initial pain becomes more intense and thus

Pain of duodenal or pancreatic origin may be referred to the back; pain from the biliary tree,

seems to radiate or travel from the initial site. It may be felt superficially or more deeply, but is usually well localized.

Pain may not only be referred from abdominal organs to nonabdominal sites; it may also be referred to the abdomen from the chest, spine, or pelvis, thus complicating the assessment of abdominal pain.

After you get the history of abdominal pain in the patient's own words, ask the patient to show you just where it is. If clothes intervene, repeat the question during your examination. Where does the pain start? Does it travel anywhere?

What is the pain like? If the patient has trouble describing it, try a multiple-choice question: "Is it aching, cramping, burning, gnawing, or what?"

How severe is the pain? Is it bearable? Does it interfere with the patient's usual activities? Does it make the patient lie down? The description of the severity of the pain may tell you something about the patient's responses to pain and its impact on the patient's life, but it is not consistently helpful in assessing cause. Sensitivity to abdominal pain varies widely among people and tends to diminish over the later years, thus masking acute abdominal problems in the elderly, especially those in or beyond their 70s.

Careful timing of the pain, on the other hand, is particularly helpful. Did it start suddenly or gradually? When did the pain begin? How long does it last? What is its pattern over a 24-hour period? over weeks and months? Are you dealing with an acute illness or a chronic or recurring one?

What aggravates or relieves the pain, with special reference to eating, antacids, alcohol, medications (including aspirin-containing and other over-the-counter drugs), emotional factors, and possibly posture? Is the pain related to bodily functions such as defecation, menstruation, and urination?

What symptoms are associated with the pain, and in what sequence do they occur?

"How is your appetite?" continues the gastrointestinal history but may also lead into other important areas. *Anorexia* refers to loss or lack of appetite. Distinguish it from intolerance to certain foods or reluctance to eat anything because of anticipated discomfort. *Nausea*, which patients often describe as "feeling sick to my stomach," may progress to retching and vomiting. *Retching* describes the spasmodic movements of the chest and diaphragm that precede and culminate in *vomiting*—the forceful expulsion of gastric contents out through the mouth.

to the right shoulder or the right posterior chest.

The pain of pleurisy or acute myocardial infarction may be referred to the upper abdomen.

See Table 2-7, Abdominal Pain, pp. 78–79.

Cramping (colicky) pain suggests a relationship to peristalsis.

Citrus fruits may aggravate the pain of reflux esophagitis. Abdominal discomfort with milk ingestion suggests lactase deficiency.

Anorexia, nausea, and vomiting accompany gastrointestinal disorders and many other conditions such as pregnancy, responses to prescribed or other drugs, diabetic acidosis, adrenal insufficiency, hypercalcemia, uremia, liver disease, emotional states, and (though without nausea) anorexia/bulimia nervosa.

Regurgitation, the raising of esophageal or gastric contents in the absence of nausea or retching, has implications quite different from vomiting.

Regurgitation may occur when the esophagus is narrowed or when the gastroesophageal sphincter is incompetent.

Assess these symptoms in the usual manner. Ask about any vomitus or regurgitated material, and inspect it yourself if possible. What color is it? What does the vomitus smell like? How much has there been? Ask specifically about blood in the vomitus and try to estimate its amount.

Gastric juice is clear or mucoid. Small amounts of yellowish or greenish bile are common and have no special significance. Brownish or blackish vomitus with small particles that look like coffee grounds suggests blood that has been altered by gastric acid. Both this (when confirmed by chemical testing) and red blood are termed *hematemesis*.

Common causes of hematemesis include duodenal or gastric ulcer, esophageal or gastric varices, and gastritis. A fecal odor suggests obstruction of the ileum or a gastrocolic fistula.

Do the symptoms or setting suggest the complications of vomiting, such as aspiration into the lungs (especially in elderly, debilitated, or obtunded patients), dehydration and electrolyte imbalance (after prolonged vomiting), or significant loss of blood?

Symptoms of blood loss (light-headedness, faintness, syncope) depend on the rate and volume of bleeding and rarely appear before 500 ml or more are lost.

To assess *bowel function*, start with some open-ended questions: "How are your bowel movements? How often do you move your bowels? Do you have any difficulties? Has there been any change in your bowel habits?" The frequency of bowel movements varies in normal adults from about three times a day to twice a week. Changes within these limits, however, may be very significant in an individual patient.

When asking details about the appearance of the stools, it may be helpful to find out if the patient looks at them. You may thus avoid being misled by confusing or negative responses.

Inquire about the color of the stools and ask about any *black stools* (suggesting *melena*) or *red blood in the stools* (*hematochezia*). If either condition is present, how long has the patient noticed it? How often? If the blood is red, how much is there? Is it pure blood, mixed in with the stool, or on the surface of it? Is there blood on the toilet paper?

See Table 2-8, Black and Bloody Stools, p. 80.

Patients vary widely in their concepts of constipation and diarrhea. **When a person complains of either symptom, determine his or her meaning for the term. What is the *constipation* like: a decrease in the frequency of bowel movements? the passage of hard and perhaps painful stools? the need to strain unusually hard? a sense of incomplete defecation or pressure in the rectum? What do the stools look like? What remedies has the patient tried? Explore the setting in which the constipation has occurred, with particular reference to**

See Table 2-9, Constipation, p. 81.

medications, emotional stress, the person's ideas of normal bowel habits, and the time and conditions available for defecation. Occasionally constipation becomes complete, with passage of neither feces nor gas. This is termed *obstipation*.

Obstipation occurs in intestinal obstruction.

Diarrhea refers to an excessive frequency in the passage of stools that are usually unformed or watery.

Try to determine the size or the volume of the stools as well as their frequency. Are they bulky or small? How often must the patient go to the toilet to pass them?

Consistently large diarrheal stools suggest a disorder in the small bowel or proximal colon; small, frequent stools with urgency to pass them suggest a disorder in the left colon or rectum.

What are the stools like qualitatively? Are they mushy or watery? What color are they? Do they look greasy or oily? frothy? Do they smell unusually foul? Is mucus, pus, or blood associated? Do they float in the toilet (because of excessive gas), and are they therefore difficult to flush?

Large, yellowish or gray, greasy, foul-smelling, and sometimes frothy or floating stools suggest *steatorrhea* (fatty stools), associated with malabsorption.

Assess the course of the diarrhea over time. Is it acute, chronic, or recurrent? Remember, however, that your patient may be experiencing the first acute episode in a chronic or recurrent illness.

See Table 2-10, Diarrhea (pp. 82–83).

Does diarrhea waken the patient at night?

Nocturnal diarrhea suggests an organic cause.

What seems to aggravate and relieve the diarrhea? Does the patient get relief from a bowel movement, or is there an intense urge, with straining, but little or no result (*tenesmus*)?

Relief by moving the bowels or passing gas suggests a disorder in the left colon or rectum. Tenesmus suggests a problem in the rectum near the anal sphincter.

In what setting has the diarrhea occurred, including travel, emotional stress, or a new medication? Do family members or companions have similar symptoms?

What are the associated symptoms?

Jaundice, or *icterus*, refers to the yellowish discoloration of the skin and eyes by an increased amount of bilirubin, a bile pigment derived chiefly from the breakdown of hemoglobin. Normally, liver cells take up this bilirubin, conjugate (or combine) it with other substances so that it becomes water soluble, and then excrete it into the bile. Bile passes normally through the biliary tree into the small intestine. Mechanisms of jaundice include:

1. Increased production of bilirubin
2. Decreased uptake of bilirubin by the liver cells

Bilirubin in the blood is predominantly unconjugated in jaundice due to any of the first three mechanisms. Causes include hemolytic anemia (increased production) and Gilbert's syndrome.

3. Decreased ability of the liver to conjugate the bilirubin, and
4. Decreased excretion of bilirubin into the bile with resulting escape of some bilirubin, now in its conjugated form, back into the blood. The cause may lie *within the liver itself,* as

    a. Hepatocellular jaundice, due to damage to the liver cells, or as
    b. Cholestatic jaundice, a more selective excretory impairment due to damage of liver cells or of intrahepatic bile ducts.

When excretion of bilirubin is impaired, the bilirubin in the blood is predominantly conjugated. Causes include:
a. Viral hepatitis, cirrhosis
b. Drug-induced cholestasis (oral contraceptives, methyl testosterone, chlorpromazine) or primary biliary cirrhosis

Alternatively, the cause may lie in *obstruction of the extrahepatic bile ducts.*

Obstruction of the common bile duct by gallstones or cancer of the pancreas

As you interview the jaundiced patient, pay special attention to the associated symptoms and the setting in which the illness occurred.

What color was the urine as the patient became ill? and now? When conjugated bilirubin increases in the blood it may appear in the urine, darkening it into a yellowish brown or tea-like color. Unconjugated bilirubin is not excreted in the urine.

Dark urine stained by bilirubin indicates impaired excretion of bilirubin into the gastrointestinal tract.

How about the color of the stools? When excretion of bile into the intestine is completely obstructed, the stools become light-colored and gray (or *acholic,* without bile).

Acholic stools may occur briefly in viral hepatitis and are common in obstructive jaundice.

Does the skin itch without other obvious explanation?

Itching favors cholestatic or obstructive jaundice.

Is there associated pain? What is its pattern? Have there been past and repeated attacks of pain?

Are there factors in the patient's setting that increase the risks of liver disease, such as

Consider the aching pain of a distended liver capsule; the persistent pain of pancreatic cancer; and episodes of biliary colic.

1. **Hepatitis: travel in areas of poor sanitation, known contacts with jaundiced persons, sexual contacts with carriers of hepatitis B, ingestion of raw clams or oysters, use of inadequately sterilized needles or syringes (as in drug addiction), treatment with blood transfusions or blood products or exposure to them (as in laboratories, dental offices, or dialysis units)**
2. **Cirrhosis and other alcohol-related liver disease. (Interview the patient carefully about the consumption of alcohol.)**
3. **Toxic liver damage, as produced by medications and industrial exposure**
4. **Gallbladder disease, its symptoms, or gallbladder surgery that might have contributed to extrahepatic biliary obstruction**
5. **Hereditary disorders. (Review the family history.)**

THE URINARY TRACT

Disorders of the urinary tract may cause pain in either the back or the abdomen. *Kidney pain* is felt at or below the costal margin posteriorly, near the costovertebral angle. It may radiate anteriorly toward the umbilicus.

Kidney pain occurs in acute pyelonephritis.

Kidney pain is a visceral pain that is usually produced by sudden distention of the renal capsule and is typically dull, aching, and steady. Dramatically different is *ureteral pain* (*ureteral or renal colic*), a severe colicky pain that often originates in the costovertebral angle and radiates around the trunk into the lower quadrant of the abdomen and possibly on into the upper thigh and testicle or labium. Ureteral pain results from sudden distention of the ureter and associated distention of the renal pelvis.

Renal or ureteral colic is caused by sudden obstruction of a ureter, as by urinary stones or blood clots.

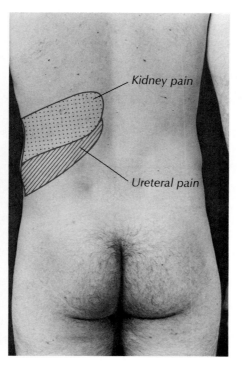

Bladder disorders may cause suprapubic pain. Pain associated with bladder infection, if present at all in the abdomen, is typically dull and steady. Pain associated with sudden overdistention of the bladder is often agonizing, while chronic bladder distention is usually painless. *Prostatic pain* is felt in the perineum and occasionally in the rectum.

Pain of sudden overdistention in acute urinary retention

*Pain on urination** accompanies inflammation or irritation of either the bladder or the urethra and is usually felt as a burning sensation. Men typically feel it in or proximal to the glans penis, while women perceive it in one of two ways: as an internal urethral discomfort, sometimes described as pressure, or as an external burning caused by urine as it flows across irritated or inflamed labia.

Cystitis and urethritis commonly cause painful urination. Consider also stones, foreign bodies or tumors in the bladder, and acute prostatitis. In women, internal burning sug-

* Clinicians often refer to painful urination as *dysuria*. Some authorities, however, prefer to define dysuria as any difficulty in voiding.

Several symptoms other than pain may accompany voiding. *Urinary urgency* is an unusually intense and immediate desire to void. It sometimes leads to involuntary voiding (*urge incontinence*). In a man with partial obstruction to urinary outflow from the bladder, a cluster of symptoms often develops: *hesitancy* in starting the urinary stream, *straining* to void, *reduced caliber and force of the urinary stream,* and *dribbling* as he tries to complete the voiding process.

Urinary urgency suggests infection or irritation of the bladder. In men, pain on urination without frequency or urgency suggests urethritis.

Three terms describe important alterations in the patterns of voiding urine. *Polyuria* refers to a significant increase in 24-hour urinary volume, roughly defined as exceeding 3 liters. It must be distinguished from *urinary frequency,* abnormally frequent voiding. Although urinary frequency may be secondary to polyuria and is then associated with a high volume of urine with each voiding, frequency is often associated instead with relatively small volumes at each passage. *Nocturia* refers to urinary frequency at night, sometimes defined as when the bladder wakens the patient more than once. A change in nocturnal voiding patterns as well as the number of trips to the toilet should be considered in assessing this symptom. Like frequency itself, nocturia may be associated with large or small volumes of urine. *Polydipsia* is an abnormally high intake of water or other fluids and is commonly associated with polyuria.

Polyuria indicates an abnormally high production of urine by the kidneys. Frequency without polyuria (during the day or night) suggests either a disorder of the urinary bladder or impairment to flow at or below the bladder neck.

See Table 2-11, Polyuria, Frequency, and Nocturia, pp. 84–85.

Blood in the urine is an important symptom known as *hematuria,* often identified only by urinalysis. When visible to the naked eye it is called *gross hematuria.* Blood may give the urine a pinkish or brownish cast or in larger amounts may make it look frankly bloody. Be sure not to mistake menstrual bleeding for hematuria. If urine is reddish, inquire about the ingestion of beets or medications that sometimes discolor the urine. Test the urine with dipstick and microscopic examination before settling on the term hematuria.

Causes of hematuria include cystitis, malignancy of the bladder or kidney, stones, trauma, tuberculosis, and acute glomerulonephritis. Bilirubin may color the urine yellowish brown.

Drugs that may color the urine reddish include phenolphthalein (common in over-the-counter laxatives) and phenazopyridine (Pyridium).

Urinary incontinence refers to an involuntary loss of urine that has become a social or hygienic problem. It usually points to a disorder in the urinary bladder or urethra, in the structures that support or surround them, or in the neural regulatory mechanisms that control urination.

The normal adult bladder is a hollow muscular organ that can expand to accommodate roughly 300 ml of urine at relatively low pressures. As distention continues it stimulates the smooth muscle of the bladder (the detrusor muscle) to contract, pressure in the bladder rises, and the urge to void becomes conscious. If the setting is inconvenient for voiding, higher centers in the brain can inhibit detrusor contractions until the normal

Incontinence may result when detrusor contractions are too strong (*urge incontinence*), when intraurethral pressure is too low (*stress incontinence*), and when the bladder is grossly enlarged

bladder capacity of 400 ml to 500 ml is reached. Pressure within the urethra that exceeds that in the bladder holds the accumulating urine within the bladder reservoir and prevents incontinence. Factors contributing to intraurethral pressure include smooth muscle in the urethra (the internal urethral sphincter), the thickness of normal urethral mucosa, and, in women, sufficient muscular support of the bladder and proximal urethra to maintain the proper geometric relations between them. Striated muscle around the urethra can contract voluntarily to interrupt the voiding process.

because of outlet obstruction (*overflow incontinence*). Incontinence may also be due to poor general health, to environmental factors (*functional incontinence*), or to medications. See Table 2-12, Urinary Incontinence, pp. 86–87.

Neuroregulatory control of the bladder functions at several levels. In an infant, the bladder empties by a reflex mechanism at the sacral level of the spinal cord. Adult voluntary control of urination depends also on higher centers within the brain and on motor and sensory pathways between the brain and the sacral cord.

General questions for a urinary history include: "Do you have any difficulty passing your urine? How often do you go? Do you get up at night to go? How often? How much do you pass at a time? Is there any pain or burning? Do you have to go so badly that you sometimes have trouble getting to the toilet in time? Do you ever leak any urine? . . . or wet yourself?" If the patient has been incontinent, ask when it happens and how often. Can the patient sense when the bladder is full? and when voiding occurs? Ask women specifically if sudden coughing, sneezing, or laughing makes them lose urine (*stress incontinence*). Roughly half of even young women who have not borne children report this experience.

Unawareness of a full bladder or of wetness suggests a sensory or mental deficit.

Occasional leakage of small amounts of urine is not necessarily significant.

What color is the urine? Has it ever been reddish, or brownish? If it seems relevant inquire about pain in the abdomen or back, but in the absence of urinary symptoms you may prefer to cover these topics in your gastrointestinal and musculoskeletal histories.

Ask additional questions of middle-aged or elderly men. "Do you have trouble getting your stream started? Do you have to stand closer to the toilet than you used to? Have you noticed a change in the force or size of your stream? Do you have to strain down in order to void? Do you hesitate or stop in the middle of voiding? Do you dribble after you're through?"

The most common cause of these symptoms is partial obstruction of the bladder outlet due to benign prostatic hyperplasia. A urethral stricture may also cause them.

THE GENITAL SYSTEM—FEMALE

Questions in this section focus on menstruation, pregnancy and related topics, vulvovaginal symptoms, and sexual function.

For the menstrual history, ask the patient how old she was when her monthly, or menstrual, periods began (age at *menarche*). When did her last period start, and, if possible, the one before that? How often do the periods come (as measured by the first day of successive periods)? How regular or irregular are they? How long do they last? How heavy is the flow? What color is it? Flow can be assessed roughly by the number of pads or tampons used daily. Because women vary in their assessments of when sanitary equipment should be changed, however, ask the patient whether she usually soaks a pad or tampon, spots it lightly, or what. Further, does she use more than one at a time? Does she have any bleeding between periods? any bleeding after intercourse or after douching?

The dates of previous periods may alert you to possible pregnancy or menstrual irregularities.

Unlike the normal dark red menstrual discharge, excessive flow tends to be bright red and may include "clots" (not true fibrin clots).

Does the patient have any discomfort or pain before or during her periods? If so, what is it like, how long does it last, and does it interfere with her usual activities? Are other symptoms associated? Ask a middle-aged or older woman if she has stopped menstruating. When? Did any symptoms accompany her change? Has she had any bleeding since?

Questions about menarche, menstruation, and menopause may give you excellent opportunities to explore the patient's need for information, her self-image, and her attitude toward her body. When talking with an adolescent girl, for example, opening questions might include: "How did you first learn about monthly periods? How did you feel when they started? Many girls worry when their periods aren't regular or come late. Has anything like that bothered you?" For a middle-aged woman, "How did (do) you feel about not having your periods any more? Has it affected your life in any way?"

Girls in the United States usually begin to menstruate between the ages of 9 and 16 years, and often take a year or more before they settle into a reasonably regular pattern. Age at menarche varies with several factors. One is the age at which women in the adolescent's parents' families began to menstruate. Another is race: white girls on the average have earlier menarche than black girls. A third is nutritional status: well nourished girls start to menstruate earlier than those who are poorly nourished. The interval between periods ranges roughly from 24 to 32 days; the flow lasts from 3 to 7 days.

Amenorrhea refers to the absence of periods. Failure to initiate periods is called *primary amenorrhea*, while the cessation of periods after they have been established is termed *secondary amenorrhea*. Pregnancy, lactation, and menopause are physiologic forms of the secondary type. *Oligomenorrhea* refers to infrequent periods, which may also be irregular. This pattern is common for as long as 2 years after menarche and it also occurs before menopause.

Other causes of secondary amenorrhea include low body weight from any cause, including malnutrition and anorexia nervosa; stress; chronic illness; and hypothalamic–pituitary–ovarian dysfunctions.

Polymenorrhea means abnormally frequent periods, and *menorrhagia* refers to an increased amount or duration of flow. Bleeding may also

Increased frequency, increased flow, or bleeding between pe-

occur between periods (variously termed *metrorrhagia* or *intermenstrual bleeding*), after intercourse (*postcoital bleeding*), or after other vaginal contact such as occurs with douches.

riods may have organic causes or may be dysfunctional. Postcoital bleeding suggests cervical disease (*e.g.*, polyps, cancer) or, in an older woman, atrophic vaginitis.

Menopause, the cessation of menses, usually occurs between the ages of 45 and 52 years, but the range of normal is wider. *Postmenopausal bleeding* is defined as bleeding that occurs after 6 months without periods. The only symptoms clearly associated with menopause are *hot flushes* (or *flashes*), the sweating associated with them, and sometimes the disturbance of sleep that they may cause.

Postmenopausal bleeding raises the question of endometrial cancer, although it also has other causes.

Dysmenorrhea refers to pain with menstruation and is usually felt as a bearing down, aching, or cramping sensation in the lower abdomen and pelvis. *Premenstrual syndrome* (*PMS*) refers to several symptoms noted by some women during the 4 to 10 days before a period. These include tension, nervousness, irritability, depression, and mood swings; weight gain, abdominal bloating, edema, and tenderness of the breasts; and headaches. Though usually mild, the symptoms may be severe and disabling.

Standard questions related to pregnancies include: "Have you ever been (or how often have you been) pregnant? Have you ever had a miscarriage or an abortion? How often? How many living children do you have?" Inquire about any difficulties with the pregnancies and the timing and circumstances of any abortion (spontaneous or induced). What kind of birth control methods, if any, have the patient and her partner used, and how satisfied is she with them?

If amenorrhea suggests a pregnancy now, inquire about its possibility (history of intercourse) and about common early symptoms: tenderness, tingling, or increased size of the breasts; urinary frequency; nausea and vomiting; easy fatigability; and feelings that the baby is moving (the last usually noted at about 20 weeks). Be alert to the patient's feelings in discussing all these topics, and explore them as seems indicated. (See Chapter 14, The Pregnant Woman.)

Amenorrhea followed by heavy bleeding suggests a threatened abortion or dysfunctional uterine bleeding related to lack of ovulation.

The most common vulvovaginal symptoms are *vaginal discharge* and local *itching*. **Follow your usual approach. If the patient reports a discharge, inquire about its amount, color, consistency, and odor. Ask too about any local *sores* or *lumps* in the vulvar area. Are they painful or not? Because patients vary in their understanding of anatomic terms here, be prepared with some alternative phrasing: "Any itching (or other symptom) near your vagina? . . . between your legs? . . . in your privates?"**

See Table 13-5, Vaginitis, p. 405.

See Table 13-1, Lesions of the Vulva, p. 401.

Local symptoms or findings on physical examination may raise the possibility of sexually transmitted diseases. After establishing the

usual attributes of any symptoms, inquire about sexual contacts and past history of venereal disease. "Have you ever had herpes? . . . any other problems such as gonorrhea? . . . syphilis? . . . pelvic infections?" Continue with the more general questions suggested on page 22.

If the patient seems to have a sexual problem, ask her to tell you about it. Direct questions help you to assess each phase of the sexual response: desire, arousal, and orgasm. "Have you maintained an interest in (appetite for) sex?" inquires about the desire phase. For the orgasmic phase, "Are you able to reach a climax (reach an orgasm or 'come')? Is it important for you to reach a climax?" And for arousal, "Do you get sexually aroused? Do you lubricate easily (get wet)? Do you stay too dry?"

Sexual dysfunctions are classified according to the phase of sexual response. A woman may lack desire (*hypoactive sexual desire disorder*), she may fail to become aroused and to attain adequate lubrication of her vagina (*female sexual arousal disorder*), or she may be unable to reach orgasm much or all of the time (*inhibited female orgasm*).

Further, "Are you satisfied with your sex life as it is now? Has there been any significant change in the last few years? Are you satisfied with your ability to perform sexually? How satisfied do you think your partner is? Do you feel that your partner is satisfied with the frequency of sexual activity?"

In addition to ascertaining the nature of a sexual problem, ask about its onset, severity (persistent or sporadic), setting, and factors, if any, that make it better or worse. What does the patient think is the cause of the problem, what has she tried to do about it, and what does she hope for? The setting of a sexual dysfunction is an important but complicated topic, involving the patient's general health, medications and drugs including alcohol, her partner's and her own knowledge of sexual practices and techniques, her attitudes, values, and fears, the relationship and communication between her and her partner(s), and the environment in which sexual activity takes place.

Ask also about any discomfort or pain on intercourse (*dyspareunia*). If she has had it, try to localize the symptom. Is it near the outside, occurring at the start of intercourse, or does she feel it farther in, when her partner's penis (or other objects) are pushing deeper? *Vaginismus* refers to an involuntary spasm of the muscles surrounding the vaginal orifice that makes penetration during intercourse painful or impossible.

Superficial pain suggests local inflammation, atrophic vaginitis, or inadequate lubrication; deeper pain may be due to pelvic disorders or pressure on a normal ovary. The cause of vaginismus may be physical or psychological.

THE GENITAL SYSTEM—MALE

For men, questions about the genital system follow naturally after those dealing with the urinary system. They focus on local symptoms and on sexual function.

Ask about any *discharge from the penis*, dripping, or staining of the underwear. If discharge is present, ascertain the amount, its color and

A penile discharge suggests urethritis.

consistency, and any associated symptoms. Inquire about *sores* or *growths on the penis* and any *swelling or pain in the scrotum*. **These symptoms raise the question of sexually transmitted diseases. Ask about previous symptoms or a past history of diseases such as herpes, gonorrhea, and syphilis. Continue with the more general questions suggested on page 22.**

See Table 12-1, Abnormalities of the Penis (p. 379) and Table 12-2, Abnormalities in the Scrotum (pp. 380–381). Many skin conditions other than sexually transmitted diseases affect the genitalia, and a sexually transmitted disease may be present without symptoms or signs.

Because sexually transmitted diseases may involve other parts of the body, additional questions are often indicated. An introductory explanation may be useful. **"Sexually transmitted diseases can involve any bodily opening where you have sex. It's important for you to tell me which openings you use." And further, as needed, "Do you have oral sex? . . . anal sex?" If the answers to these questions are affirmative, ask about symptoms such as diarrhea, rectal bleeding, anal itching or pain, and sore throat.**

Infections from oral–penile transmission include gonorrhea, *Chlamydia*, syphilis, and herpes. Symptomatic or asymptomatic proctitis caused by one or more microorganisms may follow anal intercourse.

If the patient seems to have a sexual problem, ask him to tell you about it. Direct questions help you to assess each phase of the sexual response. "Have you maintained an interest in (appetite for) sex?" asks about the desire phase.

Lack of desire, not due to another disorder, is termed *hypoactive sexual desire disorder*.

To assess the arousal phase, ask, "Are you able to achieve and maintain an erection?" If there seems to be a problem here, ask the patient how firm the penis becomes. Is the problem constant or sporadic? Are there circumstances in which erection is normal: with other partners? on awakening during the night or in the morning? with masturbation? Were there any changes in his relationship with his partner or in his life situation at the time when the problem began?

In an *erectile dysfunction* (impotence) a man cannot attain and maintain an erection sufficient for penetration. Causes are organic, psychogenic, or both. Consistent dysfunction in all circumstances favors an organic cause. Consider medications, other drugs, diabetes mellitus, arterial insufficiency, and neurologic problems.

Questions relating to ejaculation refer to the phase of orgasm. Either prematurity or delay may be a problem. For ejaculation that is premature (too soon and out of control), ask "About how long does intercourse last? Do you come too soon? Do you feel you have any control over it? Do you think your partner would like intercourse to last longer?" For delayed ejaculation, "Do you sometimes find that you can't come (ejaculate, have an orgasm) even though your erection is all right?" Inquire about the frequency of the problem, medications, and other circumstances in which the problem developed.

Premature ejaculation is very common, especially in young men.

Delayed ejaculation (*inhibited male orgasm*) is less common and usually affects middle-aged and older men. It may be psychogenic, organic, or both.

Further, "Are you satisfied with your sex life as it is now? Has there been any significant change over the last few years? How satisfied do

you think your partner is? Do you feel that your partner is satisfied with the frequency of sexual activity?"

As with women, inquire about the onset, severity, and setting of any problem. What does the patient think has caused it, what has he tried to do about it, and what does he hope for?

THE PERIPHERAL VASCULAR SYSTEM

Pain in the arms and legs may arise from the skin, the peripheral vascular system, the musculoskeletal system, or the nervous system. In addition, visceral pain, such as that from myocardial infarction, may be referred to the extremities.

Symptoms associated with the pain often give clues to its vascular nature. *Swelling of the feet and legs*, for example, may signify venous disease, although it has many other causes, and *coldness* and *numbness* often accompany arterial disorders. The *redness*, *swelling*, and *tenderness* of local inflammation are seen in some vascular disorders as well as in other conditions that may mimic them. In contrast, relatively brief leg cramps that commonly occur at night in otherwise healthy people do not indicate a circulatory problem, and cold hands and feet are so common in healthy people that they have relatively little predictive value.

See Table 2-13, Painful Peripheral Vascular Disorders and Their Mimics, pp. 88–89. Local inflammation is seen in superficial thrombophlebitis, lymphangitis, cellulitis, and erythema nodosum. The origin of the common leg cramp is poorly understood.

For most patients, inquiry about two symptoms suffices for screening: swelling of the feet and legs, and pain or discomfort in the legs. "Do your fingertips change color in the cold? How?" may also be useful.

Severe pallor of the fingers, often followed by cyanosis and then redness, indicates Raynaud's disease or phenomenon.

With middle-aged and older people you should also ask about *intermittent claudication*, a specific pattern of pain that accompanies impairment of arterial flow. "How far can you walk without stopping to rest?" is a good opening question. Then determine what makes the patient stop and how quickly relief is felt.

Aching, cramping, and possibly numbness or severe fatigue that appear with walking and disappear promptly with rest typify intermittent claudication.

THE MUSCULOSKELETAL SYSTEM

"Have you had any *pains in your joints*?" turns the interview explicitly to the musculoskeletal system. An affirmative answer to this question may indicate, however, a problem not only in the joints but also in bones, muscles, and tissues around the joints. Either now or during the examination, ask the patient to show you as clearly as possible where the pain is felt. Where did it start? What then? Pain originating in the small joints of the hands and feet is more sharply localized than that from the larger joints. Pain from the hip joint is especially deceptive. Although it is typically felt in the groin or the buttock, it is sometimes felt in the anterior thigh or partly or solely in the knee.

Problems in tissues around joints include inflammation of bursae (*bursitis*), tendons (*tendonitis*), or tendon sheaths (*tenosynovitis*), and stretching or tearing of ligaments (*sprains*).

"Hip pain" felt near the greater trochanter of the femur suggests trochanteric bursitis.

Determine whether the pain has involved one joint or its adjacent tissues or whether several joints have been affected. If the latter, in what pattern has the involvement spread? Has the pain disappeared from the one or more joints initially involved only to migrate to others, or has the initial pain persisted while pain has progressed to other joints? Is the involvement symmetrical, affecting similar joints on both sides of the body?

Pain in only one joint area suggests bursitis, tendonitis, monoarticular arthritis, or an injury. Rheumatic fever and early gonococcal arthritis often have a migratory pattern of spread; rheumatoid arthritis typically shows a progressive or additive pattern and is symmetrical.

Assess the quality and severity of the pain.

Timing is particularly important. Did the pain develop rapidly over the course of a few hours, or insidiously over weeks or even months? Has the course been one of slow progression, or have there been periods of improvement and worsening? How long has the pain lasted? What is it like over the course of a day? in the morning? and as the day wears on?

Unusually severe and rapidly developing pain in a swollen joint, not explained by injury, suggests acute gouty or septic arthritis. In children, especially consider osteomyelitis that involves bone contiguous to a joint.

What aggravates and relieves the pain, with special reference to exercise, rest, and treatments? In what setting did the pain develop? Was there an acute injury or excessive use of the body part?

What symptoms are associated? Here there are three relevant categories. First, are there *other symptoms in the involved joint(s)*—specifically, swelling, stiffness, limitation of motion, tenderness, warmth, or redness? Pains in the joints without objective evidence of arthritis such as swelling, tenderness, or warmth are called *arthralgias*. Pains in the muscles are called *myalgias*. **Inquire about *swelling* in your usual manner, trying to localize it as accurately as possible.**

See Table 2-14, Patterns of Chronic Pain In or Around the Joints, pp. 90–91.

For *limitation of motion,* ask about activities with which the joint problems have interfered. When relevant, specifically inquire about the patient's ability to walk, stand, lean over, sit, sit up, rise from a sitting position, climb, pinch, grasp, turn a page, open a door or jar, and care for his or her own bodily needs, such as combing hair, brushing teeth, feeding, dressing, and washing, including washing hard-to-reach areas such as the perineum.

Stiffness is often difficult to assess because people use the term in different ways. Stiffness in the musculoskeletal interview refers to the subjective perception of tightness or resistance to movement, the opposite of feeling limber. It is often associated with discomfort or pain. If the patient has not volunteered a sense of stiffness, ask about it. **Two good questions are "What time do you get up in the morning?" and "What time do you feel about as loose as you are going to get?"** Then calculate the duration of the patient's stiffness. Stiffness, together with muscular soreness, is felt by healthy people after unusually strenuous muscular exertion and peaks in intensity around the second day after exertion.

Stiffness after inactivity is common in degenerative joint disease but usually lasts only a few minutes. This is sometimes called *gelling*. Stiffness in rheumatoid arthritis and other inflammatory arthritides often lasts 30 minutes or longer. Stiffness also accompanies the "fibrositis" syndrome and polymyalgia rheumatica.

Tenderness, warmth, and redness are often best detected on examination, but patients can sometimes give you this information and guide you to points of tenderness.

Tenderness, warmth, and redness in a joint suggest acute gout, septic arthritis, or possibly rheumatic fever.

The second category of associated symptoms includes *generalized symptoms* such as *fever, chills, fatigue, anorexia, weight loss*, and *weakness*.

Generalized symptoms are common in rheumatoid and other inflammatory arthritides. High fever and chills suggest an infectious cause.

Third, are there *symptoms elsewhere in the body that give important clues as to the nature of the problem?* These include

- *Skin conditions* such as
    A butterfly rash on the cheeks

    Systemic lupus erythematosus

    The scaly rash and pitted nails of psoriasis

    Psoriatic arthritis

    A few red macules, papules, pustules, or vesicles on the distal extremities

    Gonococcal arthritis

    An expanding erythematous patch early in an illness

    Lyme disease

    Hives

    Serum sickness, drug reaction

    Erosions or scales on the penis and crusted scaling papules on the soles and palms

    Reiter's syndrome, which also includes arthritis, urethritis, and conjunctivitis

    The maculopapular rash of rubella

    Arthritis of rubella

    Clubbing of the fingernails (see p. 149)

    Hypertrophic osteoarthropathy

- Red, burning, and itchy eyes (*conjunctivitis*)

    Reiter's syndrome

- Preceding *sore throat*

    Acute rheumatic fever or gonococcal arthritis

- *Diarrhea* and *abdominal pain*

    Arthritis with ulcerative colitis or regional enteritis

- Symptoms of *urethritis*

    Reiter's syndrome or possibly gonococcal arthritis

Even if the patient denies joint pain, specifically ask about *backache*, a very common symptom. Use your usual interviewing method to

See Table 2-15, Low Back Pain, p. 92.

develop a clear picture of the problem. If pain radiates into the legs, ask about numbness, tingling, or weakness that may be associated.

Associated numbness, tingling, or weakness suggests involvement of nerve roots.

Pain in the neck **is also common. Approach it in the same manner. When neck pain is chronic, be alert for manifestations of pressure on the spinal cord: weakness, loss of sensation, and, in late stages, loss of bladder and bowel control.**

See Table 2-16, Pains in the Neck, p. 93.

THE NERVOUS SYSTEM

"Have you ever fainted or passed out?" turns the discussion to *loss of consciousness.* **Get as complete and unbiased a description of the event as you can. Try to determine what seems to have precipitated the attack(s), what kind of warning, if any, the patient felt before passing out, how long the unconsciousness lasted, and how the patient felt after recovery. Was the patient standing, sitting, or lying down when the attack started? What was the patient's appearance just before and during the attack? Patients may have learned from others about their appearance and activities while they were unconscious, but if the nature of the problem is unclear try to talk with someone who has observed the event.**

In young people with temporary loss of consciousness, consider especially vasodepressor syncope, hyperventilation, and tonic–clonic (grand mal) seizures. In elderly patients, think first of cardiac causes and postural hypotension. When temporary loss of consciousness lasts more than a few minutes, think of hypoglycemia, hypocapnia from hyperventilation, and hysterical fainting.

Syncope refers to the sudden but temporary loss of consciousness that occurs when blood flow to the brain becomes insufficient. It is commonly described as fainting. The symptoms of an impending faint, including muscular weakness, lightheadedness, and other premonitory feelings without actual loss of consciousness, are called *near syncope* or *pre-syncope.* These are assessed in the usual manner. Syncope must be distinguished from generalized seizures—a task sometimes made difficult by the fact that a severe syncopal attack can occasionally produce a few clonic movements and even urinary incontinence. Syncope is not usually associated, however, with a fully developed tonic–clonic (grand mal) seizure or with fecal incontinence.

See Table 2-17, Syncope and Similar Disorders, pp. 94–95.

In contrast with syncope, a tonic–clonic (grand mal) seizure usually starts more quickly, lasts longer, is more likely to involve injury and incontinence, and is followed by a slower recovery.

A *seizure* is a paroxysmal disorder that may or may not involve a loss of consciousness, and may also involve abnormal sensations, movements, feelings, or thought processes. It is caused by a sudden, excessive electrical discharge in the cerebral cortex or its underlying structures. **"Have you ever had any seizures or spells? . . . any fits or convulsions?"** opens the discussion. As with syncope, get as full a description as possible, including precipitating circumstances, warnings, behavior and feelings during the attack, duration of the attack, and feelings after it. Ask about age at onset, the frequency of seizures, any recent change in frequency, and use of medications. Is there a history of prior head injury or other conditions that may be causally related?

See Table 2-18, Seizure Disorders, pp. 96–97.

To assess motor performance, ask about *weakness* of any part of the body and about *paralysis,* an inability to move a part. Did the weakness start slowly or suddenly? Has it progressed and how? What bodily parts are involved? Does the weakness affect one or both sides? What movements are affected? Try to distinguish between distal and proximal weakness. For distal weakness in the arms, inquire about hand movements such as opening a jar or can or using hand tools such as scissors, pliers, or a screwdriver. For distal weakness in the legs, ask about frequent tripping. For proximal weakness, ask about combing hair, trying to reach something on a high shelf, and difficulty in rising from a chair or taking a high step up. Does the weakness increase with repeated effort and improve after rest? Are there associated sensory or other symptoms?

Local weakness may result from abnormalities in the upper motor neurons, the lower motor neurons, the neuromuscular junctions, or the muscles themselves. If it does not follow a neuroanatomic pattern and is unexplained otherwise, consider a conversion reaction. Bilateral, predominantly distal weakness suggests a polyneuropathy; bilateral proximal weakness, a myopathy. Weakness made worse with repeated effort and improved with rest suggests myasthenia gravis and related syndromes.

Tremors and other *involuntary movements* occur with or without additional neurologic manifestations. **Ask about trembling, shakiness, or bodily movements that the patient seems unable to control.**

See Table 18-6, Involuntary Movements, pp. 554–556.

Pain may stem from neurologic causes and is usually reported in other parts of the systems review, such as the head and musculoskeletal system.

Other sensory symptoms include lost or altered sensation. **Ask about numbness, tingling, pins-and-needles sensations, or other peculiar or unpleasant feelings in the body. If a patient reports numbness, try to determine the real meaning—a** *loss of sensation,* **an inability to move the part, or an altered sensation. Use your usual style of questioning, paying particular attention to location.**

Loss of sensation, paresthesias, and dysesthesias occur with lesions involving the peripheral nerves, sensory roots, spinal cord, and higher centers. Paresthesias in the hands and around the mouth commonly accompany hyperventilation.

Paresthesias are peculiar sensations of various kinds that have no obvious stimulus. They include tingling, prickling, and feelings of warmth, coldness, and pressure. Paresthesias are what everyone feels when an arm or a leg "goes to sleep" after the compression of a nerve. *Dysesthesias* are distorted sensations in response to a stimulus, and may last longer than the stimulus itself. For example, a person may perceive a light touch or a pinprick as an unpleasant burning or tingling sensation.

Distinct from these symptoms is an almost indescribable *restlessness of the legs* that typically develops at rest and is accompanied by an urge to move about. Walking gives relief.

These symptoms suggest the common but often overlooked restless legs syndrome.

THE HEMATOLOGIC SYSTEM

The assessment of hematologic disorders depends heavily on physical examination and the laboratory, but symptoms too have some value.

Anemia must become moderate or severe before producing symptoms. It then decreases exercise tolerance and leads to dyspnea and palpitations. In persons with atherosclerosis, it may decrease the threshold for angina pectoris, intermittent claudication, or transient ischemic attacks. Patients with severe anemia may report a variety of symptoms that may lead you astray: headache, dizziness, vertigo, syncope, anorexia, nausea, intolerance to cold, amenorrhea, menorrhagia, loss of libido, and impotence.

Spontaneous bleeding and bleeding disproportionate to an injury suggest a generalized bleeding disorder. It may be congenital or acquired. Normal hemostasis depends on three mechanisms: (1) vasoconstriction following a vascular injury, (2) formation of a platelet plug, and (3) formation of a fibrin clot. The most common bleeding disorders result from deficits in the last two categories. Platelet plugs are essential for prompt hemostasis, especially in the capillaries of the skin and mucous membranes. Fibrin clots are especially important as a second line of defense, particularly in larger vessels such as arterioles or venules.

Congenital bleeding disorders, involving the clotting mechanism, are most common in males. The family history is often positive.

A platelet disorder, therefore, is likely to cause capillary bleeding into the skin or mucous membranes. When the bleeding is initiated by injury, it tends to occur without delay. In contrast, a clotting disorder tends to cause bleeding deep in the tissues. After an injury, bleeding tends to appear several hours later. Bleeding due to a vascular defect tends to resemble that of a platelet disorder and may be associated with it.

Petechiae (see p. 151) in the skin and mucous membranes and small bruises are common in platelet disorders. Large bruises, deep *hematomas* (local masses of extravasated blood), and *hemarthroses* (blood in the joints) are seen in clotting disorders.

"Do you bleed or bruise easily?" opens this discussion. Further, "Have you ever bled a lot (or too much) after having a tooth pulled? . . . or after an operation? How about nosebleeds?" If there is a history of bleeding, try to distinguish between a localized problem and a more general bleeding tendency. If the latter is present, determine the sites of bleeding, timing in relation to possible injury, duration, frequency, and severity. Has the patient needed blood transfusions? Ask about medications, including aspirin and "blood thinners," and, if you have not already specifically done so, carefully review the family history for bleeding problems. Are there reasons to suspect a deficiency in vitamin C or K?

Spontaneous bleeding, bleeding with minor trauma, and bleeding in several sites suggest a general disorder.

Inadequate diet, malabsorption

THE ENDOCRINE SYSTEM

The assessment of endocrine function depends not so much on additional symptoms as on pulling together the data already gathered and recognizing the underlying pattern of an endocrine disorder. When you begin to recognize such a pattern, ask about symptoms that you know might be relevant but try to avoid leading the patient. When you suspect Addison's disease, for example, "Have you noticed any change in the color of your skin?" is better than "Has your skin become darker?"

(Text continues on p. 70)

Obesity, weakness, fatigue, easy bruising, ankle edema, and decreased or absent menstrual periods suggest Cushing's syndrome (adrenal cortical hyperfunction), while weakness, weight loss, nausea, vomiting, darkened skin, and symptoms of postural hypotension

Table 2-1   Headaches

Table 2-1   Headaches

PROBLEM	PROCESS	LOCATION	QUALITY AND SEVERITY	TIMING	
				ONSET	DURATION
TENSION HEADACHES	Unclear, may be related to sustained muscle contraction	Usually bilateral; may be generalized or localized to the back of the head and upper neck or to the frontotemporal area	Mild and aching or a nonpainful tightness and pressure	Gradual	Variable: hours or days, but often weeks or months
MIGRAINE HEADACHES (*"Classic migraine" is distinguished from "common migraine" by visual or neurologic symptoms during the half hour before the headache.*)	Dilatation of arteries outside or inside the skull, possibly of biochemical origin; often familial	Typically frontal or temporal, one or both sides, but also may be occipital or generalized. "Classic migraine" is typically unilateral.	Throbbing or aching; variable in severity	Fairly rapid, reaching a peak in 1–2 hr	Several hours to 1–2 dy
TOXIC VASCULAR HEADACHES *due to fever, toxic substances, or drug withdrawal*	Dilatation of arteries, mainly inside the skull	Generalized	Aching, of variable severity	Variable	Depends on cause
CLUSTER HEADACHES	Unclear	One-sided; high in the nose, and behind and over the eye	Steady, severe	Abrupt, often 2–3 hr after falling asleep	Roughly 1–2 hr
HEADACHES WITH EYE DISORDERS **ERRORS OF REFRACTION** (*farsightedness and astigmatism, but not nearsightedness*)	Probably the sustained contraction of the extraocular muscles, and possibly of the frontal, temporal, and occipital muscles	Around and over the eyes, may radiate to the occipital area	Steady, aching, dull	Gradual	Variable
ACUTE GLAUCOMA	Sudden increase in intraocular pressure (see p. 178)	In and around one eye	Steady, aching, often severe	Often rapid	Variable, may depend on treatment
HEADACHES WITH ACUTE PARANASAL SINUSITIS	Mucosal inflammation of the paranasal sinuses and their openings	Usually above the eye (frontal sinus) or in the cheekbone area (maxillary sinus), one or both sides	Aching or throbbing, variable in severity	Variable	Often several hours at a time, recurring over days or longer

Blanks appear in these tables when the categories are not applicable or are not usually helpful in assessing the problem.

Table 2-1 Headaches

COURSE	ASSOCIATED SYMPTOMS	FACTORS THAT AGGRAVATE OR PROVOKE	FACTORS THAT RELIEVE	CONVENIENT CATEGORIES OF THOUGHT
Often recurrent or persistent over long periods	Symptoms of anxiety, tension, and depression may be present.	Sustained muscular tension, as in driving or typing; emotional stress	Variable	The two most common kinds of headache
Often begins between childhood and early adulthood. Typically recurrent at intervals of weeks, months, or years, usually decreasing with pregnancy and advancing age	Often nausea and vomiting. A minority of patients have preceding visual disturbances (local flashes of light, blind spots) or neurologic symptoms (local weakness, sensory disturbances, and other symptoms).	May be provoked by alcohol, certain foods, or tension. More common premenstrually. Aggravated by noise and bright light	Quiet, dark room; sleep; sometimes transient relief from pressure on the involved artery, if early in the course	Vascular headaches
Depends on cause	Depends on cause	Fever, carbon monoxide, hypoxia, withdrawal of caffeine, other causes	Depends on cause	
Typically clustered in time, with several each day or week and then relief for weeks or months	Unilateral stuffy, runny nose, and reddening and tearing of the eye	During a cluster, may be provoked by alcohol		
Variable	Eye fatigue, "sandy" sensations in the eyes, redness of the conjunctivas	Prolonged use of the eyes, particularly for close work	Rest of the eyes	Face pains
Variable, may depend on treatment	Diminished vision, sometimes nausea and vomiting	Sometimes provoked by drops that dilate the pupils		
Often recurrent in a repetitive daily pattern: starting in the morning (frontal) or in the afternoon (maxillary)	Local tenderness, nasal congestion, discharge, and fever	May be aggravated by coughing, sneezing, or jarring the head	Nasal decongestants	

(Table continues on next page) ➡

Table 2-1 Headaches

Table 2-1 (Cont'd.)

PROBLEM	PROCESS	LOCATION	QUALITY AND SEVERITY	TIMING	
				ONSET	DURATION
TRIGEMINAL NEURALGIA	Mechanism variable, often unknown	Cheek, jaws, lips, or gums (second and third divisions of the trigeminal nerve)	Sharp, short, brief, lightninglike jabs; very severe	Abrupt	Each jab is transient, but jabs recur in clusters at intervals of seconds or minutes.
GIANT CELL ARTERITIS	Chronic inflammation of the cranial arteries, cause unknown, often associated with polymyalgia rheumatica	Localized near the involved artery (most often the temporal, also the occipital); may become generalized	Aching, throbbing, or burning, often severe	Gradual or rapid	Variable
CHRONIC SUBDURAL HEMATOMA	Bleeding into the subdural space after trauma, followed by slow accumulation of fluid that compresses the brain	Variable	Steady, aching	Gradual onset weeks to months after the injury	Often depends on surgical intervention
POSTCONCUSSION SYNDROME	Mechanism unclear	May be localized to the injured area, but not necessarily	Variable	Within a few hours of the injury	Weeks, months, or even years
MENINGEAL IRRITATION, *as from infection (meningitis) or blood (subarachnoid hemorrhage)*	Inflammation of the meninges and related pain-sensitive structures within the skull	Generalized; particularly severe at the base of the skull	Steady and severe; may be throbbing in meningitis	Fairly rapid (meningitis) or abrupt, peaking in 1–2 min (subarachnoid hemorrhage)	Variable, usually days
BRAIN TUMOR	Displacement of or traction on pain-sensitive arteries and veins or pressure on nerves, all within the skull	Varies with the location of the tumor	Aching, steady, variable in intensity	Variable	Often brief

Table 2-1   Headaches

COURSE	ASSOCIATED SYMPTOMS	FACTORS THAT AGGRAVATE OR PROVOKE	FACTORS THAT RELIEVE	CONVENIENT CATEGORIES OF THOUGHT
Pain may be troublesome for months, then disappears for months, but often recurs. It is uncommon at night.	Exhaustion from recurrent pain	Typically triggered by touching certain areas of the lower face or mouth, or by chewing, talking, or brushing teeth		
Recurrent or persistent over weeks to months	Tenderness of the adjacent scalp; fever, malaise, fatigue, and anorexia; muscular aches and stiffness; visual loss or blindness			Consider these three in older adults
Progressively severe but may be obscured by clouded consciousness	Alterations in consciousness, changes in personality, and hemiparesis (weakness on one side of the body). The injury is often forgotten.			
Tends to diminish over time	Giddiness or vertigo, irritability, restlessness, tenseness, fatigue, and difficulty concentrating	Mental and physical exertion, straining, stooping, emotional excitement, alcohol	Rest	Headaches following head trauma
Persistent single headache in an acute illness	An acute febrile illness (meningitis) or headache and sudden collapse, often with loss of consciousness (hemorrhage). Vomiting and fever may accompany either.			Acute, severe illnesses
Often intermittent, but progressive	Neurologic and mental symptoms and nausea and vomiting may develop.	May be aggravated by coughing, sneezing, or sudden movements of the head		An underlying concern of patient and clinician alike

suggest Addison's disease (adrenal insufficiency).

(Text continued from p. 65)
There are, however, a few additional symptoms that are important in an endocrine evaluation. These relate primarily to diabetes mellitus and to thyroid dysfunction.

Polyuria, already described in the section on the urinary tract, is a frequent symptom of diabetes mellitus. It is then typically associated with excessive *thirst* and with *polydipsia* (an increased intake of fluids). *Polyphagia* (increased food intake) may also occur.

Other symptoms that often accompany the onset of diabetes mellitus include weakness, fatigue, weight loss, and blurred vision.

An assessment of thyroid function involves questions concerning *temperature intolerance* and *sweating*. **Opening questions include "Do you prefer hot or cold weather? Do you generally dress more warmly or less warmly than most people? Do you use more blankets or fewer blankets than others at home? Do you sweat (or perspire) more or less than most people?"** As people grow older, they sweat less, tolerate cold less well, and tend to prefer warmer environments. For other symptoms that may be related to abnormal thyroid function, see Table 7-24, Thyroid Enlargement and Function (p. 229).

Intolerance to cold, preferences for warm clothing and many blankets, and decreased sweating suggest hypothyroidism; the opposites suggest hyperthyroidism.

Episodic sweating and heat intolerance often occur during menopause.

SCREENING FOR MENTAL STATUS

In the course of the interview you often identify clues to emotional or other psychiatric problems. It is usually wise to inquire about these when the patient mentions them. A few screening questions about *nervousness, tensions, mood,* and possibly *memory* should be included in most histories. This subject is sufficiently important, however, to warrant its own chapter.

Table 2-2   Vertigo

Table 2-2   Vertigo

PROBLEM	TIMING			HEARING	TINNITUS	OTHER ASSOCIATED SYMPTOMS
	ONSET	DURATION	COURSE			
BENIGN POSITIONAL VERTIGO	Sudden, on rolling over onto the affected side or tilting the head up	Brief, a few seconds to minutes	Persists a few weeks, may recur	Not affected	Absent	Sometimes nausea and vomiting
VESTIBULAR NEURONITIS *(acute labyrinthitis)*	Sudden	Hours to days, up to 2 wk	May recur over 12–18 mo	Not affected	Absent	Nausea, vomiting
MENIERE'S DISEASE	Sudden	Several hours to a day or more	Recurrent	Sensorineural hearing loss that improves and recurs, eventually progresses; one or both sides*	Present, fluctuating*	Nausea, vomiting, pressure or fullness in the affected ear
DRUG TOXICITY *(as from aminoglycosides or alcohol intoxication)*	Insidious or acute	May or may not be reversible. Partial adaptation occurs.		May be impaired, both sides	May be present	Nausea, vomiting
TUMOR, PRESSING ON THE 8TH NERVE	Insidious**	Variable	Variable	Impaired, one side	Present	Those of pressure on the 5th, 6th, and 7th cranial nerves

Additional disorders of the brainstem or cerebellum may also cause vertigo. These include ischemia secondary to atherosclerosis, tumors, and multiple sclerosis. Additional neurologic symptoms and signs are usually present.

* Hearing impairment, tinnitus, and rotary vertigo do not always develop concurrently. Time is often required to make this diagnosis.

** Persistent unsteadiness is more common but vertigo may occur.

Table 2-3   Chest Pain

Table 2-3   Chest Pain

PROBLEM	PROCESS	LOCATION	QUALITY	SEVERITY
ANGINA PECTORIS	Temporary myocardial ischemia, usually secondary to narrowed arteries due to coronary atherosclerosis	Retrosternal or across the anterior chest, sometimes radiating to the shoulders, arms, neck, lower jaw, or upper abdomen	Pressing, squeezing, tight, heavy, occasionally burning	Mild to moderate, sometimes perceived as discomfort rather than pain
MYOCARDIAL INFARCTION	Prolonged myocardial ischemia, resulting in irreversible muscle damage (necrosis)	Same as in angina	Same as in angina	Often but not always a severe pain
PERICARDITIS	1. Irritation of parietal pleura adjacent to the pericardium	Precordial, may radiate to the tip of the shoulder and to the neck	Sharp, knifelike	Often severe
	2. Mechanism unclear	Retrosternal, may radiate to the neck and shoulders	Crushing	Severe
DISSECTING AORTIC ANEURYSM	A splitting within the layers of the aortic wall, allowing the passage of blood to dissect a channel	Anterior chest, radiating to the neck, back, or abdomen	Ripping, tearing	Very severe
TRACHEOBRONCHITIS	Inflammation of the trachea and large bronchi	Upper sternal or on either side of the sternum	Burning	Mild to moderate
PLEURAL PAIN	Irritation of the parietal pleura, as from acute pleurisy, pneumonia, pulmonary infarction, or neoplasm	Chest wall overlying the process	Sharp, knifelike	Often severe
REFLUX ESOPHAGITIS	Inflammation of the esophageal mucosa by reflux of gastric acid	Retrosternal, may radiate to the back	Burning, may be squeezing	Mild to severe
DIFFUSE ESOPHAGEAL SPASM	Motor dysfunction of the esophageal muscle	Retrosternal, may radiate to the back, arms, and jaw	Usually squeezing	Mild to severe
CHEST WALL PAIN	Variable, often unclear	Often below the left breast or along the costal cartilages, also elsewhere	Stabbing, sticking, or dull, aching	Variable
ANXIETY	Unclear	Precordial, below the left breast, or across the anterior chest	Stabbing, sticking, or dull, aching	Variable

Note: Remember that chest pain may be referred from extrathoracic structures such as the neck (arthritis) and abdomen (biliary colic, acute cholecystitis). Pleural pain may be due to abdominal conditions such as subdiaphragmatic abscess.

Table 2-3   Chest Pain

TIMING	FACTORS THAT AGGRAVATE	FACTORS THAT RELIEVE	ASSOCIATED SYMPTOMS
Usually 1–3 min but up to 10 min. Prolonged episodes up to 20 min	Effort, especially in the cold; meals; emotional stress. May occur at rest	Rest, nitroglycerine	Sometimes dyspnea, nausea, sweating
20 min to several hr			Nausea, vomiting, sweating, weakness
Persistent	Breathing, coughing, lying down, sometimes swallowing	Sitting up may relieve it.	Of the underlying illness
Persistent			Of the underlying illness
Persistent, maximal at the onset			Syncope, hemiplegia, paraplegia
Variable	Coughing		Cough
Persistent	Breathing, coughing, movements of the trunk	Lying on the involved side may relieve it.	Of the underlying illness
Variable	Large meal; bending over, lying down	Antacids, sometimes belching	Sometimes regurgitation, dysphagia
Variable	Swallowing of food or cold liquid; emotional stress	Sometimes nitroglycerine	Dysphagia
Fleeting to hours or days	Movement of chest, trunk, arms		Often local tenderness
Fleeting to hours or days	May follow effort, emotional stress		Breathlessness, palpitations, weakness, anxiety

Table 2-4 Dyspnea

Table 2-4 Dyspnea

PROBLEM	PROCESS	TIMING
LEFT-SIDED HEART FAILURE *(left ventricular failure or mitral stenosis)*	Elevated pressure in the pulmonary capillary bed with transudation of fluid into the interstitial spaces and alveoli, decreased compliance (increased stiffness) of the lungs, and increased work of breathing	Dyspnea may progress slowly, or suddenly as in acute pulmonary edema.
CHRONIC BRONCHITIS*	Excessive mucus production in the bronchi, followed by chronic obstruction of the airways	Chronic productive cough followed by slowly progressive dyspnea
PULMONARY EMPHYSEMA*	Overdistention of the air spaces distal to the terminal bronchioles, with destruction of the alveolar septa and chronic obstruction of the airways	Slowly progressive dyspnea; relatively mild cough later
BRONCHIAL ASTHMA	Airways narrowed by smooth muscle contraction, edema of the bronchial walls, and secretions	Acute episodes, separated by symptom-free periods
DIFFUSE INFILTRATIVE LUNG DISEASES *(such as sarcoidosis, widespread pulmonary neoplasms, and coal workers' pneumoconiosis)*	Abnormal and widespread infiltration of cells, fluid, and collagen into the interstitial spaces. Many causes	Progressive dyspnea, which varies in its rate of development with the cause
PNEUMONIA	Inflammation of the lung parenchyma from the respiratory bronchioles to the alveoli	An acute illness, the timing of which varies with the etiologic agent
SPONTANEOUS PNEUMOTHORAX	Leakage of air into the pleural space through blebs on the visceral pleura, with resulting partial or complete collapse of the lung	Sudden onset of dyspnea
ACUTE PULMONARY EMBOLISM	Sudden occlusion of all or part of the pulmonary arterial tree by a blood clot that usually originates in the deep veins of the legs or pelvis	Sudden onset of dyspnea
ANXIETY WITH HYPERVENTILATION	Overbreathing, with resultant respiratory alkalosis and fall in the partial pressure of carbon dioxide in the blood	Episodic, often recurrent

* Chronic bronchitis and emphysema often coexist.

Table 2-4   Dyspnea

FACTORS THAT AGGRAVATE	FACTORS THAT RELIEVE	ASSOCIATED SYMPTOMS	SETTING
Exertion, lying down	Rest, sitting up, though dyspnea may become persistent	Often cough, orthopnea, paroxysmal nocturnal dyspnea; sometimes wheezing	History of heart disease or its predisposing factors
Exertion, inhaled irritants, respiratory infections	Expectoration; rest, though dyspnea may become persistent	Chronic productive cough, recurrent respiratory infections; wheezing may develop	History of smoking, air pollutants, recurrent respiratory infections
Exertion	Rest, though dyspnea may become persistent	Cough, with scant mucoid sputum	History of smoking, air pollutants, sometimes a familial deficiency in alpha$_1$-antitrypsin
Variable, including allergens, irritants, respiratory infections, exercise, and emotion	Separation from aggravating factors	Wheezing, cough	Environmental and emotional conditions
Exertion	Rest, though dyspnea may become persistent	Often weakness, fatigue. Cough less common than in other lung diseases	Variable
		Pleuritic pain, cough, sputum, fever	Variable
		Pleuritic pain	Often a previously healthy young adult
		Often none. Retrosternal oppressive pain if the occlusion is massive. Pleuritic pain, cough, and hemoptysis may follow an embolism if pulmonary infarction ensues. Symptoms of anxiety (see below).	Postpartum or postoperative periods; prolonged bed rest; congestive heart failure, chronic lung disease, and fractures of hip or leg; thrombophlebitis
More often occurs at rest than after exercise. An upsetting event may not be evident.	Breathing in and out of a paper or plastic bag sometimes helps the associated symptoms.	Sighing, lightheadedness, numbness or tingling of the hands and feet, palpitations, chest pain	Other manifestations of anxiety may be present.

Table 2-5   Cough and Hemoptysis

Table 2-5   Cough and Hemoptysis*

PROBLEM	COUGH AND SPUTUM	ASSOCIATED SYMPTOMS AND SETTING
ACUTE INFLAMMATIONS		
LARYNGITIS	Dry cough (without sputum), may become productive of variable amounts of sputum	An acute, fairly minor illness with hoarseness. Often associated with viral nasopharyngitis
TRACHEOBRONCHITIS	Dry cough, may become productive (as above)	An acute illness, often with burning retrosternal discomfort. Often associated with viral syndromes, as above
MYCOPLASMA AND VIRAL PNEUMONIAS	Dry cough, often becoming productive of mucoid sputum	An acute febrile illness, possibly dyspnea
BACTERIAL PNEUMONIAS	Pneumococcal: sputum mucoid or purulent; may be blood-streaked, diffusely pinkish, or rusty	An acute illness with chills, high fever, dyspnea, and chest pain. Pneumococcal pneumonia often is preceded by acute upper respiratory infection.
	Klebsiella: similar; or sticky, red, and jellylike	*Klebsiella* pneumonia typically occurs in older alcoholic men.
CHRONIC INFLAMMATIONS		
CHRONIC BRONCHITIS	Chronic cough; sputum mucoid to purulent, may be blood-streaked or even bloody	Often long-standing cigarette smoking. Recurrent superimposed infections. Wheezing and dyspnea may develop.
BRONCHIECTASIS	Chronic cough; sputum purulent, often copious and foul-smelling; may be blood-streaked or bloody	Recurrent bronchopulmonary infections common; sinusitis may coexist.
PULMONARY TUBERCULOSIS	Cough dry or sputum that is mucoid or purulent; may be blood-streaked or bloody	Early, no symptoms. Later, anorexia, weight loss, fatigue, fever, and night sweats
LUNG ABSCESS	Sputum purulent and foul-smelling; may be bloody	A febrile illness. Often poor dental hygiene and a prior episode of impaired consciousness
BRONCHIAL ASTHMA	Cough, with thick mucoid sputum, especially near the end of an attack	Episodic wheezing and dyspnea, but the cough may occur alone. Often a history of allergy
NEOPLASM		
CANCER OF THE LUNG	Cough dry to productive; sputum may be blood-streaked or bloody	Usually a long history of cigarette smoking. Associated manifestations are numerous.
CARDIOVASCULAR DISORDERS		
LEFT VENTRICULAR FAILURE OR MITRAL STENOSIS	Often dry, especially on exertion or at night; may progress to the pink frothy sputum of pulmonary edema or to frank hemoptysis	Dyspnea, orthopnea, paroxysmal nocturnal dyspnea
PULMONARY EMBOLI	Dry to productive; may be dark, bright red, or mixed with blood	Dyspnea, anxiety, chest pain, fever; factors that predispose to deep venous thrombosis
TRAUMA AND PHYSICAL AGENTS		
IRRITATING PARTICLES, CHEMICALS, OR GASES	Variable. There may be a latent period between exposure and symptoms.	Exposure to irritants. Eyes, nose, and throat may be affected.
FOREIGN BODY LODGED IN THE LOWER AIRWAY	Acute: dry. Later: productive	Acute: choking (may be forgotten). Later: dyspnea and wheezing
EXTERNAL CHEST TRAUMA	Sputum blood-streaked or grossly bloody	Puncture, laceration, or contusion of the lung

* Characteristics of hemoptysis are printed in red.

Table 2-6 Dysphagia

Table 2-6 Dysphagia

PROCESS AND PROBLEM	TIMING	FACTORS THAT AGGRAVATE	FACTORS THAT RELIEVE	ASSOCIATED SYMPTOMS AND CONDITIONS
TRANSFER DYSPHAGIA, *due to motor disorders affecting the pharyngeal muscles*	Acute or gradual onset and a variable course, depending on the underlying disorder	Attempts to start the swallowing process		Aspiration into the lungs or regurgitation into the nose with attempts to swallow. Neurologic evidence of stroke, bulbar palsy, or other neuromuscular condition
ESOPHAGEAL DYSPHAGIA MECHANICAL NARROWING				
• *Mucosal rings and webs*	Intermittent	Solid foods	Regurgitation of the bolus of food	Usually none
• *Esophageal stricture*	Intermittent, may become slowly progressive	Solid foods	Regurgitation of the bolus of food	A long history of heartburn and regurgitation
• *Esophageal cancer*	May be intermittent at first; progressive over months	Solid foods, with progression to liquids	Regurgitation of the bolus of food	Pain in the chest and back and weight loss, especially late in the course of illness
MOTOR DISORDERS • *Diffuse esophageal spasm*	Intermittent	Solids or liquids	Maneuvers described below; sometimes nitroglycerine	Chest pain that mimics angina pectoris or myocardial infarction and lasts minutes to hours; possibly heartburn
• *Scleroderma*	Intermittent, may progress slowly	Solids or liquids	Repeated swallowing, movements such as straightening the back, raising the arms, or a Valsalva maneuver (straining down against a closed glottis)	Heartburn. Other manifestations of scleroderma
• *Achalasia*	Intermittent, may progress	Solids or liquids		Regurgitation, often at night when lying down, with nocturnal cough; possibly chest pain precipitated by eating

Table 2-7   Abdominal Pain

Table 2-7   Abdominal Pain

PROBLEM	PROCESS	LOCATION	QUALITY
PEPTIC ULCER AND DYSPEPSIA *(These disorders cannot be reliably differentiated by symptoms and signs.)*	Peptic ulcer refers to a demonstrable ulcer, usually in the duodenum or stomach. Dyspepsia causes similar symptoms but no ulceration.	Epigastric, may radiate to the back	Variable: gnawing, burning, boring, aching, pressing, or hungerlike
CANCER OF THE STOMACH	A malignant neoplasm	Epigastric	Variable
ACUTE PANCREATITIS	An acute inflammation of the pancreas	Epigastric, sometimes radiating to the back or other parts of the abdomen; may be poorly localized	Usually steady
CHRONIC PANCREATITIS	Fibrosis of the pancreas secondary to recurrent inflammation	Epigastric, radiating through to the back	Steady, deep
CANCER OF THE PANCREAS	A malignant neoplasm	Epigastric, with pain in either upper quadrant, depending on the location of the cancer; often radiates to the back	Steady, deep
BILIARY COLIC	Sudden obstruction of the cystic duct or common bile duct by a gallstone	Epigastric or right upper quadrant; may radiate to the right scapula and shoulder	Steady, aching; *not* colicky
ACUTE CHOLECYSTITIS	Inflammation of the gallbladder usually triggered by persisting obstruction of the cystic duct by a gallstone	Right upper quadrant or upper abdominal; may radiate to the right scapular area	Steady, aching
ACUTE DIVERTICULITIS	Acute inflammation of a colonic diverticulum, a saclike mucosal outpouching through the colonic muscle	Left lower quadrant	May be cramping at first but becomes steady
ACUTE APPENDICITIS	Acute inflammation of the appendix with distention or obstruction	1. Poorly localized *periumbilical pain* followed usually by 2. *Right lower quadrant pain*	1. Mild but increasing, possibly cramping 2. Steady and more severe
ACUTE MECHANICAL INTESTINAL OBSTRUCTION	Obstruction of the bowel lumen, most commonly caused by (1) adhesions or hernias (small bowel), or (2) cancer or diverticulitis (colon)	1. *Small bowel:* periumbilical or upper abdominal 2. *Colon:* lower abdominal or generalized	1. Cramping 2. Cramping

Table 2-7   Abdominal Pain

TIMING	FACTORS THAT MAY AGGRAVATE	FACTORS THAT MAY RELIEVE	ASSOCIATED SYMPTOMS AND SETTING
Intermittent. Duodenal ulcer is more likely than gastric ulcer or dyspepsia to cause pain that (1) wakes the patient at night, and (2) occurs intermittently over a few weeks, then disappears for months, and then recurs.	Variable	Food and antacids may bring relief, but not necessarily in any of these disorders and least commonly in gastric ulcer.	Nausea, vomiting, belching, bloating; heartburn (more common in duodenal ulcer); weight loss (more common in gastric ulcer). Dyspepsia is more common in the young (20–29 yr), gastric ulcer in the older (over 50 yr), and duodenal ulcer in those from 30–60 yr.
The history of pain is typically shorter than in peptic ulcer. The pain is persistent and slowly progressive.	Often food	*Not* relieved by food or antacids	Anorexia, nausea, easy satiety, weight loss, and sometimes bleeding. Most common in ages 50–70
Acute onset, persistent pain	Lying supine	Leaning forward with trunk flexed	Nausea, vomiting, abdominal distention, fever. Often a history of previous attacks and of alcohol abuse or gallstones
Chronic or recurrent course	Alcohol, heavy or fatty meals	Possibly leaning forward with trunk flexed; often intractable	Symptoms of decreased pancreatic functions may appear: diarrhea with fatty stools (steatorrhea) and diabetes mellitus.
Persistent pain; relentlessly progressive illness		Possibly leaning forward with trunk flexed; often intractable	Anorexia, nausea, vomiting, weight loss, and jaundice. Emotional symptoms, including depression
Rapid onset over a few minutes, lasts one to several hours and subsides gradually. Often recurrent			Anorexia, nausea, vomiting, restlessness
Gradual onset; course longer than in biliary colic	Jarring, deep breathing		Anorexia, nausea, vomiting, and low fever
Often a gradual onset			Fever, constipation. There may be initial brief diarrhea.
1. Lasts roughly 4–6 hr 2. Depends on intervention	1. 2. Movement or cough	1. 2. If it subsides temporarily, suspect perforation of the appendix.	Anorexia, nausea, possibly vomiting, which typically follow the onset of pain; low fever
1. Occurs in paroxysms; may decrease over time as bowel mobility is impaired 2. Occurs in paroxysms, but typically milder than in small bowel obstruction			1. Vomiting of bile and mucus (with high obstruction) or foul-smelling fecal material (with low obstruction). Obstipation develops. 2. Vomiting late if at all. Obstipation occurs early. Prior symptoms of the underlying cause, such as a change in bowel habits or bleeding

Table 2-8   Black and Bloody Stools

Table 2-8   Black and Bloody Stools

PROBLEM	SELECTED CAUSES	ASSOCIATED SYMPTOMS AND SETTING
MELENA Melena refers to the passage of black, tarry (sticky and shiny) stools. Tests for occult blood are positive. Melena signifies the loss of at least 60 ml of blood into the gastrointestinal tract (less in infants and children), usually from the esophagus, stomach, or duodenum. Less commonly, when intestinal transit is slow, the blood may originate in the jejunum, ileum, or ascending colon. In infants, melena may result from swallowing blood during the birth process.	Peptic ulcer	Often, but not necessarily, a history of epigastric pain
	Gastritis or stress ulcers	Recent ingestion of alcohol, aspirin, or other anti-inflammatory drugs; recent bodily trauma, severe burns, surgery, or increased intracranial pressure
	Esophageal or gastric varices	Cirrhosis of the liver or other cause of portal hypertension
	Reflux esophagitis	History of heartburn
BLACK, NONSTICKY STOOLS Black stools may result from other causes and then usually give negative results when tested for occult blood. (Ingestion of iron or other substances, however, may cause a positive test result in the absence of blood.) These stools have no pathologic significance.	Ingestion of iron, bismuth salts as in Pepto-Bismol, licorice, or even commercial chocolate cookies	
RED BLOOD IN THE STOOLS Red blood usually originates in the colon, rectum, or anus, and much less frequently in the jejunum or ileum. Upper gastrointestinal hemorrhage, however, may also cause red stools. The amount of blood lost is then usually large (more than a liter). Transit time through the intestinal tract is accordingly rapid, thus giving insufficient time for the blood to turn black.	Cancer of the colon	Often a change in bowel habits
	Benign poylps of the colon	Often no other symptoms
	Diverticula of the colon	Often no other symptoms
	Inflammatory conditions of the colon and rectum • Ulcerative colitis	See Table 2-10, Diarrhea.
	• Infectious dysenteries	See Table 2-10, Diarrhea.
	• Proctitis in homosexual men (various causes)	Rectal urgency, tenesmus
	Ischemic colitis	Lower abdominal pain and sometimes fever or shock in persons over 50 yr
	Hemorrhoids	Blood on the toilet paper, on the surface of the stool, or dripping into the toilet
	Anal fissure	Blood on the toilet paper or on the surface of the stool; anal pain
REDDISH BUT NONBLOODY STOOLS	The ingestion of beets	Pink urine, which usually precedes the reddish stool

Table 2-9   Constipation

Table 2-9   Constipation

PROBLEM	PROCESS	SETTING AND ASSOCIATED SYMPTOMS
LIFE ACTIVITIES AND HABITS		
INADEQUATE TIME OR SETTING FOR THE DEFECATION REFLEX	Ignoring the sensation of a full rectum inhibits the defecation reflex.	Hectic schedules, unfamiliar surroundings, bed rest
FALSE EXPECTATIONS OF BOWEL HABITS	Expectations of "regularity" or more frequent stools than a person's norm	Beliefs, treatments, and advertisements that promote the use of laxatives
DIET DEFICIENT IN FIBER	Decreased fecal bulk	Other factors such as debilitation and constipating drugs may contribute.
IRRITABLE BOWEL SYNDROME	A common disorder of bowel motility	Small, hard stools, often with mucus. Periods of diarrhea. Cramping abdominal pain. Stress may aggravate.
MECHANICAL OBSTRUCTION		
CANCER OF THE RECTUM OR SIGMOID COLON	Progressive narrowing of the bowel lumen	Change in bowel habits; often diarrhea, abdominal pain, and bleeding. In rectal cancer, tenesmus and pencil-shaped stools
FECAL IMPACTION	A large, firm, immovable fecal mass, most often in the rectum	Rectal fullness, abdominal pain, and diarrhea around the impaction. Common in debilitated, bedridden, and often elderly patients
OTHER OBSTRUCTING LESIONS (*such as diverticulitis, volvulus, intussusception, or hernia*)	Narrowing or complete obstruction of the bowel	Colicky abdominal pain, abdominal distention, and in intussusception, often "currant jelly" stools (red blood and mucus)
PAINFUL ANAL LESIONS	Pain may cause spasm of the external sphincter and voluntary inhibition of the defecation reflex.	Anal fissures, painful hemorrhoids, perirectal abscesses
DRUGS	A variety of mechanisms	Opiates, anticholinergics, antacids containing calcium or aluminum, and many others
DEPRESSION	A disorder of mood. See Table 3-3, Distinguishing Features of Depressive Disorders.	Fatigue, feelings of depression, and other somatic symptoms
NEUROLOGIC DISORDERS	Interference with the autonomic innervation of the bowel	Spinal cord injuries, multiple sclerosis, Hirschsprung's disease, and other conditions
METABOLIC CONDITIONS	Interference with bowel motility	Pregnancy, hypothyroidism, hypercalcemia

Table 2-10   Diarrhea

Table 2-10   Diarrhea

PROBLEM	PROCESS	CHARACTERISTICS OF STOOL
ACUTE DIARRHEA		
NONINFLAMMATORY INFECTIONS	Infection by viruses, toxin-producing bacteria (such as *Escherichia coli, Staphylococcus aureus*) or *Giardia lamblia*	Watery, without blood, pus, or mucus
INFLAMMATORY INFECTIONS	Invasion of the intestinal mucosa by organisms such as *Shigella, Salmonella, Campylobacter,* and invasive *E. coli*	Loose to watery, often with blood, pus, or mucus
DRUG-INDUCED DIARRHEA	Action of many drugs such as magnesium-containing antacids, antibiotics, antineoplastic agents, and laxatives	Loose to watery
CHRONIC OR RECURRENT DIARRHEA		
NONSPECIFIC DIARRHEAL SYNDROMES		
• *Irritable bowel syndrome*	A disorder of bowel motility	Loose; may show mucus but no blood. Small, hard stools with constipation
• *Cancer of the sigmoid colon*	Partial obstruction by a malignant neoplasm	May be blood-streaked
INFLAMMATORY DIARRHEAS		
• *Ulcerative colitis*	Inflammation of the mucosa and submucosa of the rectum and colon with ulceration; cause unknown	From soft to watery, often containing blood
• *Crohn's disease of the small bowel (regional enteritis) or colon (granulomatous colitis)*	Chronic inflammation of the bowel wall, typically involving the terminal ileum and/or proximal colon	Small, soft to loose or watery, usually free of gross blood (enteritis) or with less bleeding than ulcerative colitis (colitis)
VOLUMINOUS DIARRHEAS		
• *Malabsorption syndromes*	Defective absorption of fat and other substances including fat-soluble vitamins, with excessive excretion of fat (steatorrhea); many causes	Typically bulky, soft, light yellow to gray, mushy, greasy or oily, and sometimes frothy; particularly foul-smelling; usually float in the toilet
• *Osmotic diarrheas* *Lactose intolerance*	Deficiency in intestinal lactase	Watery diarrhea of large volume
Abuse of osmotic purgatives	Laxative habit, often surreptitious	Watery diarrhea of large volume
• *Secretory diarrheas, associated with a number of uncommon conditions, such as the Zollinger–Ellison syndrome*	Variable	Watery diarrhea of large volume

Table 2-10 Diarrhea

TIMING	ASSOCIATED SYMPTOMS	SETTING, PERSONS AT RISK
Duration of a few days, possibly longer. Lactase deficiency may lead to a longer course.	Nausea, vomiting, periumbilical cramping pain. Temperature normal or slightly elevated	Often travel, a common food source, or an epidemic
An acute illness or varying duration	Lower abdominal cramping pain and often rectal urgency, tenesmus; fever	Travel, contaminated food or water. Male homosexuals at higher risk (anal intercourse)
Acute, recurrent, or chronic	Possibly nausea; usually little if any pain	Prescribed or over-the-counter medications
Often worse in the morning. Diarrhea rarely wakes the patient at night.	Crampy lower abdominal pain, abdominal distention, flatulence, nausea, constipation	Young and middle-aged adults, especially women
Variable	Change in usual bowel habits, crampy lower abdominal pain, constipation	Middle-aged and older adults, especially over 55 yr
Onset ranges from insidious to acute. Typically recurrent, may be persistent. Diarrhea may wake the patient at night.	Crampy lower or generalized abdominal pain, anorexia, weakness, fever	Often young people
Insidious onset, chronic or recurrent. Diarrhea may wake the patient at night.	Crampy periumbilical or right lower quadrant (enteritis) or diffuse (colitis) pain, with anorexia, low fever, and/or weight loss. Perianal or perirectal abscesses and fistulas.	Often young people, especially in the late teens, but also in the middle years. More common in Jews
Onset of illness typically insidious	Anorexia, weight loss, fatigue, abdominal distention, often crampy lower abdominal pain. Symptoms of nutritional deficiencies such as bleeding (vitamin K), bone pain and fractures (vitamin D), glossitis (vitamin B), and edema (protein)	Variable, depending on cause
Follows the ingestion of milk and milk products; is relieved by fasting	Crampy abdominal pain, abdominal distention, flatulence	Blacks, Asians, Native Americans
Variable	Often none	Persons with anorexia nervosa or bulimia nervosa
Variable	Weight loss, dehydration, nausea, vomiting, and cramping abdominal pain	Variable, depending on cause

Table 2-11 Polyuria, Frequency, and Nocturia

Table 2-11 Polyuria, Frequency, and Nocturia

PROBLEM	MECHANISMS	SELECTED CAUSES	ASSOCIATED SYMPTOMS
POLYURIA	Deficiency in antidiuretic hormone (diabetes insipidus)	A disorder of the posterior pituitary and hypothalamus	Thirst and polydipsia, often severe and persistent; nocturia
	Renal unresponsiveness to antidiuretic hormone (nephrogenic diabetes insipidus)	A number of kidney diseases, including hypercalcemic and hypokalemic nephropathy; drug toxicity, *e.g.*, from lithium	Thirst and polydipsia, often severe and persistent; nocturia
	Solute diuresis • Electrolytes, such as sodium salts	Large saline infusions, potent diuretics, certain kidney diseases	Variable
	• Nonelectrolytes, such as glucose	Uncontrolled diabetes mellitus	Thirst, polydipsia, and nocturia
	Excessive water intake	Primary polydipsia	Polydipsia tends to be episodic. Thirst may not be present. Nocturia is usually absent.
FREQUENCY WITHOUT POLYURIA	Decreased capacity of the bladder		
	• Increased bladder sensitivity to stretch because of inflammation	Cystitis, bladder stones, tumor, or foreign body	Burning on urination, urinary urgency, sometimes gross hematuria
	• Decreased elasticity of the bladder wall	Infiltration by scar tissue or tumor	Symptoms of associated inflammation (see above) are common.
	• Decreased cortical inhibition of bladder contractions	Upper motor neuron disease	Urinary urgency; symptoms of upper motor neuron disease such as weakness and paralysis
	Impaired emptying of the bladder, with residual urine in the bladder		
	• Partial mechanical obstruction of the bladder neck or proximal urethra	Most commonly benign prostatic hyperplasia; also urethral stricture and other obstructive lesions of the bladder or prostate	Prior obstructive symptoms: hesitancy in starting the urinary stream, straining to void, reduced size and force of the stream, and dribbling during or at the end of urination
	• Loss of lower motor or sensory nerve supply to the bladder	Neurologic disease affecting the sacral nerves or nerve roots, *e.g.*, diabetic neuropathy	Weakness or sensory defects

Table 2-11   Polyuria, Frequency, and Nocturia

PROBLEM	MECHANISMS	SELECTED CAUSES	ASSOCIATED SYMPTOMS
NOCTURIA			
WITH HIGH VOLUMES	Most types of polyuria (see p. 84)		
	Decreased concentrating ability of the kidney with loss of the normal decrease in nocturnal urinary output	Chronic renal insufficiency due to a number of diseases	Possibly other symptoms of renal insufficiency
	Excessive fluid intake before bedtime	Habit, especially involving alcohol and coffee	
	Fluid-retaining, edematous states. Dependent edema accumulates during the day and is excreted when the patient lies down at night.	Congestive heart failure, nephrotic syndrome, hepatic cirrhosis with ascites, chronic venous insufficiency	Edema and other symptoms of the underlying disorder. Urinary output during the day may be reduced as fluid reaccumulates in the body. See Table 15-3, Mechanisms and Patterns of Edema.
WITH LOW VOLUMES	Frequency without polyuria (see p. 84)		
	Voiding while up at night without a real urge, a "pseudo-frequency"	Insomnia	Variable

Table 2-12   Urinary Incontinence

Table 2-12   Urinary Incontinence

PROBLEM	MECHANISMS
STRESS INCONTINENCE The urethral sphincter is weakened so that transient increases in intra-abdominal pressure raise the bladder pressure to levels that exceed urethral resistance.	In women, most often a weakness of the pelvic floor with inadequate muscular support of the bladder and proximal urethra and a change in the angle between the bladder and the urethra. Suggested causes include childbirth and surgery. Local conditions affecting the internal urethral sphincter, such as postmenopausal atrophy of the mucosa and urethral infection, may also contribute.
URGE INCONTINENCE Detrusor contractions are stronger than normal and overcome the normal urethral resistance. The bladder is typically small.	1. Decreased cortical inhibition of detrusor contractions, as by strokes, brain tumors, dementia, and lesions of the spinal cord above the sacral level 2. Hyperexcitability of sensory pathways, caused by, for example, bladder infections, tumors, and fecal impaction 3. Deconditioning of voiding reflexes, caused by, for example, frequent voluntary voiding at low bladder volumes
OVERFLOW INCONTINENCE Detrusor contractions are insufficient to overcome urethral resistance. The bladder is typically large, even after an effort to void.	1. Obstruction of the bladder outlet, as by benign prostatic hyperplasia or tumor 2. Weakness of the detrusor muscle associated with lower motor neuron disease at the sacral level 3. Impaired bladder sensation that interrupts the reflex arc, as from diabetic neuropathy
FUNCTIONAL INCONTINENCE This is a functional inability to get to the toilet in time because of impaired health or environmental conditions.	Problems in mobility resulting from weakness, arthritis, poor vision, or other conditions. Environmental factors such as an unfamiliar setting, distant bathroom facilities, bedrails, or physical restraints
INCONTINENCE SECONDARY TO MEDICATIONS Drugs may contribute to any type of incontinence listed.	Sedatives, tranquilizers, anticholinergics, sympathetic blockers, and potent diuretics

Patients may have more than one kind of incontinence. Many women with stress incontinence also have some degree of urge incontinence, for example, and an elderly person may be incontinent for several different reasons.

Table 2-12 Urinary Incontinence

SYMPTOMS	PHYSICAL SIGNS
Momentary leakage of small amounts of urine concurrent with stresses such as coughing, laughing, and sneezing while the person is in an upright position. A desire to urinate is not associated with pure stress incontinence.	The bladder is not detected on abdominal examination. Stress incontinence may be demonstrable, especially if the patient is examined before voiding and in a standing position. Atrophic vaginitis may be evident.
Incontinence preceded by an urge to void. The volume tends to be moderate. Urgency Frequency and nocturia with small to moderate volumes If acute inflammation is present, pain on urination Possibly "pseudo-stress incontinence"—voiding 10–20 sec after stresses such as a change of position, going up or down stairs, and possibly coughing, laughing, or sneezing	The bladder is not detectable on abdominal examination. When cortical inhibition is decreased, signs of upper motor neuron disease or mental deficits are often, though not necessarily, present. When sensory pathways are hyperexcitable, signs of local pelvic problems or a fecal impaction may be present.
A continuous dripping or dribbling incontinence Decreased force of the urinary stream Prior symptoms of partial urinary obstruction or symptoms of neurologic disease may be present.	The bladder is often found enlarged on abdominal examination and may be tender. Other possible signs include prostatic enlargement, signs of lower motor neuron disease, a decrease in sensation including perineal sensation, and diminished to absent reflexes.
Incontinence on the way to the toilet or only in the early morning	The bladder is not detectable on physical examination. Look for physical or environmental clues to the likely cause.
Variable. A careful history and chart review are important.	Variable

Table 2-13   Painful Peripheral Vascular Disorders and Their Mimics

Table 2-13   Painful Peripheral Vascular Disorders and Their Mimics

PROBLEM	PROCESS	LOCATION
ARTERIAL DISORDERS		
ARTERIOSCLEROSIS OBLITERANS		
• *Intermittent claudication*	Episodic muscular ischemia induced by exercise, due to obstruction of large or middle-sized arteries by atherosclerosis	Usually the calf, but may also be felt in the buttock, hip, thigh, or foot, depending on the level of obstruction
• *Rest pain*	Ischemia even at rest	Distal pain, in the toes or forefoot
ACUTE ARTERIAL OCCLUSION	Embolism or thrombosis, possibly superimposed on arteriosclerosis obliterans	Distal pain, usually involving the foot and leg
VENOUS DISORDERS		
SUPERFICIAL THROMBOPHLEBITIS	Clot formation and acute inflammation in a superficial vein	Pain in a local area along the course of a superficial vein, most often in the saphenous system
DEEP VENOUS THROMBOSIS	Clot formation in a deep vein	Pain, if present, is usually in the calf, but the process more often is painless.
CHRONIC VENOUS INSUFFICIENCY (DEEP)	Chronic venous engorgement secondary to venous occlusion or incompetency of venous valves	Diffuse aching of the leg(s)
ACUTE LYMPHANGITIS	Acute bacterial infection (usually streptococcal) spreading up the lymphatic channels from a portal of entry such as an injured area or an ulcer	An arm or a leg
THROMBOANGIITIS OBLITERANS (*Buerger's disease*)	Inflammatory and thrombotic occlusions of small arteries and also of veins, occurring in smokers	1. Intermittent claudication, particularly in the arch of the foot 2. Rest pain in the fingers or toes
RAYNAUD'S DISEASE (*and phenomenon*)	Episodic spasm of the small arteries and arterioles, without organic occlusion. When the syndrome is secondary to other conditions (and then called Raynaud's phenomenon), occlusion may occur.	Distal portions of one or more fingers. Pain is usually not prominent unless fingertip ulcers develop. Numbness and tingling are common.
MIMICS*		
ACUTE CELLULITIS	Acute bacterial infection of the skin and subcutaneous tissues	Arms, legs, or elsewhere
ERYTHEMA NODOSUM	Inflammatory lesions associated with a variety of systemic disorders	Anterior surfaces of both lower legs

* Mistaken primarily for acute superficial thrombophlebitis

Table 2-13   Painful Peripheral Vascular Disorders and Their Mimics

TIMING	FACTORS THAT AGGRAVATE	FACTORS THAT RELIEVE	ASSOCIATED MANIFESTATIONS
Fairly brief: pain usually forces the patient to rest.	Exercise such as walking	Rest usually stops the pain in 1–3 min.	Local fatigue, numbness, diminished pulses, often signs of arterial insufficiency (see p. 453)
Persistent, often worse at night	Elevation of the feet, as in bed	Sitting with legs dependent	Numbness, tingling, signs of arterial insufficiency (see p. 453)
Sudden onset; associated symptoms may occur without pain.			Coldness, numbness, weakness, absent distal pulses
An acute episode lasting days or longer			Local redness, swelling, tenderness, a palpable cord, possibly fever
Often hard to determine because of lack of symptoms			Possibly swelling of the foot and calf and local calf tenderness; often nothing
Chronic, increasing as the day wears on	Prolonged standing	Elevation of the leg(s)	Chronic edema, pigmentation, possibly ulceration (see pp. 453–454)
An acute episode lasting days or longer			Red streak(s) on the skin, with tenderness, enlarged tender lymph nodes, and fever
1. With exercise 2. Chronic, persistent, may be worse at night		Permanent cessation of smoking (but patients seldom stop)	Distal coldness, sweating, numbness, and cyanosis; ulceration and gangrene at the tips of fingers or toes; migratory thrombophlebitis
Relatively brief (minutes) but recurrent	Exposure to cold, emotional upset	Warm environment	Color changes in the distal fingers: severe pallor (essential for the diagnosis) followed by cyanosis and then redness
An acute episode lasting days or longer			A local area of diffuse swelling, redness, and tenderness with enlarged, tender lymph nodes and fever; no palpable cord
Pain associated with a series of lesions over several weeks			Raised, red, tender swellings recurring in crops; often malaise, joint pains, and fever

Table 2-14   Patterns of Chronic Pain in and Around the Joints

Table 2-14   Patterns of Chronic Pain in and Around the Joints

PROBLEM	PROCESS	COMMON LOCATIONS	PATTERN OF SPREAD	ONSET	PROGRESSION AND DURATION
RHEUMATOID ARTHRITIS	Chronic inflammation of synovial membranes with secondary erosion of adjacent cartilage and bone, and damage to ligaments and tendons	Hands (proximal interphalangeal and metacarpophalangeal joints), feet (metatarsophalangeal joints), wrists, knees, elbows, and ankles	Symmetrically additive: progresses to other joints while persisting in the initial ones	Usually insidious	Often chronic with remissions and exacerbations
OSTEOARTHRITIS *(degenerative joint disease)*	Degeneration and progressive loss of cartilage within the joints, damage to underlying bone, and the formation of new bone at the margins of the cartilage	Knees, hips, hands (distal and sometimes proximal interphalangeal joints), cervical and lumbar spine, and wrists (the first carpometacarpal joint); also joints previously injured or diseased	Additive; however, only one joint may be involved.	Usually insidious	Slowly progressive with temporary exacerbations after periods of overuse
GOUTY ARTHRITIS					
ACUTE GOUT	An inflammatory reaction to microcrystals of sodium urate	Base of the big toe (the first metatarsophalangeal joint), the instep or dorsum of feet, the ankles, knees, and elbows	Early attacks are usually confined to one joint.	Sudden, often at night, often after injury, surgery, fasting, or excessive food or alcohol intake	Occasional isolated attacks lasting days up to 2 wk; they may get more frequent and severe, with persisting symptoms.
CHRONIC TOPHACEOUS GOUT	Multiple local accumulations of sodium urate in the joints and other tissues (tophi), with or without inflammation	Feet, ankles, wrists, fingers, and elbows	Additive, not so symmetrical as rheumatoid arthritis	Gradual development of chronicity with repeated attacks	Chronic symptoms with acute exacerbations
POLYMYALGIA RHEUMATICA	A disease of unclear nature seen in people over 50 yr, especially women; may be associated with giant cell arteritis	Muscles of the hip girdle and shoulder girdle; symmetrical		Insidious or abrupt, even appearing overnight	Chronic but ultimately self-limiting
THE "FIBROSITIS" SYNDROME	Muscular aching and stiffness with specific, tender "trigger areas." May accompany other diseases. Mechanisms unclear	"All over" but especially in the neck, shoulders, elbows, hands, low back, and knees	Shifts unpredictably or worsens in response to immobility, excessive use, or chilling	Variable, may follow an upsetting event	Chronic, with "ups and downs"

The vagueness of these characteristics is in itself a clue to the fibrositis syndrome.

Table 2-14 Patterns of Chronic Pain in and Around the Joints

ASSOCIATED SYMPTOMS				
SWELLING	REDNESS, WARMTH, AND TENDERNESS	STIFFNESS	LIMITATION OF MOTION	GENERALIZED SYMPTOMS
Frequent swelling of synovial tissue in joints or tendon sheaths; also subcutaneous nodules	Tender, often warm, but seldom red	Prominent, often for an hour or more in the mornings, also after inactivity	Often develops	Weakness, fatigue, weight loss, and low fever are common.
Small effusions in the joints may be present, especially in the knees; also bony enlargement.	Possibly tender, seldom warm, and rarely red	Frequent but brief (usually 5–10 min), in the morning and after inactivity	Often develops	Usually absent
Present, within and around the involved joint	Hot, red, and exquisitely tender	Not evident	Motion is limited primarily by pain.	Fever may be present.
Present, as tophi, in joints, bursae, and subcutaneous tissues	Tenderness, warmth, and redness may be present during exacerbations.	Present	Present	Possibly fever; patient may also develop symptoms of renal failure and renal stones.
None	Muscles often tender, but not warm or red	Prominent, especially in the morning	Usually none	Malaise, a sense of depression, possibly anorexia, weight loss, and fever, but no true weakness
None	Specific tender "trigger areas," often not recognized until examination	Present, especially in the morning	Absent, though stiffness is greater at the extremes of movement	Fatigue and a disturbance of sleep are usually associated.

Table 2-15   Low Back Pain

Table 2-15   Low Back Pain

PATTERNS	POSSIBLE CAUSES	POSSIBLE PHYSICAL SIGNS
COMMON LOW BACK PAIN Acute, often recurrent, or possibly chronic aching pain in the lumbosacral area, possibly radiating into the posterior thighs but not below the knees. The pain is often precipitated or aggravated by moving, lifting, or twisting motions and is relieved by rest. Spinal movements are typically limited by pain. This is the back pain common from the teenage years through the 40s.	The exact cause cannot usually be proven. Intervertebral disc disease is probably involved in many cases. Congenital disorders of the spine, such as spondylolisthesis, may be present in a small percentage. In older women or in persons on long-term corticosteroid therapy, consider osteoporosis complicated by a collapsed vertebra.	Local tenderness, muscle spasm, pain on movement of the back, and loss of the normal lumbar lordosis, but no motor or sensory loss or reflex abnormalities. In osteoporosis there may be a thoracic kyphosis, percussion tenderness over a spinous process, or fractures elsewhere such as in the thoracic spine or in a hip.
SCIATICA A radicular (nerve root) pain, usually superimposed on low back pain. The sciatic pain is shooting and radiates down one or both legs, usually to below the knee(s) in a dermatomal distribution, often with associated numbness and tingling and possibly local weakness. The pain is usually worsened by spinal movement such as bending and by sneezing, coughing, or straining.	A herniated intervertebral disc with compression or traction of nerve root(s) is the most common cause in persons under age 50 yr. The nerve roots of L5 or S1 are most often affected. Spinal cord tumors or abscesses are much less common causes. Compared to a disc, they tend to affect more nerve roots and to produce more neurologic deficits.	Pain on straight leg raising (see pp. 489–490), tenderness of the sciatic nerve, loss of sensation in a dermatomal distribution, local muscular weakness and atrophy, and decreased to absent reflex(es), especially affecting the ankle jerks. Dermatomal signs and reflex changes may be absent when only a single root is affected.
BACK PAIN OR SCIATICA WITH PSEUDOCLAUDICATION Pseudoclaudication is a pain in the back or legs that worsens with walking and improves with flexing of the spine, as by sitting or bending forward.	Lumbar stenosis, which is a combination of degenerative disc disease and osteoarthritis that creates pressure or traction on the spinal nerves. It is a common cause of pain after age 60.	The posture may become flexed forward.
CHRONIC PERSISTENT LOW BACK STIFFNESS	Ankylosing spondylitis, a chronic inflammatory polyarthritis, most common in young men.	Loss of the normal lumbar lordosis, muscle spasm, and limitation of anterior and lateral flexion.
	Diffuse idiopathic skeletal hyperostosis (DISH), which affects middle-aged and older men	Possible decrease in spinal mobility
ACHING NOCTURNAL BACK PAIN, UNRELIEVED BY REST	Consider metastatic malignancy in the spine, as from cancer of the prostate, breast, lung, thyroid, and kidney, and multiple myeloma.	Variable with the source. Local bone tenderness may be present.
BACK PAIN REFERRED FROM THE ABDOMEN OR PELVIS Usually a deep, aching pain, the level of which varies with the source	Peptic ulcer, pancreatitis, pancreatic cancer, chronic prostatitis, endometriosis, dissecting aortic aneurysm, retroperitoneal tumor, and other causes	Spinal movements are not painful and range of motion is not affected. Look for signs of the primary disorder.

Table 2-16   Pains in the Neck

Table 2-16   Pains in the Neck

Classifications of neck pain vary considerably, partly because pathologic or other presumably definitive criteria are usually lacking. While "simple stiff neck" is very common, for example, people who have it seldom seek care for it.

PATTERNS	POSSIBLE CAUSES	POSSIBLE PHYSICAL SIGNS
"SIMPLE STIFF NECK" Acute, episodic, localized pain in the neck, often appearing on awakening and lasting 1–4 dy. No dermatomal radiation	The mechanisms are not understood.	Local muscular tenderness and pain on certain movements
ACHING NECK A persistent dull aching in the back of the neck, often spreading to the occiput. This is common with postural strain, as with prolonged typing or studying, and may also accompany tension and depression.	Poorly understood; may be related to sustained muscle contraction, as in muscle tension headaches (see Table 2-1, Headaches).	Local muscular tenderness. When areas of pain and tenderness are also present elsewhere in the body, consider the fibrositis syndrome (see Table 2-14, Patterns of Chronic Pain In and Around the Joints).
"CERVICAL SPRAIN" Acute and often recurrent neck pains that are often more severe and last longer than "simple stiff neck." There may be a precipitating factor such as a whiplash injury, heavy lifting, or a sudden movement, but there is no dermatomal radiation.	Poorly understood	Local tenderness and pain of movement
NECK PAIN WITH DERMATOMAL RADIATION* Neck pain as in "cervical sprain" but with radiation of the pain to the shoulder, back, or arm in a dermatomal distribution. This radicular pain is typically sharp, burning, or tingling in quality.	Compression of one or more nerve roots caused by either a herniated cervical disc or degenerative disease of the intervertebral discs with bony spurring	Muscle tenderness and spasm, a limited range of neck motion, increase in the pain on coughing or straining, and possible sensory loss, weakness, muscular atrophy, and decreased reflexes in the areas involved
NECK PAIN WITH SYMPTOMS SUGGESTING COMPRESSION OF THE CERVICAL SPINAL CORD* Associated here is weakness or paralysis of the legs, often with a decrease in or loss of sensation. These symptoms may occur in addition to the radicular symptoms or by themselves. The neck pain may be mild or even absent.	Compression of the spinal cord in the neck caused by either a herniated cervical disc or degenerative disease of the intervertebral discs with bony spurring	Limited range of motion in the neck, weakness or paralysis in the legs of the upper motor neuron type, Babinski responses, loss of position and vibration sense in the legs, and, less commonly, loss of pain and temperature sensation. Radicular signs in the arms may also be present.

* Tumors or abscesses of the cervical spinal cord, though less common, should also be considered.

Table 2-17 Syncope and Similar Disorders

Table 2-17 Syncope and Similar Disorders

PROBLEM	MECHANISM	PRECIPITATING FACTORS
VASODEPRESSOR SYNCOPE *(the common faint)*	Sudden peripheral vasodilatation, especially in the skeletal muscles, without a compensatory rise in cardiac output. Blood pressure falls.	A strong emotion such as fear or pain
POSTURAL *(orthostatic)* **HYPOTENSION**	1. *Inadequate vasoconstrictor reflexes* in both arterioles and veins, with resultant venous pooling, decreased cardiac output, and low blood pressure	1. Standing up
	2. *Hypovolemia,* a diminished blood volume insufficient to maintain cardiac output and blood pressure, especially in the upright position	2. Standing up after hemorrhage or dehydration
COUGH SYNCOPE	Several possible mechanisms associated with increased intrathoracic pressure	Severe paroxysm of coughing
MICTURITION SYNCOPE	Unclear	Emptying the bladder after getting out of bed to void
CARDIOVASCULAR DISORDERS ARRHYTHMIAS	Decreased cardiac output secondary to rhythms that are too fast (usually more than 180) or too slow (less than 35–40)	A sudden change in rhythm
AORTIC STENOSIS AND HYPERTROPHIC CARDIOMYOPATHY	Vascular resistance falls with exercise, but cardiac output cannot rise.	Effort
MYOCARDIAL INFARCTION	Sudden arrhythmia or decreased cardiac output	Variable
MASSIVE PULMONARY EMBOLISM	Sudden hypoxia or decreased cardiac output	Variable
DISORDERS RESEMBLING SYNCOPE HYPOCAPNIA *(decreased carbon dioxide)* DUE TO HYPERVENTILATION	Constriction of cerebral blood vessels secondary to hypocapnia that is induced by hyperventilation	Possibly a stressful situation
HYPOGLYCEMIA	Insufficient glucose to maintain cerebral metabolism; secretion of epinephrine contributes to symptoms.	Variable, including fasting
HYSTERICAL FAINTING DUE TO A CONVERSION REACTION*	The symbolic expression of an unacceptable idea through body language	Stressful situation

* Important diagnostic observations in hysterical fainting include normal skin color and normal vital signs, sometimes bizarre and purposive movements, and occurrence in the presence of other people.

Table 2-17 Syncope and Similar Disorders

PREDISPOSING FACTORS	PRODROMAL MANIFESTATIONS	POSTURAL ASSOCIATIONS	RECOVERY
Fatigue, hunger, a hot, humid environment	Restlessness, weakness, pallor, nausea, salivation, sweating, yawning	Usually occurs when standing, possibly when sitting	Prompt return of consciousness when lying down, but pallor, weakness, nausea, and slight confusion may persist for a time.
1. Peripheral neuropathies and disorders affecting the autonomic nervous system; drugs such as antihypertensives and vasodilators; prolonged bed rest	1. Often none	1. Occurs soon after the person stands up	1. Prompt return to normal when lying down
2. Bleeding from the GI tract or trauma, potent diuretics, vomiting, diarrhea, polyuria	2. Lightheadedness and palpitations (tachycardia) on standing up	2. Usually occurs soon after the person stands up	2. Improvement on lying down
Chronic bronchitis in a muscular man	Often none except for cough	May occur in any position	Prompt return to normal
Nocturia, usually in elderly or adult men	Often none	Standing to void	Prompt return to normal
Organic heart disease and old age decrease the tolerance to abnormal rhythms.	Often none	May occur in any position	Prompt return to normal unless brain damage has resulted
The cardiac disorders	Often none	Occurs with or after exercise	Usually a prompt return to normal
Coronary artery disease	Often none	May occur in any position	Variable
Deep venous thrombosis	Often none	May occur in any position	Variable
A predisposition to anxiety attacks and hyperventilation	Dyspnea, palpitations, chest discomfort, numbness and tingling of the hands and around the mouth lasting for several minutes. Consciousness is often maintained.	May occur in any position	Slow improvement as hyperventilation ceases
Insulin therapy and a variety of metabolic disorders	Sweating, tremor, palpitations, hunger; headache, confusion, abnormal behavior, coma. True syncope is uncommon.	May occur in any position	Variable, depending on severity and treatment
Hysterical personality traits	Variable	A slump to the floor, often from a standing position without injury	Variable, may be prolonged, often with fluctuating responsiveness

Table 2-18 Seizure Disorders

Table 2-18   Seizure Disorders

Partial seizures are those that start with focal manifestations. They may or may not become generalized. They are further divided into *simple partial seizures,* which do not impair consciousness, and *complex partial seizures,* which do. Either of these two may progress into a third type, *partial seizures that become generalized.* Partial seizures of all kinds usually indicate a structural lesion in the cerebral cortex, such as a scar, tumor, or infarction. The quality of such seizures helps the clinician to localize the causative lesion in the brain.

PROBLEM	CLINICAL MANIFESTATIONS	POSTICTAL *(POSTSEIZURE)* STATE
PARTIAL SEIZURES		
SIMPLE PARTIAL SEIZURES		
• *With motor symptoms* *Jacksonian*	Tonic and then clonic movements that start unilaterally in the hand, foot, or face and spread to other body parts on the same side	Normal consciousness
Other motor	Turning of the head and eyes to one side, or tonic and clonic movements of an arm or leg without the Jacksonian spread	Normal consciousness
• *With sensory symptoms*	Numbness, tingling; simple visual, auditory, or olfactory hallucinations such as flashing lights, buzzing, or odors	Normal consciousness
• *With autonomic symptoms*	A "funny feeling" in the epigastrium, nausea, pallor, flushing, lightheadedness	Normal consciousness
• *With psychic symptoms*	Anxiety or fear; feelings of familiarity (déjà vu) or unreality; dreamy states; fear or rage; flashback experiences; more complex hallucinations	Normal consciousness
COMPLEX PARTIAL SEIZURES These may start with simple partial seizures or with impaired consciousness. Automatisms may develop.	The seizure may or may not start with autonomic or psychic symptoms. Consciousness is impaired and the person appears confused. Automatisms include automatic motor behaviors such as chewing, smacking the lips, walking about, and unbuttoning clothes; also more complicated and skilled behaviors such as driving a car.	The patient may remember initial autonomic or psychic symptoms (then termed an *aura*) but is amnesic for the rest of the seizure. Temporary confusion and headache may occur.
PARTIAL SEIZURES THAT BECOME GENERALIZED	Partial seizures that become generalized resemble tonic–clonic seizures (see p. 97). Unfortunately, the patient may not recall the focal onset and observers may overlook it.	As in a tonic–clonic seizure. Two attributes indicate a partial seizure that has become generalized: (1) the recollection of an aura, and (2) a unilateral neurologic deficit during the postictal period.

Table 2-18   Seizure Disorders

Generalized seizures, in contrast to partial ones, begin with either bilateral bodily movements or impairment of consciousness, or both. They suggest a widespread, bilateral cortical disturbance that may be either hereditary or acquired. When generalized seizures of the tonic–clonic (grand mal) variety start in childhood or young adulthood, they are often hereditary. When tonic–clonic seizures begin after the age of 30, suspect either a partial seizure that has become generalized or a general seizure caused by a toxic or metabolic problem. Toxic and metabolic causes include withdrawal from alcohol or other sedative drugs, uremia, hypoglycemia, hyperglycemia, hyponatremia and water intoxication, and bacterial meningitis.

PROBLEM	CLINICAL MANIFESTATIONS	POSTICTAL (POSTSEIZURE) STATE
GENERALIZED SEIZURES		
TONIC–CLONIC CONVULSION (*grand mal*)*	The person loses consciousness suddenly, sometimes with a cry, and the body stiffens into tonic extensor rigidity. Breathing stops and the person becomes cyanotic. A clonic phase of rhythmic muscular contraction follows. Breathing resumes and is often noisy, with excessive salivation. Injury, tongue biting, and urinary incontinence may occur.	Confusion, drowsiness, fatigue, headache, muscular aching, and sometimes the temporary persistence of bilateral neurologic deficits such as hyperactive reflexes and Babinski responses. The person has amnesia for the seizure and recalls no aura.
ABSENCE	A sudden brief lapse of consciousness, with momentary blinking, staring, or movements of the lips and hands but no falling. Two subtypes are recognized. *Petit mal absences* last less than 10 sec and stop abruptly. *Atypical absences* may last more than 10 sec.	No aura recalled. In petit mal absences, a prompt return to normal; in atypical absences, some postictal confusion
ATONIC SEIZURE, OR DROP ATTACK	Sudden loss of consciousness with falling but no movements. Injury may occur.	Either a prompt return to normal or a brief period of confusion
MYOCLONUS	Sudden, brief, rapid jerks, involving the trunk or limbs. Associated with a variety of disorders	Variable
PSEUDOSEIZURES		
These may mimic seizures but are due to a conversion reaction (a psychological disorder).	The movements may have personally symbolic significance and often do not follow a neuroanatomic pattern. Injury is uncommon.	Variable

* *Febrile convulsions* that resemble brief tonic–clonic seizures may occur in infants and young children. They are usually benign but occasionally may be the first manifestation of a seizure disorder.

Chapter 3
Mental Status

Components of Mental Function

In every body system, clinicians have selected certain readily observable characteristics with which to assess the structure and function of that system, to distinguish a healthy from a pathologic state, and to diagnose disease. While symptoms, heart sounds, pressures, and pulse waves serve these purposes in the cardiovascular system, for example, various components of mental function do so for the mind. Although these components in no way encompass all the aspects of human thought and feeling, they serve as useful clinical tools.

Level of consciousness refers to people's alertness and state of awareness of their environment. *Attention* refers to the ability to focus or concentrate over time on one task or activity. An inattentive or distractible person whose consciousness is clouded is grossly impaired in giving a history or responding to questions. *Memory*, too, contributes importantly to such responses. A person first must register or record material in the mind—a function usually tested by asking for immediate repetition of material. Information must then be stored or retained in memory. *Recent* (or *short-term*) *memory* refers to memory over an interval of minutes, hours, or days, while *remote* (or *long-term*) *memory* refers to intervals of years. *Orientation* depends on both memory and attention. It refers to people's awareness of who or what they are in relation to time, place, and other people.

A person becomes aware of objects in the environment and their qualities and interrelationships through sensory *perceptions*. While most perceptions are initiated by external stimuli, others, like dreams and hallucinations, arise in the mind itself.

Thought processes refers to the sequence, logic, coherence, and relevance of a person's thought as it leads to selected goals. While thought processes describe how people think, *thought content* refers to what they think about. Thought includes insight and judgment. In the context of a mental status examination, *insight* refers to a person's awareness that his or her symptoms or disturbed behaviors are abnormal. One person may realize that the hallucinations experienced are mental figments, for example, while another, lacking this insight, is convinced that they are real external phenomena. In making *judgments*, a person compares and evaluates alternatives for purposes of deciding on a course of action. Inherent in judgment is a set of values that may or may not be based on reality and may or may not conform to societal norms.

In contrast to thought, affect and mood describe how people feel. *Affect* is an immediately observable, usually episodic feeling tone expressed through voice, facial expression, or demeanor, while *mood* is a more sustained emotion that may color a person's view of the world. As weather is to climate, so affect is to mood.

People communicate with each other through *language,* a complex symbolic system of expressing, receiving, and comprehending words. Like consciousness, attention, and memory, language is essential to other mental functions; significant impairment here makes assessment of certain other functions difficult or even impossible.

Higher cognitive functions include a person's *vocabulary,* fund of *information,* and abilities to *think abstractly, calculate* numbers, and *copy or construct objects* that have two or three dimensions.

None of the functions described in this chapter deals directly with personality, psychodynamics, or personal experiences. These other, very important aspects are explored during the interview. By integrating and correlating all the relevant data, the clinician tries to understand the person as a whole.

CHANGES WITH AGE

Adolescence marks a time of continuing intellectual maturation during which a person's fund of information and vocabulary continue to grow —a process that began in childhood. At approximately 12 years of age, adolescents begin to think abstractly—to use generalizations, make hypotheses, develop theories, reason logically, and consider future plans, risks, and possibilities. Given intelligence, education, and experience, among other requisites, judgment develops along with an underlying set of values. This maturational process, however, like height, weight, and puberty, varies in its time of onset, pace, and duration and cannot be predicted by chronological age alone. Some individuals never achieve the levels customarily defined as normal adult function.

Lack of ability to think abstractly and to weigh consequences affects health-related behaviors such as sexual activity, the use of tobacco, alcohol, or other drugs, and taking risks that lead to accidents. In a society in which such behaviors are emphasized in the media and elsewhere, they are all prevalent among adolescents. In addition, some psychological problems may appear during the teenage years. These include concerns over a changing body, panic attacks, rage reactions, depression, suicidal behaviors, and psychotic disorders, including schizophrenia.

Aging. Age-related losses may take their toll on the mental function of an elderly person. These include the deaths of loved ones and friends, retirement from valued employment, diminution in income, decreased physical capacities including impairments in vision and hearing, and perhaps decreased stimulation or growing isolation. In addition, biological changes affect the aging brain. Brain volume and the number of cortical brain cells decrease, and both microanatomic and biochemical changes have been identified. Nevertheless, most men and women adapt well to getting older. They maintain their self-esteem, they alter their activities in ways that are appropriate to their changing capacities and circumstances, and eventually they ready themselves for death.

Most elderly people do well on a mental status examination but functional impairments may become evident, especially at advanced ages. Many older people complain of their memories. "Benign forgetfulness" is the usual explanation and may occur at any age. This term refers to a difficulty in recalling the names of people or objects or certain details of specific events. Naming this common phenomenon, when appropriate, may help to reassure a person who is worried that it signifies Alzheimer's disease. In addition to this circumscribed forgetfulness, elderly people retrieve and process data more slowly, and they take more time to learn new material. Their motor responses may slow, and their ability to perform complex tasks may become impaired.

The clinician must often try to distinguish these age-related changes from the manifestations of specific mental disorders, some of which are more prevalent in old age. The dementia associated with Alzheimer's disease has been estimated to affect about 5 percent of people over 65 and 20 percent of those who are 85 or older, but its prevalence may be even higher. Depression is quite common in elderly patients who are hospitalized, but not in those who are living at home. Delirium is an important disorder among the aged. Elderly people are especially susceptible to this temporary confusional state, and the clinician must recognize it promptly in order to treat it properly and protect the patient from harm. Further, delirium may be the first clue to a physical illness, such as a myocardial infarction or pneumonia.

Techniques of Examination

Most of the mental status examination should be done in the context of the interview. As you talk to the patient and listen to the story, you should assess level of consciousness, general appearance and affect, and ability to pay attention, remember, understand, and speak. By noting the patient's vocabulary and general fund of information in the context of cultural and educational background you can often make a rough estimate of intelligence, while the patient's responses to illness and circumstance often tell you much about insight and judgment. If the patient has unusual thoughts, preoccupations, beliefs, or perceptions, you should explore them as the subject arises. Moreover, if you suspect a problem in orientation or memory, you can check these too as part of the interview. "Let's see, your last clinic appointment was when? . . . and the date today is . . . ?"

For many patients, such an evaluation is sufficient. For others, however, you need to go further. All patients with documented or suspected brain lesions, those with psychiatric symptoms, and those in whom family members or friends have reported vague behavioral symptoms need further careful, specific assessment. Patients who seem unable to take their medications properly, whose attention to home or business responsibilities seems to be slipping, and who are losing interest in their usual activities may be showing signs of dementia. The patient who is behaving strangely after surgery or during an acute illness may be delirious. Each problem should be identified as expeditiously as possible. Mental function, moreover, importantly influences a person's ability to find and hold a job and thus may constitute the critical component in evaluating disability.

For these kinds of patients, and others as well, you will need to supplement your interview with questions in specific areas. In doing so, give simple introductory explanations, be tactful, and show the same acceptance and respect for the patient as in other portions of the examination.

Many students feel insecure in performing mental status examinations and are reluctant to do them. They may worry about upsetting patients, invading their privacy, and labeling their thoughts or behavior as pathologic. It may be helpful to discuss these concerns or some of the issues they raise with your instructor or other experienced clinicians. As in other parts of the assessment process, your skills and confidence will improve with practice and rewards will follow. Many patients will appreciate an understanding listener, and some will owe their health, their safety, or even their lives to your attention.

The format that follows should help to organize your observations but it is not intended as a step-by-step guide. When a full examination is indicated, you should be flexible in your approach while thorough in your coverage. In some situations, however, sequence is important. If during your initial interview the patient's consciousness, attention, comprehension of words, or ability to speak seems impaired, assess this attribute promptly. A person so impaired cannot give a reliable history and you will not be able to test most of the other mental functions.

APPEARANCE AND BEHAVIOR

Use here all the relevant observations made throughout the course of your history and examination. Include:

LEVEL OF CONSCIOUSNESS. Is the patient awake and alert? Does the patient seem to understand your questions and respond appropriately and reasonably quickly, or is there a tendency to lose track of the topic and fall silent or even asleep?

See Table 3-1, Levels of Consciousness (p. 113). Loss of consciousness may result from extensive impairment of the cerebral cortex or of the arousal mechanisms in the brainstem. The cause may be structural (as in a cerebrovascular accident or a tumor) or metabolic (as in hypoglycemia, hypoxia, and poisoning).

If the patient does not respond to your questions, escalate the stimulus in steps:

1. Give a command to see if the patient can follow it. ("Open your eyes. Squeeze my hand.")
2. Call the patient's name.
3. Touch the arm.
4. Shake the shoulder, or
5. Produce pain. For example, you can press the bony ridges above the eyes with your thumb or pinch the side of the neck. Avoid undue roughness that might cause bruising or other injury.

Impaired hearing may also cause lack of response to verbal commands.

Note both the stimulus required and the patient's response to it, including opening the eyes, other bodily movements, and vocal responses. Observe what happens when the stimulus stops.

POSTURE AND MOTOR BEHAVIOR. Does the patient lie in bed, or prefer to walk about? Note bodily posture and the patient's ability to relax. Observe the pace, range, and character of movements. Do they seem to be made under voluntary control? Are certain parts immobile? Do posture and motor activity change with topics under discussion or with activities or people around the patient?

Tense posture, restlessness, and fidgetiness of anxiety; crying, pacing, and handwringing of agitated depression; hopeless, slumped posture and slowed movements of depression; bizarre or sustained posture in schizophrenia; singing, dancing and expansive movements of a manic episode; oral–facial dyskinesias (p. 556)

DRESS, GROOMING, AND PERSONAL HYGIENE. How is the patient dressed? Is clothing clean, pressed, and properly fastened? How does it compare with clothing worn by people of comparable age and social group? Note the patient's hair, nails, teeth, skin, and, if present, beard. How are they groomed? How do the person's grooming and hygiene compare with those of other people of comparable age, lifestyle, and socioeconomic group? Compare one side of the body with the other.

Deterioration in grooming and personal hygiene may occur in depression, schizophrenia, and organic brain syndromes, but always consider the norms of a person's group. Excessive fastidiousness may be seen in an obsessive–compulsive disorder. One-sided neglect may result from a lesion in the opposite parietal cortex, usually the non-dominant side.

FACIAL EXPRESSION. Observe the face, both at rest and when the patient is interacting with others. Watch for variations in expression with topics under discussion. Are they appropriate? Or is the face relatively immobile throughout?

Expressions of anxiety, depression, apathy, anger, elation. Facial immobility of parkinsonism

MANNER, AFFECT, AND RELATIONSHIP TO PERSONS AND THINGS. Using your observations of facial expression, voice, and bodily movements, assess the patient's affect. Does it vary appropriately with topics under discussion? Does one consistent affect prevail, or is the affect labile, blunted, or flat? Does it seem inappropriate or extreme at certain points? If so, how? Note the patient's openness, approachability, and reactions to others and to the surroundings. Does the patient seem to hear or see things that you do not or seem to be conversing with someone who is not there?

Anger, hostility, suspiciousness, or evasiveness of paranoid patients. Elation and euphoria of the manic syndrome. Flat affect and remoteness of schizophrenia. Apathy (dulled affect with detachment and indifference) in organic brain syndromes. Anxiety, depression

SPEECH AND LANGUAGE

Throughout the interview, note the characteristics of the patient's speech, including:

QUANTITY. Is the patient talkative or relatively silent? Are comments spontaneous or only in response to direct questions?

RATE. Is speech fast or slow?

Slow speech of depression; rapid loud speech in a manic syndrome

VOLUME (LOUDNESS)

FLUENCY, which includes not only the rate but also the ability to speak smoothly, clearly, and with appropriate inflections. Be alert to specific abnormal patterns such as:

See Table 3-2, Disorders of Speech, p. 114.

● *Poor articulation of words.* What sounds are especially affected?

Dysarthria

● *Disturbed rhythm and inflection,* such as hesitancy and speaking in a monotone

● *Circumlocutions,* in which phrases or sentences are substituted for a word the person cannot think of, as "what you write with" for "pen"

Monotonous, slow, weak voice in parkinsonism. Hesitancy and searching for words in aphasia

● *Paraphasias,* in which words are malformed ("I write with a den"), wrong ("I write with a bar"), or invented ("I write with a dar")

Circumlocutions and paraphasias are noted in aphasic disorders.

SPECIAL TESTING FOR APHASIA. If your observations of the patient's spontaneous speech suggest a possible disorder of language (*aphasia*), proceed with further specific testing. When language is seriously im-

Aphasia may lead to incoherent, unintelligible speech and may then be mistaken for a

paired, taking a history from the patient and assessing cognitive functions may be impossible. Although these additional observations are not part of a routine examination, they will help you to identify and differentiate among the several kinds of aphasias.

psychotic illness unless the language deficit is recognized.

Testing for Aphasia

WORD COMPREHENSION	You can test a person's comprehension of spoken language by two methods. First, ask the patient to point to objects in the room or to specify body parts as you name them. "Will you please point to your nose . . . the telephone . . . the bedspread." Second, ask a series of questions that can be answered with "yes" or "no" or with an appropriate head movement. "Are you sitting on a chair? Can dogs fly?"	Word comprehension is impaired in some but not all kinds of aphasia. Deficiencies in vision, hearing, and intellectual capacity may also affect performance.
REPETITION	Ask the patient to repeat items of increasing length and complexity, from monosyllabic words to sentences. Note the fluency and accuracy of the responses.	Repetition is impaired in some but not all kinds of aphasia.
NAMING	Ask the patient to name a series of objects or colors as you point them out. Gradually increase the difficulty of the questions—from "hat" and "red," for example, to "belt buckle" and "purple." Note the fluency and accuracy of the responses.	Naming is impaired in some but not all kinds of aphasia.
READING COMPREHENSION	Write several simple commands, each on a separate paper in large clear print. "CLOSE YOUR EYES" and "RAISE YOUR HAND." A person's prior reading ability and educational experience affect performance here.	Failure in reading comprehension often accompanies failure in word comprehension, but each may occur independently.
WRITING	Ask the patient to make up and write a sentence about a topic such as the room, the patient's job, or family. Note whether the sentence makes sense, has a subject and verb, and is correctly spelled.	Writing, like speech, is affected by some forms of aphasia. Motor impairment, such as hemiplegia, may affect performance.

MOOD

You should assess mood during the interview by exploring the patient's own perceptions of it. Find out about the patient's usual mood level and how it has varied with life events. "How did you feel about that?", for example, or, more generally, "How are your spirits?" The reports of relatives and friends may be of great value in making this assessment.

Moods include sadness and deep melancholy; contentment, joy, euphoria, and elation; anger and rage; anxiety and worry; and detachment and indifference.

What has the patient's mood been like? How intense has it been? Has it been labile or fairly unchanging? How long has it lasted? Is it appropriate to the patient's circumstances? In case of depression, have there also been episodes of an elevated mood, suggesting a bipolar disorder?

For depressive and bipolar disorders, see Table 3-3, Disorders of Mood, p. 115.

If you suspect depression, assess its depth and any associated risk of suicide. A series of questions such as the following is useful, proceeding as far as the patient's positive answers warrant.

Do you get pretty discouraged (or depressed or blue)?
How low do you feel?
What do you see for yourself in the future?
Do you ever feel that life isn't worth living? Or that you would just as soon be dead?

Have you ever thought of doing away with yourself?
How did (do) you think you would do it?
What would happen after you were dead?

Although many student clinicians feel uneasy about exploring thoughts of suicide, most patients can discuss their thoughts and feelings about it freely with you, sometimes with considerable relief. By such discussion, you demonstrate your interest and concern for what may well be the patient's most serious and threatening problem. By avoiding the issue, you may miss the most important feature of the patient's illness.

THOUGHT AND PERCEPTIONS

THOUGHT PROCESSES. Assess the logic, relevance, organization, and coherence of the patient's thought processes as they are revealed in words and speech throughout the interview. Does speech progress in a

Variations and Abnormalities in Thought Processes

CIRCUMSTAN-TIALITY	Speech characterized by indirection and delay in reaching the point because of unnecessary detail, although the components of the description have a meaningful connection. Many people without mental disorders are circumstantial.	Observed in persons with compulsive personality disorders
LOOSENING OF ASSOCIATIONS	Speech in which a person shifts from one subject to others that are unrelated or only obliquely related without realizing that the subjects are not meaningfully connected	Observed in schizophrenia, manic episodes, and other psychiatric disorders
FLIGHT OF IDEAS	An almost continuous flow of accelerated speech in which a person changes abruptly from topic to topic. Changes are usually based on understandable associations, plays on words or distracting stimuli, but the ideas do not progress to sensible conversation.	Most frequently noted in manic episodes, but may also be present in organic mental disorders and schizophrenia
NEOLOGISMS	Invented or distorted words, or words with new and highly idiosyncratic meanings	Observed in schizophrenia, other psychotic disorders, and aphasia
INCOHERENCE	Speech that is largely incomprehensible because of illogic, lack of meaningful connections, abrupt changes in topic, or disordered grammar or word use. Both loosening of associations and flight of ideas, when severe, may produce incoherence.	Observed in severely disturbed psychotic persons (usually schizophrenic) and also in persons with aphasia
BLOCKING	Sudden interruption of speech in mid-sentence or before completion of an idea. The person attributes this to losing the thought. Blocking occurs in normal people.	Blocking may be striking in schizophrenia.
CONFABULATION	Fabrication of facts or events in response to questions, to fill in the gaps in an impaired memory	Common in the organic amnestic syndrome
PERSEVERATION	Persistent repetition of words or ideas	Occurs in organic mental disorders, schizophrenia, and other psychotic disorders
ECHOLALIA	Repetition of the words and phrases of others	Occurs in organic mental disorders and schizophrenia
CLANGING	Speech in which a person chooses a word on the basis of sound rather than meaning, as in rhyming and punning speech. For example, "Look at my eyes and nose, wise eyes and rosy nose. Two to one, the ayes have it!"	Clanging occurs in schizophrenia and manic episodes.

logical manner toward a goal? Here you are using the patient's speech as a window into the patient's mind. Listen for patterns of speech that suggest disorders of thought processes, as outlined on the previous page.

THOUGHT CONTENT. You should ascertain most of the information relevant to thought content during the interview. Follow appropriate leads as they occur rather than using stereotyped lists of specific questions. For example, "You mentioned a few minutes ago that a neighbor was responsible for your entire illness. Can you tell me more about that?" Or, in another situation, "What do you think about at times like these?"

You may need to make more specific inquiries. If so, couch them in tactful and accepting terms. "When people are upset like this, they sometimes can't keep certain thoughts out of their minds," or ". . . things seem unreal. Have you experienced anything like this?"

In these ways find out about any of the patterns shown in the following table.

Abnormalities of Thought Content

COMPULSIONS	Repetitive acts that a person feels driven to perform in order to produce or prevent some future state of affairs, although expectation of such an effect is unrealistic	Compulsions, obsessions, phobias, and anxieties are often associated with neurotic disorders. See Table 3-4, Anxiety Disorders (p. 116).
OBSESSIONS	Recurrent, uncontrollable thoughts, images, or impulses that a person considers unacceptable and alien	
PHOBIAS	Persistent, irrational fears, accompanied by a compelling desire to avoid the stimulus	
ANXIETIES	Apprehensions, fears, tensions, or uneasiness that may be focused (phobia) or free-floating (a general sense of ill-defined dread or impending doom)	
FEELINGS OF UNREALITY	A sense that things in the environment are strange, unreal, or remote	Delusions and feelings of unreality or depersonalization are more often associated with psychotic disorders. See Table 3-5, Psychotic Disorders (p. 117).
FEELINGS OF DEPERSONALIZATION	A sense that one's self is different, changed, or unreal, or has lost identity	
DELUSIONS	False, fixed, personal beliefs that are not shared by other members of the person's culture or subculture. Examples include: • *Delusions of persecution* • *Grandiose delusions* • *Delusional jealousy* • *Delusions of reference* in which a person believes that external events, objects, or people have a particular and unusual personal significance (for example, that the radio or television might be commenting on or giving instructions to the person) • *Delusions of being controlled* by an outside force • *Somatic delusions* of having a disease, disorder, or physical defect • *Systematized delusions*, a single delusion with many elaborations or a cluster of related delusions around a single theme, all systematized into a complex network	

PERCEPTIONS. Inquire about false perceptions in a manner similar to that used for thought content. For example, "When you heard the voice speaking to you, what did it say? How did it make you feel?" Or, "After you've been drinking a lot, do you ever see things that aren't really there?" Or, "Sometimes after major surgery like this, people hear peculiar or frightening things. Have you experienced anything like that?" In these ways find out about the following abnormal perceptions.

Abnormalities of Perception	
ILLUSIONS	Misinterpretations of real external stimuli
HALLUCINATIONS	Subjective sensory perceptions in the absence of relevant external stimuli. The person may or may not recognize the experiences as false. Hallucinations may be auditory, visual, olfactory, gustatory, tactile, or somatic. (False perceptions associated with dreaming, falling asleep, and awakening are not classified as hallucinations.)

Illusions and hallucinations are usually associated with psychotic disorders such as schizophrenia and delirium. See Table 3-5, Psychotic Disorders (p. 117).

INSIGHT AND JUDGMENT. These attributes are usually best assessed during the interview.

Insight. Some of your very first questions of the patient often yield important information about insight: "What brings you to the hospital?" "What seems to be the trouble?" "What do you think is wrong?" More specifically, note whether or not the patient is aware that a particular mood, thought, or perception is abnormal or part of an illness.

Patients with psychotic disorders often lack insight into their illness. Denial of impairment may accompany some neurologic disorders.

Judgment. You can usually assess judgment by noting the patient's responses to family situations, jobs, use of money, and interpersonal conflicts. "How do you plan to get the help you'll need after leaving the hospital?" "How are you going to manage if you lose your job?" "If your husband starts to abuse you again, what will you do?" "Who will attend to your financial affairs while you are in the nursing home?"

Judgment may be poor in organic brain disease, mental retardation, and psychotic states. Judgment is affected also by intelligence, education, socioeconomic options, and cultural values.

Note whether decisions and actions are based on reality or, for example, on impulse, wish fulfillment, or disordered thought content. What values seem to underlie the patient's decisions and behavior? Allowing for cultural variations, how do these compare with mature adult standards? Because judgment is part of the maturational response, it may be variable and unpredictable during adolescence.

MEMORY AND ATTENTION

ORIENTATION. By skillful questioning you can often determine the patient's orientation in the context of the interview. For example, you can ask quite naturally for specific dates and times, the patient's address and telephone number, the names of family members, or the route taken to

Disorientation occurs especially when memory and attention are impaired, as in organic mental syndromes. See Table

the hospital. At times—when rechecking the status of a delirious patient, for example—simple, direct questions may be indicated. "Can you tell me what time it is now . . . and what day is it?" In either of these ways, determine the patient's orientation for:

- *Time* (*e.g.,* the time of day, day of the week, month, season, date and year, duration of hospitalization)
- *Place* (*e.g.,* the patient's residence, the names of the hospital, city, and state)
- *Person* (*e.g.,* the patient's own name, and the names of relatives and professional personnel)

ATTENTION. Tests of attention include:

Digit Span. Explain that you would like to test the patient's ability to concentrate, perhaps adding that people tend to have trouble with that when they are in pain, or ill, or feverish, or whatever. Recite a series of digits, starting with two at a time and speaking each number clearly at a rate of about one per second. Ask the patient to repeat the numbers back to you. If this repetition is accurate, try a series of three numbers, then four, and so on as long as the patient responds correctly. Jotting down the numbers as you say them helps to assure your own accuracy. If the patient makes a mistake, try once more with another series of the same length. Stop after a second failure in a single series.

Poor performance of digit span is characteristic of organic brain syndromes such as delirium and dementia. Performance is also limited by mental retardation and by performance anxiety.

In choosing digits you may use street numbers, zip codes, telephone numbers, and other numerical sequences that are familiar to you, but avoid consecutive numbers, easily recognized dates, and sequences that are possibly familiar to the patient.

Now, starting again with a series of two ask the patient to repeat the numbers to you backwards.

Normally, a person should be able to repeat correctly at least five to eight digits forward and four to six backwards.

Serial 7s. Instruct the patient, "Starting from a hundred, subtract 7, and keep subtracting 7. . . ." Note the effort required and the speed and accuracy of the responses. (Writing down the answers helps you keep up with the arithmetic.) Normally, a person can complete serial 7s in 1½ minutes, with fewer than four errors. If the patient cannot do serial 7s, try 3s or counting backward.

Poor performance may be secondary to organic brain syndromes such as delirium and dementia, but also occurs with mental retardation, lack of education, loss of calculating ability, anxiety, and depression.

Spelling Backward can substitute for serial 7s. Say a five-letter word, spell it, *e.g.,* W-O-R-L-D, and ask the patient to spell it backward.

REMOTE MEMORY. Inquire about birthdays, anniversaries, social security number, names of schools attended, jobs held, or past historical events such as wars relevant to the patient's past.

Remote memory may be impaired in the late stages of dementia.

RECENT MEMORY (*e.g.,* the events of the day). Ask questions with answers that you can check against other sources so that you will know whether or not the patient is confabulating (making up facts to compensate for a defective memory). These might include the day's weather, today's appointment time in the clinic, and medications or laboratory tests taken during the day. (Asking what the patient had for breakfast is a waste of time unless you can easily check the accuracy of the answer.)

Recent memory, including new learning ability, is impaired in organic brain syndromes such as dementia, delirium, and the amnestic syndrome. Impairments in attention produced by anxiety, depression, and mental retardation also impair recent memory. See Table 3-6, Organic Mental Syndromes and Disorders (p. 118).

NEW LEARNING ABILITY. Give the patient three or four words such as "83 Water Street and blue," or "table, flower, green, and hamburger." Ask the patient to repeat them so that you know that the information has been heard and registered. (This step, like digit span, tests registration and immediate recall.) Then proceed to other parts of the examination. After about 3 to 5 minutes, ask the patient to repeat the words. Note the accuracy of the response, awareness of whether or not it is correct, and any tendency to confabulate. Normally, a person should be able to remember the words.

HIGHER COGNITIVE FUNCTIONS

INFORMATION AND VOCABULARY

Information and vocabulary, when observed clinically, enable a rough estimate of a person's intelligence. Assess them during the interview. Ask a student, for example, about favorite courses, or inquire about a person's work, hobbies, reading, favorite television programs, or current events. Explore such topics first with simple questions, then with more difficult ones. Note the person's grasp of information, the complexity of the ideas expressed, and the vocabulary used.

More directly, you can ask about specific facts, such as

    The name of the president, vice president, or governor
    The names of the last four or five presidents
    The names of five large cities in the country

If considered against the patient's cultural and educational background, information and vocabulary are fairly good indicators of intelligence. They are relatively unaffected by any but the most severe psychiatric disorders and may be helpful in distinguishing mentally retarded adults (whose information and vocabulary are limited) from those with mild or moderate dementia (whose information and vocabulary are fairly well preserved).

CALCULATING ABILITY. Test the patient's ability to do arithmetical calculations, starting at the rote level with simple addition ("What is 4 + 3? . . . 8 + 7?") and multiplication ("What is 5×6? . . . 9×7?"). The task can be made more difficult by using two-digit numbers ("15 + 12" or "25 $\times$ 6") or longer, written examples.

Poor performance may be a useful sign of dementia or may accompany aphasia, but it must be assessed in terms of the patient's intelligence and education.

Alternatively, pose practical and functionally important questions, such as "If something costs 78 cents and you give the clerk one dollar, how much should you get back?"

ABSTRACT THINKING. The capacity to think abstractly can be tested in two ways.

Proverbs. Ask the patient what people mean when they use some of the following proverbs:

A stitch in time saves nine.
Don't count your chickens before they're hatched.
The proof of the pudding is in the eating.
A rolling stone gathers no moss.
The squeaking wheel gets the grease.

Note the relevance of the answers and their degree of concreteness or abstractness. For example, "You should sew a rip before it gets bigger" is concrete, while "Prompt attention to a problem prevents trouble" is abstract. Average patients should give abstract or semi-abstract responses.

Similarities. Ask the patient to tell you how the following are alike:

An orange and an apple   A church and a theater
A cat and a mouse   A piano and a violin
A child and a dwarf   Wood and coal

Note the accuracy and relevance of the answers and their degree of concreteness or abstractness. For example, "A cat and a mouse are both animals" is abstract, "They both have tails" is concrete, and "A cat chases a mouse" is not relevant.

CONSTRUCTIONAL ABILITY. The task here is to copy figures of increasing complexity onto a piece of blank unlined paper. Show each figure one at a time and ask the patient to copy it as well as possible.

Concrete responses are often given by persons with mental retardation, delirium, or dementia, but may also be simply a function of little education. Schizophrenics may respond concretely or with personal, bizarre interpretations.

The three diamonds below are rated poor, fair, and good (but not excellent).

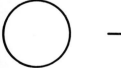 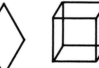 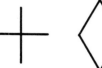 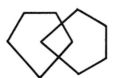 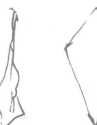 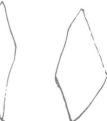

(Strub RL, Black FW: The Mental Status Examination in Neurology, 2nd ed, p 107. Philadelphia, FA Davis, 1985)

In another approach, ask the patient to draw a clock face complete with numbers and hands. The example below is rated excellent.

These three clocks are poor, fair, and good.

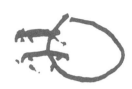

(Strub RL, Black FW: The Mental Status Examination in Neurology, 2nd ed, p 114. Philadelphia, FA Davis, 1985)

If vision and motor ability are intact, poor performance in constructional ability suggests organic brain disease such as dementia or parietal lobe damage. Mental retardation may also impair performance.

Tables 3-3 through 3-6 summarize the manifestations of selected disorders. They demonstrate how the data collected can be used diagnostically, and will help you to recognize and think about certain patterns of illness.

These tables are based, with permission, chiefly on the *Diagnostic and Statistical Manual of Mental Disorders*, Third Edition—Revised, Washington, D.C., American Psychiatric Association, 1987. For further details and criteria for these diagnoses and for other disorders, the reader should consult this manual, its successor, or comprehensive textbooks of psychiatry.

Table 3-1 Levels of Consciousness

Table 3-1 Levels of Consciousness

Consciousness varies on a continuum. Descriptions of its levels differ a bit in detail, but four levels are widely recognized: normal consciousness, drowsiness or obtundation, stupor, and coma. Delirium also frequently involves a reduced level of consciousness. Because of its additional characteristics, however, it does not fall neatly on this continuum and is classified separately (see p. 118).

NORMAL CONSCIOUSNESS	Normally conscious persons are alert, awake, and aware of both self and the environment, and respond to external stimuli.
DROWSINESS OR OBTUNDATION	Drowsy (obtunded) persons are not fully alert to their environment. Consciousness is clouded and attentiveness impaired. They think more slowly and less clearly. Spontaneous movement is diminished. Although responsive to stimuli such as questions or commands, they tend to fall asleep afterward.
STUPOR	Stuporous persons show a marked reduction in mental and physical activity. Vigorous stimuli such as pain are needed to elicit responses, and these responses are markedly reduced, slowed, inadequate, or even absent. They may, for example, consist only of mumbling, groans, or restless movements. Reflex activity is preserved.
COMA	Comatose persons are completely unconscious and cannot be aroused even by painful stimuli. There are no voluntary movements. In light coma some reflex activity is preserved, but in deep coma it is lost. For further evaluation of the comatose patient see pp. 543–547.

Specific observations about a patient's appearance, behavior, and responses to stimuli are much more valuable clinically than a single word such as "stupor." Such words, though useful in quickly summarizing an assessment, are inevitably ambiguous and preclude evaluation of slight but important changes over time. The Glasgow Coma Scale,* frequently used for hour-to-hour evaluation, helps to identify a condition as improving, stable, or deteriorating. The scale includes three kinds of activities: opening of the eyes, verbal responses, and motor responses. The three responses are rated numerically and summarized as a total score. Note that the term "coma" in this scale applies only when the total score is lower than 6.

The eyes open	Spontaneously	4
	To verbal stimuli	3
	To pain	2
	Never	1
Best verbal response	Oriented and converses	5
	Disoriented and converses	4
	Inappropriate words	3
	Incomprehensible sounds	2
	No response	1
Best motor response		
To verbal command	Obeys	6
To painful stimuli	Localizes pain	5
	Flexor withdrawal	4
	Flexion—abnormal (decorticate rigidity)**	3
	Extension (decerebrate rigidity)**	2
	No response	1
	Total score	3 to 15

* With permission, from Teasdale G, Jennett B: Assessment of coma and impaired consciousness. Lancet 2:81,1974.

** Decorticate and decerebrate rigidity are illustrated on p. 560.

Table 3-2 Disorders of Speech

Table 3-2 Disorders of Speech

Disorders of speech may be divided into three groups: (1) disorders of the voice, (2) disorders of articulation, and (3) disorders involving the production and comprehension of language. In the terms below, the prefix dys- implies a less severe impairment than the prefix a- (or an-), but these distinctions are not always made in practice. The term given first is the more commonly used.

Aphonia (dysphonia) refers to a *disorder of the volume, quality, or pitch of the voice* secondary to disease of the larynx or its nerve supply. The voice may be hoarse or reduced to a whisper. Articulation and language itself are unimpaired. Causes include laryngitis, laryngeal tumors, and a unilateral vocal cord paralysis (10th cranial nerve).

Dysarthria (anarthria) refers to *defective articulation* secondary to a motor deficit involving the lips, tongue, palate, or pharynx. Words may be nasal, slurred, or indistinct. There may be special difficulty with consonants formed by the lips (*m, b, p*), the tongue (*d, t, l*), or the pharynx (*k* and hard *g* as in got). Causes include disorders of the upper or lower motor neurons, the cerebellum, the extrapyramidal system, or the muscles.

Aphasia (dysphasia) refers to a *disorder of language* itself. The cause usually lies in the left cerebral cortex. Two of the several kinds of aphasia are compared below.

	BROCA'S APHASIA *(Expressive)*	**WERNICKE'S APHASIA** *(Receptive)*
QUALITIES OF SPONTANEOUS SPEECH	Nonfluent; slow, with few words and laborious effort. Inflection and articulation are impaired, but words are meaningful with nouns, transitive verbs, and important adjectives. Small grammatical words are often dropped.	Fluent; often rapid, voluble and effortless. Inflection and articulation are good but sentences lack meaning and words are malformed (paraphasias) or invented (neologisms). Speech may be totally incomprehensible.
COMPREHENSION	Fairly good	Impaired
REPETITION	Impaired (as in spontaneous speech)	Impaired
NAMING	Impaired, though the patient recognizes objects	Impaired
READING COMPREHENSION	Fairly good	Impaired
WRITING	Impaired	Impaired

Table 3-3   Disorders of Mood

Table 3-3   Disorders of Mood

Mood disorders are divided into two groups. For the diagnosis of a *depressive disorder,* the patient must have had one or more periods of depression but no manic or hypomanic episodes.* In a *bipolar disorder,* in contrast, the patient must have had one or more manic or hypomanic episodes, and usually has had a major depressive episode. In each case, an organic cause must be excluded. The characteristics of major depressive and manic episodes are summarized below. In addition, two other less severe but more chronic conditions —*dysthymia* and *cyclothymia*—are described briefly, and some other causes of mood disturbances are given.

Depression in an elderly patient is sometimes mistaken for dementia (p. 118) because of the person's apathy, indifference, decreased movements and speech, and lack of self-care. Attributes that help to distinguish these conditions conclude this table.

MAJOR DEPRESSIVE EPISODE

Essential features. For at least 2 wk either (1) a depressed mood most of the time (or possibly an irritable mood in children or adolescents), or (2) loss of interest or pleasure in almost all activities.

Other symptoms during this time must include at least four of the following (or three if both essential features are present):
• Significant weight gain or weight loss (not due to dieting)
• Insomnia or hypersomnia
• Psychomotor agitation or retardation
• Fatigue or loss of energy
• Feelings of worthlessness or inappropriate guilt
• Decreased ability to think or concentrate, or indecisiveness
• Recurrent thoughts of death or suicide, or a suicide attempt

In severe cases, hallucinations and delusions may occur.

MANIC EPISODE

Essential features. A distinct period of an abnormally and persistently elevated, expansive, or irritable mood, marked enough to impair work, social activities, or relationships or to require hospitalization for the protection of self or others.

Other symptoms during this time must include at least three of the following (or four if the mood is irritable):
• Inflated self-esteem or grandiosity
• Decreased need for sleep
• Increased talkativeness or pressure to keep talking
• Flight of ideas or racing thoughts
• Distractibility
• Increased goal-directed activity or psychomotor agitation
• Excessive involvement in pleasurable, high-risk activities

In severe cases, hallucinations and delusions may occur.

DYSTHYMIA

A chronic mood disturbance of at least 2 yr duration, with depression and associated symptoms most of the time. In children and adolescents, an irritable mood may be present and the minimal duration of symptoms is one year.

CYCLOTHYMIA

A chronic mood disturbance of at least 2 yr duration (1 yr for children and adolescents), with frequent periods of hypomanic and depressed moods or loss of interest and pleasure

OTHER CAUSES OF DEPRESSION

Depression may also accompany (1) an organic mood syndrome with depression, (2) dementia, (3) schizophrenia, (4) schizoaffective disorder, and (5) uncomplicated bereavement.

OTHER CAUSES OF MANIA/HYPOMANIA

An elevated mood may also accompany (1) an organic mood syndrome with mania (due to drugs such as amphetamines or corticosteroids), or (2) schizophrenia of the paranoid type.

DISTINGUISHING FEATURES OF DEPRESSION AND DEMENTIA IN THE ELDERLY

DEPRESSION	DEMENTIA
Affect constricted	Affect inappropriate, shallow, or labile
Orientation fairly good	Orientation poor
Memory for major events and political figures good	Memory for major events and political figures poor
Answers to questions are slow and reluctant, with ''I don't know'' responses, but the person, if cooperative, understands words and follows commands.	Answers to questions approximate, with possible perseveration or confabulation. The person has difficulty understanding words and following commands.
The person emphasizes failures, disabilities, and poor memory.	The person may emphasize trivial accomplishments.
Symptoms are not worse in the evening or night.	Symptoms are worse in the evening or night.

* A hypomanic episode resembles a manic episode but causes less impairment and does not necessitate hospitalization.

Table 3-4   Anxiety Disorders

Table 3-4   Anxiety Disorders

Anxiety disorders are very common. Their key features are anxious feelings and avoidance behaviors. These disorders can be clustered according to the presence of panic attacks, specific fears, obsessions or compulsions, and specific precipitating stresses. Anxiety may also be due to psychotic or organic mental disorders, but these should be classified separately.

WITH PANIC ATTACKS

PANIC DISORDER WITH OR WITHOUT AGORAPHOBIA	Unexpected and recurrent intense fear or discomfort, lasting minutes or hours, and at times associated with symptoms such as dyspnea, dizziness or faintness, palpitations or rapid heart rate, trembling, sweating, choking, nausea or abdominal distress, feelings of unreality or depersonalization, numbness or tingling, flushes or chills, chest pain, and fears of dying, doing something uncontrolled, or going crazy. The attack may be accompanied by *agoraphobia*, a fear of being in a place or situation where escape or help might not be possible.

WITH SPECIFIC FEARS

SEPARATION ANXIETY DISORDER	Excessive anxiety concerning separation from those to whom a child under 18 years is attached. The anxiety must have lasted for at least 2 wk.
AVOIDANCE DISORDER OF CHILDHOOD OR ADOLESCENCE	Excessive shrinking from contact with unfamiliar people, experienced by a child or adolescent for at least 6 mo. Relations with familiar people are warm.
SOCIAL PHOBIA	Persisting fear of being humiliated or embarrassed by acting in certain ways, *e.g.,* speaking or eating in public. The fear interferes with work, social activities, or relationships or causes marked distress.
SIMPLE PHOBIA	Persisting fear of objects (such as snakes or dogs) or of situations (such as heights or air travel). The fear interferes with work, social activities, or relationships or causes marked distress.

WITH OBSESSIONS OR COMPULSIONS

OBSESSIVE-COMPULSIVE DISORDER	Obsessions or compulsions that are markedly distressing or time-consuming or that interfere with work, social activities, or relationships

WITH PRECIPITATING STRESSORS

POSTTRAUMATIC STRESS DISORDER	Intense fears and avoidance behaviors following an extremely distressing event such as a threat to life, rape, military combat, or disaster. Reliving the event through distressing recollections, illusions, hallucinations, flashbacks, or dreams occurs and the person tries to avoid it. Decreased responsiveness to the external world and symptoms of arousal are associated.
ADJUSTMENT DISORDER WITH ANXIOUS MOOD	Nervousness, worry, and jitteriness in response to stressors. The symptoms (1) are excessive and (2) impair function in school, work, social activities, or relationships. They must start within 3 mo of the stressor and last not more than 6 mo.

WITHOUT PRECIPITATING STRESSORS

GENERALIZED ANXIETY DISORDER, *or if the person is <18 yr,* **OVERANXIOUS DISORDER**	Unrealistic or excessive anxiety that involves at least two life circumstances and that lasts for at least 6 mo. A variety of other symptoms are associated, including those of motor tension, autonomic hyperactivity, and vigilance (*e.g.,* insomnia, irritability, an exaggerated startle response, and feeling keyed up).

Table 3-5   Psychotic Disorders

Table 3-5   Psychotic Disorders

Psychotic symptoms indicate gross impairment in reality testing. They include delusions, hallucinations, incoherence, a marked loosening of associations, and bizarre or grossly disorganized behaviors. Specific diagnosis depends on the nature and the duration of the symptoms.

SCHIZOPHRENIA	Manifestations during the *active stage* of schizophrenia include disordered thought processes, delusions that are often bizarre, hallucinations, a flat or inappropriate affect, a disturbed sense of self, bizarre psychomotor behavior, and impaired personal and social function. Impaired function often develops in a *prodromal phase* and persists in a later *residual phase*. Six mo of symptoms or impairment are required for this diagnosis.
SCHIZOPHRENIFORM DISORDER	Manifestations of a schizophreniform disorder resemble those of schizophrenia but last less than 6 mo.
BRIEF REACTIVE PSYCHOSIS	Psychotic symptoms in a brief reactive psychosis last from a few hours to one month and are associated with emotional turmoil. They appear after a markedly stressful event, and the person eventually returns to his or her previous level of function.
MOOD DISORDERS WITH PSYCHOTIC FEATURES	Both depressive and bipolar disorders may be associated with delusions and hallucinations. To diagnose a mood disorder with psychotic features, the delusions and hallucinations must not be present without the mood symptoms.
SCHIZOAFFECTIVE DISORDER	A schizoaffective disorder has features of both schizophrenia and a mood disturbance. To make this diagnosis, the delusions or hallucinations should be present for at least 2 wk without prominent mood symptoms.
DELUSIONAL DISORDER *(Paranoid)*	A delusional (paranoid) disorder is characterized by a persistent delusion that is not bizarre. Instead, it involves real life situations, such as having a disease or infection or being deceived by a spouse or lover. Hallucinations, if present, are not prominent. The person usually functions well at work and behaves quite normally unless the delusional ideas are being discussed or acted upon. Social and marital relations are often disturbed.
ORGANIC MENTAL SYNDROMES AND DISORDERS	Always consider the possibility that there is an organic cause of psychotic symptoms. See Table 3-6, Organic Mental Syndromes and Disorders.

Table 3-6   Organic Mental Syndromes and Disorders

Table 3-6   Organic Mental Syndromes and Disorders

Organic mental syndromes and disorders are identified by their psychological and behavioral characteristics and by demonstrating (or at times inferring) an organic cause.

GLOBAL IMPAIRMENTS

DELIRIUM   The two key features of delirium involve attention and thought. The patient's ability to pay appropriate attention to external stimuli and to shift attention to new external stimuli is reduced. Thought is disorganized: rambling, irrelevant, or incoherent.

In addition, at least two of the following should also be present for this diagnosis: (1) a reduced level of consciousness, (2) disturbed perceptions (*e.g.*, illusions and hallucinations), (3) sleep disturbances (insomnia or daytime sleepiness), (4) increased or decreased psychomotor activity, (5) disorientation, and (6) impaired memory.

Delirium typically develops over hours or days, and the symptoms fluctuate during the day. Causes are multiple, including drug intoxication, systemic infection, metabolic disorders, and postoperative states.

DEMENTIA   The key feature of dementia is an impaired memory. Recent memory usually decreases first, then remote memory. Other symptoms develop, at least one of which is needed for the diagnosis: (1) impairment in abstracting ability, (2) impaired judgment, (3) other disturbances of cortical functions such as those that involve language, recognition of objects, or constructional ability, and (4) a change in personality.

Causes are multiple. *Primary degenerative dementia of the Alzheimer type*—the most common form—is a diagnosis reached by excluding other causes. It typically has an insidious onset and a progressive course. A *multi-infarct dementia*, due to cerebrovascular disease, usually has an abrupt onset and a stepwise course.

SELECTIVE IMPAIRMENTS

AMNESTIC SYNDROME   The key feature of the amnestic syndrome is an impaired recent and remote memory. The patient is usually disoriented and may confabulate, but the more global deficits of delirium and dementia are not present. Of the several causes, the most common is thiamine deficiency associated with the chronic use of alcohol.

ORGANIC HALLUCINOSIS   The key feature of organic hallucinosis is prominent and persistent or recurrent hallucinations. Some patients recognize that these originate in their minds; others are delusionally convinced of their reality. This delusion, if present, is limited to the hallucinations. Causes include hallucinogens, the chronic use of alcohol, sensory deprivation, and seizures.

ORGANIC SYNDROMES THAT MAY MIMIC OTHER MENTAL DISORDERS

ORGANIC DELUSIONAL SYNDROME   The key feature of this syndrome is prominent delusions. Hallucinations, if present, are not prominent. The symptoms may suggest schizophrenia. Causes include amphetamines, cannabis, hallucinogens, and certain brain diseases.

ORGANIC MOOD SYNDROME   The key feature of an organic mood syndrome is a prominent and persistently depressed, elevated, or expansive mood. The mood and associated symptoms may suggest a major depressive or manic episode. Causes of an organic depressive syndrome include reserpine, methyldopa, viral illness, and strokes. Thyroid and adrenal dysfunction can cause either a depressive or a manic syndrome.

ORGANIC ANXIETY SYNDROME   The key feature of an organic anxiety syndrome is either prominent and recurrent panic attacks or generalized anxiety. For this diagnosis, the impaired attention of delirium should not be associated. Causes include endocrine disorders (*e.g.*, fasting hypoglycemia, hypercortisolism), intoxication (as from caffeine, amphetamines, cocaine), and withdrawal from alcohol or sedatives.

PERSONALITY DISTURBANCE

ORGANIC PERSONALITY SYNDROME   The key feature of this syndrome is a persistent personality disturbance (life-long, accentuated, or recent) that involves at least one of the following: (1) affective instability, (2) recurrent outbursts of aggression or rage, (3) markedly impaired social judgment, (4) marked apathy and indifference, (5) suspiciousness or paranoid ideation. Delirium and dementia must be excluded. The usual cause is structural brain damage, as from a tumor, trauma, or cerebrovascular disease.

Chapter 4
Physical Examination: Approach and Overview

GENERAL APPROACH

Most patients view a physical examination with at least some anxiety. They feel vulnerable, physically exposed, apprehensive about possible pain, and uneasy over what the clinician may find. At the same time, they often appreciate detailed concern for their problems and may even enjoy the attention they receive.

Mindful of such feelings, the skillful clinician is thorough without wasting time, systematic without being rigid, gentle yet not afraid to cause discomfort if this should be required. By listening, looking, touch, or smell, the skillful clinician examines each body part and at the same time senses the whole patient, notes the wince or worried glance, and calms, explains, and reassures.

Early in their experience students, like patients, are apprehensive. They feel uneasy in their ambiguous roles as student-professionals and uncertain of their newfledged competencies. Touching intimate areas of a patient's body and making a patient uncomfortable typically cause special concern. Anxieties are unavoidable.

Over time, however, competence and self-confidence grow. Through study and repetitive practice, the flow of the examination becomes smooth, and you can gradually shift your attention from where to place your hands or instruments to what you hear, see, and feel. At the same time you become accustomed to the physical contact, skilled in minimizing discomfort, and more conscious of the patient's reactions than of your own feelings. Before long, you will be able to accomplish in 5 to 10 minutes what first took an hour or two. Continuing progress should be a lifetime goal.

Despite inevitable insecurities as you begin to examine patients, you should take command of your own demeanor and affect. Try to look calm, organized, and competent, even when you do not exactly feel that way. If you forget a portion of your examination, as you undoubtedly will, you do not need to get flustered. Simply do that part out of sequence—smoothly. If you have already left the patient, return and ask if you can check one more thing. Avoid expressions of disgust, alarm, distaste, or other negative reactions. They have no place at the bedside, even when you come upon an ominous mass, a deep and smelly ulcer, or even a pubic louse.

As in the interview, be sensitive to the patient's feelings. The patient's facial expression or an apparently casual question such as "Is it okay?" may give you clues to previously unexpressed worries. Ascertain them when you can. Pay attention to the patient's physical comfort as well. Adjust the slant of the bed or examining table according to the patient's needs insofar as possible, and use pillows for comfort or blankets for warmth as necessary. Assure as much privacy as possible by using drapes appropriately and closing doors.

As an examiner you too should be comfortable, because awkward positions may impair your perceptions. Adjust the bed to a convenient height, and ask the patient to move toward you if this will help you reach a body part more comfortably.

Good lighting and a quiet environment contribute importantly to what you can see and hear but may be remarkably hard to find in a hospital. Do the best you can. If a nearby patient's television is interfering with your ability to hear the sounds in your patient's chest, politely ask the neighbor to lower the volume. Most people cooperate readily. Remember to thank them when you are through.

As you proceed with your examination, keep the patient informed as to what you intend to do, especially when you anticipate possible embarrassment or discomfort. Patients vary considerably in their knowledge of examination procedures and hence in their need for information. Some people want to know what you are doing when you listen to the lungs or feel for a liver, while others already know or do not care. By words or gestures, be as clear as possible in your instructions. When telling patients what to do, be courteous rather than authoritarian. "I would like to examine your heart now. Would you please lie down" carries a different and better message than "I'm going to examine your heart now. Lie down on the table." Authority stems from competence and personal relationship, not from command.

Clinicians differ in how and when they report their findings to their patients. Beginning students should avoid almost all such interpretive statements because they do not yet carry the primary responsibility for the patient and may give conflicting or erroneous information. As experience and responsibility increase, however, sharing findings with the patient becomes appropriate. If you know or suspect that the patient has specific concerns, it may be helpful to make a reassuring comment as you finish examining the relevant area. A steady series of reassuring comments, however, presents at least one potential problem: what to say when you find an unexpected abnormality. You may wish you had maintained judicious silence earlier.

All students, however, should develop one habit with which they can reassure their patients and avoid unnecessary alarm. As a beginner, you may spend much more time with some procedures, such as the ophthalmoscopic examination or cardiac auscultation, than does the experienced clinician. Whenever you realize you are doing this, pause and explain. "I would like to spend a long time examining your heart because I want to listen to each of the heart sounds carefully. It does not mean that I hear anything wrong." Be forthright with the patient about your status as a student. Such openness will clarify your relationship and probably reduce anxieties on both sides.

How Complete Should an Examination Be? No simple answer can be given to this common question. The outline below summarizes a fairly comprehensive examination suitable for an adult patient who is ill or has several complaints or who wants a thorough checkup. It also summarizes a clinician's basic repertory of examining skills.

For patients who have symptoms restricted to a specific body system or region, a more limited examination may be more appropriate. Here, as in the history, you select the relevant methods to assess the problem as precisely and efficiently as possible. The patient's symptoms and demographic characteristics such as age and sex all influence this selection and help you decide what to do. So does your knowledge of disease patterns. Out of all the patients you might see with a sore throat, for example, you will need to decide who has a common cold and does not need a careful examination of the abdomen and, in contrast, whose liver and spleen you should try to feel because of the likelihood of infectious mononucleosis. The clinical thinking that underlies and guides such decisions is discussed in Chapter 20.

The utility of a comprehensive "periodic physical examination" to detect and prevent disease in asymptomatic men and women has been challenged in recent years. Techniques that in randomized trials have been shown clearly to reduce the subsequent morbidity and mortality in such people are few indeed: assessment of blood pressure and palpation of a woman's breasts. Additional techniques, supported by nonrandomized trials, include listening to the heart for evidence of valvular disease and a pelvic examination with Papanicolaou smears. The list of recommended examinations can be expanded somewhat further on the basis of expert opinion and clinical experience, but it is not a lengthy list.

A thorough examination, however, does more than prevent sickness and prolong the lives of apparently healthy men and women. Most people who seek health care have health-related worries or symptoms. The physical examination may help both to identify such concerns and to explain the symptoms. It gives information with which to answer the patient's questions, offers opportunities for health education, provides baseline data for future use, and increases both the credibility and the conviction of the clinician's advice or reassurance. The physical contact involved often enhances the clinician–patient relationship. Furthermore, students must repeatedly perform such examinations in order to gain proficiency, and clinicians must do them periodically in order to maintain their skills. How best to divide one's usually limited time with a patient between listening, discussion, or counseling on the one hand and the physical examination on the other may be a complicated judgment.

Sequence. The sequence of the comprehensive examination is designed to minimize the patient's movements and maximize the examiner's efficiency. Variations in order are possible, of course, and you may wish to develop a method of your own. If so, avoid distasteful or unhygienic sequences such as moving from a patient's feet, genitalia, or rectum to the face or mouth or from rectum to vagina.

The Examiner's Position and Handedness. This book recommends examining a supine patient from the patient's right side, moving to the foot of the bed or to the other side as necessary. Accustoming yourself to working chiefly from one side helps you to master the skills more quickly and promotes the efficiency of your examination, although it admittedly may limit the ease with which you can adapt to unusual circumstances.

The right side has several advantages over the left: the jugular veins on the right are more reliable for estimating venous pressure, the palpating hand rests more comfortably on the apical impulse, the right kidney is more frequently palpable than the left, and examining tables are sometimes placed against one wall to favor this right-handed approach.

Left-handed students will understandably find this position awkward at first but are encouraged to practice it. Unless they are reasonably ambidextrous, however, most will find it easier to use the left hand while percussing or while holding instruments such as an otoscope or a reflex hammer.

OVERVIEW OF A COMPREHENSIVE EXAMINATION

You may wish to skim the following outline now to get an overview of the physical examination. Subsequent chapters deal with individual body regions or systems, each considered in isolation. After you have completed the study and practice involved in one or more chapters, reread this overview to see how each component of the examination fits into an integrated whole.

GENERAL SURVEY. Observe the general state of health, stature and habitus, and sexual development. Weigh the patient, if possible. Note posture, motor activity, and gait; dress, grooming, and personal hygiene; and any odors of body or breath. Watch the patient's facial expressions and note manner, affect, and reactions to the persons and things in the environment. Listen to the patient's speech and note state of awareness or level of consciousness.

The survey continues throughout the history and examination.

VITAL SIGNS. Count the pulse and respiratory rate. Measure the blood pressure and, if indicated, the body temperature.

SKIN. Observe the skin and its characteristics. Identify any lesions, noting their location, distribution, arrangement, type, and color. Inspect and palpate the hair and nails. Study the patient's hands.

The patient is sitting on the edge of the bed or examining table, unless this position is contraindicated. You should be standing in front of the patient, moving to either side as you need to.

Begin your assessment of the skin with the exposed areas—the hands, forearms, and face. Continue it as you examine other body regions such as the thorax, abdomen, genitalia, and limbs.

HEAD. Examine the hair, scalp, skull, and face.

EYES. Check visual acuity and, if indicated, the visual fields. Note the position and alignment of the eyes. Observe the eyelids and inspect the sclera and conjunctiva of each eye. With oblique lighting, inspect each cornea, iris, and lens. Compare the pupils and test their reactions to light. Assess the extraocular movements. With an ophthalmoscope, inspect the ocular fundi.

The room should be darkened for the ophthalmoscopic examination.

EARS. Inspect the auricles, canals, and drums. Check auditory acuity. If acuity is diminished, check lateralization (Weber test) and compare air and bone conduction (Rinne test).

NOSE AND SINUSES. Examine the external nose, and with aid of a light and speculum inspect the nasal mucosa, septum, and turbinates. Palpate for tenderness of the frontal and maxillary sinuses.

MOUTH AND PHARYNX. Inspect the lips, buccal mucosa, gums, teeth, roof of the mouth, tongue, and pharynx.

NECK. Inspect and palpate the cervical lymph nodes. Note any masses or unusual pulsations in the neck. Feel for any deviation of the trachea. Observe the sound and effort of the patient's breathing. Inspect and palpate the thyroid gland.

BACK. Inspect and palpate the spine and muscles of the back. Check for costovertebral angle tenderness.

Move behind the sitting patient to feel the thyroid gland and to examine the back, posterior thorax, and lungs.

POSTERIOR THORAX AND LUNGS. Inspect, palpate, and percuss the chest. Identify the level of diaphragmatic dullness on each side. Listen to the breath sounds, identify any adventitious sounds, and, if indicated, listen to the transmitted voice sounds.

BREASTS, AXILLAE, AND EPITROCHLEAR NODES. In a woman, inspect the breasts with her arms relaxed and then elevated, and then with her hands pressed on her hips. In either sex, inspect the axillae and feel for the axillary nodes. Feel for the epitrochlear nodes.

Move to the front again.

By this time you have examined the patient's hands, surveyed the back, and, at least in women, made a fair estimate of the range of motion at the shoulders. Your examination of the anterior thorax will include inspection of additional musculoskeletal structures. Use these observations, together with the patient's history and ease of movement throughout the examination, in deciding whether or not to continue with a full musculoskeletal examination.

If you need to do a more complete musculoskeletal examination, it is convenient to examine the hands, arms, shoulders, neck, and jaw while the patient is still in the sitting position. Inspect and palpate the joints and check their range of motion.

BREASTS. Palpate the breasts, while at the same time continuing your inspection.

Ask the patient to lie down. You should stand at the right side of the patient's bed.

ANTERIOR THORAX AND LUNGS. Inspect, palpate, and percuss the chest. Listen to the breath sounds, any adventitious sounds, and, if indicated, transmitted voice sounds.

CARDIOVASCULAR SYSTEM. Inspect and palpate the carotid pulsations. Listen for carotid bruits. Observe the jugular venous pulsations, and measure the jugular venous pressure in relation to the sternal angle.

Inspect and palpate the precordium. Note the location, diameter, amplitude, and duration of the apical impulse. Listen at the apex and the lower sternal border with the bell of a stethoscope. Listen at each auscultatory area with the diaphragm. Listen for physiologic splitting of the second heart sound and for any abnormal heart sounds or murmurs.

Elevate the head of the bed to about 30° for the cardiovascular examination, adjusting it as necessary to see the jugular venous pulsations. The patient should roll partly onto the left side while you listen at the apex. Then have the patient lie back while you listen to the rest of the heart. The patient should sit, leaning forward, and exhale while you listen for the murmur of aortic regurgitation.

ABDOMEN. Inspect, auscultate, and percuss the abdomen. Palpate lightly, then deeply. Try to feel the liver, spleen, kidneys, and aorta.

Lower the head of the bed to the flat position. The patient should be supine.

RECTAL EXAMINATION IN MEN. Inspect the sacrococcygeal and perianal areas. Palpate the anal canal, rectum, and prostate. If the patient cannot stand, examine the genitalia before doing the rectal examination.

The patient is lying on his left side for the rectal examination.

GENITALIA AND RECTAL EXAMINATION IN WOMEN. Examine the external genitalia, vagina, and cervix. Obtain Pap smears. Palpate the uterus and the adnexa. Do a rectovaginal and rectal examination.

The patient is supine in the lithotomy position. You should be seated at first, then standing at the foot of the examining table.

LEGS. Inspect the legs, assessing the

The patient is supine.

Peripheral Vascular System. Note any swelling, discoloration, or ulcers. Palpate for pitting edema. Feel the dorsalis pedis, posterior tibial, and femoral pulses, and, if indicated, the popliteal pulses. Palpate the inguinal lymph nodes.

Musculoskeletal System. Note any deformities or enlarged joints. If indicated, palpate the joints and check their range of motion.

Neurologic System. Observe the muscle bulk, the position of the limbs, and any abnormal movements.

MUSCULOSKELETAL SYSTEM. Examine the alignment of the spine and its range of motion, the alignment of the legs, and the feet.

The patient is standing. You should sit on a chair or stool.

PERIPHERAL VASCULAR SYSTEM. Inspect for varicose veins.

GENITALIA AND HERNIAS IN MEN. Examine the penis and scrotal contents and check for hernias.

SCREENING NEUROLOGIC EXAMINATION. Observe the patient's gait and ability to walk heel-to-toe, walk on the toes, walk on the heels, hop in place, and do shallow knee bends. Check for a pronator drift and do a Romberg test. Assess the strength of the grip and of the vertically raised arms. Look for winging as the arms are lowered.

Check the deep tendon reflexes and plantar responses.

The patient is sitting or supine.

Assess sensory function by testing pain and vibration in the hands and feet, light touch on the limbs, and stereognosis in the hands.

ADDITIONAL NEUROLOGIC EXAMINATION. If indicated, go on to a more thorough examination, including:

Cranial Nerves not already examined: sense of smell, strength of the temporal and masseter muscles, corneal reflexes, facial movements, gag reflex, and strength of the trapezii and sternomastoid muscles.

Motor. Muscle tone, strength, and coordination

Abdominal Reflexes

Sensory. Pain, temperature, light touch, position, vibration, and discrimination

MENTAL STATUS. If indicated and not done during the interview, assess the patient's mood, thought processes, thought content, abnormal perceptions, insight and judgment, memory and attention, information and vocabulary, calculating abilities, abstract thinking, and constructional ability.

When you have completed your examination, tell the patient what to do and what to expect next. If you are examining a hospitalized patient, rearrange the immediate environment to suit the patient. If you initially found the bed rails up, put them back in this position unless you are sure that they are not necessary. Lower the bed so that the patient can get in and out easily without risking falls. When you have finished, wash your hands and clean your equipment or dispose of it properly.

Examining the Supine Patient. Under certain circumstances, the sequence of the examination must differ from the one described. Some patients, for example, are unable to sit up in bed or stand. You can examine the head, neck, and anterior chest of such persons as they lie supine. Then roll the patient onto each side to listen to the lungs, examine the back, and inspect the skin. The remainder of the examination is completed with the patient supine.

Tangential Lighting. Tangential lighting is recommended for the inspection of several structures such as the jugular venous pulse, the thyroid gland, and the apical impulse of the heart. This is a method of casting light along the edge of a surface in order to create shadows. As shown on the left below, these shadows help to reveal any elevations or indentations—moving or stationary—on that surface.

The patient is supine.

The patient is sitting or supine.

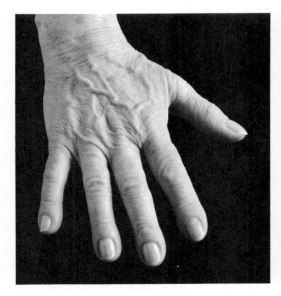

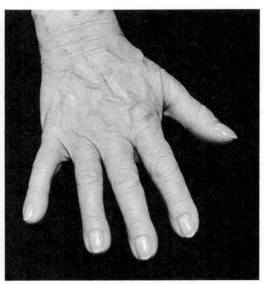

TANGENTIAL LIGHTING   **PERPENDICULAR LIGHTING**

When light is perpendicular to the surface or diffuse, as shown on the right above, shadows are reduced and subtle undulations in the surface are lost. Experiment with focused, tangential lighting across the tendons and veins on the back of your hand, and try to see the pulsations of the radial artery at your wrist.

Chapter 5
The General Survey

Anatomy and Physiology

Most of the specific anatomy and physiology relevant to the general survey may be found in later chapters. This section deals briefly with the more general topics of body height, weight, and habitus, and introduces the concept of sexual maturity ratings.

In all these attributes, people vary importantly according to the region of the world in which they live, socioeconomic status, nutrition, genetic makeup, early illnesses, gender, and the era in which they were born. The apparent shortening of aging Americans, for example, is partly illusory. Although people do shrink with age, their heights also vary according to the year of their birth. Young adults today on the average have grown taller than their parents, and the parents taller than the grandparents. This section cannot deal with all the variations of "normal" resulting from these many factors, but the clinician should be extremely cautious in applying the norms of one group to a person of another.

HEIGHT, GROWTH, AND HABITUS. Persons grow in height from birth to late adolescence. When the annual gain in height is measured and charted, one can readily discern an *adolescent growth spurt*, which in girls peaks relatively early in puberty, approximately at the age of 12, and in boys relatively late, approximately at the age of 14. Musculoskeletal proportions change during this growth spurt, with variations in degree and timing according to gender. A boy's shoulders, for example, broaden more than a girl's, while a girl's hips widen more than a boy's. These changes are summarized in the illustration on the next page.

Toward the other end of the lifespan, other changes occur. People decrease in height, and posture may become somewhat stooped as the thoracic spine becomes more convex and the knees and hips fail to extend fully. Fat tends to concentrate near the hips and lower abdomen and, together with weakening of the abdominal muscles, often produces a potbelly. The figure on page 131 illustrates some of the changes occurring in persons ranging in age from 78 to 94. These and other changes with age are further detailed in subsequent chapters.

SEXUAL MATURITY RATINGS. Changes in an adolescent's reproductive organs and secondary sex characteristics are closely related to the growth

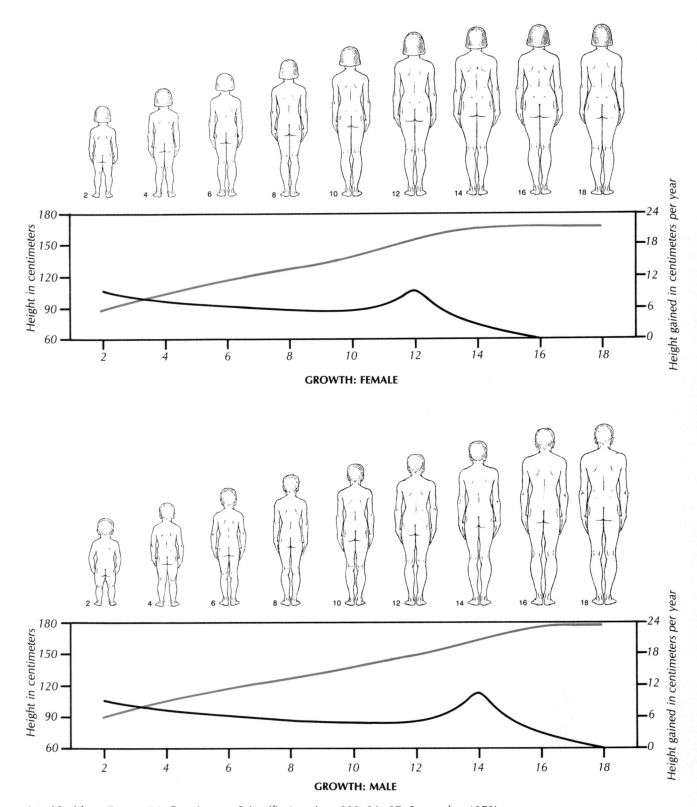

(Modified from Tanner JM: Growing up. Scientific American 229: 36–37, September 1973)

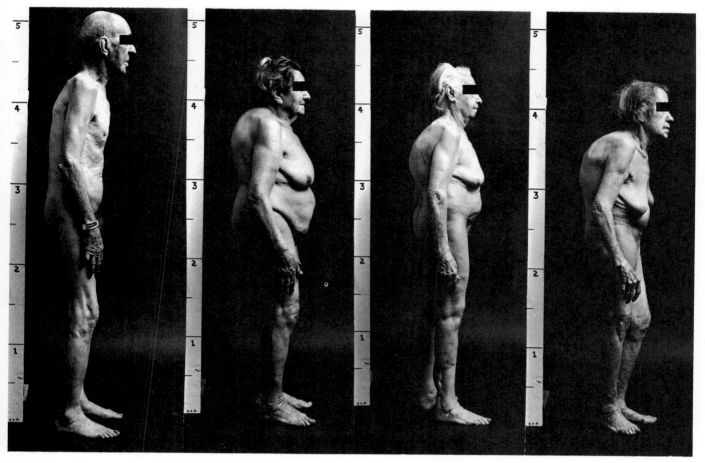

A man, age 82, and three women, ages 78, 79, and 94, respectively. (Rossman I: Clinical Geriatrics, 3rd ed, p 4. Philadelphia, JB Lippincott, 1986)

spurt. Later chapters describe sexual maturity ratings by which the clinician can assess sexual development: in breasts and pubic hair of girls and in genitalia and pubic hair of boys. The interrelationships between these sexual characteristics and the adolescent growth spurt give the clinician a biological yardstick with which to assess an adolescent's growth and development and to identify significant deviations from normal patterns. They also help the clinician to interpret for the adolescent whether growth and sexual maturation are proceeding normally and to predict what further changes may be expected.

During your initial survey of the adolescent patient, you measure only one of these variables—height. You may also make a few preliminary observations of breast and muscular development, pitch of voice, and facial hair. The full meaning of these observations, however, does not emerge until you correlate them with other data: the patient's body habitus, growth pattern over time, muscular development, sexual maturity ratings, and psychosexual feelings, attitudes, and knowledge. During the assessment process, you will bring these interrelated variables together and try to understand the patient's development and any related problems as well as you can.

WEIGHT. Definitions of appropriate weights for adults remain controversial. They are influenced by aesthetic preferences, cultural attitudes, and medical specialty, among other factors, and there are scientific arguments over the interpretation and applicability of available data. The 1983 Metropolitan figures for height and weight, shown in Table 5-1, are based on actuarial data from 25 insurance companies in the United States and Canada. The weights listed are associated with the lowest mortality rates for men and women between the ages of 25 and 59, during the years from 1954 to 1972.

Table 5-1   Height/Weight Table for Adults
(Weight in Pounds Without Clothes)

HEIGHT WITHOUT SHOES		MEN AGED 25–59 YEARS			WOMEN AGED 25–59 YEARS		
FEET	INCHES	SMALL FRAME	MEDIUM FRAME	LARGE FRAME	SMALL FRAME	MEDIUM FRAME	LARGE FRAME
4	9				99–108	106–118	115–128
4	10				100–110	108–120	117–131
4	11				101–112	110–123	119–134
5	0				103–115	112–126	122–137
5	1	123–129	126–136	133–145	105–118	115–129	125–140
5	2	125–131	128–138	135–148	108–121	118–132	128–144
5	3	127–133	130–140	137–151	111–124	121–135	131–148
5	4	129–135	132–143	139–155	114–127	124–138	134–152
5	5	131–137	134–146	141–159	117–130	127–141	137–156
5	6	133–140	137–149	144–163	120–133	130–144	140–160
5	7	135–143	140–152	147–167	123–136	133–147	143–164
5	8	137–146	143–155	150–171	126–139	136–150	146–167
5	9	139–149	146–158	153–175	129–142	139–153	149–170
5	10	141–152	149–161	156–179	132–145	142–156	152–173
5	11	144–155	152–165	159–183			
6	0	147–159	155–169	163–187			
6	1	150–163	159–173	167–192			
6	2	153–167	162–177	171–197			
6	3	157–171	166–182	176–202			

(Derived from 1983 Metropolitan Height and Weight Tables: Stat Bull Metrop Life Found 64, No. 1:6–7, 1983)

Body frame, as used in Table 5-1, is determined by *elbow breadth*: the distance between the medial and lateral epicondyles of the elbow (see p. 462), with the forearm flexed to 90° and held in front of the body. The figures in Table 5-2 show elbow breadths (preferably measured with calipers) calculated for persons of medium frame in five different height groups. Elbow breadths that are greater or smaller than the given ranges for a specific height indicate large and small frames respectively.

Table 5-2   Medium Body Frame by Height and Elbow Breadth

MEN		WOMEN	
HEIGHT WITHOUT SHOES (in Feet & Inches)	ELBOW BREADTH (in Inches)	HEIGHT WITHOUT SHOES (in Feet & Inches)	ELBOW BREADTH (in Inches)
5'1"–5'2"	2½"–2⅞"	4'9"–4'10"	2¼"–2½"
5'3"–5'6"	2⅝"–2⅞"	4'11"–5'2"	2¼"–2½"
5'7"–5'10"	2¾"–3"	5'3"–5'6"	2⅜"–2⅝"
5'11"–6'2"	2¾"–3⅛"	5'7"–5'10"	2⅜"–2⅝"
6'3"	2⅞"–3¼"	5'11"	2½"–2¾"

(Derived from 1983 Metropolitan Height and Weight Tables: Stat Bull Metrop Life Found 64, No. 1:5, 1983)

Techniques of Examination

Begin your observations from the first moment you see the patient. Does the patient hear you when called in the waiting room? rise with ease? walk easily or stiffly? If hospitalized when you first meet, what is the patient doing: sitting up and enjoying television? or lying in bed? What occupies the bedside table: a magazine? a flock of "get well" cards? a Bible or rosary? an emesis basin? or nothing at all? Each of these observations should raise one or more tentative hypotheses and guide your further assessments. Continue your observation throughout the interview and examination.

Speech and all the attributes of appearance and behavior that were described in Chapter 3, Mental Status, are relevant to this general survey. Level of consciousness, manner, affect, and relationship to persons and things, though not discussed again in this chapter, should also be kept in mind. Speech, posture, motor activity, dress, grooming, and personal hygiene are included but with different kinds of examples from those used in Chapter 3.

APPARENT STATE OF HEALTH. This judgment is an evaluative summary that should be supported by specific observations. Try to define the attributes that substantiate your conclusions. Thinness and weakness in an octogenarian with a tottering gait and a quavery voice suggest frailty, for example, while an ashen, sweaty face suggests an acute illness such as shock.

Acutely or chronically ill, frail, feeble; robust, vigorous

SIGNS OF DISTRESS. For example,

- Cardiorespiratory distress

  Labored breathing, wheezing, cough

- Pain

  Wincing, sweating, protectiveness of a painful part

- Anxiety

  Anxious face, fidgety movements, cold moist palms

SKIN COLOR AND POSSIBLE LESIONS. See Chapter 6 for further details.

Pallor, cyanosis, jaundice, changes in pigmentation

STATURE AND HABITUS. If possible, measure the patient's height in stocking feet. Is the patient unusually short or tall? Is the build slender and lanky, muscular, or stocky? Is the body symmetrical? Note the general bodily proportions and look for any deformities.

Very short stature in Turner's syndrome and in achondroplastic, renal, and hypopituitary dwarfism; long limbs in proportion to the trunk in hypogonadism and Marfan's syndrome

SEXUAL DEVELOPMENT. Are the voice, facial hair, and breast size appropriate to the patient's age and gender?

Delayed or precocious puberty, hypogonadism, virilism

WEIGHT. Is the patient emaciated, slender, plump, obese, or somewhere in between? If obese, is the fat distributed rather evenly or does it concentrate in the trunk?

Generalized fat in simple obesity; truncal fat with relatively thin limbs in Cushing's syndrome

If possible, weigh the patient. Weight provides one index of caloric sufficiency, and changes over time give other valuable diagnostic data. Remember that weight may rise or fall with changes in body fluids as well as in fat or muscle.

Causes of weight loss include malignancy, diabetes mellitus, hyperthyroidism, chronic infection, depression, diuresis, and successful dieting.

POSTURE, GAIT, AND MOTOR ACTIVITY. What is the patient's preferred posture?

Preference for sitting up in left-sided heart failure, and for leaning forward with arms braced in chronic obstructive pulmonary disease

Is the patient restless or quiet? How often does the patient move about? How fast are the movements?

Fast, frequent movements of hyperthyroidism; slowed activity of myxedema

Are there apparently involuntary motor activities, or are some bodily parts immobile? What parts are involved?

Tremors or other involuntary movements; paralyses. See Table 18-4, Involuntary Movements (pp. 554–556).

Does the patient walk easily, with comfort, self-confidence, and good balance, or is there a limp, discomfort on walking, fear of falling, loss of balance, or abnormality in motor pattern?

See Table 18-3, Abnormalities of Gait and Posture (pp. 552–553).

DRESS, GROOMING, AND PERSONAL HYGIENE. How is the patient dressed? Is clothing appropriate to the temperature and weather? Is it clean, properly buttoned, and zipped? How does it compare with clothing worn by people of comparable age and social group?

Dress may reflect the cold intolerance of hypothyroidism, the hiding of a skin rash or needle marks, or personal preferences in lifestyle.

Glance at the patient's shoes. Have holes been cut in them? Are the laces tied? Or is the patient wearing slippers?

Cut-out holes or slippers may indicate gout, bunions, or other painful foot conditions. Untied laces or slippers also suggest edema.

Is the patient wearing any unusual jewelry?

Copper bracelets are sometimes worn for arthritis.

Note the patient's hair and fingernails, together with any use of cosmetics.

Nail polish and hair coloring that have "grown out" suggest loss of interest in personal appearance and may even help you estimate its duration.

Do personal hygiene and grooming seem appropriate to the patient's age, lifestyle, occupation, and socioeconomic group? There are, of course, wide variations in norms.

Unkempt appearance may be seen in depression and chronic organic brain disease, but this appearance must be compared with the patient's probable norm.

ODORS OF BODY OR BREATH. Although odors may give important diagnostic clues, avoid one common mistake: never assume that alcohol on a patient's breath explains neurologic or mental status findings. Alcoholics may have other serious and potentially correctable problems such as hypoglycemia or a subdural hematoma, and an alcoholic breath does not necessarily mean alcoholism.

Breath odors of alcohol, acetone (diabetes), pulmonary infections, uremia, or liver failure

FACIAL EXPRESSION. Observe facial expression at rest, during conversation about specific topics, during the physical examination, and in interaction with others.

The stare of hyperthyroidism; the immobile face of parkinsonism

SPEECH. Listen for the pace of speech and its pitch, clarity, and spontaneity.

Fast speech of hyperthyroidism; slow, thick, hoarse voice of myxedema

VITAL SIGNS. Note the pulse, blood pressure, respiratory rate, and temperature. You may choose to make these measurements at the beginning of the examination or to integrate them with your cardiovascular and thoracic assessments. If you do them now, count the radial pulse. Then, with your fingers still on the patient's wrist, count the respiratory rate without the patient's realizing it. (Breathing may change when a person becomes conscious that someone is watching.) Check the blood pressure; if it is high, repeat your measurement later in the examination.

See Table 9-15, Abnormalities of the Arterial Pulse (p. 308). See Table 8-1, Abnormalities in Rate and Rhythm of Breathing (p. 256).

Although measurement of temperature may be omitted in many ambulatory visits, take it if symptoms or signs suggest a possible abnormality. Oral thermometers are more convenient and more acceptable to patients than rectal ones, but oral glass thermometers should not be used when patients are unconscious, restless, or unable to close their mouths.

Hyperpyrexia refers to extreme elevation in body temperature, above 41.1° C (106° F). *Fever* or *pyrexia* refers to an elevated temperature, while *hypothermia* refers to an abnormally low temperature, below 35° C (95° F) rectally.

To take an *oral temperature* with a glass thermometer, shake the thermometer down to below 35.5° C (96° F), insert it under the tongue, instruct the patient to close both lips, and wait 3 to 5 minutes. Then read the thermometer, reinsert it for a minute, and read it again. If the temperature is still rising, repeat this procedure until the reading remains stable.

Causes of fever include infections, trauma (such as surgery or crushing injury), malignancies, infarctions, blood disorders (such as acute hemolytic anemia), and immune disorders (such as drug fevers and collagen diseases).

To take a *rectal temperature*, select a rectal thermometer (with a stubby tip), lubricate it, and insert it about 3 cm to 4 cm (1½ inches) into the anal canal, in a direction pointing toward the umbilicus. Remove and read it after 3 minutes.

Electronic thermometers with disposable probe covers are available for both rectal and oral temperatures. They shorten the time required to record an accurate temperature to about 10 seconds.

Whether an oral temperature is taken with a glass or an electronic thermometer, drinking hot or cold liquids may alter it artifactually. Wait 10 to 15 minutes before measurement.

The average oral temperature, usually quoted at 37° C (98.6° F), fluctuates considerably and must be interpreted accordingly. In the early morning hours it may be as low as 35.8° C (96.4° F), in the late afternoon or evening as high as 37.3° C (99.1° F). Rectal temperatures average 0.4° to 0.5° C (0.7° to 0.9° F) higher than oral readings, but this difference varies considerably.

The chief cause of hypothermia is exposure to cold. Other predisposing causes include decreased muscular movement (as from paralysis), interference with vasoconstriction (as from alcohol and sepsis), starvation, hypothyroidism, and hypoglycemia. Elderly people are especially susceptible to hypothermia and are less likely to develop fever.

Rapid respiratory rates tend to increase the discrepancy between oral and rectal temperatures. Rectal measurements are then more reliable.

Chapter 6
The Skin

Barbara Bates, with the assistance of Shelley Schuler

Anatomy and Physiology

The skin is composed of three layers: the epidermis, the dermis, and the subcutaneous tissues.

The most superficial layer, the *epidermis*, is thin, devoid of blood vessels, and itself divided into two layers: an outer horny layer of dead keratinized cells, and an inner cellular layer where both melanin and keratin are formed.

The epidermis depends on the underlying *dermis* for its nutrition. The dermis is well supplied with blood. It contains connective tissue, the sebaceous glands, and some of the hair follicles. It merges below with the *subcutaneous tissues*, which contain fat, the sweat glands, and the remainder of the hair follicles.

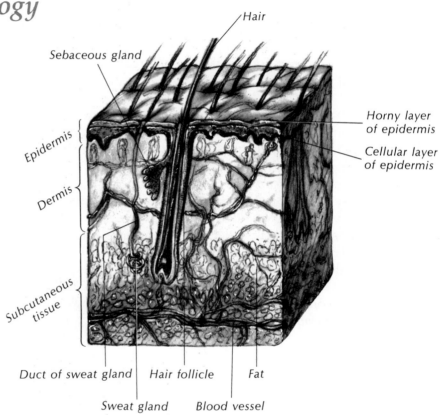

Hair — Sebaceous gland — Epidermis — Dermis — Subcutaneous tissue — Horny layer of epidermis — Cellular layer of epidermis — Duct of sweat gland — Sweat gland — Hair follicle — Blood vessel — Fat

Hair, nails, and sebaceous and sweat glands are considered appendages of the skin. Adults have two types of hair: vellus and terminal. Vellus hair is short, fine, inconspicuous, and unpigmented, while terminal hair in contrast is coarser, thicker, more conspicuous, and usually pigmented. Scalp hair and eyebrows are examples of terminal hair.

Sebaceous glands secrete a protective fatty substance which gains access to the skin surface through the hair follicles. These glands are present on all skin surfaces except for the palms and soles. Sweat glands are of two types: eccrine and apocrine. The eccrine glands are widely distributed, open directly onto the skin surface, and by their sweat production help to control body temperature. In contrast, the apocrine glands are found chiefly in the axillary and genital regions, usually open into hair follicles, and are stimulated by emotional stress. Bacterial decomposition of apocrine sweat is responsible for adult body odor.

The color of normal skin depends primarily on four pigments: melanin, carotene, oxyhemoglobin, and deoxyhemoglobin. The amount of *melanin*, the brownish pigment of the skin, is genetically determined and is increased by sunlight. *Carotene* is a golden yellow pigment that exists in subcutaneous fat and in heavily keratinized areas such as the palms and soles.

Hemoglobin, which circulates in the red cells and carries most of the oxygen of the blood, exists in two forms. *Oxyhemoglobin,* a bright red pigment, predominates in the arteries and capillaries. An increase in blood flow through the arteries to the capillaries of the skin causes a reddening of the skin, while the opposite change usually produces pallor. The skin of light-colored persons is normally redder on the palms, soles, face, neck, and upper chest.

As blood passes through the capillary bed, some of the oxyhemoglobin loses its oxygen to the tissues and thus changes to *deoxyhemoglobin*—a darker, less red, and somewhat bluer pigment. An increased concentration of deoxyhemoglobin in cutaneous blood vessels gives the skin a bluish cast known as *cyanosis.* Although cyanosis may signal serious disease, it may merely reflect a normal vascular response to various stimuli. When a person is anxious or exposed to a cold environment, for example, cutaneous blood flow decreases and slows, allowing the tissues to extract relatively more oxygen. The nailbeds then look bluish while the hands look pale and feel cool. When cyanosis results from increased tissue extraction of oxygen, it is called *peripheral* cyanosis. When it results from increased concentrations of deoxygenated hemoglobin in arterial blood, it is called *central* cyanosis.

In dark-skinned persons, melanin may mask the other pigments, making it difficult to identify pallor, unusual redness, or cyanosis. The palms, soles, fingertips, and nailbeds of dark-skinned persons contain less melanin than other areas, and it may be helpful to inspect these areas when making this assessment.

Skin color is affected not only by pigments but also by the scattering of light as it is reflected back through the turbid superficial layers of the skin or vessel walls. This scattering makes the color look more blue and less red. The bluish color of a subcutaneous vein is due to this effect, for example; it is much bluer than the venous blood obtained on venipuncture.

CHANGES WITH AGE

Adolescence. During the pubertal years coarse, or terminal, hair appears in new places: the face in boys, and the axillae and pubic areas in both sexes. Hair on the trunk and limbs increases through and after puberty, more obviously in men. During puberty apocrine glands enlarge, axillary sweating increases, and the characteristic adult body odor appears.

Aging. As people age their skin wrinkles, becomes lax, and loses turgor. The vascularity of the dermis decreases and the skin of white persons tends to look paler and more opaque. Comedones (blackheads) often appear on the cheeks or around the eyes. Where skin has been exposed to the sun it looks weatherbeaten: thickened, yellowed, and deeply furrowed. Skin on the backs of the hands and forearms appears thin, fragile, loose, and transparent, and may show whitish, depigmented patches known as pseudoscars. Well demarcated, vividly purple macules or patches, termed senile purpura, may also appear in the same areas, fading after several weeks. These purpuric spots come from blood that has leaked through poorly supported capillaries and has spread within the dermis. Dry skin (asteatosis)—a common problem—is flaky, rough, and often itchy. It is frequently shiny, especially on the legs, where a network of shallow fissures often creates a mosaic of small polygons.

Brown macules known as liver spots, or senile lentigines, frequently appear on the backs of the hands and forearms or, less commonly, on the face (see p. 153). Unlike the familiar freckles, they do not fade spontaneously when protected from the sun. Also common are seborrheic keratoses—pigmented, raised, warty, and often slightly greasy lesions that develop most often on the trunk but also occur on the face and hands (see p. 152). Actinic (or senile) keratoses, which are less common, develop on exposed surfaces, first as small reddened areas and then as raised, rough, yellow to brown lesions (see p. 152).

From middle life on, sebaceous hyperplasia may become evident on the face, especially on the forehead and nose. Hyperplastic sebaceous glands, which must be differentiated from basal cell epitheliomas, are yellowish, flattened papules with central depressions. They often look like diminutive doughnuts and range in size from 1 mm to 3 mm or more in diameter.

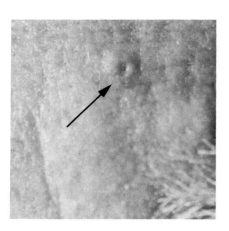

Sebaceous hyperplasia in a 53-year-old woman.

Cherry angiomas are very common, first appearing fairly early in adulthood (see p. 151). Most frequently found on the trunk, they have no significance.

While all these changes occur so frequently that they may be considered part of normal aging, two less common findings in older people are distinctly abnormal: squamous cell carcinoma, which sometimes develops in an actinic keratosis, and basal cell epithelioma. (See Color Plate 6-2, Skin Tumors, p. 152.)

Nails lose some of their luster with age and may yellow and thicken, especially on the toes.

Hair on the scalp loses its pigment, producing the well known graying. At as early as 20 years of age a man's hairline may start to recede at the temples; hair loss at the vertex follows. Many women show loss of hair in a similar pattern, but it is less severe. Balding in this distribution is genetically determined. In both sexes, the number of scalp hairs decreases in a generalized, more subtle pattern, and the diameter of each hair diminishes.

Less familiar, but probably more important clinically, is the normal hair loss elsewhere on the body: the trunk, pubic areas, axillae, and limbs. These changes will be discussed, where relevant, in later chapters. Coarse facial hairs appear on the chin and upper lip of many women by about the age of 55, but do not increase further thereafter.

Many of the observations described here pertain to white persons and do not necessarily apply to other racial groups. For example, Native American men have relatively little facial and body hair compared to that of white men and should not be evaluated by white norms.

Techniques of Examination

Begin your observation of the skin and related structures during the general survey and continue it throughout the rest of your examination. The entire skin surface should be inspected in good light, preferably natural light or artificial light that resembles it. Correlate your findings with observations of the mucous membranes. Specific diseases may manifest themselves in both areas, and both are necessary for the assessment of skin color. Techniques of examining these membranes are described in later chapters.

SKIN. Inspect and palpate the skin. Note its:

Color. Patients may be more sensitive to a change in their own skin color than the clinician is. Ask about it. Look for increased pigmentation (brownness), loss of pigmentation, redness, pallor, cyanosis, and yellowing of the skin.

The red color of oxyhemoglobin and the pallor due to a lack of it are best discerned where the horny layer of the epidermis is thinnest and causes the least scatter: the fingernails, the lips, and the mucous membranes, particularly those of the mouth and the palpebral conjunctiva. Inspect these areas in particular for pallor. In dark-skinned persons, the palms and soles may also be useful.

The conjunctiva is not very helpful in assessing cyanosis, and the nailbeds are so frequently affected by peripheral factors that they may be misleading. The lips, buccal mucosa, and tongue are usually best for the assessment of central cyanosis, although even the lips can become blue in the cold. Further, melanin pigment in the lips may give a false impression of cyanosis in some persons with dark complexions, especially those of Mediterranean heritage. The nails and the skin of the extremities are helpful in identifying peripheral cyanosis.

Look for the yellow color of excessive carotene in the palms, soles, and face. For the yellow color of jaundice, in contrast, look particularly in the bulbar conjunctiva against the background of the white sclera. Look for it also in the palpebral conjunctiva, the lips, and the hard palate, under the tongue, and in the skin itself. To see jaundice more easily in the lips, blanch out the red color by pressure with a glass slide.

Moisture. For example, dryness, sweating, oiliness

Artificial light often distorts colors and masks jaundice.

See Table 6-1, Variations in Skin Color (pp. 145–146).

Pallor due to decreased redness is seen in anemia and in decreased blood flow, as in fainting or arterial insufficiency.

Causes of peripheral cyanosis include anxiety, cold exposure, and venous obstruction. Causes of central cyanosis include advanced lung disease, congenital heart disease, and abnormal hemoglobins. Cyanosis in congestive heart failure is usually peripheral, reflecting decreased blood flow, but in pulmonary edema it may also be central.

Carotenemia

Jaundice suggests liver disease or excessive hemolysis of red blood cells.

Dryness in hypothyroidism; oiliness in acne

Techniques of Examination	Examples of Abnormalities

Temperature. Use the backs of your fingers to make this assessment. In addition to identifying generalized warmth or coolness of the skin, note the temperature of any red areas.

Generalized warmth in fever, hyperthyroidism; coolness in hypothyroidism. Local warmth of inflammation

Texture. For example, roughness, smoothness

Roughness in hypothyroidism

Mobility and Turgor. Lift a fold of skin and note the ease with which it is moved (mobility) and the speed with which it returns into place (turgor).

Decreased mobility in edema, scleroderma; decreased turgor in dehydration

Lesions. Observe any lesions of the skin.

1. First, identify the *anatomic location* of the lesions and their *distribution* over the entire surface of the body. Are they generalized or localized? Do they, for example, involve only the exposed surfaces, or the intertriginous (skin fold) areas, or areas exposed to specific allergens or irritants such as wrist bands, rings, or industrial chemicals?

Many skin diseases have typical distributions. Acne affects the face, upper chest, and back; psoriasis, the knees and elbows (among other areas); and *Candida* infections, the intertriginous areas.

2. Then note the *grouping or arrangement* of the lesions. They may be, for example, linear, clustered, annular (in a ring), arciform (in an arc), or dermatomal (covering a skin band that corresponds to a sensory nerve root; see pp. 509–510).

Vesicles in a unilateral dermatomal pattern are typical of herpes zoster.

3. Then try to identify the *type of skin lesions* (*e.g.*, macules, papules, vesicles). If possible, find representative and recent lesions that have not been traumatized by scratching or otherwise altered. Inspect them carefully and feel them.

See Table 6-2, Basic Types of Skin Lesions (pp. 147–148); Color Plate 6-1, Vascular and Purpuric Lesions of the Skin (p. 151); and Color Plate 6-2, Skin Tumors (p. 152).

4. Note the *color* of the lesions.

NAILS. Inspect and palpate the fingernails and toenails. Note their color and shape, and any lesions. Longitudinal bands of pigment may be seen in the nails of normal black persons.

See Table 6-3, Abnormalities and Variations of the Nails (p. 149).

HAIR. Inspect and palpate the hair. Note its quantity, distribution, and texture.

Alopecia refers to hair loss—diffuse, patchy, or total.

The differential diagnosis of skin abnormalities is beyond the scope of this book. After familiarizing yourself with the basic types of lesions, review their appearances in Table 6-6 and in a relatively brief but well illustrated textbook of dermatology. Whenever you see a skin lesion, make a consistent habit of looking it up in such a text. The type of lesions, their location, and their distribution, together with other information from the history and the examination, should equip you well for this search and, in time, for arriving at specific dermatologic diagnoses.

See Color Plate 6-3, Skin Lesions in Context (pp. 153–154).

Table 6-1   Variations in Skin Color

Table 6-1   Variations in Skin Color

COLOR	PROCESS	SELECTED CAUSES	TYPICAL LOCALIZATION
BROWN	Deposition of melanin	Sunlight	Exposed area
		Pregnancy	Face (mask of pregnancy, also called melasma or chloasma), nipples, areolae, linea nigra, vulva
		Addison's disease and some pituitary tumors	Exposed areas, points of pressure and friction, nipples, genitalia, palmar creases (normally darker in black persons), recent scars; often generalized
GRAYISH TAN OR BRONZE	Deposition of melanin and hemosiderin	Hemochromatosis	Exposed areas, genitalia, scars; often generalized
BLUE (*Cyanosis*)	Increased amount of deoxyhemoglobin secondary to hypoxia. This may be either—		
	• Peripheral (capillary), or	Anxiety or cold environment	Nails, sometimes lips
	• Central (arterial)	Heart or lung disease	Lips, buccal mucosa, tongue, nails
	Abnormal hemoglobin	Congenital or acquired methemoglobinemia; sulfhemoglobinemia	Lips, buccal mucosa, tongue, nails
REDDISH BLUE	Combination of an increase in the total amount of hemoglobin, an increase in reduced hemoglobin, and capillary stasis	Polycythemia	Face, conjunctiva, mouth, hands, feet
RED	Increased visibility of normal oxyhemoglobin because of—		
	• Dilatation or increased number of superficial blood vessels or increased blood flow	Fever, blushing, alcohol intake, local inflammation	Face and upper chest or local area of inflammation
	• Decreased oxygen use in the skin	Cold exposure	The areas exposed to the cold (*e.g.,* ears)

➡ Continued

Table 6-1 Variations in Skin Color

Table 6-1 (Cont'd.)

COLOR	PROCESS	SELECTED CAUSES	TYPICAL LOCALIZATION
YELLOW			
JAUNDICE	Increased bilirubin levels	Liver disease, red blood cell hemolysis	Conjunctiva, then other mucous membranes and generalized
CAROTENEMIA	Increased levels of carotene	Increased intake of carotene-containing vegetables and fruits; myxedema, hypopituitarism, diabetes mellitus, anorexia nervosa	Palms, soles, face; does not involve conjunctiva or other mucous membranes
CHRONIC UREMIA	A subtle pale-yellowish hue due to the retention of urinary chromogens, superimposed on the pallor of anemia; increased melanin may also contribute.	Chronic renal disease	Most evident in exposed areas, may be generalized; does not involve conjunctiva or other mucous membranes
DECREASED COLOR	Decreased melanin • Congenital inability to form melanin	Albinism	Generalized lack of pigment in skin, hair, eyes
	• Acquired loss of melanin	Vitiligo	Patchy, symmetrical, often involving the exposed areas
		Tinea versicolor (a common fungus infection that decreases skin exposure to sunlight in the involved areas)	Chest, upper back, neck
	Decreased visibility of oxyhemoglobin • Decreased blood flow in superficial vessels	Syncope, shock, some normal variations	Most evident in face, conjunctiva, mouth, nails
	• Decreased amount of oxyhemoglobin	Anemia	Most evident in face, conjunctiva, mouth, nails
	Edema. (Edema of the skin masks the colors of melanin and hemoglobin and prevents the appearance of jaundice.)	Nephrotic syndrome	The edematous areas

Table 6-2   Basic Types of Skin Lesions

Table 6-2   Basic Types of Skin Lesions

PRIMARY LESIONS (*May Arise From Previously Normal Skin*)

CIRCUMSCRIBED, FLAT, NONPALPABLE CHANGES IN SKIN COLOR

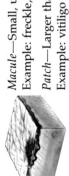

Macule—Small, up to 1 cm.* Example: freckle, petechia

Patch—Larger than 1 cm. Example: vitiligo

PALPABLE ELEVATED SOLID MASSES

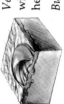

Papule—Up to 0.5 cm. Example: an elevated nevus

Plaque—A flat, elevated surface larger than 0.5 cm, often formed by the coalescence of papules

Nodule—0.5 cm to 1–2 cm; often deeper and firmer than a papule

Tumor—Larger than 1–2 cm

Wheal—A somewhat irregular, relatively transient, superficial area of localized skin edema. Example: mosquito bite, hive

CIRCUMSCRIBED SUPERFICIAL ELEVATIONS OF THE SKIN FORMED BY FREE FLUID IN A CAVITY WITHIN THE SKIN LAYERS

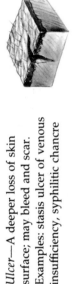

Vesicle—Up to 0.5 cm; filled with serous fluid. Example: herpes simplex

Bulla—Greater than 0.5 cm; filled with serous fluid. Example: 2nd-degree burn

Pustule—Filled with pus. Examples: acne, impetigo

SECONDARY LESIONS (*Result From Changes in Primary Lesions*)

LOSS OF SKIN SURFACE

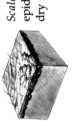

Erosion—Loss of the superficial epidermis; surface is moist but does not bleed. Example: moist area after the rupture of a vesicle, as in chickenpox

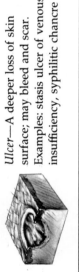

Ulcer—A deeper loss of skin surface; may bleed and scar. Examples: stasis ulcer of venous insufficiency, syphilitic chancre

Fissure—A linear crack in the skin. Example: athlete's foot

MATERIAL ON THE SKIN SURFACE

Crust—The dried residue of serum, pus, or blood. Example: impetigo

Scale—A thin flake of exfoliated epidermis. Examples: dandruff, dry skin, psoriasis

➤ *Continued*

Table 6-2   Basic Types of Skin Lesions

Table 6-2   (Cont'd)

MISCELLANEOUS LESIONS

Lichenification—Thickening and roughening of the skin with increased visibility of the normal skin furrows. Example: atopic dermatitis

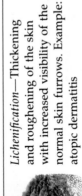

Scar—Replacement of destroyed tissue by fibrous tissue

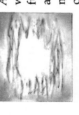

Keloid—A hypertrophied scar

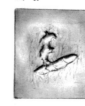

Atrophy—Thinning of the skin with loss of the normal skin furrows; the skin looks shinier and more translucent than normal. Example: arterial insufficiency

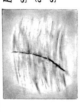

Excoriation—An abrasion or scratch mark. It may be linear, as illustrated, or rounded, as in a scratched insect bite.

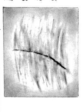

Burrow of Scabies—A person with scabies has intense itching. Skin lesions include small papules, pustules, lichenified areas, and excoriations. With a magnifying lens, look for the *burrow* of the mite that causes it. A burrow is a minute, slightly raised tunnel in the epidermis and is commonly found on the finger webs and on the sides of the fingers. It looks like a short (5–15 mm), linear or curved, gray line and may end in a tiny vesicle.

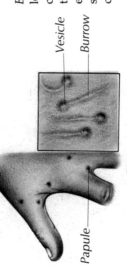

Vesicle

Burrow

Papule

Several additional terms deserve mention. A *comedo* is the common blackhead and marks the plugged opening of a sebaceous gland. Comedones are one of the hallmarks of acne. *Telangiectasias* are dilated small vessels that look either red or bluish. They can appear by themselves or as parts of other lesions such as a basal cell carcinoma or radiodermatitis (skin injury from ionizing radiation). The common mole—a flat to slightly elevated, round, evenly pigmented lesion—is technically called a *nevus*, although there are other nevi that look quite different.

* Authorities vary somewhat in their definitions of skin lesions by size. Dimensions given in this table should be considered approximate, not rigid.

Table 6-3   Abnormalities and Variations of the Nails

Table 6-3   Abnormalities and Variations of the Nails

CLUBBING OF THE NAILS
NORMAL

Normal angle 160°

The angle between the normal finger nail and the nail base is about 160°. When palpated, the nail base feels firm.

EARLY CLUBBING

Springy, floating   *Straightened angle (180°)*

In early clubbing, the angle between nail and nail base straightens out. The nail base gives a springy or floating sensation when palpated. You can simulate this by squeezing your middle finger from each side between your thumb and ring finger of the same hand, just behind the nail. Then palpate the nail base with the index finger of the opposite hand.

LATE CLUBBING

Angle greater than 180°   *Swollen, springy, floating*

In late clubbing, the base of the nail becomes visibly swollen and the angle between nail and nail base exceeds 180°. Clubbing has many causes, including hypoxia and lung cancer.

CURVED NAILS

Curved nail   *Normal angle*

Curved nails, a variant of normal, should not be confused with clubbing. Here, although the nails may show a convex curve as they may in clubbing, the normal angle between nail and nail base is preserved.

SPOON NAILS *(koilonychia)*

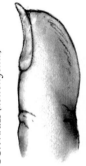

Spoon nails are characterized by concave curves. Spoon nails are sometimes seen in iron-deficiency anemia, although they are not specific for this disorder.

BEAU'S LINES

Beau's lines are transverse depressions in the nails associated with acute severe illness. Appearing some weeks later, they grow out with the nail gradually over several months.

PARONYCHIA

The term paronychia refers to inflammation of the skin around the nail. It is characterized by swelling and sometimes redness and tenderness.

SPLINTER HEMORRHAGES

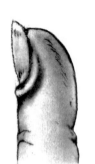

Splinter hemorrhages are red or brown linear streaks in the nail bed, parallel to the long axis of the fingers. Although traditionally associated with subacute bacterial endocarditis and trichinosis, they are nonspecific, often occurring with minor trauma or without apparent cause. They have been described in from 10% to 20% of hospitalized adults.

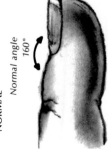
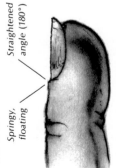

Color Plate 6-1   Vascular and Purpuric Lesions of the Skin

| | VASCULAR | | | PURPURIC | |
	SPIDER ANGIOMA	VENOUS STAR	CHERRY ANGIOMA	PETECHIA/PURPURA	ECCHYMOSIS
COLOR	Fiery red	Bluish	Bright or ruby red; may become brownish with age	Deep red or reddish purple, fading away over time	Purple or purplish blue, fading to green, yellow, and brown with time
SIZE	From very small to 2 cm	Variable, from very small to several inches	1–3 mm	Petechiae, 1–3 mm; purpura, larger	Variable, larger than petechiae
SHAPE	Central body, sometimes raised, surrounded by erythema and radiating legs	Variable. May resemble a spider or be linear, irregular, cascading	Round, flat or sometimes raised, may be surrounded by a pale halo	Rounded, sometimes irregular; flat	Round, oval, or irregular; may have a central subcutaneous flat nodule (a hematoma)
PULSATILITY	Often demonstrable in the body of the spider, when pressure with a glass slide is applied	Absent	Absent	Absent	Absent
EFFECT OF PRESSURE	Pressure on the body causes blanching of the spider.	Pressure over the center does not cause blanching, but diffuse pressure blanches the veins.	May show partial blanching, especially if pressure is applied with the edge of a pinpoint	None	None
DISTRIBUTION	Face, neck, arms, and upper trunk; almost never below the waist	Most often on the legs, near veins; also anterior chest	Trunk, also extremities	Variable	Variable
SIGNIFICANCE	Liver disease, pregnancy, vitamin B deficiency; also occurs in some normal people	Often accompanies increased pressure in the superficial veins, as in varicose veins	None; increase in size and numbers with aging	Blood outside the vessels; may suggest a bleeding disorder or, if petechiae, emboli to skin	Blood outside the vessels; often secondary to trauma; also seen in bleeding disorders

(Sources of photos: *Spider Angioma*—Marks R: Skin Disease in Old Age. Philadelphia, JB Lippincott, 1987; *Petechia/Purpura*—Kelley WN: Textbook of Internal Medicine. Philadelphia, JB Lippincott, 1989)

Color Plate 6-2   Skin Tumors

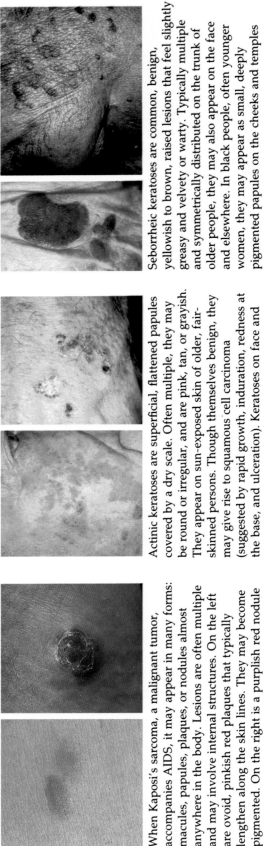

BASAL CELL EPITHELIOMA

A basal cell epithelioma, though malignant, grows slowly and seldom metastasizes. It is most common in fair-skinned adults over 40, and usually appears on the face. An initial translucent nodule spreads, leaving a depressed center and a firm, elevated border. Telangiectatic vessels are often visible, as in this lesion on the eyelid.

SQUAMOUS CELL CARCINOMA

Squamous cell carcinoma usually appears on sun-exposed skin of fair-skinned adults over 60. It may develop in an actinic keratosis. It usually grows more quickly than a basal cell epithelioma, is firmer, and looks redder. The face and the back of the hand are often affected, as shown here.

MALIGNANT MELANOMA

Noticeable growth or color change in a benign nevus (mole) warns of possible malignant melanoma, a highly malignant tumor most common in fair-skinned people. Suggestive signs are variation in color, an irregular perimeter, a raised and irregular surface, ulceration, and crusting. Two forms are illustrated: superficial spreading (left) and nodular (right).

KAPOSI'S SARCOMA IN AIDS

When Kaposi's sarcoma, a malignant tumor, accompanies AIDS, it may appear in many forms: macules, papules, plaques, or nodules almost anywhere in the body. Lesions are often multiple and may involve internal structures. On the left are ovoid, pinkish red plaques that typically lengthen along the skin lines. They may become pigmented. On the right is a purplish red nodule on the foot.

ACTINIC KERATOSIS

Actinic keratoses are superficial, flattened papules covered by a dry scale. Often multiple, they may be round or irregular, and are pink, tan, or grayish. They appear on sun-exposed skin of older, fair-skinned persons. Though themselves benign, they may give rise to squamous cell carcinoma (suggested by rapid growth, induration, redness at the base, and ulceration). Keratoses on face and hand, typical locations, are shown.

SEBORRHEIC KERATOSIS

Seborrheic keratoses are common, benign, yellowish to brown, raised lesions that feel slightly greasy and velvety or warty. Typically multiple and symmetrically distributed on the trunk of older people, they may also appear on the face and elsewhere. In black people, often younger women, they may appear as small, deeply pigmented papules on the cheeks and temples (dermatosis papulosa nigra).

(Sources of photos: *Basal Cell Epithelioma, Squamous Cell Carcinoma, Actinic Keratosis,* and *Seborrheic Keratosis*—Sauer GC: Manual of Skin Diseases, 5th ed. Philadelphia, JB Lippincott, 1985; *Malignant Melanoma*—Balch CM, Milton GW [eds]: Cutaneous Melanoma. Philadelphia, JB Lippincott, 1985; *Kaposi's Sarcoma in AIDS*—DeVita VT Jr, Hellman S, Rosenberg SA [eds]: AIDS: Etiology, Diagnosis, Treatment, and Prevention. Philadelphia, JB Lippincott, 1985)

Color Plate 6-3   Skin Lesions in Context

This table shows a variety of primary and secondary skin lesions. Try to identify them, including those indicated by letters, before reading the accompanying text.

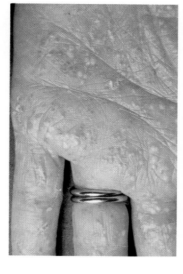

Macules on the dorsum of the hand, wrist, and forearm (senile lentigines or freckles)

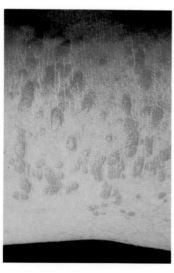

Papules on the knee (in lichen planus)

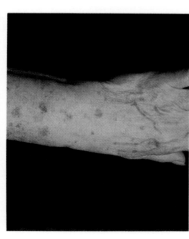

Pustules on the palm (in pustular psoriasis)

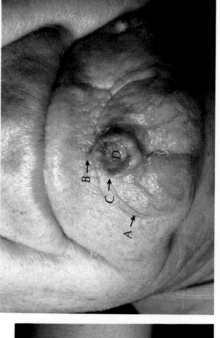
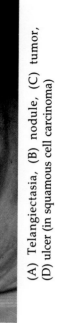
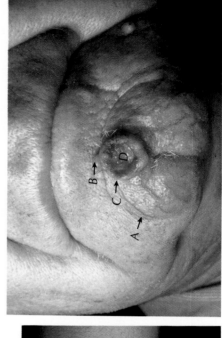

(A) Telangiectasia, (B) nodule, (C) tumor, (D) ulcer (in squamous cell carcinoma)

(A) Bulla and (B) target (or iris) lesion (in erythema multiforme)

Vesicles on the chin (in pemphigus)

► *Continued*

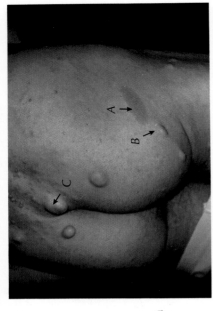

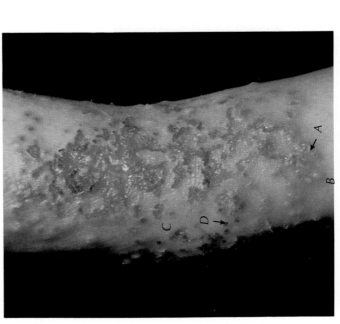

(A) Excoriation and (B) lichenification on the leg (in atopic dermatitis)

Wheals (or urticaria) (in a drug eruption in an infant)

(A) Patch, (B) nodule, (C) tumor—a combination typical of neurofibromatosis. A patch of this color is called a café-au-lait spot.

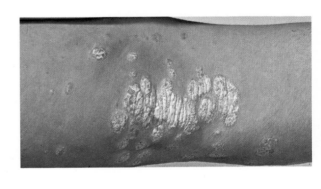

Plaques with scales on the front of a knee (in psoriasis)

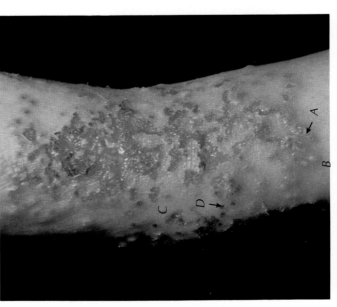

(A) Vesicle, (B) pustule, (C) erosions, (D) crust, on the back of a knee (in infected atopic dermatitis)

(Source of all photos except for *Macules*: Sauer GC: Manual of Skin Diseases, 5th ed. Philadelphia, JB Lippincott, 1985)

Chapter 7
The Head and Neck

Anatomy and Physiology

THE HEAD

Regions of the head take their names from the underlying bones (*e.g.*, frontal area, occipital area). Knowledge of the anatomy of the skull is thus helpful in localizing and describing physical findings.

Two salivary glands can be examined clinically: the parotid gland, which when enlarged is sometimes visible and palpable superficial to and behind the mandible, and the submaxillary (submandibular) gland, which is located deep to the mandible. Feel for the latter as you press your tongue against your upper incisors. Its lobular surface can often be felt against the tightened muscle. The openings of the parotid and submaxillary ducts are visible within the oral cavity.

The superficial temporal artery passes upward just in front of the ear, where it is readily palpable. In many normal people, especially thin and elderly ones, the tortuous course of one of its branches can be traced across the forehead.

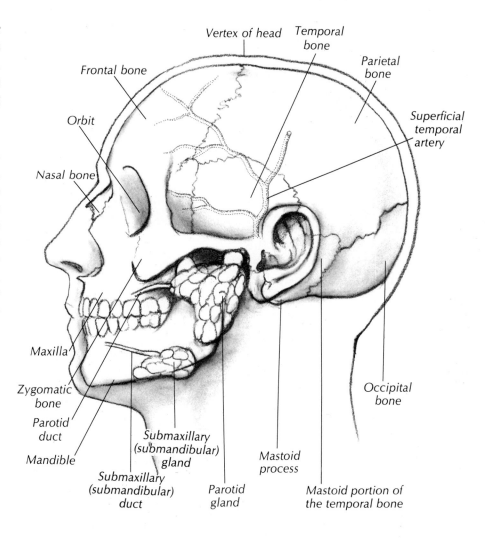

THE EYE

GROSS ANATOMY. Identify the structures illustrated. Note that the upper eyelid covers a portion of the iris but does not normally overlap the pupil. The opening between the eyelids is called the palpebral fissure. The white sclera may look somewhat buff-colored at its extreme periphery. This color should not be mistaken for the yellow of jaundice.

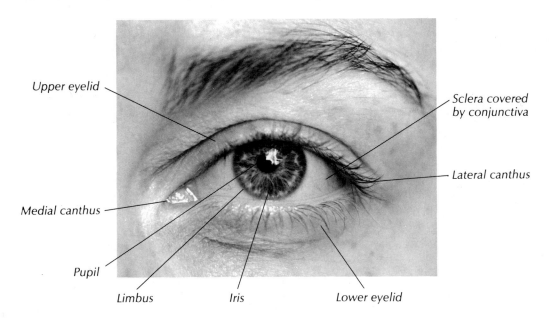

Except for the cornea, the parts of the eyeball visible anteriorly are covered by the conjunctiva. At the margin of the cornea (limbus), the conjunctiva merges with the corneal epithelium. A portion of the conjunctiva with its vessels lies loosely on the surface of the sclera and is called the bulbar conjunctiva. Above and below, it forms a deep recess and then folds forward to join the tissues of the eyelids (palpebral conjunctiva). The eyelids themselves are given form and consistency by thin strips of connective tissue known as the tarsal plates. Within each tarsal plate lies a row of parallel meibomian glands which open on the lid margin posteriorly. The levator palpebrae muscle, which raises the upper eyelid, has a dual innervation: from the oculomotor nerve (3rd cranial nerve) and from the sympathetic system.

A three-layered film of tear fluid protects the conjunctiva and cor-

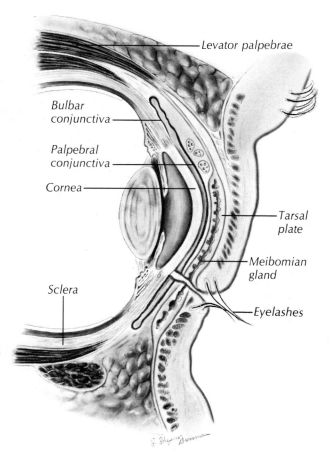

SAGITTAL SECTION OF ANTERIOR EYE WITH LIDS CLOSED

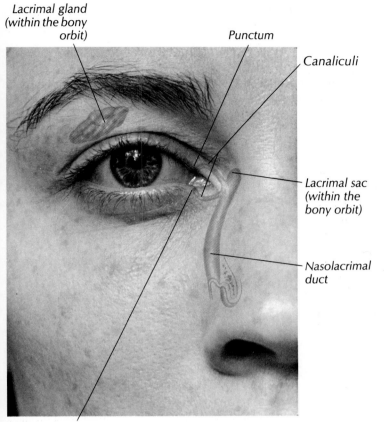

Lacrimal gland (within the bony orbit)

Punctum

Canaliculi

Lacrimal sac (within the bony orbit)

Nasolacrimal duct

Punctum

nea from drying, inhibits microbial growth, and gives a smooth optical surface to the cornea. The oily outermost layer of this fluid is secreted by the meibomian glands. The other two layers originate in conjunctival glands and in the lacrimal gland. The lacrimal gland lies mostly within the bony orbit above and lateral to the eyeball. The tear fluid spreads across the eye and drains medially through two tiny holes called lacrimal puncta. Each punctum can be found on a small elevation of the lid margin. The tears then pass through canaliculi into the lacrimal sac and on into the nose through the nasolacrimal duct. The lacrimal sac lies protected in a small bony depression inside the bony orbit.

especially in black people. Patches of it may occur in the conjunctiva, and tiny brown dots may be seen in the sclera. The latter lie about 0.5 cm from the limbus, at points where vessels or nerves penetrate the sclera. They may mimic foreign bodies.

The eyeball itself is a spherical structure designed to focus a controlled amount of light on the neurosensory elements within the retina. Muscles within the iris control pupillary size. Muscles of the ciliary body control the thickness of the lens, enabling the normal eye to focus in turn on objects near and far away. At the posterior pole of the eye the retinal surface shows a slight depression—the fovea centralis—which marks the point of central vision. The retina immediately around it is called the mac-

Brown pigment may be seen against the white of the sclera,

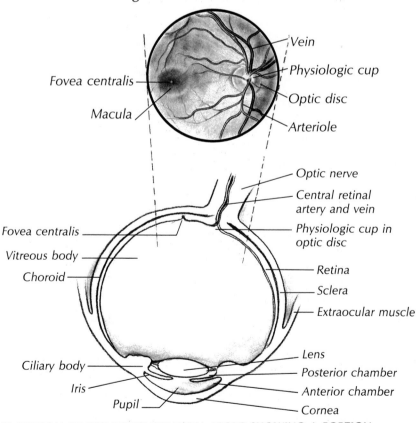

Fovea centralis

Macula

Vein

Physiologic cup

Optic disc

Arteriole

Optic nerve

Central retinal artery and vein

Physiologic cup in optic disc

Retina

Sclera

Extraocular muscle

Fovea centralis

Vitreous body

Choroid

Ciliary body

Iris

Pupil

Lens

Posterior chamber

Anterior chamber

Cornea

CROSS SECTION OF THE RIGHT EYE FROM ABOVE SHOWING A PORTION OF THE FUNDUS COMMONLY SEEN WITH THE OPHTHALMOSCOPE

ula. The optic nerve with its retinal vessels joins the eye somewhat medial to this point. It is visible ophthalmoscopically as the optic disc. The portion of the eye posterior to the lens is termed the fundus of the eye. It includes most of the structures normally inspected with the ophthalmoscope: retina, choroid, fovea, macula, optic disc, and retinal vessels. The most anterior parts of the retina and the ciliary body are visible only by special techniques.

A clear liquid called *aqueous humor* fills the anterior and posterior chambers of the eye. Aqueous humor is produced by the ciliary body, circulates from the posterior chamber through the pupil into the anterior chamber, and then drains out through the canal of Schlemm. Pressure within the eye depends primarily upon this circulatory system.

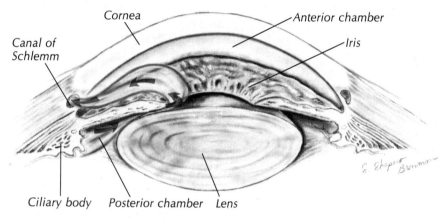

CIRCULATION OF AQUEOUS HUMOR

The vitreous body, a transparent mass of gelatinous material, fills the eyeball behind the lens and helps to maintain the shape of the eye.

VISUAL PATHWAYS. For a clear visual image, reflected light from an object must pass through the cornea, aqueous humor, lens, and vitreous, and be focused on the retina. Images so formed are upside down and reversed right to left. An object in the upper temporal visual field, therefore, strikes the lower nasal quadrant of the retina. An oval blind spot in

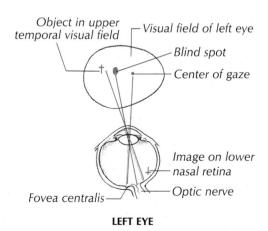

LEFT EYE

the visual field of each eye, 15° temporal to the line of gaze, is explained by the lack of retinal receptors overlying the optic disc.

In response to a light stimulus, nerve impulses are conducted through the retina, the optic nerve, and the optic tract to the midbrain, and thence to the visual cortex of the occipital lobe. The spatial arrangements of nerve fibers in the retina are preserved in the optic nerves: temporal fibers run laterally in the nerve; nasal fibers run medially. At the optic chiasm, however, the nasal or medial fibers cross over so that the left optic tract contains fibers only from the left half of each retina and the right optic tract contains fibers only from the right half.

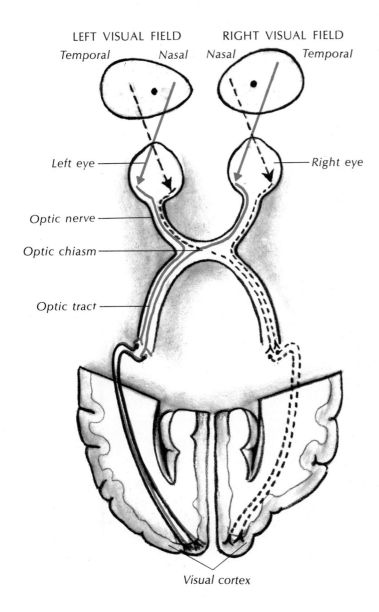

PUPILLARY REACTIONS. Pupillary size changes in response to light and to the effort of focusing on a near object.

The Light Reaction. A light beam shining onto the retina causes pupillary constriction in both that eye (the *direct reaction* to light) and the opposite eye (the *consensual reaction*).

The initial sensory pathways are similar to those described on page 159: retina, optic nerve, and optic tract. The pathways diverge, however, in the midbrain, and through a series of synapses impulses are transmitted through the oculomotor nerve (3rd cranial nerve) and thence to the constrictor muscles of the iris on each side.

The Near Reaction. When a person shifts gaze from a far object to a close one, the eyes respond in three ways: the pupils constrict (the near reaction), the eyes converge, and the lenses become more convex (accommodation).

Pupillary constriction with near gaze, like that in response to light, is mediated by the oculomotor nerve. *Convergence* is also mediated by the oculomotor nerve, as described below under Extraocular Movements. The response of the lenses, called *accommodation,* is not visible. Their increased convexity, caused by contraction of the ciliary muscles, brings near objects into focus.

AUTONOMIC NERVE SUPPLY TO THE EYES. Fibers traveling in the oculomotor nerve and producing pupillary constriction are part of the parasympathetic nervous system. The iris is also supplied by sympathetic fibers. When these are stimulated, pupillary dilation and some elevation of the eyelid result. The sympathetic pathway starts in the hypothalamus, passes down

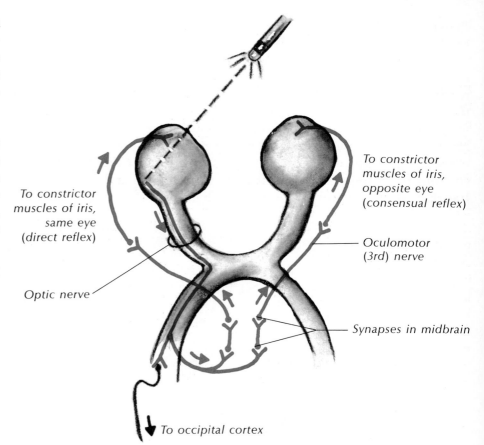

To constrictor muscles of iris, same eye (direct reflex)

To constrictor muscles of iris, opposite eye (consensual reflex)

Oculomotor (3rd) nerve

Optic nerve

Synapses in midbrain

To occipital cortex

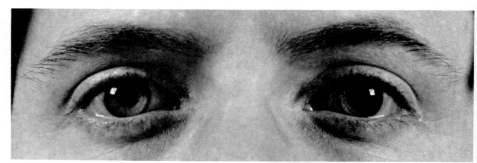

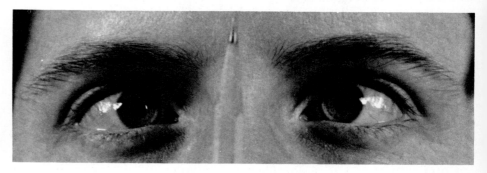

THE NEAR REACTION

through the brainstem and cervical cord, and continues out to the sympathetic trunk and ganglia of the neck. Sympathetic fibers then follow a nerve plexus around the carotid artery and its branches into the orbit.

EXTRAOCULAR MOVEMENTS. The movement of each eye is controlled by the coordinated action of six muscles, the four rectus and two oblique muscles. The function of each muscle, together with that of the nerve that supplies it, may be tested by asking the patient to move the eye in the direction predominantly controlled by that muscle. There are six such *cardinal directions,* indicated by the red lines. When a person looks down and to the right, for example, the right inferior rectus (3rd cranial nerve) is principally responsible for moving the right eye while the left superior oblique (4th cranial nerve) is principally responsible for moving the left. If one of these muscles is paralyzed, deviation of the eyes from their normal conjugate, or parallel, positions will be most obvious in this direction of gaze.

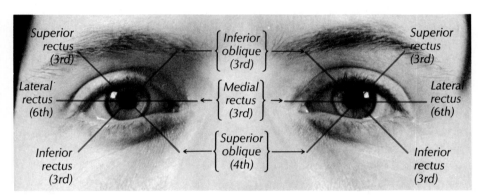

THE EAR

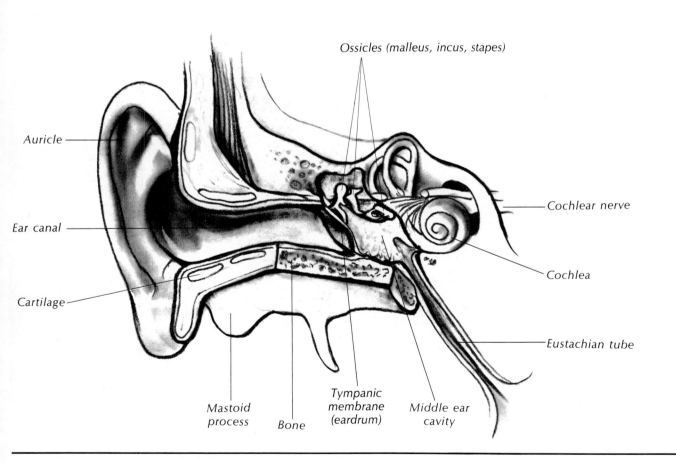

ANATOMY. The ear has three compartments: the external ear, the middle ear, and the inner ear.

The external ear comprises the auricle and ear canal. The auricle consists chiefly of cartilage covered by skin and has a firm, elastic consistency.

The ear canal opens behind the tragus and curves inward about 24 mm. Its outer portion is surrounded by cartilage. The skin in this outer portion is hairy and contains glands that produce cerumen (wax). The inner portion of the canal is surrounded by bone and lined by thin, hairless skin. Pressure on this latter area causes pain —a point to remember when you examine the ear.

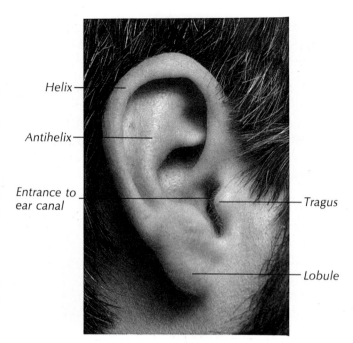

The bone behind and below the ear canal is the mastoid part of the temporal bone. The lowest portion of this bone, the mastoid process, is palpable behind the lobule.

At the end of the ear canal lies the tympanic membrane or eardrum, marking the lateral limits of the middle ear. The middle ear is an air-filled cavity across which sound is transmitted by way of three tiny bones, the ossicles. It is connected by the eustachian tube to the nasopharynx.

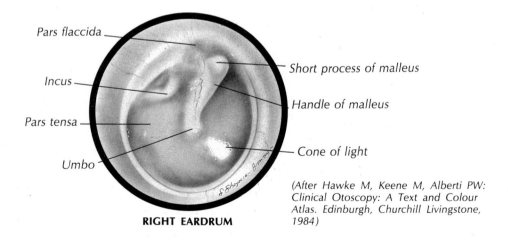

RIGHT EARDRUM

(After Hawke M, Keene M, Alberti PW: *Clinical Otoscopy: A Text and Colour Atlas.* Edinburgh, Churchill Livingstone, 1984)

The eardrum may be visualized as an oblique membrane pulled inward at its center by one of the ossicles, the malleus. Find the handle and the short process of the malleus—the two chief landmarks. From the umbo, where the eardrum meets the tip of the malleus, a light reflection called the cone of light fans downward and anteriorly. Above the short process lies a small portion of the eardrum called the pars flaccida. The remainder of the drum is the pars tensa. Anterior and posterior malleolar folds, which extend obliquely upward from the short process, separate the pars flaccida from the pars tensa but are usually invisible unless the eardrum is retracted. A second ossicle, the incus, can sometimes be seen through the drum.

Much of the middle ear and all of the inner ear are inaccessible to direct examination. Some inferences concerning their condition can be made, however, by testing auditory function.

PATHWAYS OF HEARING. Vibrations of sound pass through the air of the external ear and are transmitted through the eardrum and ossicles of the middle ear into the cochlea, a part of the inner ear.

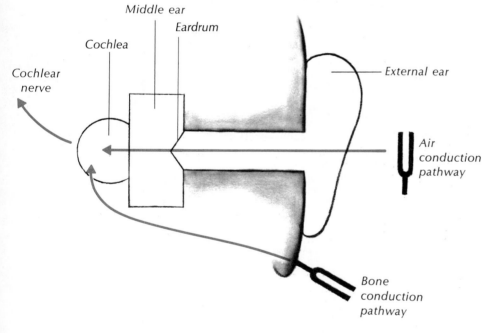

Here nerve impulses are initiated and sent to the brain by way of the cochlear nerve (a portion of the 8th cranial nerve). This pathway is the usual one in normal hearing. An alternate pathway used for testing purposes bypasses the external and middle ear by setting the bone of the skull into vibration and thereby stimulating the inner ear directly.

Hearing over the usual pathways, including the air-filled external and middle ear, is called air conduction. Hearing dependent upon sound transmitted through bone to the inner ear is called bone conduction. In the normal person, the usual pathway (*i.e.,* air conduction) is the more sensitive.

EQUILIBRIUM. The labyrinth within the inner ear senses the position and movements of the head and helps to maintain balance.

THE NOSE AND PARANASAL SINUSES

Review the terms used to describe the external anatomy of the nose.

Approximately the upper third of the nose is supported by bone, the lower two thirds by cartilage. Air enters the nasal cavity by way of the anterior naris on either side, then passes into a widened area known as the vestibule and on through the slitlike nasal passage to the nasopharynx. The medial wall of each nasal cavity is formed by the nasal septum which, like the external nose, is supported by both bone and cartilage. It is covered by a mucous membrane well supplied with blood. The vestibule, unlike the rest of the nasal cavity, is lined with hair-bearing skin, not mucosa.

Laterally, the anatomy is more complex. Curving bony structures, the turbinates, covered by a highly vascular mucous membrane, protrude into the nasal cavity. Below each turbinate is a groove, or meatus, each named according to the turbinate above it. Into the inferior meatus drains the nasolacrimal duct; into the middle meatus drain most of the paranasal sinuses. Their openings are not usually visible.

The additional surface area provided by the turbinates and the mucosa covering them aids the nasal cavities in their principal functions: cleansing, humidification, and temperature control of inspired air.

Inspection of the nasal cavity through the anterior naris is usually limited to the vestibule, the

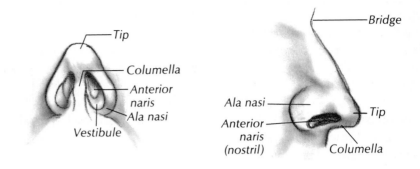

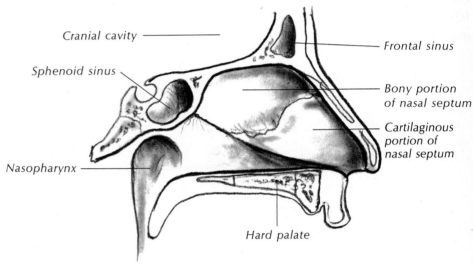

MEDIAL WALL—RIGHT NASAL CAVITY
(Mucous membrane removed to show the structure of the nasal septum)

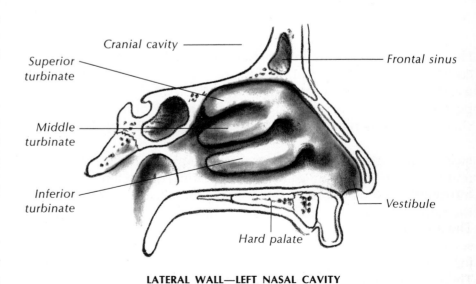

LATERAL WALL—LEFT NASAL CAVITY

anterior portion of the septum, and the lower and middle turbinates. Examination by means of a naso-pharyngeal mirror is required for detection of posterior abnormalities. It is beyond the scope of this book.

The paranasal sinuses are air-filled cavities within the bones of the skull. Like the nasal cavities into which they drain, they are lined with mucous membrane. Their locations are diagrammed below. Only the frontal and maxillary sinuses are readily accessible to clinical examination.

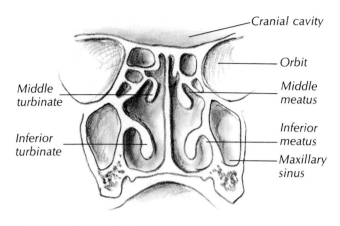

Cranial cavity

Orbit

Middle meatus

Middle turbinate

Inferior meatus

Inferior turbinate

Maxillary sinus

CROSS SECTION OF NASAL CAVITY—ANTERIOR VIEW

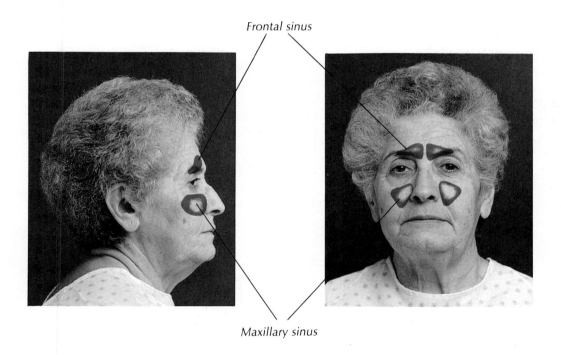

Frontal sinus

Maxillary sinus

THE MOUTH AND THE PHARYNX

Structures in the mouth and pharynx are illustrated on page 166.

The dorsum of the tongue is covered with papillae, giving it a roughened surface. A thin white coating is found frequently and is normal. Often just visible toward the back of the tongue are the large vallate papillae. These should not be confused with tumor nodules.

Above and behind the tongue rises an arch formed by the anterior and posterior pillars, soft palate, and uvula. The tonsils can be seen in the fossae, or cavities, between the anterior and posterior pillars. In adults, however, the tonsils are often small or absent because of normal atrophy or surgical removal. A normal posterior pharynx may show small blood vessels and patches of lymphoid tissue on its surface.

The undersurface of the tongue is relatively smooth. At its base the ducts of the submaxillary gland (Wharton's ducts) pass forward to their openings near the midline. Each parotid duct (Stensen's duct) opens onto the buccal mucosa near the upper 2nd molar, where its location is frequently marked by a small papilla.

A full complement of 32 adult teeth (16 in each jaw) is identified below.

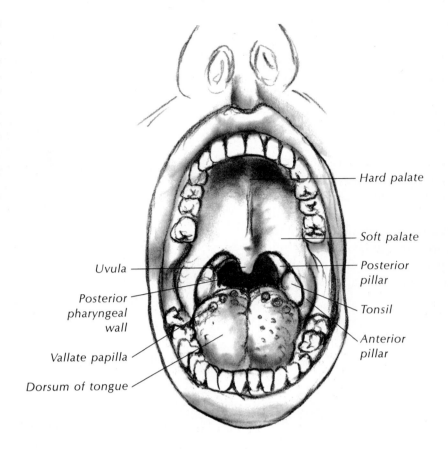

Hard palate

Soft palate

Posterior pillar

Tonsil

Anterior pillar

Uvula

Posterior pharyngeal wall

Vallate papilla

Dorsum of tongue

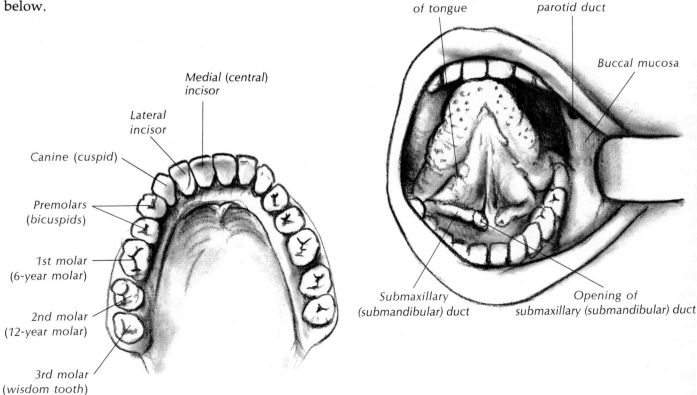

Medial (central) incisor

Lateral incisor

Canine (cuspid)

Premolars (bicuspids)

1st molar (6-year molar)

2nd molar (12-year molar)

3rd molar (wisdom tooth)

Undersurface of tongue

Opening of parotid duct

Buccal mucosa

Submaxillary (submandibular) duct

Opening of submaxillary (submandibular) duct

THE NECK

For descriptive purposes, each side of the neck can be seen as divided into two triangles by the sterno-mastoid (sternocleidomastoid) muscle. The anterior triangle is bounded above by the mandible, laterally by the sternomastoid, and medially by the midline of the neck. The posterior triangle extends from the sternomastoid to the trapezius and is bounded below by the clavicle. A portion of the omohyoid muscle crosses the lower portion of the posterior triangle and can be mistaken by the uninitiated for a lymph node or mass.

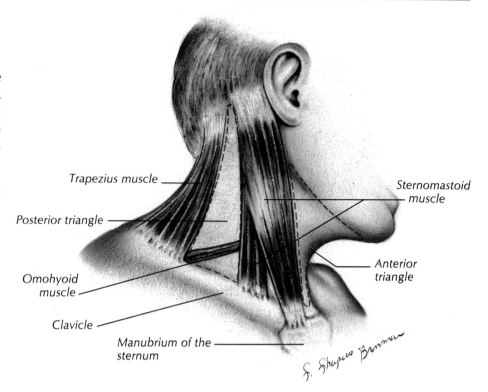

From above down, identify the following midline structures: (1) the mobile hyoid bone just below the mandible, (2) the thyroid cartilage, readily identified by the notch on its superior edge, (3) the cricoid cartilage, (4) the tracheal rings, and (5) the softer thyroid isthmus, which lies across the trachea below the cricoid. The lateral lobes of the thyroid curve posteriorly around the sides of the trachea and the esophagus. Except in the midline, the thyroid gland is covered by thin straplike muscles, among which only the sternomastoids are visible.

Women have larger and more easily palpable glands than do men.

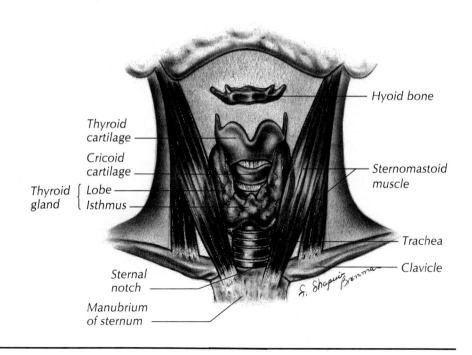

Deep to the sternomastoids run the great vessels of the neck: the carotid artery and internal jugular vein. The external jugular vein passes diagonally over the surface of the sternomastoid.

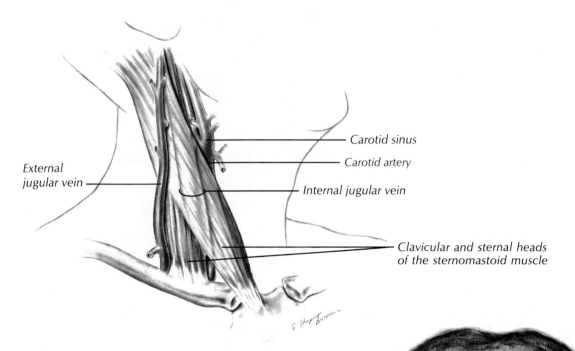

External jugular vein

Carotid sinus

Carotid artery

Internal jugular vein

Clavicular and sternal heads of the sternomastoid muscle

The lymph nodes of the head and neck have been classified in a variety of ways. One classification is shown here, together with the directions of lymphatic drainage. The deep cervical chain is largely obscured by the overlying sternomastoid muscle, but at its two extremes the tonsillar node and the supraclavicular nodes may be palpable. The submaxillary nodes lie superficial to the submaxillary gland, from which they should be differentiated. Nodes are normally round or ovoid, smooth, and smaller than the gland. The gland is larger and has a lobulated, slightly irregular surface (see p. 155).

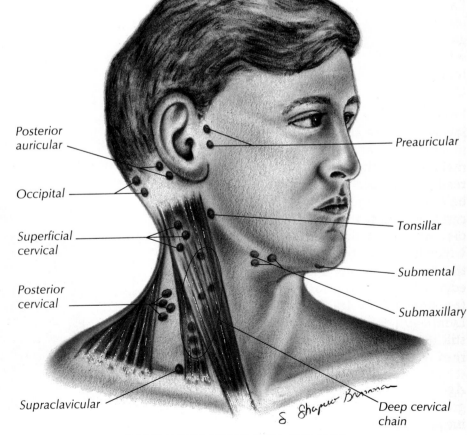

Posterior auricular

Occipital

Superficial cervical

Posterior cervical

Supraclavicular

Preauricular

Tonsillar

Submental

Submaxillary

Deep cervical chain

LYMPH NODES OF THE HEAD AND NECK

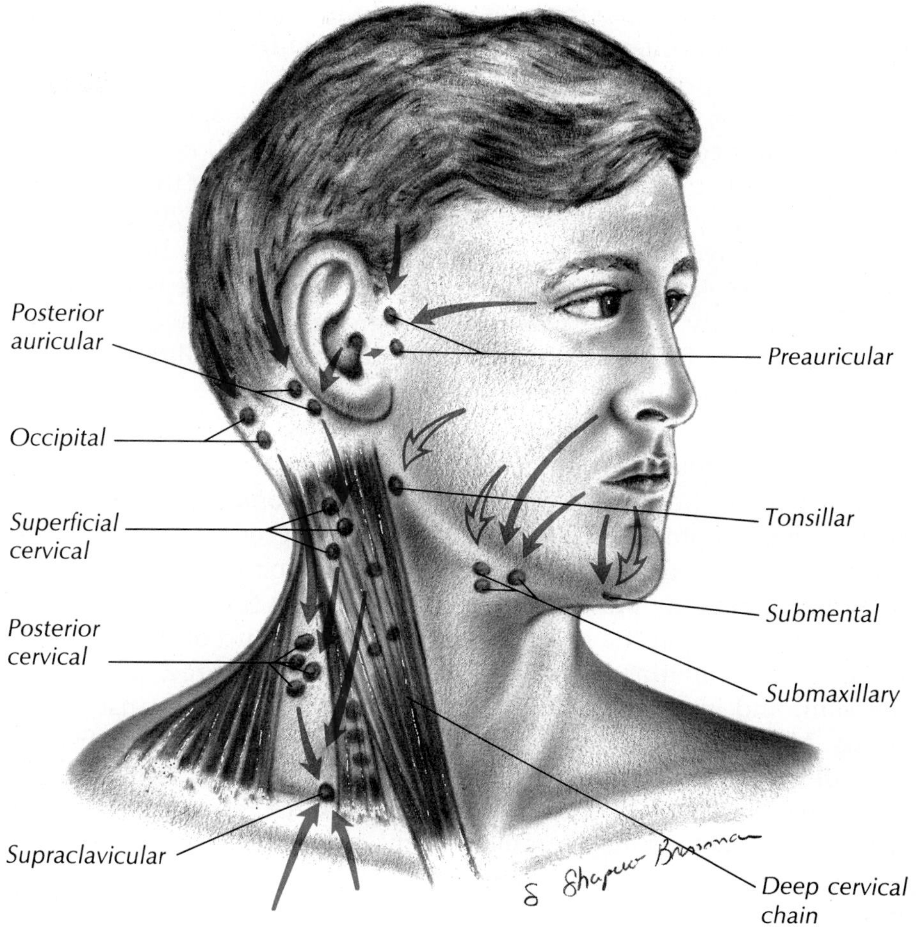

LYMPHATIC DRAINAGE OF THE HEAD AND NECK

External lymphatic drainage
Internal lymphatic drainage (eg. from mouth and throat)

Note that the tonsillar, submaxillary, and submental nodes drain portions of the mouth and throat as well as the more superficial tissues of the face.

Knowledge of the lymphatic system is important to a sound clinical habit: whenever a malignant or inflammatory lesion is observed, look for involvement of the regional lymph nodes that drain it; whenever a node is enlarged or tender, look for a source in the area that it drains.

CHANGES WITH AGE

Adolescence. Several changes in the head and neck accompany adolescence. In boys the voice begins to deepen and the thyroid cartilage enlarges perceptibly during the adolescent growth spurt. Facial hair appears on the upper lip, then on the cheeks and the lower lip, and finally on the chin. The facial contours of both boys and girls change subtly as children turn into young adults. Lengthening of the eyeballs in their anteroposterior diameter may cause or accentuate myopia, or nearsightedness. The comedones (black-heads) and pustules of acne appear on the face so commonly that they are almost considered an adolescent norm. Lymphoid tissues, which grow rapidly in late childhood (see p. 561), are still relatively prominent in adolescents, and cervical lymph nodes are readily palpable in most teenagers.

Aging. Tonsils, which are also composed of lymphoid tissue, become gradually smaller after the age of 5 years. In adulthood, they become inconspicuous or invisible. The frequency of palpable cervical nodes gradually diminishes with age and, according to one study, falls below

50% some time between the ages of 50 and 60. In contrast to the lymph nodes, the submaxillary glands become easier to feel in older people.

The eyes, ears, and mouth bear the brunt of old age. Visual acuity remains fairly constant between the ages of 20 and 50 and then diminishes, gradually until about age 70 and more rapidly after that. Nevertheless, most elderly people retain good to adequate vision—20/20 to 20/70 as measured by standard charts. Near vision, however, begins to blur noticeably for virtually everyone. From childhood on, the lens gradually loses its elasticity and the eye grows progressively less able to focus on nearby objects. This loss of accommodative power, called presbyopia, usually becomes noticeable in one's 40s.

Just as aging alters function of the eyes, it also alters structure. In some elderly people the fat that surrounds and cushions the eye within the bony orbit atrophies, allowing the eyeball to recede somewhat in the orbit. The skin of the eyelids becomes wrinkled, occasionally hanging in loose folds. Fat may push the fascia of the eyelids forward, creating soft bulges, especially in the lower lids and the inner third of the upper ones (p. 199). Combinations of a weakened levator palpebrae, relaxation of the skin, and increased weight of the upper eyelid may cause a senile ptosis. More important, the lower lid may fall outward away from the eyeball or turn inward onto it, resulting in ectropion and entropion, respectively (p. 199). Because their eyes produce fewer lacrimal secretions, aging patients may complain of dryness of the eyes.

Corneal arcus, or arcus senilis, is common in elderly persons and in them has no clinical significance (p. 202). The corneas lose some of their luster. The pupils become smaller—a characteristic that makes it more difficult to examine the fundi of elderly people. The pupils may also become slightly irregular but should continue to respond to light and near effort. Except for possible impairment in upward gaze, extraocular movements should remain intact.

Lenses thicken and yellow with age, impairing the passage of light to the retinas, and elderly people need more light to read and do fine work. When the lens of an elderly person is examined with a flashlight it frequently looks gray, as if it were opaque, when in fact it permits good visual acuity and looks clear on ophthalmoscopic examination. Do not depend on your flashlight alone, therefore, to make a diagnosis of cataract—a true opacity of the lens (p. 202). Cataracts do become relatively common, however, affecting 1 out of 10 people in their 60s and 1 out of 3 in their 80s. Because the lens continues to grow over the years, it may push the iris forward, narrowing the angle between iris and cornea and increasing the risk of narrow-angle glaucoma (p. 178).

Ophthalmoscopic examination reveals fundi that have lost their youthful shine and light reflections. The arterioles look narrowed, paler, straighter, and less brilliant (p. 124). Drusen (colloid bodies) may be seen

(p. 210). On a somewhat more anterior plane you may be able to see some vitreous floaters—degenerative changes that may cause annoying specks or webs in the field of vision. You may also find evidence of other, more serious, conditions that occur more often in elderly people than in younger ones: senile macular degeneration, glaucoma, retinal hemorrhages, or possibly retinal detachment.

Acuity of hearing, like that of vision, usually diminishes with age. Early losses, which start in young adulthood, involve primarily the high-pitched sounds beyond the range of human speech and have relatively little functional significance. Gradually, however, loss continues and begins to encroach on sounds in the middle and lower ranges. When a person fails to catch the upper tones of words while hearing the lower ones, words sound distorted and conversation is difficult to understand, especially in noisy environments. Hearing loss associated with aging, known as presbycusis, becomes increasingly evident, usually after the age of 50.

Diminished salivary secretions and a decreased sense of taste have been attributed to aging, but recent studies suggest that medications or various diseases probably account for most of these changes. Teeth may wear down or become abraded over time, or they may be lost to dental caries or other conditions (pp. 225–226). Periodontal disease is the chief cause of tooth loss in most adults (p. 225). If a person has no teeth, the lower portion of the face looks small and sunken, with accentuated "purse-string" wrinkles radiating out from the mouth. Overclosure of the mouth may lead to maceration of the skin at the corners—angular stomatitis (p. 222). The bony ridges of the jaws that once surrounded the tooth sockets are gradually resorbed, especially in the lower jaw.

Techniques of Examination

THE HEAD

Because abnormalities covered by the hair are so easily missed, ask if the patient has noticed anything wrong with the scalp or hair. If you note a hairpiece or wig, ask the patient to remove it.

Examine:

THE HAIR. Note its quantity, distribution, pattern of loss if any, and texture. Identify nits (the eggs of lice) if present, differentiating them from dandruff.

Fine hair in hyperthyroidism; coarse hair in hypothyroidism. Tiny white ovoid nits adherent to hairs; loose white flakes of dandruff

THE SCALP. Part the hair in several places and look for scaliness, lumps, or other lesions.

Redness and scaling in seborrheic dermatitis, psoriasis

THE SKULL. Observe the general size and contour of the skull. Note any deformities, lumps, or tenderness. Familiarize yourself with the irregularities in a normal skull, such as those near the suture lines between the parietal and occipital bones.

Enlarged skull in hydrocephalus, Paget's disease of bone

THE FACE. Note the patient's facial expression and contours. Observe for asymmetry, involuntary movements, edema, and masses.

See Table 7-1, Selected Facies (p. 197).

THE SKIN. Observe the skin, noting its color, pigmentation, texture, thickness, hair distribution, and any lesions.

Acne in many adolescents. Hirsutism (excessive facial hair) in some women

THE EYES

TESTING VISION

Visual Acuity is a test of central vision. If possible, use a Snellen eye chart and light it well. Position the patient 20 feet from the chart. Patients who use glasses other than reading glasses should wear them. Ask the patient to cover one eye with a card (to prevent peeking through the fingers) and to read the smallest line of print possible. Coaxing to attempt the next line may improve performance. A patient who cannot read the largest letter should be positioned closer to the chart and the distance from it noted. Determine the smallest line of print from which the patient can identify more than half the letters. Record the visual acuity designated at the side of this line, together with the use of glasses, if any. Visual acuity is expressed as two numbers (*e.g.,* 20/30), in which the first indicates the distance of the patient from the chart and the second, the distance at which a normal eye can read the line of letters.

Vision of 20/200 means that the patient can read print at 20 feet that a person with normal vision could read at 200 feet. The larger the second number, the worse the vision. "20/40 corrected" means the patient could read the 40 line with glasses (a correction).

Myopia refers to impaired far vision.

Testing near vision with a hand-held card in patients older than 45 years is important in order to identify the need for reading glasses or bifocals. Hand-held cards also enable you to test visual acuity at the bedside. The card should be held about 13 inches from the patient's eyes. Patients who have reading glasses should wear them for this test.

If you have no charts, screen visual acuity with any available print. If patients cannot read even the largest letters, test their ability to count your upraised fingers and distinguish light (such as your flashlight) from dark.

Presbyopia refers to the impaired near vision found in middle-aged and older people.

In the United States, a person is usually considered legally blind when vision in the better eye, corrected by glasses, is 20/200 or less. Legal blindness also results from a constricted field of vision: 20° or less in the better eye.

Visual Fields. A visual field is the entire area seen by an eye when its gaze is fixed on a central point. Visual fields are conventionally diagrammed separately, from the patient's point of view. The central point of each circle represents the focus of gaze; the circumference of the circle is 90° from the line of gaze as measured from the corneal surface. The visual field, shown by the white areas below, is divided into quadrants.

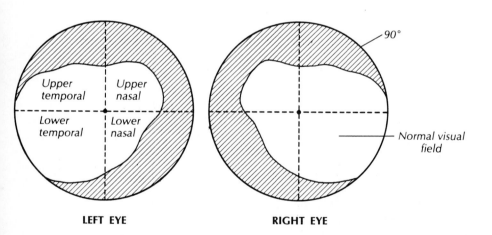

LEFT EYE   RIGHT EYE

Visual fields are normally limited above by the brows, below by the cheeks, and medially by the nose, as shown by the shaded areas.

One method of testing visual fields is by *confrontation*. Although this can be omitted in routine examinations, it is indicated if you suspect a visual or neurologic defect. Face the patient directly from about 2 feet away, with your eyes on the same level. Ask the patient to cover one eye by hand or card and to look at your eye directly opposite. Close your other eye.

As you and the patient look at each other's eyes, your visual fields should roughly mirror each other. On a plane midway between you, your fields should be much the same and you can assess the patient's field accordingly. Temporally and inferotemporally, however, both the patient's field and your own field extend beyond the reach of your testing hand. Accept this limitation.

Abnormalities detectable by confrontation may be diagrammed simply, as follows:

A horizontal defect

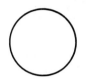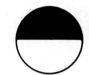

Homonymous hemianopsia, a loss of vision on the same side of each field

See Table 7-2, Visual Field Defects Produced by Selected Lesions in the Visual Pathways (p. 198).

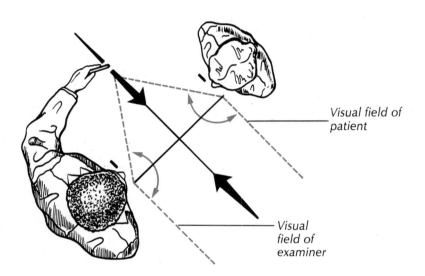

Visual field of patient

Visual field of examiner

Slowly bring a pencil or other test object from the periphery into the field of vision on the plane midway between you and the patient. Ask the patient to say "now" as soon as it appears. Use this stimulus in the eight directions shown, and estimate the patient's visual field.

Repeat these steps with the other eye.

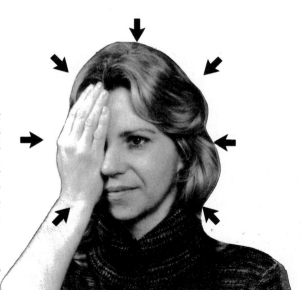

Another technique may help to define hemianoptic or horizontal visual defects. After the patient has covered one eye as before, simultaneously present similar test objects in two separate visual fields. Ask the patient (1) which object is seen, and (2) whether both objects are seen equally clearly.

Not seeing one object or seeing it less clearly suggests a visual defect.

POSITION AND ALIGNMENT OF THE EYES. From in front of the patient, survey the eyes for their position and alignment with each other. If you note unusually prominent eyes, especially on one side, inspect them from above. Stand behind the seated patient, draw the upper lids gently upward, and note the relationship of the corneas to the lower lids.

Exophthalmos refers to an abnormal protrusion of the eyeball. Bilateral exophthalmos suggests Graves' disease. Unilateral involvement suggests a tumor or an inflammatory lesion of the orbit but may also be seen in Graves' disease.

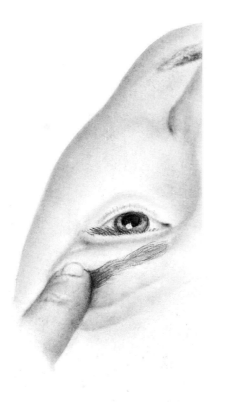
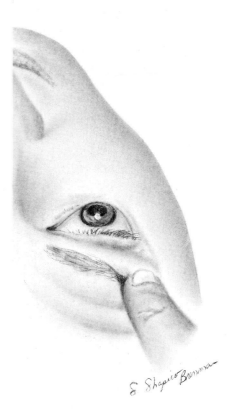

EYEBROWS. Inspect the eyebrows, noting their quantity and distribution and any scaliness of the underlying skin.

Scaliness in seborrheic dermatitis.

EYELIDS. Note the position of the lids in relation to the eyeballs. Inspect for:

- Width of the palpebral fissues
- Edema of the lids
- Color of the lids (*e.g.,* redness)
- Lesions
- Condition and direction of the eyelashes
- Adequacy with which the eyelids close. Look for this especially when the eyes are unusually prominent, when there is facial paralysis, or when the patient is unconscious.

See Table 7-3, Abnormalities of the Eyelids (p. 199). *Blepharitis* is an inflammation of the eyelids along the lid margins, often with crusting or scales.

Failure of the eyelids to close exposes the corneas to serious damage.

LACRIMAL APPARATUS. Briefly inspect the regions of the lacrimal gland and lacrimal sac for swelling.

See Table 7-4, Lumps and Swellings In and Around the Eyes (p. 200).

Look for excessive tearing or dryness of the eyes. The proper assessment of dryness may require special testing, as described in texts of ophthalmology.

Excessive tearing may result from increased tear production due to conjunctival inflammation or corneal irritation or from inadequate drainage due to ectropion (p. 199) or nasolacrimal duct obstruction.

Special Technique for Nasolacrimal Duct Obstruction. Ask the patient to look up. Press on the lower lid close to the medial canthus, just *inside* the rim of the bony orbit. You are thus compressing the lacrimal sac.

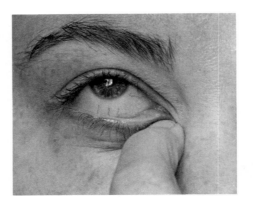

Look for fluid regurgitated out of the puncta into the eye. Avoid this test if the area is inflamed and tender.

Regurgitation of mucopurulent fluid from the puncta suggests an obstructed nasolacrimal duct.

CONJUNCTIVA AND SCLERA. Ask the patient to look up as you depress both lower lids with your thumbs, exposing the sclera and conjunctiva. Inspect the sclera and palpebral conjunctiva for color, and note the vascular pattern against the white scleral background. Look for any nodules or swelling.

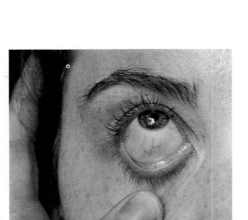

An apparently yellow sclera indicates jaundice. The pigment is actually in the overlying bulbar conjunctiva.

Pale palpebral conjunctiva of anemia

| Techniques of Examination | Examples of Abnormalities |

Techniques of Examination | **Examples of Abnormalities**

If you need a fuller view of the eye, rest your thumb and finger on the bones of the cheek and brow, respectively, and spread the lids.

Ask the patient to look to each side and down.

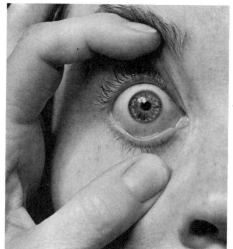

Increased number and size of visible vessels in inflammation and other disorders. See Table 7-5, Red Eyes (p. 201).

Special Technique for Inspection of the Upper Palpebral Conjunctiva. Adequate examination of the eye in search of a foreign body requires eversion of the upper eyelid. To do this:

1. Instruct the patient to <u>look down.</u>
2. Get the patient to relax the eyes —by reassurance and by gentle, assured, and deliberate movements.
3. Raise the upper eyelid slightly so that the eyelashes protrude, and then grasp the upper eyelashes and pull them gently down and forward.
4. Place a small stick such as an applicator or a tongue blade at least 1 cm above the lid margin (and therefore at the upper border of the tarsal plate). Push down on the upper eyelid, thus everting it or turning it "inside out." Do not press on the eyeball itself.
5. Secure the upper lashes against the eyebrow with your fingers and inspect the palpebral conjunctiva.
6. After your inspection, grasp the upper eyelashes and pull them gently forward. Ask the patient <u>to look up.</u> The eyelid will return to its normal position.

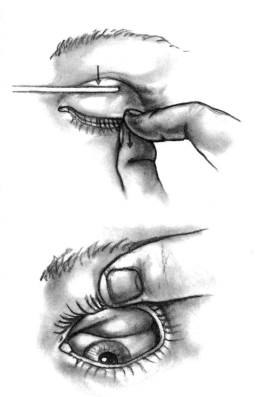

CORNEA AND LENS. With oblique lighting, inspect the cornea of each eye for opacities and note any opacities in the lens that may be visible through the pupil.

See Table 7-6, Opacities of the Cornea and Lens (p. 202).

IRIS. At the same time, inspect each iris. The markings should be clearly defined. With your light shining directly from the temporal side, look for a crescentic shadow on the medial side of the iris. Since the iris is normally fairly flat and forms a relatively open angle with the cornea, this lighting casts no shadow.

Occasionally the iris bows abnormally far forward, forming an unusually narrow angle with the cornea. The light then casts a crescentic shadow.

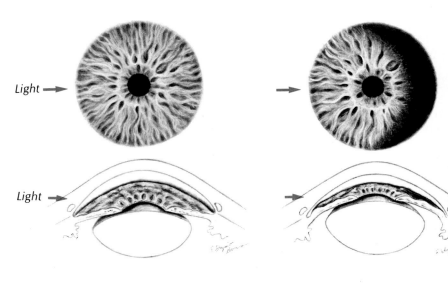

In the more common kind of glaucoma—open-angle glaucoma—the normal spatial relationship between iris and cornea is preserved and no shadow is cast, just as in a normal eye.

This narrow angle increases the risk of acute narrow-angle (angle-closure) glaucoma—a sudden increase in intraocular pressure when drainage of aqueous humor is blocked.

PUPILS. Inspect the size, shape, and equality of the pupils. Slight inequality of the pupils may be normal (benign anisocoria) but must be evaluated carefully.

Pupillary reactions are normal in benign anisocoria. Compare this entity with Horner's syndrome, oculomotor nerve paralysis, and tonic pupil. See Table 7-7, Pupillary Abnormalities (pp. 203–204).

Test the *pupillary reactions to light.* Ask the patient to look into the distance, and shine a bright light obliquely into each pupil in turn. (Both the distant gaze and the oblique lighting help to prevent a near reaction.) Look for:

● The direct reaction (pupillary constriction in the same eye)
● The consensual reaction (pupillary constriction in the opposite eye)

Always darken the room and use a bright light before deciding that a pupillary reaction is absent.

Miosis refers to constriction of the pupils, *mydriasis* to dilation.

If the reaction to light is impaired or questionable, test the *near reaction.* Testing one eye at a time makes it easier to concentrate on pupillary responses, without the distraction of extraocular movement. Hold your finger or pencil about 10 cm from the patient's eye. Ask the patient to look alternately at it and into the distance directly behind it. Watch for pupillary constriction with near effort.

EXTRAOCULAR MUSCLES. Look for weakness or imbalance of the extraocular muscles. From 2 or 3 feet directly in front of the patient, shine a light onto the eyes and ask the patient to look at it. Observing from directly behind the light, inspect the reflections in the patient's corneas. They should be visible slightly nasal to the center of the pupils.

Then assess the extraocular movements. Ask the patient to follow your finger or pencil as you sweep through the six cardinal directions of gaze. Making a wide H in the air, lead the patient's gaze (1) to the patient's extreme right, (2) to the right and upward, and (3) down on the right; then (4) without pausing in the middle, to the extreme left, (5) to the left and upward, and (6) down on the left. Move your finger or pencil at a comfortable distance from the patient. Because middle-aged or older people may have difficulty focusing on near objects, it is helpful to make this distance greater for them than for young people. Pause during upward and lateral gaze to detect nystagmus. Some patients move their heads to follow your finger. If necessary, hold the head in the proper midline position.

Testing the near reaction is helpful in diagnosing Argyll Robertson and tonic (Adie's) pupils (see p. 204).

Asymmetry of the corneal reflections indicates a deviation from normal ocular alignment, which may be caused by muscle weakness. If you notice asymmetry or if a patient has complained of double vision or eyestrain, do a *cover test* (see p. 205). A cover test may bring out a latent muscle imbalance not otherwise seen.

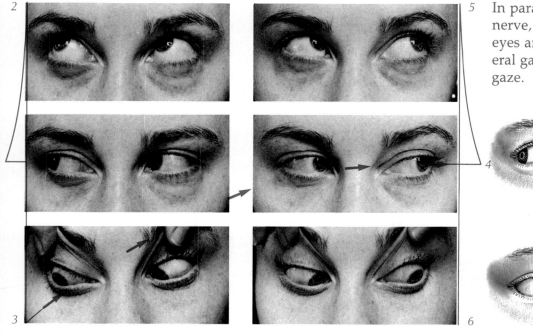

In paralysis of the left 6th nerve, illustrated below, the eyes are conjugate in right lateral gaze but not in left lateral gaze.

LOOKING RIGHT

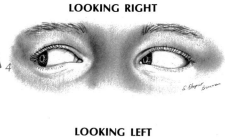

LOOKING LEFT

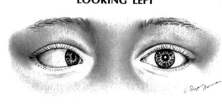

Inspect for:

- The normal conjugate, or parallel, movements of the eyes in each direction, or any deviation from normal

- *Nystagmus,* a fine rhythmic oscillation of the eyes. A few beats of nystagmus on extreme lateral gaze are within normal limits. If you see it, bring your finger in to within the field of binocular vision and look again.

- The relation of the upper eyelid to the globe as the eyes move from above downward. Normally the lid overlaps the iris slightly throughout this movement. If you suspect hyperthyroidism, ask the patient to follow your finger again as you move it slowly from up to down in the midline.

Finally, ask the patient to follow your finger or pencil as you move it in toward the bridge of the nose. Note convergence of the eyes. This is normally sustained to within 5 cm to 8 cm.

See Table 7-8, Deviations of the Eyes (p. 205).

Sustained nystagmus within the binocular field of gaze is seen in a variety of neurologic conditions. See Table 18-1, Nystagmus (pp. 548–549).

In the lid lag of hyperthyroidism a rim of sclera is seen between the upper lid and iris, and the lid appears to lag behind the globe.

Poor convergence in hyperthyroidism

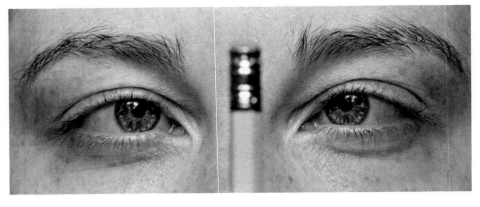

CONVERGENCE

OPHTHALMOSCOPIC EXAMINATION. In general health care, you will usually examine your patients' eyes without dilating their pupils. Your view is therefore limited to the posterior structures of the retinal surface. To see more peripheral structures, to evaluate the macula well, or to investigate unexplained visual loss, you will need to dilate the pupils unless there is a contraindication. Use an appropriate mydriatic drug such as tropicamide (Mydriacyl). The patient should understand in advance that mydriatic drops cause temporary sensitivity to light and impairment of accommodation.

If you wear glasses for marked nearsightedness or severe astigmatism, leave them on. If patients have such refractive errors and you cannot focus clearly on their fundi, it may be easier to examine them with their glasses on. Patients with contact lenses may leave them in.

Contraindications for mydriatic drops include (1) head injury and coma, in which continuing observations of pupillary reactions are important, and (2) any suspicion of narrow-angle glaucoma.

Darken the room. Switch on the ophthalmoscope light, and adjust it to the large round beam of white light.* By shining this light on the back of your hand, you can be sure that you are using the light you want and that the ophthalmoscope's electrical charge is adequate.

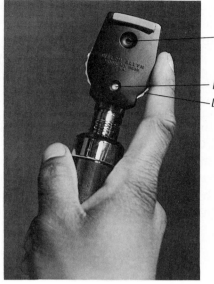

Aperture

Indicator of diopters

Lens disc

Turn the lens disc to 0 diopters (a lens that neither converges nor diverges the light rays). Keep your index finger on the lens disc so that you can focus the ophthalmoscope during the examination.

Use your *right hand* and *right eye* for the patient's *right eye;* your *left hand* and *left eye* for the patient's *left eye.* You thereby avoid facing your patient nose to nose, and your examination is closer, more mobile, and less intimate. Initially you will have difficulty using your nondominant eye, but persist. Hold your ophthalmoscope firmly braced up under the medial aspect of your bony orbit with its handle tilted laterally at about a 20° slant from the vertical. You should be able to see clearly through its aperture. Ask the patient to look slightly up and over your shoulder and gaze at a specific point on the wall.

From a position about 15 inches away from the patient and about 15° lateral to the patient's line of vision, shine the light beam on the pupil. Note the orange glow in the pupil—the *red reflex.* Also note any opacities interrupting the red reflex.

Absence of a red reflex suggests an opacity of the lens (cataract) or possibly of the vitreous. Less commonly, a detached retina or, in children, a retinoblastoma may obscure this reflex. Do not be fooled by an artificial eye, which of course has no red reflex either.

Keeping the light beam focused on the red reflex, move in on the 15° line toward the pupil until your ophthalmoscope is very close to it, almost touching the patient's eyelashes. By placing the thumb of your other hand on the patient's eyebrow you gain extra proprioceptive guidance as you come closer to the patient, but this maneuver is not essential.

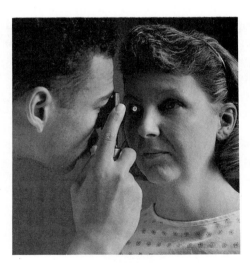

* Some clinicians like to use the large round beam for large pupils, the small round beam for small pupils. The other beams are rarely helpful. The slitlike beam is sometimes used to assess elevations or concavities in the retina, the green (or red-free) beam to detect small red lesions, and the grid to make measurements. Ignore the last three lights and practice with the large round white beam.

Try to keep both eyes open. Keep your eyes relaxed, as if gazing into the distance. You will thereby minimize the fluctuating blurriness caused by your automatic attempts to accommodate. Some patients find the light of modern ophthalmoscopes too bright. By lowering the light's intensity somewhat you can usually improve their comfort and cooperation without impairing your observations.

You should now be seeing the retina in the vicinity of the *optic disc*—a yellowish orange to creamy pink oval or round structure. The disc will probably fill your field of gaze or even exceed it. If you do not see it, follow a blood vessel centrally until you do. You can tell which direction is central by noting the angles at which vessels branch and the progressive enlargement of vessel size at each junction as you approach the disc. Some trial and error may be necessary.

When the lens has been removed surgically, its magnifying effect is lost. Retinal structures then look much smaller than usual, and you can see a much larger expanse of fundus.

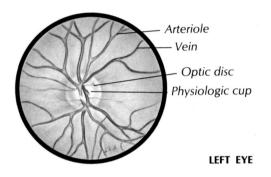

— Arteriole
— Vein
— Optic disc
— Physiologic cup

LEFT EYE

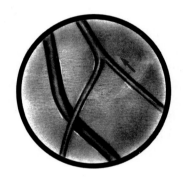

Now *bring the optic disc into sharp focus* by adjusting the lens disc. When examining a nearsighted (myopic) patient, whose eyeball is somewhat longer than normal, you will need to use a lens with a longer focus. To do this, rotate the lens disc counterclockwise to the lenses identified by the red numbers, indicating minus diopters.* When examining a farsighted patient or one whose own lens has been surgically removed, rotate the disc clockwise to the lenses of plus diopters, indicated by the black numbers. These points are illustrated below.

When the patient's eye, as well as your own, is normal in size, you can usually focus clearly on the retina with a lens of 0 diopters (clear glass).

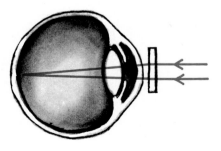

NORMAL EYE

* A diopter is a unit that measures the power of a lens to converge or diverge light.

When the patient is nearsighted, you will need a lens with a longer focus (minus diopters). When a nearsighted patient wears contact lenses, you do not need to make this adjustment.

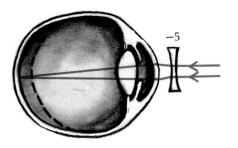

NEARSIGHTED EYE

In a nearsighted (myopic) eye, retinal structures are magnified more than usual. The disc exceeds the size of your view.

A lens with a shorter focus (*e.g.*, +1 or +2 diopters) is needed for far-sighted eyes.

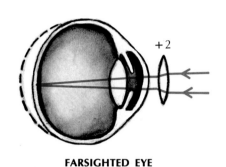

FARSIGHTED EYE

In a farsighted (hyperopic) eye, retinal structures look somewhat smaller than usual.

Note:

- The clarity of the disc outline. The nasal outline may be normally somewhat blurred.
- The color of the disc, normally yellowish orange to creamy pink
- The possible presence of normal white or pigmented rings or crescents around the disc
- The size of the central physiologic cup, if present. This cup is normally yellowish white. Its horizontal diameter is usually less than half the horizontal diameter of the disc.
- The symmetry of the eyes in terms of these observations

See Table 7-9, Normal Variations of the Optic Disc (p. 206).

See Table 7-10, Abnormalities of the Optic Disc (p. 207).

You may also see some pulsations of the veins as they cross the disc. Gentle pressure on the eye through the eyelid usually makes such pulsations evident even if you did not see them earlier. This maneuver is not, however, part of the routine examination.

The presence of venous pulsations at the disc gives some but not complete assurance that cerebrospinal fluid pressure is normal.

Identify the *arterioles and veins*. They may be distinguished by the features listed in the following table.

	ARTERIOLES	VEINS
COLOR	Light red	Dark red
SIZE	Smaller ($^2/_3$ to $^4/_5$ the diameter of veins)	Larger
LIGHT REFLEX *(or reflection)*	Bright	Inconspicuous or absent

Follow the vessels peripherally in each of four directions, noting their relative sizes and the character of the arteriovenous crossings. Identify any lesions of the surrounding *retina* and note their size, shape, color, and distribution. As you search the retina, move your head and instrument as a unit, using the patient's pupil as an imaginary fulcrum. Until you gain experience, you may repeatedly lose your view of the retina because your light falls out of the pupil. You will improve with practice.

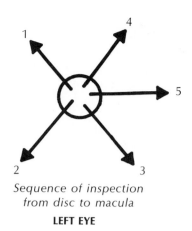

Sequence of inspection from disc to macula

LEFT EYE

See Table 7-11, Retinal Arterioles and Arteriovenous Crossings: Normal and Hypertensive (p. 208).

See Table 7-12, Red Spots and Streaks in the Fundi (p. 209).

See Table 7-13, Light-Colored Spots in the Fundi (pp. 210–211).

See Color Plate 7-1, Ocular Fundi (pp. 213–215).

Finally, by directing your light beam laterally or by asking the patient to look directly into the light, inspect the *macula*. This is an avascular area somewhat larger than the disc, with no distinct margins. Except in older people, the tiny bright reflection at its center—the fovea—helps to identify it. Shimmering light reflections in the macular area are common in young people.

The macular area is especially important because it is responsible for central vision. Senile macular degeneration is an important cause of impaired central vision in elderly people. It takes many forms, including hemorrhages, exudates, cysts, and "holes." A common form with altered pigmentation is illustrated here.

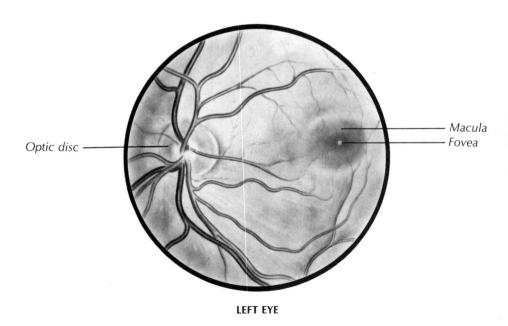

Optic disc

Macula
Fovea

LEFT EYE

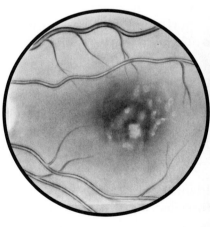

SENILE MACULAR DEGENERATION

If you suspect opacities in the *vitreous* or *lens*, inspect these normally transparent structures by rotating the lens disc progressively to diopters of around +10 or +12. This maneuver focuses on the anterior structures within the eyeball.

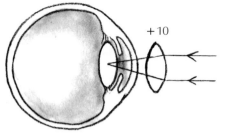

ANTERIOR STRUCTURES

Vitreous floaters may be seen as dark specks or strands at levels between the fundus and the lens. Cataracts are more anterior and more homogeneous densities in the lens.

A NOTE ON MEASUREMENT WITHIN THE EYE. Lesions of the retina can be located in relationship to the optic disc and are measured in terms of "disc diameters" and diopters. For example, among the cotton wool patches illustrated on the right there is an irregular one between 1 and 2 o'clock, less than ½ disc diameter from the disc, and measuring about 1 × ½ disc diameters.

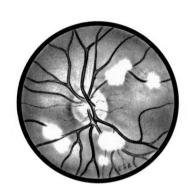

The elevated optic disc of papilledema can be measured by noting the differences in diopters of the two lenses used to focus clearly on the disc and on the uninvolved retina.

Clear focus here at +3 diopters
Clear focus here at −1 diopter

+3 − (−1) = +4, therefore a disc elevation of 4 diopters

FOR INTEREST. On ophthalmoscopic examination, the normal retina is magnified about 15 times, the normal iris about 4 times. The optic disc actually measures about 1.5 mm. At the retina, 3 diopters of elevation = 1 mm.

THE EARS

THE AURICLE. Inspect each auricle and surrounding tissues for deformities, lumps, or skin lesions.

See Table 7-14, Nodules In and Around the Ears (p. 219).

If ear pain, discharge, or inflammation is present, move the auricle up and down, press the tragus, and press firmly just behind the ear.

Movement of the auricle and tragus is painful in acute otitis externa, but not in otitis media. Tenderness behind the ear may be present in otitis media.

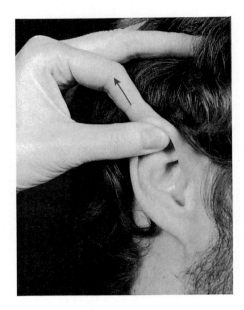

EAR CANAL AND DRUM. For the otoscopic examination, tip the patient's head to the opposite side. Grasp the auricle firmly but gently, while pulling it upward, back, and slightly out.

Insert into the canal, slightly down and forward, the largest ear speculum that the canal will accommodate. Two grips are illustrated. In the second, which is usually preferable, your hand is braced against the patient's head so that it can follow unexpected movements of the patient's head and thus avoid injury to the ear canal.

Nontender nodular swellings covered by normal skin deep in the ear canals suggest *osteomas*. These are nonmalignant overgrowths, which may obscure the drum.

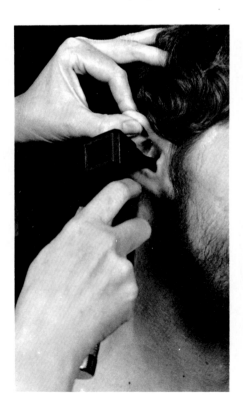
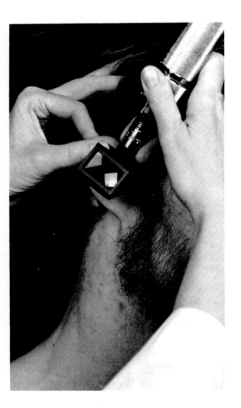

Identify any discharge or foreign bodies in the ear canal and note any redness or swelling. Cerumen, which varies in color and consistency from yellow and flaky to brown and sticky or even to dark and hard, may wholly or partly obscure your view.

In acute otitis externa the canal is often swollen, narrowed, moist, pale, and tender, as shown below. It may be reddened.

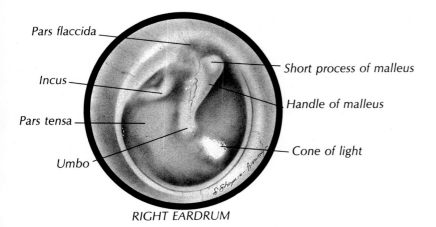

RIGHT EARDRUM

(After Hawke M, Keene M, Alberti PW: Clinical Otoscopy: A Text and Colour Atlas. Edinburgh, Churchill Livingstone, 1984)

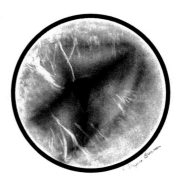

Inspect the eardrum, noting its color and contour.

In chronic otitis externa the skin of the canal is often thickened, red, and itchy.

Red bulging drum of acute purulent otitis media, amber drum of a serous effusion.

Identify the handle of the malleus, note its position, and inspect the short process. Find the cone of light.

An unusually prominent short process and a prominent handle that looks more horizontal suggest a retracted drum.

Gently move the speculum so that you can see as much of the drum as possible, including the pars flaccida superiorly and the margins of the pars tensa. Look for any perforations. The anterior and inferior margins of the drum may be obscured by the ear canal.

See Color Plate 7-2, Abnormalities of the Eardrum (pp. 216–217).

Mobility of the eardrum can be evaluated with a pneumatic otoscope. See page 603.

A serous effusion, a thickened drum, or purulent otitis media may decrease mobility.

AUDITORY ACUITY. To estimate hearing, test one ear at a time. Ask the patient to occlude one ear with a finger or, better still, occlude it yourself. When auditory acuity on the two sides is different, move your finger rapidly, but gently, in the occluded canal. The noise so produced will help to prevent the occluded ear from doing the work of the ear you wish to test. Then, standing 1 or 2 feet away, exhale fully (so as to minimize the intensity of your voice) and whisper softly toward the unoccluded ear. Choose numbers or other words with two equally accented syllables, such as "nine-four," or "baseball." If necessary, increase the intensity of your voice to a medium whisper, a loud whisper, and then a soft, medium, and loud voice. To make sure the patient does not read your lips, cover your mouth or obstruct the patient's vision.

If hearing is diminished, try to distinguish between conduction and sensorineural hearing loss. You need a quiet room and a tuning fork of 512 Hz, preferably, or possibly 1024 Hz. These frequencies fall within the range of human speech (300 Hz–3000 Hz)—the functionally most important range. Forks with lower pitches may cause you to overestimate bone conduction and may also be felt as vibration in addition to being heard. Set the fork into *light* vibration by briskly stroking it between thumb and index finger ➝ or by tapping it on your knuckles.

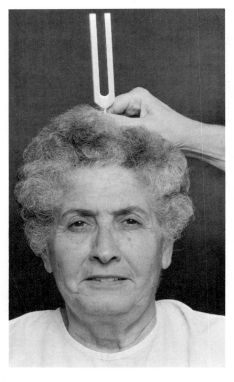

1. *Test for lateralization (Weber test).* Place the base of the lightly vibrating tuning fork firmly on top of the patient's head or on the midforehead. Ask where the patient hears it: on one or both sides. Normally the sound is heard in the midline or equally in both ears. If nothing is heard, try again, pressing the fork more firmly on the head.

In unilateral conduction hearing loss, sound is heard in, or lateralized to, the impaired ear. Visible explanations include acute otitis media, perforation of the eardrum, and obstruction of the ear canal, as by cerumen.

In unilateral sensorineural hearing loss, sound is heard in the good ear.

2. *Compare air (AC) and bone conduction (BC) (Rinne test).* Place the base of a lightly vibrating tuning fork on the mastoid bone, behind the ear and level with the canal. When the patient can no longer hear the sound, quickly place the fork close to the ear canal and ascertain whether the sound can be heard again. Here the "U" of the fork should face forward, thus maximizing its sound for the patient. Normally the sound is heard longer through air than through bone (AC > BC).

In conduction hearing loss, sound is heard through bone as long as or longer than it is through air (a negative Rinne test). In sensorineural hearing loss, sound is heard longer through air (the normal pattern and a positive Rinne test). See Table 7-15, Patterns of Hearing Loss (pp. 220–221).

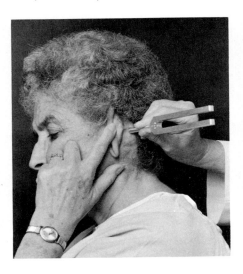
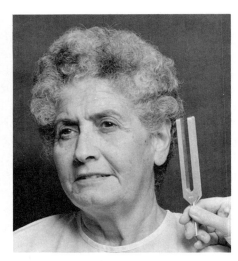

THE NOSE. Inspect the anterior and inferior surfaces of the nose. Gentle pressure on the tip of the nose with your thumb usually widens the nostrils and, with the aid of a penlight or otoscope light, you can get a partial view of each nasal vestibule.

Note any tenderness, asymmetry of the nose, or deformity. If tenderness is present, be particularly gentle and manipulate the nose as little as possible.

If you suspect nasal obstruction, test for it by pressing on each ala nasi in turn and asking the patient to breathe in.

To inspect the inside of the nose, use an otoscope, preferably equipped with a short, wide nasal speculum and a magnifying lens.* Tilt the patient's head back a bit and insert the speculum gently into the vestibule of each nostril, avoiding contact with the sensitive nasal septum. Hold the otoscope handle to one side to avoid the patient's chin and improve your mobility. By directing the speculum posteriorly, then somewhat upward, try to see both the lower and the upper portions of the nose. The passage itself is narrow and slitlike. Some asymmetry of the two sides is normal.

Tenderness of the nasal tip or alae suggests local infection (vestibulitis or furunculosis). Deviation of the lower septum is common and may be easily visible. It seldom obstructs air flow.

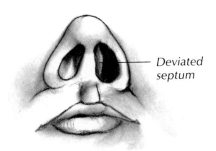

Deviated septum

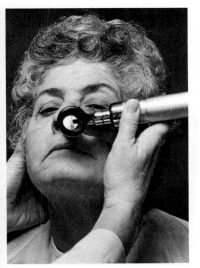

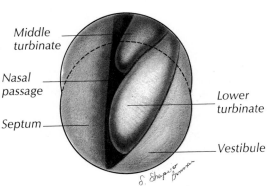

Middle turbinate

Nasal passage

Septum

Lower turbinate

Vestibule

* Unfortunately, most otoscopes that magnify do not now accept a short, wide nasal speculum. A nasal illuminator has such a speculum but lacks magnification. Some clinicians use an ear speculum in the nose, but the view is constricted. Otolaryngologists use special lighting and equipment not widely available to others.

Inspect:

1. The nasal mucosa that covers the septum and turbinates. Note its color and any swelling, bleeding, or exudate. If exudate is present, note its character: clear, mucopurulent, or purulent. The nasal mucosa is normally somewhat redder than the oral mucosa.

In viral rhinitis the mucosa is reddened and swollen; in allergic rhinitis it may be pale, bluish, or red.

2. The nasal septum. Note any deviation, inflammation, or perforation of the septum. The lower anterior portion of the septum (where the patient's finger can reach) is a common source of *epistaxis* (nosebleed).

Fresh blood or crusting may be seen. Causes of septal perforation include trauma, surgery, and the intranasal use of cocaine or amphetamines.

3. Any abnormalities such as ulcers or polyps

Polyps are pale, semitranslucent masses that usually come from the middle meatus.

Make it a habit to place all nasal and ear specula outside your instrument case after use. Then discard them or clean and disinfect them appropriately. (Check with the policies of your institution.)

THE SINUSES. Palpate for *frontal sinus tenderness* by pressing up from under the bony brow on each side. Avoid pressure on the eyes. Then press up on each *maxillary sinus.*

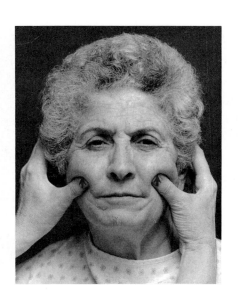

Local tenderness, together with symptoms such as pain, fever, and nasal discharge, suggests acute sinusitis involving the frontal or maxillary sinuses.

Transillumination of the Sinuses is not routine, but it is often helpful when sinus tenderness or other symptoms suggest sinusitis. The room should be thoroughly darkened. Using a strong, narrow light source, place the light snugly deep under each brow, close to the nose. Shield the

Absence of glow on one or both sides suggests a thickened mucosa or secretions in the frontal sinus, but it may also

light with your hand. Look for a dim red glow as light is transmitted through the air-filled frontal sinus to the forehead.

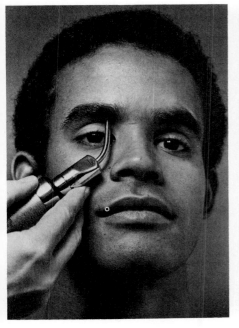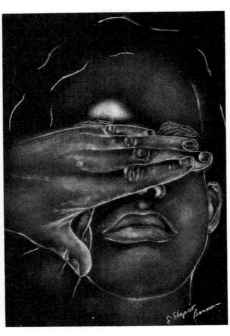

TRANSILLUMINATION OF FRONTAL SINUS

Ask the patient to tilt his or her head back with mouth opened wide. (An upper denture should first be removed.) Shine the light downward from just below the inner aspect of each eye. Look through the open mouth at the hard palate. A reddish glow indicates a normal air-filled maxillary sinus.

Absence of glow suggests thickened mucosa or secretions in the maxillary sinus. See pp. 606–607 for an alternative method of transilluminating the maxillary sinuses.

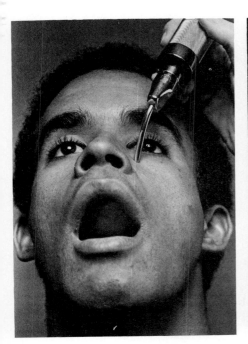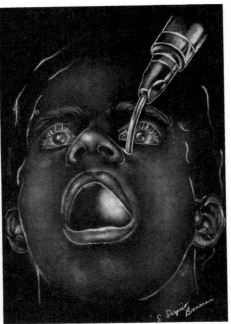

TRANSILLUMINATION OF MAXILLARY SINUS

THE MOUTH AND THE PHARYNX

If the patient wears dentures, offer a paper towel and ask the patient to remove them so that you can see the mucosa underneath. If suspicious ulcers or nodules are observed, put on a glove or finger cot and palpate the lesion, noting especially any thickening or infiltration of the tissues that might suggest malignancy.

Inspect:

THE LIPS. Observe their color and moisture, and note any lumps, ulcers, or cracking.

THE BUCCAL MUCOSA. Look into the patient's open mouth and, with a good light and the help of a tongue blade, inspect the buccal mucosa for color, pigmentation, ulcers, white patches, and nodules. Patchy brown pigmentation is normal in black people.

THE GUMS AND TEETH. Look for

● Inflammation, swelling, bleeding, retraction, or discoloration of the gums
● Loose, missing, or carious teeth and any abnormalities in the position or shape of the teeth

THE ROOF OF THE MOUTH. Inspect the color and architecture of the hard palate.

THE TONGUE. Inspect the dorsum of the tongue, including its color and papillae. Note any abnormal smoothness.

Ask the patient to put out his or her tongue, and inspect it for symmetry —a test of the 12th (hypoglossal) cranial nerve. Note its size.

Inspect the sides and the undersurface of the tongue together with the floor of the mouth. These are the areas where malignancies are most likely to develop. Note any white or reddened areas, nodules, or ulcerations. Because cancer of the tongue is more common in men over age 50, especially in those who use tobacco and drink alcohol, a further maneuver is indicated for patients in this group. Explain what you plan to do and put on gloves. Ask the patient to protrude his tongue. With your right hand, grasp the tip of the tongue with a square of gauze and gently pull it to the patient's left. Inspect the side of the tongue, and then palpate it with your gloved left hand, feeling for any induration. Reverse the procedure for the other side.

Bright red edematous mucosa underneath a denture suggests denture sore mouth. There may be ulcers or papillary granulation tissue.

Cyanosis, pallor. See Table 7-16, Abnormalities of the Lips (pp. 222–223).

See Table 7-17, Abnormalities of the Buccal Mucosa and Hard Palate (p. 224). Use of smokeless tobacco increases the risk of cancer of the buccal mucosa and gums.

See Table 7-18, Abnormalities of the Gums and Teeth (pp. 225–226).

Torus palatinus, a midline lump (see p. 224)

See Table 7-19, Abnormalities of the Tongue (p. 227).

Asymmetrical protrusion in a 12th nerve lesion and in cancer of the tongue; enlargement in myxedema and acromegaly

Cancer of the tongue is the second most common cancer of the mouth, second only to cancer of the lip. Any persistent nodule or ulcer, either red or white, must be suspect. Induration of the lesion further increases the possibility of malignancy. Cancer occurs most frequently on the side of the tongue, and next most often at its base.

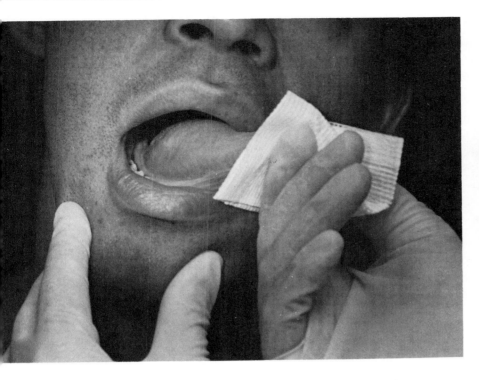

More common than cancer are *tori mandibulares*—innocuous bony nodules inside the lower jaw of some adults. At first small, tori may grow quite large, as shown below.

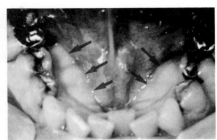

Palpate any other lesions you may have noticed in the mouth.

THE PHARYNX. Now, with the patient's mouth open but the tongue not protruded, ask the patient to say "ah" or yawn. This action may be enough to let you see the pharynx well. If not, press a tongue blade firmly down upon the midpoint of the arched tongue—far enough back to get good visualization of the pharynx but not so far that you cause gagging. Simultaneously, ask for an "ah" or a yawn. Note the rise of the soft palate—a test of the 10th cranial (vagus) nerve.

See Table 7-20, Abnormalities of the Pharynx (p. 228).

Inspect the soft palate, anterior and posterior pillars, uvula, tonsils, and posterior pharynx. Note their color and symmetry and any evidence of exudate, swelling, ulceration, or tonsillar enlargement. If possible, palpate any suspicious area for induration or tenderness. Tonsils have crypts, or deep infoldings of squamous epithelium. Whitish spots of normal exfoliating epithelium may sometimes be seen in these crypts.

White patches of exudate associated with redness and swelling, however, suggest acute exudative pharyngitis.

Break or discard your tongue blade after use.

THE NECK

SURVEY. Inspect the neck, noting its symmetry and any masses or scars. Look for enlargement of the parotid or submaxillary glands, and note any visible lymph nodes.

A scar of past thyroid surgery may be the clue to unsuspected hypothyroidism.

LYMPH NODES. Palpate the lymph nodes. Using the pads of your index and middle fingers, move the skin over the underlying tissues in each area rather than moving your fingers over the skin. The patient should be relaxed, with neck flexed slightly forward and, if needed, slightly toward the side of the examination. You can usually examine both sides at once. For the submental node, however, it is helpful to feel with one hand while bracing the top of the head with the other.

Feel in sequence for the following nodes:

1. Preauricular—in front of the ear
2. Posterior auricular—superficial to the mastoid process
3. Occipital—at the base of the skull posteriorly
4. Tonsillar—at the angle of the mandible
5. Submaxillary—midway between the angle and the tip of the mandible. These nodes are usually smaller and smoother than the lobulated submaxillary gland against which they lie.
6. Submental—in the midline a few cm behind the tip of the mandible
7. Superficial cervical—superficial to the sternomastoid
8. Posterior cervical chain—along the anterior edge of the trapezius
9. Deep cervical chain—deep to the sternomastoid and often inaccessible to examination. Hook your thumb and fingers around either side of the sternomastoid muscle to find them.
10. Supraclavicular—deep in the angle formed by the clavicle and the sternomastoid

A "tonsillar node" that pulsates is really the carotid artery.

→ *External lymphatic drainage*
⇉ *Internal lymphatic drainage (eg. from mouth and throat)*

Enlargement of a supraclavicular node, especially on the left, suggests possible metastasis from a thoracic or an abdominal malignancy.

Note their size, shape, delimitation (discrete or matted together), mobility, consistency, and any tenderness. Small, mobile, discrete, nontender nodes are frequently found in normal persons.

Tender nodes suggest inflammation; hard or fixed nodes suggest malignancy.

Enlarged or tender nodes, if unexplained, call for (1) reexamination of the regions they drain, and (2) careful assessment of lymph nodes elsewhere so that you can distinguish between regional and generalized lymphadenopathy.

Occasionally you may mistake a band of muscle or an artery for a lymph node. You should be able to roll a node in two directions: up and down, and side to side. Neither a muscle nor an artery will pass this test.

THE TRACHEA AND THE THYROID GLAND. To orient yourself to the neck, identify the thyroid and cricoid cartilages and the trachea below them. (The hyoid bone, high in the neck, should not be mistaken for a stony hard tumor.)

Inspect the trachea for any deviation from its usual midline position. Then feel for any deviation. Place your finger along one side of the trachea and note the space between it and the sternomastoid. Compare it with the other side. The spaces should be symmetrical.

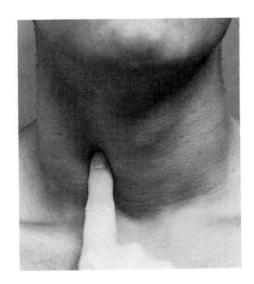

Masses in the neck may push the trachea to one side. Tracheal deviation may also signify important problems in the thorax, such as a mediastinal mass, atelectasis, or a large pneumothorax (see p. 261).

Inspect the neck for the thyroid gland. Ask the patient to bend the head back a bit. Using tangential lighting directed downward from one side of the patient's chin, inspect the region below the cricoid cartilage for the thyroid gland. Then ask the patient to take a sip from a glass of water, again extend the neck somewhat, and swallow. Watch for movement of the thyroid gland, noting its contour and symmetry.

An enlarged thyroid gland, and also many normal ones, may be visible even before swallowing. An enlarged thyroid gland is called a *goiter.*

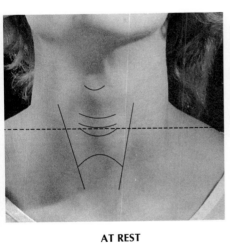

AT REST

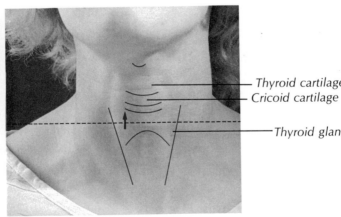

SWALLOWING

— *Thyroid cartilage*
— *Cricoid cartilage*

— *Thyroid gland*

The thyroid gland, the thyroid cartilage, and the cricoid cartilage all normally rise as the person swallows.

Now *palpate the thyroid gland.* Although there are many methods of performing this examination, palpation is probably best done from behind the patient. Because you cannot see what you are doing, you may initially find this position awkward. Orient yourself first to the patient's cricoid cartilage—the basic landmark for the examination. Feeling any thyroid tissue beforehand from in front of the patient may also guide you.

From behind, place the fingers of both hands on the patient's neck so that the index fingers are just below the cricoid. The patient's neck should be extended, but not far enough to tighten the muscles. Adjust the degree of extension as you find necessary. As the patient swallows, the thyroid isthmus should rise under your fingers. By rotating your fingers slightly downward and laterally, feel as much of the lateral lobes as possible, including their lower borders. During both maneuvers the patient should sip water as necessary to swallow as you repeat your palpation.

Although physical characteristics of the thyroid gland, such as size, shape, and consistency, are diagnostically important, they tell you little if anything about thyroid function. Assessment of thyroid function depends upon symptoms, signs elsewhere in the body, and laboratory tests. See Table 7-21, Thyroid Enlargement and Function (p. 229).

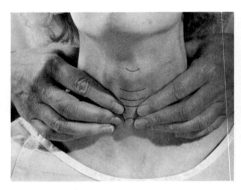
FEELING THE ISTHMUS

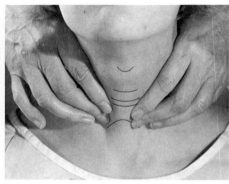
FEELING THE LATERAL LOBES

Note the size, shape, and consistency of the gland and identify any nodules or tenderness. The anterior surface of a lateral lobe is approximately the same size as the distal phalanx of the thumb; its consistency is somewhat rubbery.

The thyroid gland is usually easier to feel in a long slender neck than in a short stocky one. In the latter, further extension of the neck may help. In some persons, however, the thyroid gland is partially or wholly substernal.

If the thyroid gland is enlarged, listen over the lateral lobes with a stethoscope to detect a *bruit* (a sound similar to a cardiac murmur but of noncardiac origin).

A localized systolic or continuous bruit may be heard in hyperthyroidism.

THE CAROTID ARTERIES AND JUGULAR VEINS. You will probably wish to defer detailed examination of the great vessels of the neck until the patient lies down for the cardiovascular examination. Jugular venous distention, however, may be visible in the sitting position and should not be overlooked. You should also be alert to unusually prominent arterial pulsations. See Chapter 9 for further discussion.

Table 7-1   Selected Facies

Table 7-1   Selected Facies

ACROMEGALY

The increased growth hormone of acromegaly produces enlargement of both bone and soft tissues. The head is elongated, with bony prominence of the forehead, nose, and lower jaw. Soft tissues of the nose, lips, and ears also enlarge. The facial features appear generally coarsened.

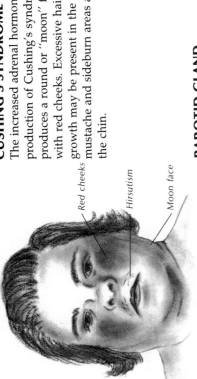

Brow prominent

Soft tissues of nose, ears, lips enlarged

Jaw prominent

CUSHING'S SYNDROME

The increased adrenal hormone production of Cushing's syndrome produces a round or "moon" face with red cheeks. Excessive hair growth may be present in the mustache and sideburn areas and on the chin.

Red cheeks

Hirsutism

Moon face

MYXEDEMA

The patient with severe hypothyroidism, or myxedema, has a dull, puffy facies. The edema, often particularly pronounced around the eyes, does not pit with pressure. The hair and eyebrows are dry, coarse, and thinned. The skin is dry.

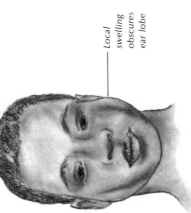

Hair dry, coarse, sparse

Lateral eyebrows thin

Periorbital edema

Puffy dull face with dry skin

PAROTID GLAND ENLARGEMENT

Chronic bilateral asymptomatic parotid gland enlargement may be associated with obesity, diabetes, cirrhosis, and other conditions. Note the swellings anterior to the ear lobes and above the angles of the jaw. Gradual unilateral enlargement suggests neoplasm. Acute enlargement is seen in mumps.

Local swelling obscures ear lobe

NEPHROTIC SYNDROME

The face is edematous and often pale. Swelling usually appears first around the eyes. The eyes may become slitlike when edema is severe.

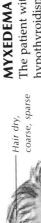

Periorbital edema

Puffy pale face

Lips may be swollen

PARKINSON'S DISEASE

Decreased facial mobility blunts expression. A masklike face may result, with decreased blinking and a characteristic stare. Since the neck and upper trunk tend to flex forward, the patient seems to peer upward toward the observer. Facial skin becomes oily, and drooling may occur.

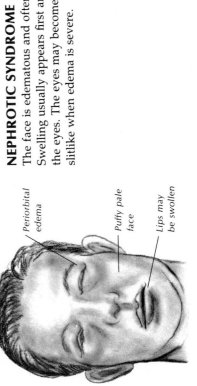
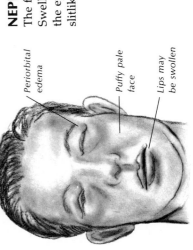

Stare

Decreased mobility

Table 7-2   Visual Field Defects Produced by Selected Lesions in the Visual Pathways

VISUAL FIELDS	BLACKENED FIELD INDICATES AREA OF NO VISION

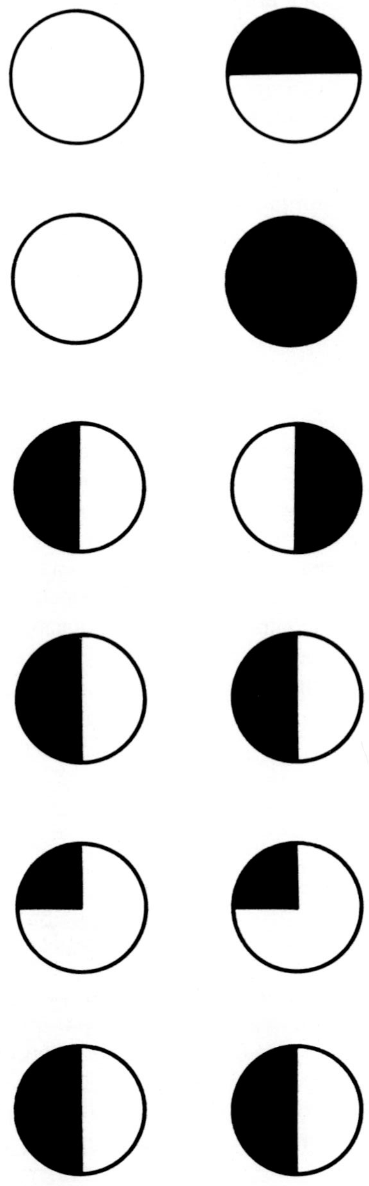

HORIZONTAL DEFECT

Occlusion of a branch of the central retinal artery may cause a horizontal (altitudinal) defect. Shown is the upper field defect associated with occlusion of the inferior branch of this artery.

BLIND RIGHT EYE (*right optic nerve*)

A lesion of the optic nerve, and of course of the eye itself, produces unilateral blindness.

BITEMPORAL HEMIANOPSIA (*optic chiasm*)

A lesion at the optic chiasm may involve only the fibers that are crossing over to the opposite side. Since these fibers originate in the nasal half of each retina, visual loss involves the temporal half of each field.

LEFT HOMONYMOUS HEMIANOPSIA (*right optic tract*)

A lesion of the optic tract interrupts fibers originating on the same side of both eyes. Visual loss in the eyes is therefore similar (homonymous) and involves half of each field (hemianopsia).

HOMONYMOUS LEFT UPPER QUADRANTIC DEFECT (*optic radiation, partial*)

A partial lesion of the optic radiation may involve only a portion of the nerve fibers, producing, for example, a homonymous quadrantic defect.

LEFT HOMONYMOUS HEMIANOPSIA (*right optic radiation*)

A complete interruption of fibers in the optic radiation produces a visual defect similar to that produced by a lesion of the optic tract.

VISUAL PATHWAYS

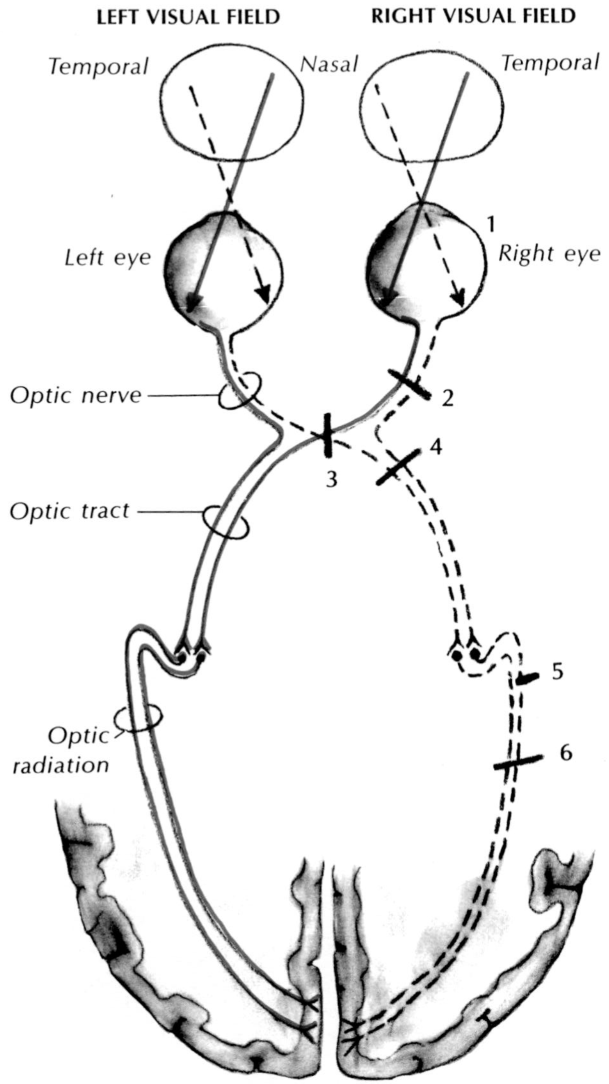

LEFT VISUAL FIELD   RIGHT VISUAL FIELD

Temporal   Nasal   Temporal

Right eye

Left eye

Optic nerve

Optic tract

Optic radiation

LEFT   RIGHT

Table 7-3   Abnormalities of the Eyelids

Table 7-3   Abnormalities of the Eyelids

PTOSIS

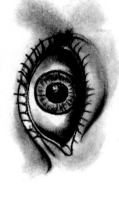

Ptosis refers to drooping of the upper eyelid. Causes include (1) muscular weakness, as in myasthenia gravis, (2) damage to the oculomotor nerve, which controls voluntary elevation of the eyelid, and (3) interference with the sympathetic nerves, which maintain smooth muscle tone of the lid (Horner's syndrome). A weakened muscle, relaxed tissues, and the weight of herniated fat may cause senile ptosis.

RETRACTION OR SPASM OF THE UPPER EYELID AND EXOPHTHALMOS

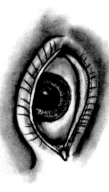

A retracted upper lid is identified by the rim of sclera between lid and iris. The eye has a stare, which often is accentuated by decreased blinking. Look for the associated lid lag when the eye moves slowly from upward to downward gaze. These signs suggest hyperthyroidism. They may simulate or accentuate exophthalmos—an actual forward protrusion of the eyeball (see p. 175).

ECTROPION

In ectropion the margin of the lid is turned outward, exposing the palpebral conjunctiva. When the punctum of the lower lid turns outward, the eye no longer drains satisfactorily and tearing occurs. Ectropion is more common in the elderly.

ENTROPION

Entropion, also more common in the elderly, is an inward turning of the lid margin. The lower lashes, which are often invisible because they are turned inward, irritate the conjunctiva and lower cornea. Asking the patient to squeeze the lids together and then open them helps to demonstrate the problem when it is not obvious.

PERIORBITAL EDEMA

Since the skin of the eyelids is loosely attached to underlying tissues, edema tends to accumulate here more easily than elsewhere. Causes are many. Consider allergies, local inflammation, myxedema, fluid-retaining states such as the nephrotic syndrome, and finally, of course, recent crying.

HERNIATED FAT

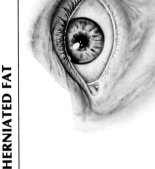

Puffy eyelids can be caused by fat as well as fluid. Fat pushes weakened fascia in the eyelids forward, producing bulges that involve the lower lids, the inner third of the upper ones, or both. Although these bulges appear more often in elderly people, they may also affect younger ones.

Table 7-4   Lumps and Swellings In and Around the Eyes

Table 7-4   Lumps and Swellings In and Around the Eyes

PINGUECULA

A yellowish triangular nodule in the bulbar conjunctiva on either side of the iris, a pinguecula is harmless. Pinguecula appear almost uniformly with aging, first on the nasal and then on the temporal side.

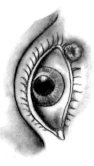
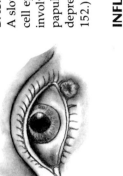

BASAL CELL EPITHELIOMA

A slowly progressive skin cancer, a basal cell epithelioma near the eye usually involves the lower lid. It appears as a papule with a pearly border and a depressed or ulcerated center. (See also p. 152.)

STY (Acute Hordeolum)

A painful, tender, red infection around a hair follicle of the eyelashes, a sty looks like a pimple or boil pointing on the lid margin.

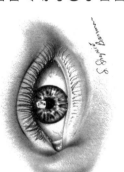

INFLAMMATION OF THE LACRIMAL SAC (Dacryocystitis)

A swelling between the lower eyelid and nose suggests inflammation of the lacrimal sac. It may be acute or chronic. An *acute* inflammation is painful, red, and tender and may have a surrounding cellulitis. *Chronic* inflammation (illustrated) is associated with obstruction of the nasolacrimal duct. Tearing is prominent and pressure on the sac produces regurgitation of material through the puncta of the eyelids.

CHALAZION

A chalazion is a chronic inflammatory lesion involving a meibomian gland. A beady nodule in an otherwise normal lid, it is usually painless. Occasionally a chalazion becomes acutely inflamed but, unlike a sty, usually points inside the lid rather than on the lid margin.

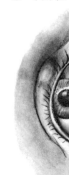

ENLARGEMENT OF THE LACRIMAL GLAND

An enlarged lacrimal gland may displace the eyeball downward, nasally, and forward. A swelling is sometimes visible above the lateral third of the upper lid, giving the lid margin an S-shaped curve. Look for the enlarged gland by raising the temporal part of the upper eyelid as the patient looks down and medially. Causes of lacrimal gland enlargement include inflammation and tumors.

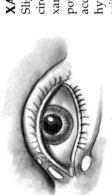
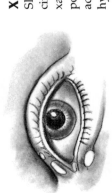

—— *Tarsal plate and conjunctiva*

—— *Lacrimal gland*

XANTHELASMA

Slightly raised, yellowish, well-circumscribed plaques in the skin, xanthelasmas appear along the nasal portions of one or both eyelids. They may accompany lipid disorders (e.g., hypercholesterolemia), but may also occur without such disorders.

Table 7-5   Red Eyes

Table 7-5   Red Eyes

	CONJUNCTIVITIS	CORNEAL INJURY OR INFECTION	ACUTE IRITIS	ACUTE GLAUCOMA	SUBCONJUNCTIVAL HEMORRHAGE
PATTERN OF REDNESS	Conjunctival injection: diffuse dilatation of conjunctival vessels with redness that tends to be maximal peripherally	Ciliary injection: dilatation of deeper vessels that are visible as radiating vessels or a reddish violet flush around the limbus. Ciliary injection is an important sign of these three conditions but may not be apparent. The eye may be diffusely red instead. Other clues of these more serious disorders are pain, decreased vision, unequal pupils, and a less than perfectly clear cornea.			Leakage of blood outside of the vessels, producing a homogeneous, sharply demarcated, red area that fades over days to yellow and then disappears
PAIN	Mild discomfort rather than pain	Moderate to severe, superficial	Moderate, aching, deep	Severe, aching, deep	Absent
VISION	Not affected except for temporary mild blurring due to discharge	Usually decreased	Decreased	Decreased	Not affected
OCULAR DISCHARGE	Watery, mucoid, or mucopurulent	Watery or purulent	Absent	Absent	Absent
PUPIL	Not affected	Not affected unless iritis develops	Small, and with time often irregular	Dilated	Not affected
CORNEA	Clear	Changes depending on cause	Clear or slightly clouded	Steamy, cloudy	Clear
SIGNIFICANCE	Bacterial, viral, and other infections; allergy; irritation	Abrasions and other injuries; viral and bacterial infections	Associated with many ocular and systemic disorders	Acute increase in intraocular pressure —an emergency	Often none. May result from trauma, bleeding disorders, or a sudden increase in venous pressure, as from cough

Table 7-6   Opacities of the Cornea and Lens

Table 7-6   Opacities of the Cornea and Lens

CORNEAL ARCUS

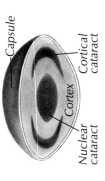

A corneal arcus is a thin grayish white arc or circle not quite at the edge of the cornea. It accompanies normal aging but may also be seen in younger people, especially blacks. In young people a corneal arcus suggests the possibility of hyperlipoproteinemia but does not prove it. Some surveys have revealed no relationship. An arcus does not interfere with vision.

CORNEAL SCAR

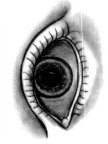

A corneal scar is a superficial grayish white opacity in the cornea, secondary to an old injury, for example, or to inflammation. Size and shape are variable. It should not be confused with the opaque lens of a cataract, visible on a deeper plane and only through the pupil.

PTERYGIUM

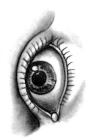

Not a true corneal opacity, a pterygium is a triangular thickening of the bulbar conjunctiva that grows slowly across the cornea, usually from the nasal side. Reddening may occur intermittently. A pterygium may interfere with vision as it encroaches upon the pupil.

CATARACTS

A cataract is an opacity of the lens and therefore can be viewed only through the pupil and on a deeper plane than corneal opacities. Cataracts are classified in many ways. When classification is by cause, old age leads the list—senile cataract. Cataracts may also be classified by location, as illustrated here in two forms—nuclear and peripheral cortical. Both are common in old age. In each of the illustrations the pupil has been widely dilated so that only a narrow rim of iris shows.

CROSS SECTION OF LENS

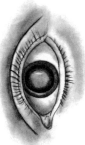

Capsule

Cortical cataract

Cortex

Nuclear cataract

A nuclear cataract forms a central gray opacity, viewed here against a black background as you might see it with a flashlight. Through the ophthalmoscope, it would appear black against the red reflex.

NUCLEAR CATARACT

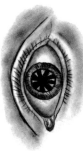

A peripheral cortical cataract produces spokelike shadows that point inward—gray against black as seen with a flashlight, or black against red with an ophthalmoscope.

PERIPHERAL CORTICAL CATARACT

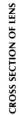

Table 7-7   Pupillary Abnormalities

Table 7-7   Pupillary Abnormalities

BLIND EYE

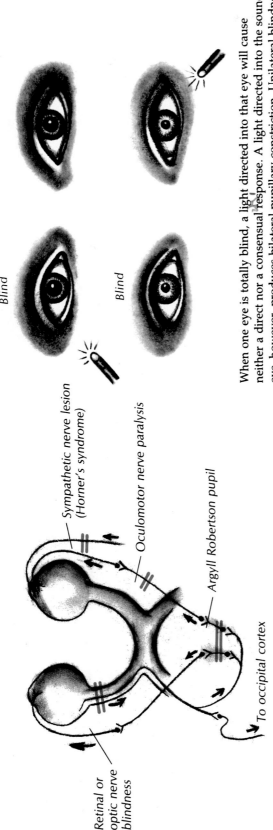

Blind

Blind

Retinal or optic nerve blindness

Sympathetic nerve lesion (Horner's syndrome)

Oculomotor nerve paralysis

Argyll Robertson pupil

To occipital cortex

karen

When one eye is totally blind, a light directed into that eye will cause neither a direct nor a consensual response. A light directed into the sound eye, however, produces bilateral pupillary constriction. Unilateral blindness does not cause pupillary inequality.

MARCUS GUNN (DEAFFERENTED) PUPIL

For illustration of a Marcus Gunn pupil, consider the blind eye above as impaired. A *swinging flashlight test* identifies this pupil. When the vision in one eye is diminished because of disease in the optic nerve, sensory input for the light reaction in that eye is decreased but not absent. A light shining into the impaired eye produces a subnormal response in both eyes alike. A light directed into the sound eye produces normal responses. When the light is swung back to the affected eye, the pupils dilate in spite of the shining light. The direct response of the impaired eye is less than the consensual response elicited immediately beforehand. This test is very useful in identifying optic nerve disease (*e.g.,* retrobulbar neuropathy) as the cause of unilaterally decreased visual acuity.

IRIDECTOMY

Complete

Peripheral

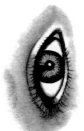

A common cause of pupillary irregularity in the elderly is iridectomy, a surgical incision in the iris, made to treat glaucoma. For cosmetic reasons it is made superiorly.

➡ *Continued*

Table 7-7 (Cont'd.)

Table 7-7 Pupillary Abnormalities

OCULOMOTOR NERVE PARALYSIS

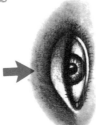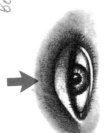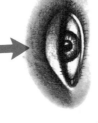

A dilated pupil that reacts neither to light nor with near effort may result from injury to the oculomotor nerve. This is called internal ophthalmoplegia. Ptosis and deviation of the eye laterally are associated when additional branches of the nerve are damaged (external ophthalmoplegia).

TONIC PUPIL (Adie's)

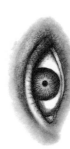

[∂ou]
Bee-Taun, oquano
as~ iaie eenu Sa

A tonic pupil is large, regular, and usually but not always unilateral. The reaction to light is diminished or absent while the near reaction, though slow and delayed, is present. Deep tendon reflexes are often decreased.

ARGYLL ROBERTSON PUPILS

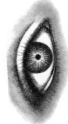

Argyll Robertson pupils are small, irregular, and bilateral. They do not react to light but do react with near effort. They are often, but not necessarily, related to central nervous system syphilis (tabes dorsalis).

HORNER'S SYNDROME

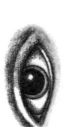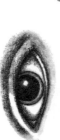

In Horner's syndrome, the sympathetic nerve supply is interrupted, most often in the neck. One pupil is small, regular, and normally reactive to light and near effort. Ptosis of the eyelid is associated, often with loss of sweating on the forehead of the involved side. In congenital Horner's syndrome, the iris on the involved side may be lighter in color than the fellow iris (heterochromia).

DILATED FIXED PUPILS

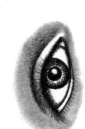

Bilaterally dilated and fixed pupils result from anticholinergic agents (e.g., atropine, mushrooms) and from glutethimide (Doriden) poisoning. Additional causes in the comatose patient include severe brain damage and profound hypoxia.

SMALL FIXED PUPILS

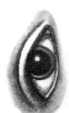

Bilaterally small, fixed, regular pupils result from morphine and related drugs, as well as from miotic drops given, for example, for glaucoma. In a comatose patient a pontine hemorrhage should also be considered.

Table 7-8   Deviations of the Eyes

Table 7-8   Deviations of the Eyes

Deviation of the eyes from their normally conjugate position is termed *strabismus* or *squint*. Strabismus may be classified into two groups: (1) *nonparalytic*, in which the deviation is constant in all directions of gaze, and (2) *paralytic*, in which the deviation varies depending on the direction of gaze.

NONPARALYTIC STRABISMUS

Nonparalytic strabismus is caused by an imbalance in ocular muscle tone. It has many causes, may be hereditary, and usually appears early in childhood. Deviations are further classified according to direction:

CONVERGENT STRABISMUS (*Esotropia*)   **DIVERGENT STRABISMUS (*Exotropia*)**

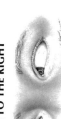

COVER TEST

A cover test is helpful. Here is what you would see in the right monocular esotropia diagrammed in the last three steps on p. 599.

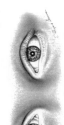

Corneal reflections are asymmetrical.

COVER

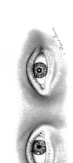

The right eye moves outward to fix on the light. (The left eye is not seen but moves inward to the same degree.)

UNCOVER

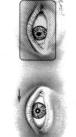

The left eye moves outward to fix on the light. The right eye deviates inward again.

PARALYTIC STRABISMUS

Paralytic strabismus is usually caused by weakness or paralysis of one or more extraocular muscles. Determine the direction of gaze that maximizes the deviation. For example:

A LEFT 6TH NERVE PARALYSIS   **LOOKING TO THE RIGHT**

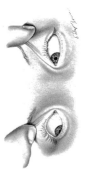

Eyes are conjugate.

LOOKING STRAIGHT AHEAD

Esotropia appears.

LOOKING TO THE LEFT

Esotropia is maximum.

A LEFT 4TH NERVE PARALYSIS   **LOOKING DOWN AND TO THE RIGHT**

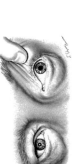

The left eye cannot look down when turned inward. Deviation is maximum in this direction.

A LEFT 3RD NERVE PARALYSIS   **LOOKING STRAIGHT AHEAD**

The eye is pulled outward by action of the 6th nerve. Upward, downward, and inward movements are impaired or lost. Ptosis and pupillary dilatation may be associated.

Table 7-9   *Normal Variations of the Optic Disc*

Table 7-9   Normal Variations of the Optic Disc

PHYSIOLOGIC CUPPING	RINGS AND CRESCENTS	MEDULLATED NERVE FIBERS

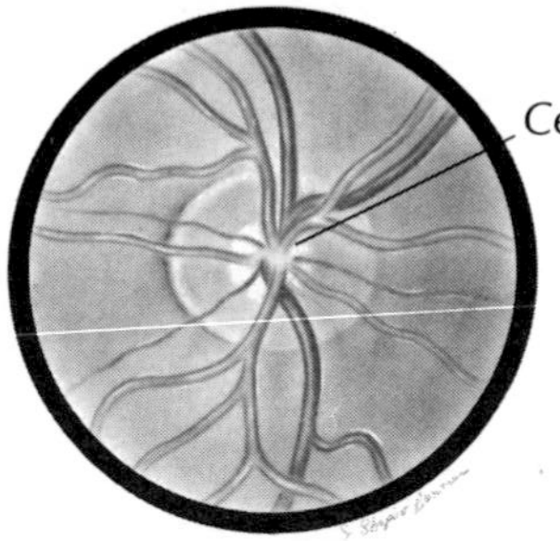

Central cup

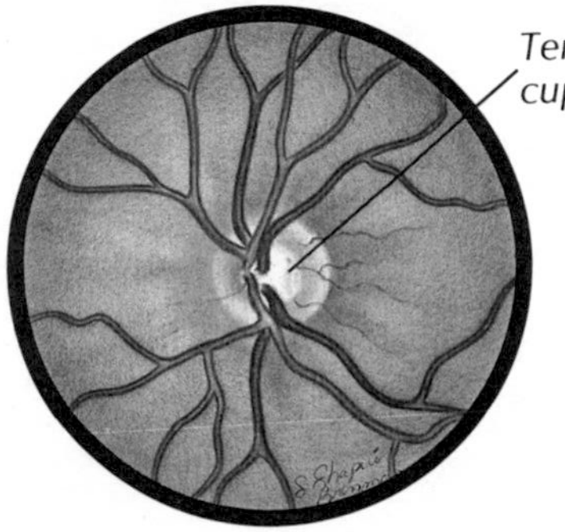

Temporal cup

The physiologic cup is a small whitish depression in the optic disc from which the retinal vessels appear to emerge. Although sometimes absent, the cup is usually visible either centrally or toward the temporal side of the disc. Grayish spots are often seen at its base.

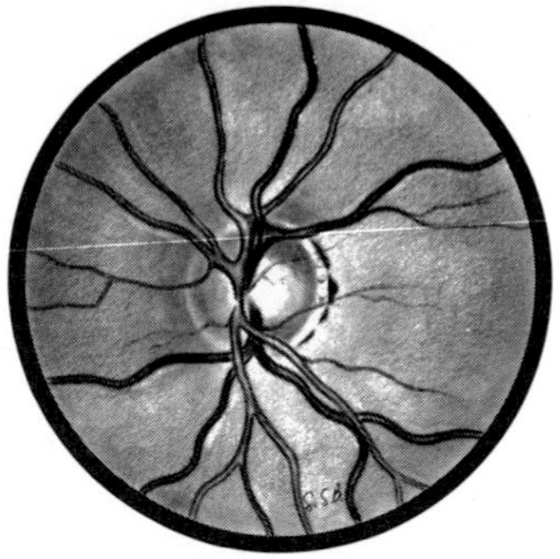

Rings and crescents are often seen around the optic disc. These are developmental variations in which you can glimpse either white sclera, black retinal pigment, or both, especially along the temporal border of the disc. Rings and crescents are not part of the disc itself and should not be included in your estimates of disc diameters.

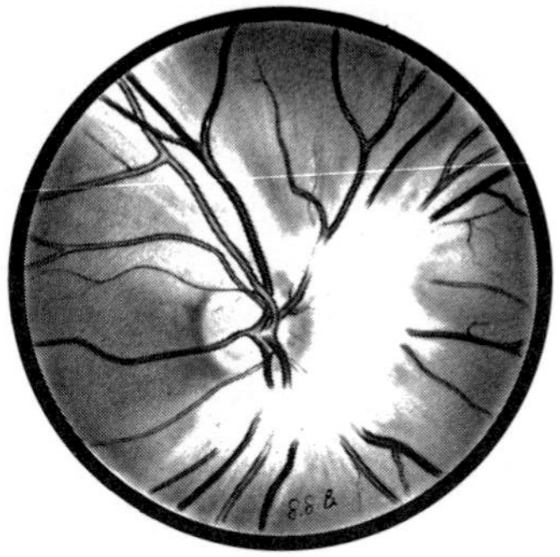

Medullated nerve fibers are a much less common but dramatic finding. Appearing as irregular white patches with feathered margins, they obscure the disc edge and retinal vessels. They have no pathologic significance.

Table 7-10   Abnormalities of the Optic Disc

Table 7-10   Abnormalities of the Optic Disc

	NORMAL	OPTIC ATROPHY	PAPILLEDEMA	GLAUCOMATOUS CUPPING
PROCESS	Tiny disc vessels give normal color to the disc.	Death of optic nerve fibers leads to loss of the tiny disc vessels.	Venous stasis leads to engorgement and swelling.	Increased pressure within the eye leads to increased cupping (backward depression of the disc) and atrophy.
APPEARANCE	Color yellowish orange to creamy pink	Color white	Color pink, hyperemic	The base of the enlarged cup is pale.
	Disc vessels tiny	Disc vessels absent	Disc vessels more visible, more numerous, curve over the borders of the disc	
	Disc margins sharp (except perhaps nasally)		Disc swollen with margins blurred	
	The physiologic cup is located centrally or somewhat temporally. It may be conspicuous or absent. Its diameter from side to side is usually less than half that of the disc.		The physiologic cup is not visible.	The physiologic cup is enlarged, occupying more than half of the disc's diameter, at times extending to the edge of the disc. Retinal vessels sink in and under it, and may be displaced nasally.

NORMAL RETINAL ARTERIOLE AND ARTERIOVENOUS (A–V) CROSSING

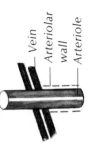

Arteriolar wall (invisible)
Column of blood
Light reflex

The normal arteriolar wall is transparent. Only the column of blood within it can usually be seen. The normal light reflex is narrow—about ¼ the diameter of the blood column.

Vein
Arteriolar wall
Arteriole

Because the arteriolar wall is transparent, a vein crossing beneath the arteriole can be seen right up to the column of blood on either side.

THE RETINAL ARTERIOLES IN HYPERTENSION

SPASM AND THICKENING OF ARTERIOLAR WALLS

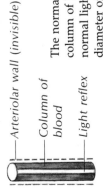

Narrowed column of blood
Narrowed light reflex

Focal narrowing

In hypertension, the arterioles may show areas of focal or generalized narrowing. The light reflex is also narrowed. Over many months or years, the arteriolar wall thickens and becomes less transparent.

COPPER WIRE ARTERIOLES

Sometimes the arterioles, especially those close to the disc, become full and somewhat tortuous and develop an increased light reflex with a bright coppery luster. Such a vessel is called a copper wire arteriole.

SILVER WIRE ARTERIOLES

Occasionally a portion of a narrowed arteriole develops such an opaque wall that no blood is visible within it. It is then called a silver wire arteriole. This change typically occurs in the smaller branches.

ARTERIOVENOUS CROSSING

When the arteriolar walls lose their transparency, changes appear in the arteriovenous crossings. Decreased transparency of the retina probably also contributes to the first two changes shown below.

CONCEALMENT OR A–V NICKING

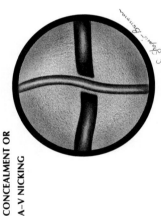

BANKING

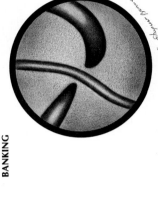

TAPERING

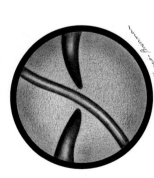

The vein appears to taper down on either side of the arteriole.

The vein appears to stop abruptly on either side of the arteriole.

The vein is twisted on the distal side of the arteriole and forms a dark, wide knuckle.

Table 7-12   Red Spots and Streaks in the Fundi

SUPERFICIAL RETINAL HEMORRHAGES

DEEP RETINAL HEMORRHAGES

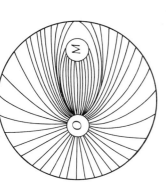

Superficial retinal hemorrhages are small, linear, flame-shaped, red streaks in the fundi. They are shaped by the superficial bundles of nerve fibers that radiate from the optic disc in the pattern illustrated (O = optic disc; M = macula). Sometimes the hemorrhages occur in clusters and then simulate a larger hemorrhage, but the linear streaking at the edges shows their true nature. Superficial hemorrhages are seen in severe hypertension, papilledema, and occlusion of the retinal vein, among other conditions.

An occasional superficial hemorrhage has a white center consisting of fibrin. White-centered retinal hemorrhages have many causes.

Deep retinal hemorrhages are small, rounded, slightly irregular red spots that are sometimes called dot or blot hemorrhages. They occur in a deeper layer of the retina than flame-shaped hemorrhages. Diabetes mellitus is a common cause.

PRERETINAL HEMORRHAGE

MICROANEURYSMS

NEOVASCULARIZATION

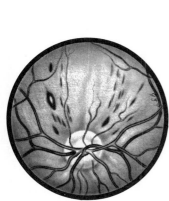

A preretinal (subhyaloid) hemorrhage develops when blood escapes into the potential space between retina and vitreous. This kind of hemorrhage is characteristically larger than retinal hemorrhages. Because it is anterior to the retina, it obscures any underlying retinal vessels. In an erect patient, gravity may cause the red cells to settle, creating a horizontal line of demarcation between plasma above and cells below. Causes include a sudden increase in intracranial pressure.

Microaneurysms are tiny, round, red spots seen commonly but not exclusively in and around the macular area. They are minute dilatations of very small retinal vessels, but the vascular connections are too small to be seen ophthalmoscopically. Microaneurysms are characteristic of diabetic retinopathy but not specific to it.

Neovascularization refers to the formation of new blood vessels. They are more numerous, more tortuous, and narrower than other blood vessels in the area and form disorderly-looking red arcades. A common cause is the late, proliferative stage of diabetic retinopathy. The vessels may grow into the vitreous, where bleeding may cause loss of vision.

Table 7-13 Light-Colored Spots in the Fundi

COTTON WOOL PATCHES (Soft Exudates)

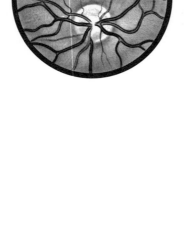

Cotton wool patches are white or grayish, ovoid lesions with irregular (thus "soft") borders. They are moderate in size but usually smaller than the disc. They result from infarcted nerve fibers and are seen with hypertension and other conditions.

HARD EXUDATES

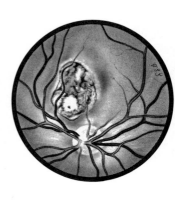

Hard exudates are creamy or yellowish, often bright lesions with well defined (thus "hard") borders. They are small and round (as shown in the lower group of exudates) but may coalesce into larger irregular spots (as shown in the upper group). They often occur in clusters or in circular, linear, or star-shaped patterns. Causes include diabetes and hypertension.

DRUSEN (Colloid Bodies)

Drusen are yellowish round spots that vary from tiny to small. They are haphazardly distributed but may concentrate at the posterior pole. Drusen appear with normal aging.

HEALED CHORIORETINITIS

Here inflammation has destroyed the superficial tissues to reveal a well defined, irregular patch of white sclera marked with dark pigment. Size varies from small to very large. Toxoplasmosis is illustrated. Multiple, small, somewhat similar-looking areas may be due to laser treatments.

Table 7-13   Light-Colored Spots in the Fundi

PROLIFERATIVE RETINOPATHY

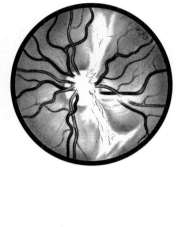

Bands or strands of white fibrous tissue develop in the late proliferative stage of diabetic retinopathy. They lie anterior to the retinal vessels and therefore obscure them. Neovascularization (p. 209) is typically associated.

COLOBOMA

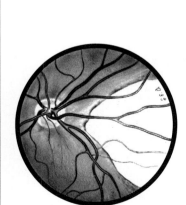

A coloboma of the choroid and retina is a developmental abnormality. A well demarcated, moderate-sized to large, white oval of sclera is visible below the disc, often extending well beyond the limits of your examination. Its borders may be pigmented.

Color Plate 7-1   Ocular Fundi

Out of a piece of paper, cut a circle about the size of an optic disc shown below. The circle simulates an ophthalmoscope's light beam. Lay it on each illustration, and inspect each fundus systematically.

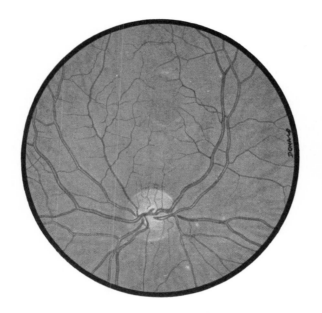 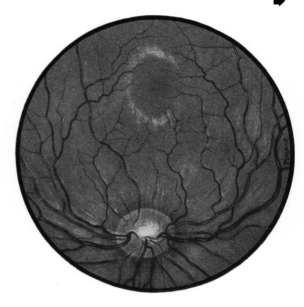

NORMAL FUNDUS OF A FAIR-SKINNED PERSON

Find and inspect the optic disc. Follow the major vessels in four directions, noting their relative sizes and the nature of the arteriovenous crossings—both normal here. Inspect the macula. The fovea is not visible in this subject. Look for any lesions in the retina. Note the striped, or tessellated, character of the fundus, especially in the lower field. This comes from normal choroidal vessels that are unobscured by pigment.

NORMAL FUNDUS OF A BLACK PERSON

Again, inspect the disc, the vessels, the macula, and the retinal background. The ring around the macula is a normal light reflection. Compare the color of the fundus to that in the illustration above. It has a grayish brownish, almost purplish cast, which comes from pigment in the retina and the choroid. This pigment characteristically obscures the choroidal vessels, and no tessellation is visible. In contrast to either of these two figures, the fundus of a white person with brunette coloring is redder.

➡ *Continued*

Color Plate 7-1 (Cont'd.)

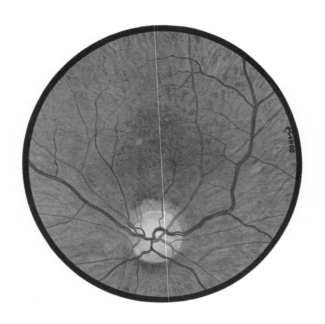

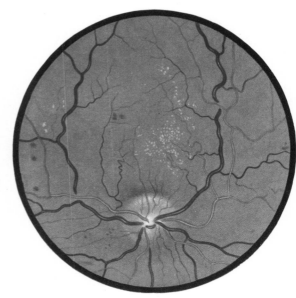

NORMAL FUNDUS OF AN AGED PERSON

Inspect the fundus as before. What differences do you observe? Two characteristics of the aging fundus can be seen in this example. The blood vessels are straighter and narrower than those in younger people, and the choroidal vessels can be seen easily. In this person the optic disc is less pink, and pigment may be seen temporal to the disc and in the macular area.

HYPERTENSIVE RETINOPATHY

Inspect the fundus as before. The nasal border of the optic disc is blurred. The light reflexes from the arterioles just above and below the disc are increased. Note the venous tapering—at the A–V crossing, about one disc diameter above the disc. Tapering and banking can be seen at 4:30 o'clock, two disc diameters from the disc. Punctate hard exudates and a few deep hemorrhages are readily visible.

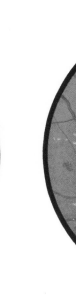

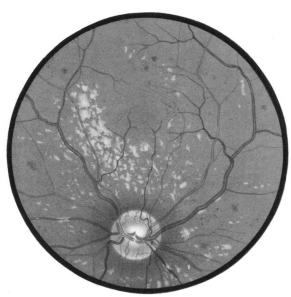

HYPERTENSIVE RETINOPATHY WITH MACULAR STAR

Punctate exudates are readily visible here. Some are scattered, while others radiate from the fovea to form a macular star. Note the two small, soft exudates about one disc diameter from the disc. A number of flame-shaped hemorrhages sweep toward 4 o'clock and 5 o'clock, and a few more may be seen toward 2 o'clock.

The changes shown in both this and the previous illustration of hypertensive retinopathy are typical of accelerated (malignant) hypertension. The other important abnormality that may accompany these changes is papilledema (p. 207).

DIABETIC RETINOPATHY

Punctate exudates have coalesced here into homogeneous, waxy-looking patches that are typical of diabetic retinopathy. What kinds of red spots can you find? Microaneurysms are most easily visible about one disc diameter below the disc. A few deep hemorrhages can also be seen, around 2 o'clock and 3 o'clock about three disc diameters from the disc.

This picture, with its combination of microaneurysms, deep hemorrhages, and hard exudates, is classified as background retinopathy. A later stage, known as proliferative retinopathy, includes neovascularization (p. 209), proliferating fibrous tissue (p. 211), and vitreous hemorrhages.

(Source of illustrations: Michaelson IC: Textbook of the Fundus of the Eye, 3rd ed, pp 52, 131, 141. Edinburgh, Churchill Livingstone, 1980)

Color Plate 7-2   Abnormalities of the Eardrum

NORMAL EARDRUM   **PERFORATION OF THE DRUM**   **TYMPANOSCLEROSIS**

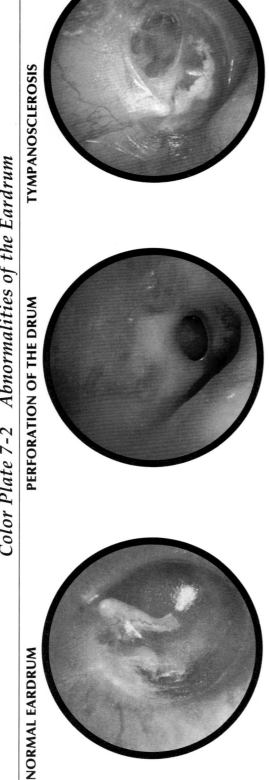

This normal right eardrum (tympanic membrane) is pinkish gray. The handle of the malleus lies in a somewhat oblique position behind the upper part of the drum. The short process of the malleus pushes the membrane laterally, creating a small white elevation. Above the short process lies a small portion of the eardrum called the pars flaccida. The remainder of the drum is the pars tensa. Anterior and posterior malleolar folds, which extend obliquely upward from the short process, separate the pars flaccida from the pars tensa, but they are often invisible unless the eardrum is retracted. From the umbo the bright cone of light fans anteriorly and downward. Other light reflections seen in this photo are artifactual. Posterior to the malleus, part of the incus is visible behind the drum. The small blood vessels that course along the handle of the malleus are within the range of normal and do not indicate inflammation. The ear canal, which surrounds the eardrum, looks flatter than it really is because of distortion inherent in the photographic technique.

Perforations are holes in the eardrum that usually result from purulent infections of the middle ear. They are classified as *central* perforations, which do not extend to the margin of the drum, and *marginal* perforations, which do involve the margin. The more common central perforation is illustrated here. In this case a reddened ring of granulation tissue surrounds the perforation, indicating a chronic infectious process. The eardrum itself is scarred and no landmarks are discernible. Discharge from the infected middle ear may drain out through such a perforation, but none is visible here.

A perforation of the eardrum often closes in the healing process, as illustrated in the next photo. The membrane covering the hole may be exceedingly thin and transparent.

In the inferior portion of this left eardrum there is a large, chalky white patch with irregular margins. It is typical of tympanosclerosis: a deposition of hyaline material within the layers of the tympanic membrane that sometimes follows a severe otitis media. It does not usually impair hearing and is seldom clinically significant.

Other abnormalities in this eardrum include a *healed perforation* (the large oval area in the upper posterior drum) and signs of a *retracted drum*. A retracted drum is pulled medially, away from the examiner's eye, and the malleolar folds are tightened into sharp outlines. The short process often protrudes sharply, and the handle of the malleus, pulled inward at the umbo, looks foreshortened and more horizontal.

BULLOUS MYRINGITIS

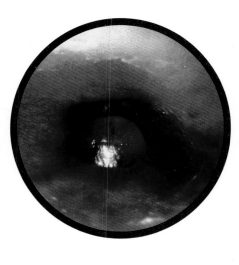

ACUTE OTITIS MEDIA WITH PURULENT EFFUSION

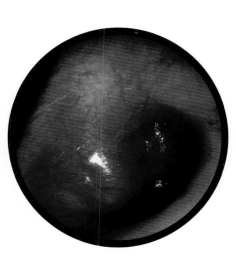

SEROUS EFFUSIONS

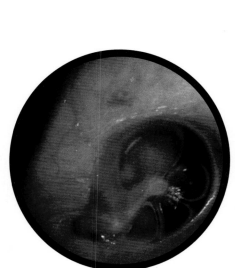

Serous effusions are usually caused by viral upper respiratory infections (*otitis media with serous effusion*) or by sudden changes in atmospheric pressure as from flying or diving (*otitic barotrauma*). The eustachian tube cannot equalize the air pressure in the middle ear with that of the outside air. Air is partly or completely absorbed from the middle ear into the bloodstream, and serous fluid accumulates there instead. Symptoms include fullness and popping sensations in the ear, mild conduction hearing loss, and perhaps some pain.

Amber fluid behind the eardrum is characteristic, as in this left drum of a patient with otitic barotrauma. A fluid level, a line between air above and amber fluid below, can be seen on either side of the short process. Air bubbles (not always present) can be seen within the amber fluid.

Acute otitis media with purulent effusion is caused by bacterial infection. Symptoms include earache, fever, and hearing loss. The eardrum reddens, loses its landmarks, and bulges laterally, toward the examiner's eye.

In this left ear the upper portion of the drum is reddened by dilated blood vessels and has begun to bulge. The short process and the handle of the malleus, though less distinct than normal, are still discernible. Later all landmarks are lost and the entire fiery red drum bulges laterally. Spontaneous rupture (perforation) of the drum may follow, with discharge of purulent material into the ear canal.

Moving the auricle and pressing on the tragus do not cause pain in otitis media as they usually do in acute otitis externa. Hearing loss is of the conduction type. Acute purulent otitis media is much more common in children than in adults.

Bullous myringitis is a viral infection characterized by painful hemorrhagic vesicles that appear on the tympanic membrane, the ear canal, or both. Symptoms include earache, blood-tinged discharge from the ear, and hearing loss of the conduction type.

In this illustration a large vesicle on the posterior wall of the right ear canal contains serous fluid (as shown by its yellowish color) together with some dark red blood peripherally. The eardrum, not well seen here, would be likely to show similar lesions. The skin of the ear canal shows hemorrhagic patches.

Several different viruses may cause this condition.

(Sources of photos: *Normal Eardrum*—Hawke M, Keene M, Alberti PW: Clinical Otoscopy: A Text and Colour Atlas, p 68. Edinburgh, Churchill Livingstone, 1984; *Eardrum abnormalities photos*—Courtesy of Michael Hawke, M.D., Toronto, Canada)

Table 7-14   Nodules In and Around the Ears

Table 7-14   Nodules In and Around the Ears

LYMPH NODES

Preauricular node

Posterior auricular node

Mastoid process

Small lymph nodes just anterior to the tragus or overlying the mastoid process are quite common. Although sometimes visible, they are best detected by palpation.

SEBACEOUS CYSTS

Cyst

Punctum

Sebaceous cysts are common, especially behind the ear. They are characteristically *in* rather than beneath the skin and often show a central black dot or punctum which identifies the opening of the blocked sebaceous gland.

KELOID

Keloids

A keloid, which is a nodular, hypertrophic mass of scar tissue, may develop in an earlobe pierced for earrings. Keloids are especially common in black people.

TOPHUS

Tophi

Tophi are deposits of uric acid crystals characteristic of gout. They appear as hard nodules in the helix or antihelix. They occasionally discharge white chalky crystals.

DARWIN'S TUBERCLE

Typical location

A small elevation in the rim of the ear, a Darwin's tubercle is a harmless congenital variation from normal—the equivalent of the tip of a mammalian ear. It should not be mistaken for a tophus.

CHONDRODERMATITIS HELICIS

Tender nodule

This entity is characterized by a small, chronic, painful, tender nodule in the helix of the ear. It usually affects men, involving the right ear more often than the left. It may be confused with a tophus or skin cancer. Biopsy is important.

Table 7-15   Patterns of Hearing Loss

Hearing loss is divided into two major types: (1) *conduction hearing loss*, in which a disorder of the external or middle ear impairs the conduction of sound to the inner ear, and (2) *sensorineural hearing loss*, in which a disorder of the inner ear, the cochlear nerve, or its central connections impairs the transmission of nerve impulses to the brain. A *mixed hearing loss* has both deficits.

	CONDUCTION LOSS	SENSORINEURAL LOSS
	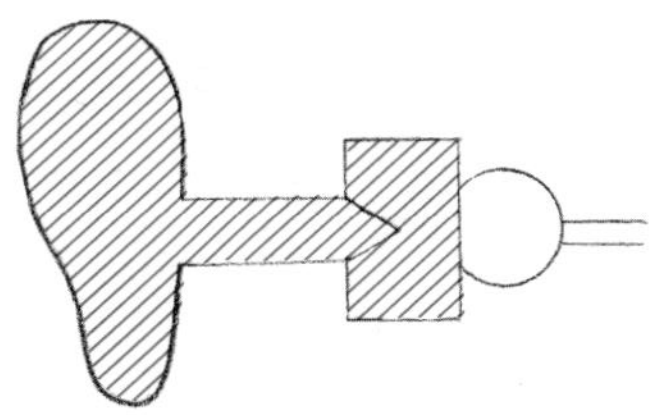	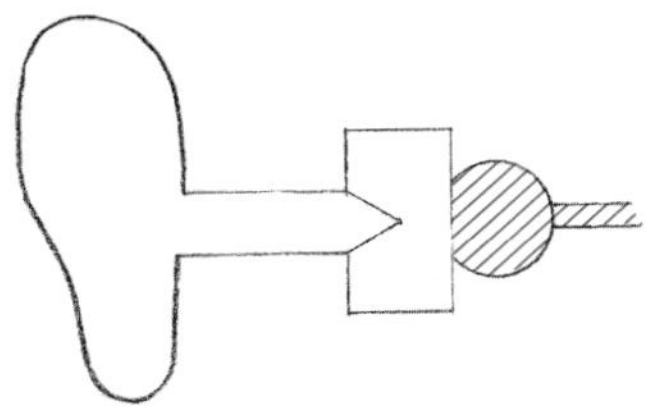
DISTORTION OF SOUNDS THAT IMPAIRS THE UNDERSTANDING OF WORDS	Relatively minor	Often present as the upper tones of words are disproportionately lost
EFFECT OF A NOISY ENVIRONMENT	Hearing may seem to improve.	Hearing typically worsens.
PATIENT'S OWN VOICE	Tends to be soft: the patient's voice is conducted through bone to a normal inner ear and cochlear nerve.	May be loud: the patient has trouble hearing his or her own voice.
USUAL AGE OF ONSET	Most often in childhood and young adulthood, up to age 40	Most often in the middle or later years
EAR CANAL AND DRUM	There is usually a visible abnormality, except in otosclerosis.	The problem is not visible.

Table 7-15   Patterns of Hearing Loss

WEBER TEST (*in unilateral hearing loss*)

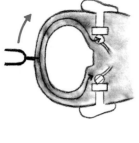

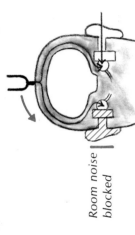

Room noise blocked

The sound lateralizes to the impaired ear. Because this ear is not distracted by room noise, it can detect vibrations better than normal. (Test yourself while occluding one ear with your finger.) This lateralization disappears in an absolutely quiet room.

The sound lateralizes to the good ear. The impaired inner ear or cochlear nerve is less able to transmit impulses no matter how the sound reaches the cochlea. The sound is therefore heard in the better ear.

RINNE TEST

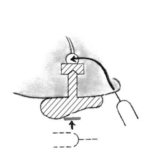

Bone conduction lasts longer than or is equal to air conduction (BC > AC or BC = AC, a negative Rinne). Pathways of normal conduction through the external or middle ear are blocked. Vibrations through bone bypass the obstruction to reach the cochlea.

Air conduction lasts longer than bone conduction (AC > BC, a positive Rinne). The inner ear or cochlear nerve is less able to transmit impulses regardless of how the vibrations reach the cochlea. The normal pattern prevails.

CAUSES INCLUDE:

Obstruction of the ear canal, otitis media, a perforated or relatively immobilized ear drum, and otosclerosis (a fixation of the ossicles by bony overgrowth)

Sustained exposure to loud noise, drugs, infections of the inner ear, trauma, tumors, congenital and hereditary disorders, and aging (presbycusis)

Further evaluation is done by audiometry and other specialized procedures.

Table 7-16 Abnormalities of the Lips

Table 7-16 Abnormalities of the Lips

HERPES SIMPLEX (*Cold Sore, Fever Blister*)

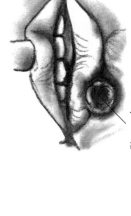

Blisters with crusting

The virus herpes simplex may produce recurrent vesicular eruptions of the lips and surrounding tissues. A small cluster of blisters develops. As these break, a crust is formed and healing ensues within 10 to 14 days.

CHANCRE

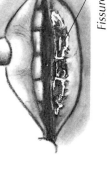

Firm ulcer

The primary lesion of syphilis may appear on the lip instead of in its more common location on the genitalia. It is a firm, buttonlike lesion which ulcerates and may become crusted. A chancre may resemble a carcinoma or a crusted cold sore. Use a glove for palpation. Dark field examination is necessary for diagnosis.

ANGULAR STOMATITIS (*Cheilosis*)

Softening, fissuring

Softening of the skin at the angles of the mouth, followed by fissuring or cracking, is called angular stomatitis or cheilosis. It may be secondary to riboflavin deficiency but it more commonly is caused by overclosure of the mouth (*e.g.*, in patients without teeth or with dentures that are too short in their vertical dimension). Saliva then wets and macerates the infolded skin, often leading to secondary infection from *Candida* or bacteria. The mucous membrane remains uninvolved.

CHEILITIS

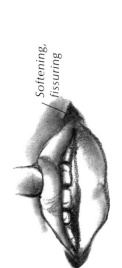

Fissures, scales, and crusts

Painful fissuring with inflammation, scaling, and crust formation characterizes cheilitis. Involving chiefly the lower lip, cheilitis is often chronic. Its causes are several and may be obscure.

Table 7-16 Abnormalities of the Lips

MUCOUS RETENTION CYST (*Mucocele*)

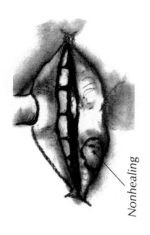

Round nodule

A round, regular, partially translucent or bluish nodule in the lip is probably a mucous retention cyst, or mucocele. This is a benign lesion, having chiefly cosmetic importance. Size varies from tiny up to 1–2 cm in diameter. The cysts may also occur inside the lower lip in the buccal mucosa.

CARCINOMA OF THE LIP

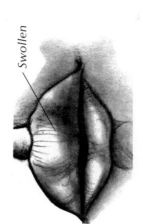

Nonhealing

Carcinoma of the lip usually involves the lower lip and may appear as a thickened plaque, ulcer, or warty growth. Much more frequent in men than in women, it is the most common form of oral cancer. Any sore or crusting lesion on the lip that does not heal must be considered suspicious.

PEUTZ–JEGHERS SYNDROME

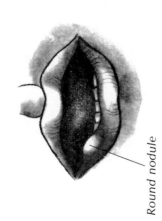

Pigmented spots

When pigmented spots on the lips are more prominent than freckling of the surrounding skin, suspect the Peutz–Jeghers syndrome. Look for abnormal pigment in the buccal mucosa to help confirm the diagnosis. Pigmented spots may also be found on the face, fingers, and hands. These findings are important because they are often associated with multiple intestinal polyps.

ANGIOEDEMA

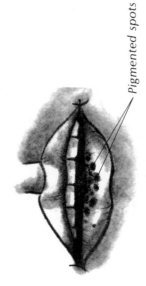

Swollen

Angioedema is a diffuse, nonpitting, tense swelling of the dermis and subcutaneous tissue. It may involve a number of structures, including the lips. It develops rather rapidly and usually disappears in a day or two. Although usually allergic in nature and sometimes associated with hives, it does not usually itch.

Table 7-17 Abnormalities of the Buccal Mucosa and Hard Palate

Table 7-17 Abnormalities of the Buccal Mucosa and Hard Palate

APHTHOUS ULCER (*Canker Sore*)

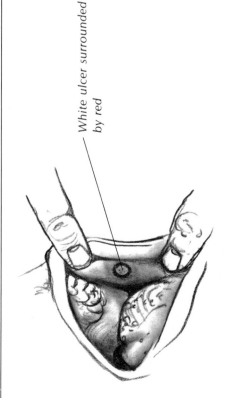

White ulcer surrounded by red

FORDYCE SPOTS (*Fordyce Granules*)

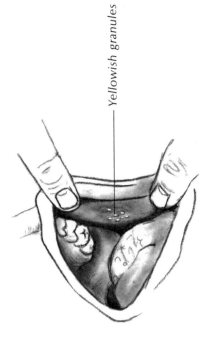

Yellowish granules

A small, round or oval, white ulcer surrounded by a halo of reddened mucosa characterizes the common aphthous ulcer. Such ulcers are painful, may be single or multiple, and are often recurrent. Any portion of the oral mucosa may be involved.

Fordyce spots are small yellowish spots visible in the buccal mucosa of most adults. They may also involve the lips. They are sebaceous glands and should not be considered an abnormality. The patient who suddenly notices and worries about them may be reassured.

TORUS PALATINUS

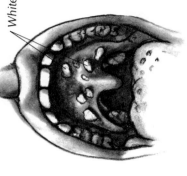

Bony

THRUSH (*Oral Candidiasis*)

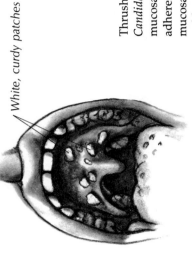

White, curdy patches

A torus palatinus is a fairly common midline bony outgrowth in the hard palate, usually developing in adulthood. Its size and lobulation vary. Although alarming at first glance, it is of no clinical consequence except perhaps in the fitting of dentures. A nodule that is not in the midline is not a torus and should suggest a tumor.

Thrush is a yeast infection due to *Candida*. It can involve the entire oral mucosa. White plaques are somewhat adherent to an often reddened mucosa; less commonly, there is only a reddened mucosa. Causes include AIDS and prolonged antibiotic or corticosteroid therapy.

Table 7-18   Abnormalities of the Gums and Teeth

Table 7-18   Abnormalities of the Gums and Teeth

NORMAL GUMS

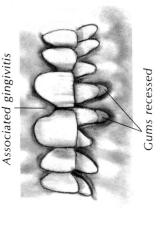

Pale red with normal stippling

Sharp interdental papilla

The gums (or gingivae) normally show a pale red stippled surface. Their margins about the teeth are sharp and the crevices between gums and teeth shallow (*e.g.*, 1–2 mm). The teeth are seated firmly in their bony sockets.

GINGIVITIS

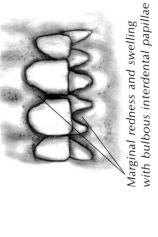

Marginal redness and swelling with bulbous interdental papillae

Redness and swelling of the margins of the gums characterize gingivitis, often the result of irritation by calculus formation. The normal stippling decreases or disappears. The gingivae between the teeth (interdental papillae) may become bulbous. The gums may bleed with light contact.

PERIODONTITIS (*Pyorrhea*)

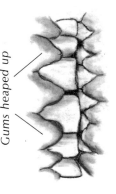

Associated gingivitis

Gums recessed

If untreated, gingivitis may progress to periodontitis, an inflammation of the deeper tissues around the teeth. This is an extremely common cause of tooth loss in adults. The crevices between the gums and teeth enlarge, and pockets containing debris and purulent material develop in these areas. The gum margins recede, exposing the necks of the teeth. The teeth may become loose.

ACUTE NECROTIZING GINGIVITIS
(*Trench Mouth, Vincent's Stomatitis*)

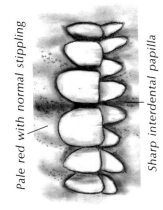

Grayish membrane over ulcerated gum margin

This is a painful gingivitis characterized by redness, swelling, and ulceration of the gingival tissues. The interdental papillae may be eroded by the ulcerative process. A grayish membrane forms over the inflamed and ulcerated gingival margins.

GINGIVAL ENLARGEMENT

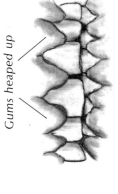

Gums heaped up

Enlargement of the gums has a variety of causes including puberty, pregnancy, Dilantin therapy, and leukemia. The gingival tissues appear heaped up and partially cover the teeth.

EPULIS

Local enlargement

Epulis is the term used to describe a localized gingival enlargement. Most are inflammatory, and some are neoplastic.

▶ *Continued*

Table 7-18   Abnormalities of the Gums and Teeth

Table 7-18 (Cont'd.)

MELANIN PIGMENTATION

Patchy brown pigment

A brownish melanin pigmentation of the gums is frequently observed. It is normal in blacks and other dark-skinned persons and may occasionally be seen even in light-skinned persons. A similar pigment pattern may be associated with Addison's disease.

DENTAL CARIES

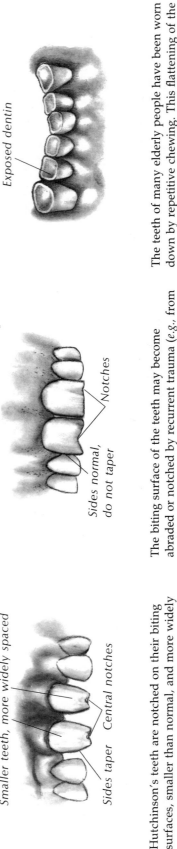

Chalky white

Discolored, with cavitation

Dental caries is first visible as a chalky white deposit in the enamel surface of the tooth. This area may then discolor to brown or black, become soft, and cavitate. Special dental techniques including x-rays are necessary for early detection.

LEAD OR BISMUTH LINE

Bluish black line

In chronic lead or bismuth poisoning, a bluish black line may appear on the gums about 1 mm from the gum margin. It does not appear where teeth are absent. Distinguish it from the much more common melanin pigmentation.

HUTCHINSON'S TEETH

Smaller teeth, more widely spaced

Sides taper   Central notches

Hutchinson's teeth are notched on their biting surfaces, smaller than normal, and more widely spaced. Their sides taper in. The upper central incisors are most often affected: the permanent, rather than deciduous, teeth are involved. They are a sign of congenital syphilis.

ABRASION OF TEETH WITH NOTCHING

Notches

Sides normal, do not taper

The biting surface of the teeth may become abraded or notched by recurrent trauma (*e.g.*, from opening bobby pins with one's teeth, or holding nails between the teeth). Unlike Hutchinson's teeth, the sides of these teeth show their normal contours; size and spacing are unaffected.

ATTRITION OF TEETH

Exposed dentin

The teeth of many elderly people have been worn down by repetitive chewing. This flattening of the biting surfaces is called attrition. The enamel may be worn away, exposing the underlying dentin. The latter often takes on a yellow or brownish stain.

Table 7-19 Abnormalities of the Tongue

Table 7-19 Abnormalities of the Tongue

SMOOTH TONGUE

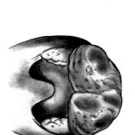

A smooth, slick, and often sore tongue that has lost its papillae suggests a deficiency in riboflavin, niacin, folic acid, vitamin B_{12}, pyridoxine, or iron. Specific diagnosis is often difficult. Anticancer drugs may also be responsible.

HAIRY TONGUE

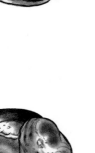

The "hair" of hairy tongue consists of elongated papillae on the dorsum of the tongue and is yellowish to brown to black. Hairy tongue may follow antibiotic therapy but may also occur spontaneously. Its cause is unknown. It is harmless.

GEOGRAPHIC TONGUE

Geographic tongue is characterized by scattered red areas on the dorsum of the tongue that are denuded of their papillae and are smooth. The contrast of these areas with the normal roughened and coated surface gives a maplike pattern which changes over time. Of unknown cause, the condition is benign.

FISSURED TONGUE

Fissures may appear in the tongue with increasing age and at times become numerous. Their appearance gives rise to the alternate term "scrotal tongue." Although food debris may accumulate in the crevices and become irritating, the fissured tongue usually has little significance.

12TH NERVE PARALYSIS

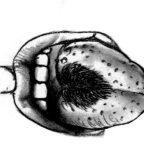

Paralysis of the 12th cranial (hypoglossal) nerve produces atrophy and fasciculations of the involved half of the tongue. Deviation toward the paralyzed side occurs when the tongue is protruded.

VARICOSE VEINS OF THE TONGUE

Small purplish or blue black round swellings may appear under the tongue with age and have aptly been called "caviar lesions." They have no significance. As with several other tongue findings, familiarity with them pays dividends when the patient or the examiner first notices them. Reassurance is in order.

LEUKOPLAKIA

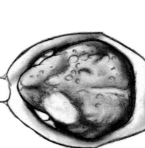

Leukoplakia is a term applied to a thickened white patch adherent to the mucous membrane. Its appearance has been likened to dried white paint. Although tongue involvement is illustrated here, leukoplakia may involve any part of the oral mucosa. Its primary significance lies in the fact that it may be premalignant.

CARCINOMA

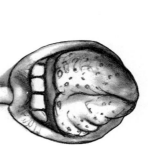

Carcinoma of the tongue is uncommon on the dorsum of the tongue, where it might be most readily noticed. Look for it at the base or edges of the tongue. Any ulcer or nodule that fails to heal in 2 to 3 weeks must be considered suspicious.

Table 7-20   Abnormalities of the Pharynx

VIRAL PHARYNGITIS

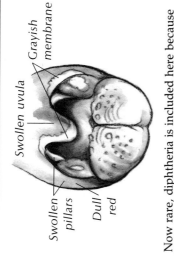

Slight redness

Prominent lymphoid patches

Viral pharyngitis may show few if any signs. Mild redness, slight swelling of the pillars, and prominent lymphoid patches on the posterior pharynx are frequent. Signs that suggest infectious mononucleosis as the cause of sore throat are petechiae on the palate and enlargement or tenderness of the posterior auricular, inguinal, and (if marked) axillary lymph nodes.

STREPTOCOCCAL PHARYNGITIS

Swollen uvula

Red

Enlarged tonsils with white patches

Classically, streptococcal infection produces redness and swelling of the tonsils, pillars, and uvula, with white or yellow patches of exudate on the tonsils. Accurate clinical diagnosis is frequently impossible, however, since streptococcal pharyngitis may occur without exudate and some viral illnesses, including infectious mononucleosis, may produce an exudative pharyngitis.

DIPHTHERIA

Swollen uvula

Grayish membrane

Swollen pillars

Dull red

Now rare, diphtheria is included here because without prompt diagnosis and treatment it may prove fatal. The throat is dull red and swollen. A thick exudate forms on the tonsils and, unlike a streptococcal exudate, may spread over the soft palate and uvula. The throat is less painful than might be expected from the severity of the patient's illness.

TONSILLAR HYPERTROPHY

Enlarged tonsils

The tonsils may be enlarged without being infected. They may protrude medially beyond the edges of the pillars even to the midline when the tongue is protruded. The size of the tonsils is not in itself an indicator of disease.

PARALYSIS OF THE 10TH CRANIAL (*Vagus*) NERVE

Failure to rise

Deviated to left

When the patient says "ah" the soft palate on the paralyzed side fails to rise. The uvula deviates to the uninvolved side.

PERITONSILLAR ABSCESS (*Quinsy Sore Throat*)

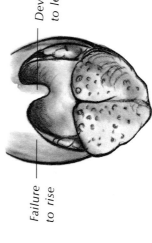

Uvula displaced

Red, tense, bulging

Peritonsillar abscess occasionally complicates acute tonsillitis. Usually caused by streptococci or staphylococci, the infection spreads from tonsil to adjacent soft tissue, producing a very painful, usually unilateral, red bulge that may extend beyond the midline. Painful swallowing may cause drooling.

Table 7-21 Thyroid Enlargement and Function

Table 7-21 Thyroid Enlargement and Function

Evaluation of the thyroid gland includes a description of the gland and a functional assessment.

DIFFUSE ENLARGEMENT	MULTINODULAR GOITER	SINGLE NODULE
A diffusely enlarged gland, or goiter, includes the isthmus and the lateral lobes, but there are no discretely palpable nodules. Causes include Graves' disease, Hashimoto's thyroiditis, and endemic goiter (related to iodine deficiency, now uncommon in the United States). Sporadic goiter refers to an enlarged gland with no apparent cause.	This term refers to an enlarged thyroid gland that contains two or more identifiable nodules. Multiple nodules suggest a metabolic rather than a neoplastic process, but irradiation during childhood, a positive family history, enlarged cervical nodes, or continuing enlargement of one of the nodules raises the suspicion of malignancy.	A clinically single nodule may be a cyst, a benign tumor, or one nodule within a multinodular gland, but it also raises the question of a malignancy. Prior irradiation, hardness, rapid growth, fixation to surrounding tissues, enlarged cervical nodes, and occurrence in males increase the probability of malignancy.

SYMPTOMS OF THYROID DYSFUNCTION

HYPERTHYROIDISM	HYPOTHYROIDISM
Nervousness	Fatigue, lethargy
Weight loss despite an increased appetite	Modest weight gain with anorexia
Excessive sweating and heat intolerance	Dry, coarse skin and cold intolerance
Palpitations	Swelling of face, hands, and legs
Frequent bowel movements	Constipation
Muscular weakness of the proximal type and tremor	Weakness, muscle cramps, arthralgias, paresthesias, impaired memory and hearing

SIGNS OF THYROID DYSFUNCTION

HYPERTHYROIDISM	HYPOTHYROIDISM
Tachycardia or atrial fibrillation	Bradycardia and, in late stages, hypothermia
Increased systolic and decreased diastolic blood pressures	Decreased systolic and increased diastolic blood pressures
Hyperdynamic cardiac pulsations with an accentuated S_1	Intensity of heart sounds sometimes decreased
Warm, smooth, moist skin	Dry, coarse, cool skin, sometimes yellowish from carotene, with nonpitting edema and loss of hair
Tremor and proximal muscle weakness	Impaired memory, mixed hearing loss, somnolence, peripheral neuropathy, carpal tunnel syndrome
With Graves' disease, eye signs such as stare, lid lag, and exophthalmos	Periorbital puffiness

Chapter 8
The Thorax and Lungs

Anatomy and Physiology

Review the *anatomy of the chest wall,* identifying the structures illustrated.

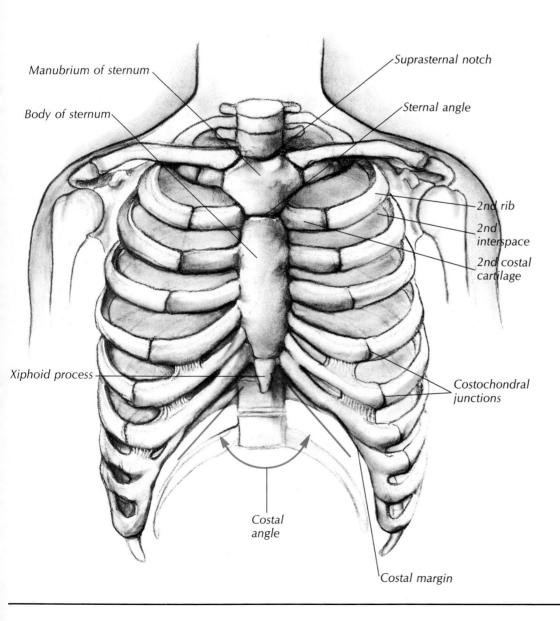

Manubrium of sternum

Body of sternum

Xiphoid process

Suprasternal notch

Sternal angle

2nd rib

2nd interspace

2nd costal cartilage

Costochondral junctions

Costal angle

Costal margin

To localize and describe a finding in relation to the chest wall you must be able to number the ribs and the interspaces between them accurately. The sternal angle (or angle of Louis) is the best guide. To find it, first identify the suprasternal notch, then move your finger down about 5 cm or a little more to find the horizontal bony ridge that joins the manubrium to the body of the sternum. Then move your finger laterally and find the adjacent 2nd rib and costal cartilage. The interspace immediately below is the 2nd interspace. From here, using two fingers, you can "walk down the interspaces," one space at a time, on an oblique line illustrated by the red numbers below. Do not try to count interspaces along the lower edge of the sternum because the ribs there are too close together. To find the interspaces in a woman with large breasts, either displace the breast laterally or palpate a little more medially than illustrated. Avoid pressing too hard on tender breast tissue.

Note that the costal cartilages of only the first seven ribs articulate with the sternum. Those of the 8th, 9th, and 10th ribs articulate instead with the costal cartilages just above them. The 11th and 12th ribs, the so-called floating ribs, have no anterior attachments. The cartilaginous tip of the 11th rib can usually be felt laterally, and the 12th rib may be felt posteriorly. Costal cartilages are not distinguishable from ribs by palpation.

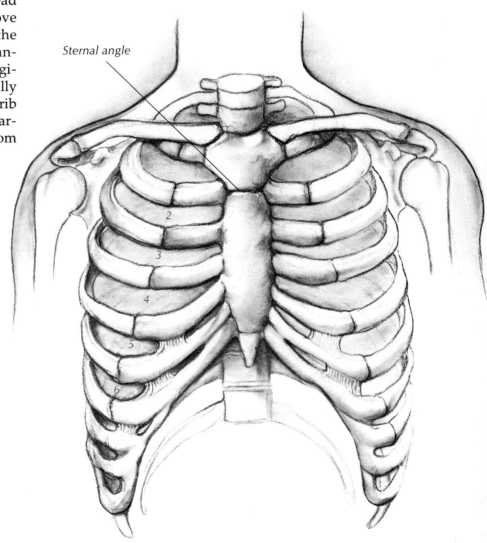

Sternal angle

Posteriorly the 11th and 12th ribs give you another possible starting point for counting ribs and interspaces. This is especially helpful in localizing findings in the lower posterior chest, but is also useful occasionally when the anterior approach is unsatisfactory. First, with the fingers of one hand, press inward and up against the lower border of the rib cage, roughly in the area indicated by the red arrow. Identify the 12th rib. Then "walk" upward in the interspaces on the red numbers or, alternatively, obliquely upward and around to the front of the chest.

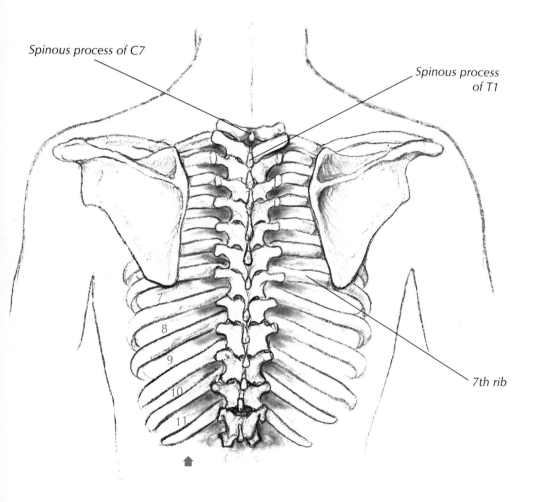

Spinous process of C7

Spinous process of T1

7th rib

Other bony landmarks and relationships are sometimes useful. The inferior angle of the scapula lies approximately at the level of the 7th rib or interspace. Findings may also be localized according to their relationship to the spinous processes of the vertebrae. When a person flexes the neck forward, the most prominent process (the vertebra prominens) is usually that of the 7th cervical. When two processes appear equally prominent, they are the 7th cervical and 1st thoracic. The processes below them can often be felt and counted, especially when the spine is flexed.

Localization of findings depends upon their relationship not only to ribs and vertebrae but also to imaginary lines drawn on the chest. Become familiar with the lines illustrated. Estimation of the midclavicular line requires accurate identification of the lateral end of the clavicle. For this refer to p. 463.

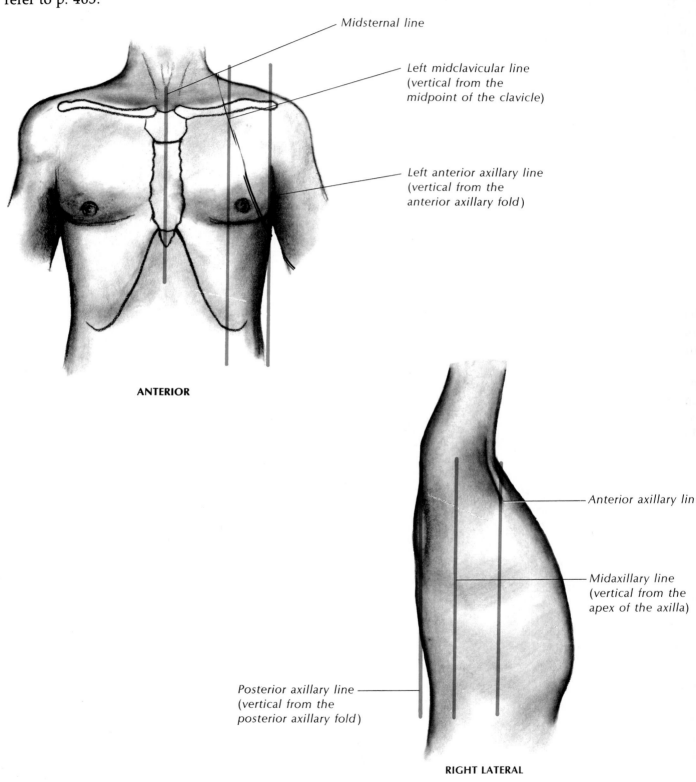

Midsternal line

Left midclavicular line (vertical from the midpoint of the clavicle)

Left anterior axillary line (vertical from the anterior axillary fold)

ANTERIOR

Anterior axillary lin

Midaxillary line (vertical from the apex of the axilla)

Posterior axillary line (vertical from the posterior axillary fold)

RIGHT LATERAL

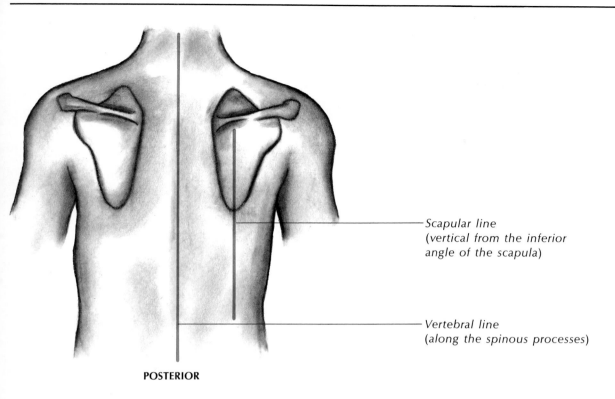

Scapular line
(*vertical from the inferior
angle of the scapula*)

Vertebral line
(*along the spinous processes*)

POSTERIOR

More general terms are also helpful: supraclavicular (above the clavicle), infraclavicular (below the clavicle), interscapular (between the scapulae), and infrascapular (below the scapula).

While examining the chest, keep in mind the probable location of the underlying lungs and their lobes. These locations can be projected mentally onto the chest wall. Key points in these surface projections include the following:

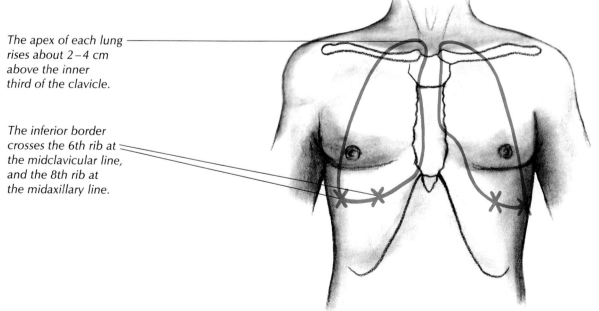

*The apex of each lung
rises about 2–4 cm
above the inner
third of the clavicle.*

*The inferior border
crosses the 6th rib at
the midclavicular line,
and the 8th rib at
the midaxillary line.*

ANTERIOR

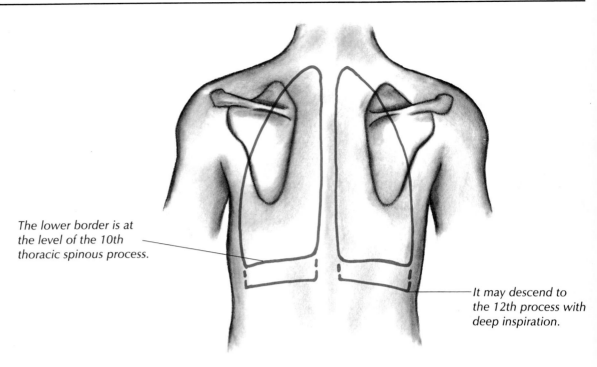

The lower border is at the level of the 10th thoracic spinous process.

It may descend to the 12th process with deep inspiration.

POSTERIOR

Each lung is divided approximately in half by an oblique (or major) fissure. Posteriorly the locations of the oblique fissures are approximated by lines drawn from the 3rd thoracic spinous process obliquely down and laterally. These lines are close to the vertebral borders of the scapulae when a person's hands are placed on top of the head. They divide upper from lower lobes.

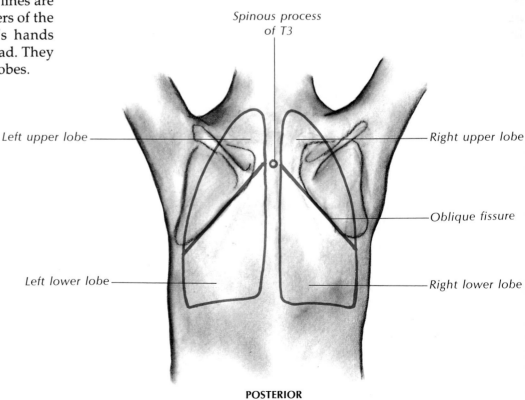

Spinous process of T3

Left upper lobe

Right upper lobe

Oblique fissure

Left lower lobe

Right lower lobe

POSTERIOR

Note that the lower lobes also have surface projections laterally and anteriorly.

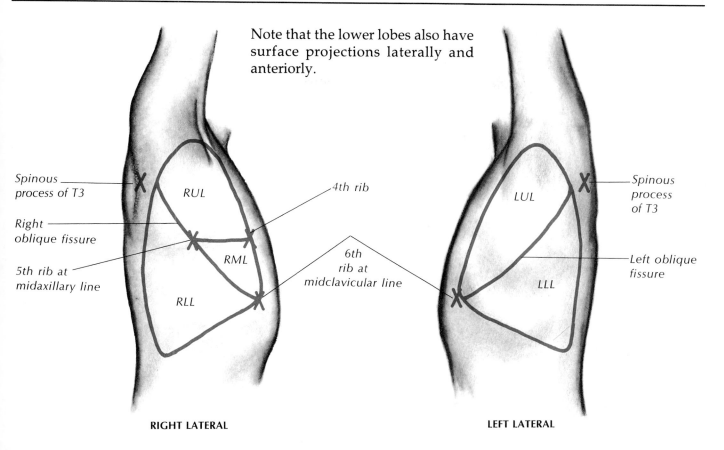

Spinous process of T3

RUL

4th rib

Right oblique fissure

5th rib at midaxillary line

RML

6th rib at midclavicular line

RLL

LUL

Spinous process of T3

Left oblique fissure

LLL

RIGHT LATERAL

LEFT LATERAL

The right lung is divided further by the horizontal (or minor) fissure into the right upper and right middle lobes. This fissure runs from the right midaxillary line at the level of the 5th rib across anteriorly at the level of the 4th rib.

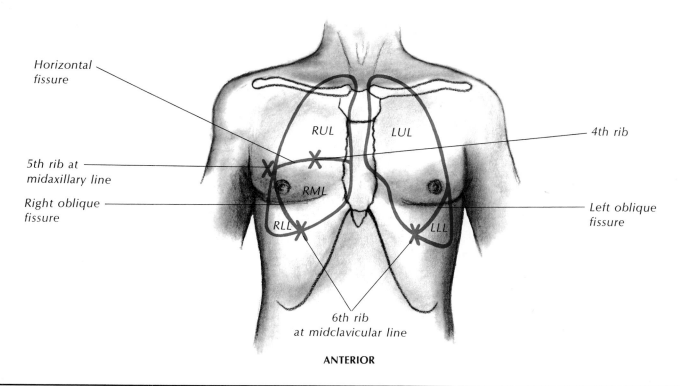

Horizontal fissure

5th rib at midaxillary line

Right oblique fissure

RUL

LUL

4th rib

RML

RLL

LLL

Left oblique fissure

6th rib at midclavicular line

ANTERIOR

Although you should be mindful of the probable location of lung lobes when examining a patient's chest and when making correlations with radiologic findings, you should usually describe your physical findings in terms that are less explicit anatomically: upper, middle, and lower lung fields, for example, or the bases (lowermost portions) of the lungs. You may then infer what lobes are involved. Signs in the right upper lung field, for example, probably originate in the right upper lobe, while those at the left base almost certainly come from the left lower lobe. Signs in the right middle lung field laterally, however, could come from any of three different lobes.

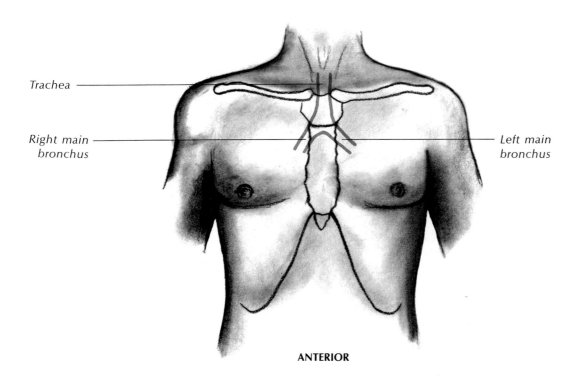

Trachea

Right main bronchus

Left main bronchus

ANTERIOR

Because certain physical findings in the chest are influenced by the closeness of the chest wall to the trachea and large bronchi, the location of these structures should also be familiar. Note that the trachea bifurcates at about the level of the sternal angle anteriorly and of the 4th thoracic spinous process posteriorly (see p. 239).

Breathing is largely an automatic act, controlled in the brainstem and mediated by the muscles of respiration. The dome-shaped diaphragm is the primary muscle of inspiration. By contracting, it lowers and flattens, thus enlarging the thoracic cavity. At the same time, it compresses the

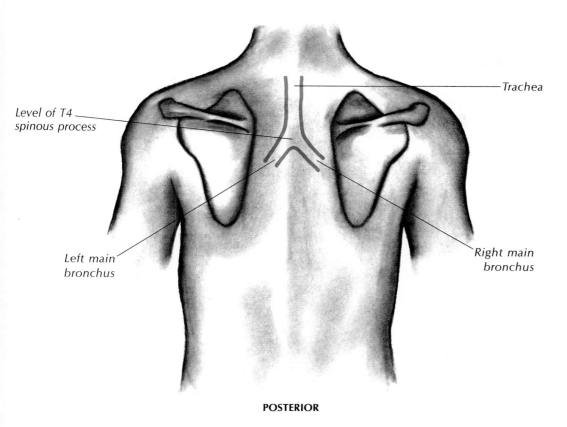

Level of T4 spinous process

Trachea

Left main bronchus

Right main bronchus

POSTERIOR

abdominal contents and the abdominal wall moves outward. Muscles in the rib cage and neck (primarily the parasternals and scalenes respectively) contribute to thoracic enlargement during inspiration.* They move the chest wall upward, anteriorly, and laterally. The thoracic expansion caused by these movements decreases intrathoracic pressure, draws air through the tracheobronchial tree into the alveoli (the distal air sacs), and expands the lungs. Oxygen diffuses into the blood of adjacent pulmonary capillaries, and carbon dioxide diffuses from the blood into the alveoli.

After the inspiratory effort stops, the lungs recoil, the diaphragm rises passively, air flows outward, the chest wall returns to its resting position, and the abdominal wall moves inward.

Normal breathing is quiet and easy—barely audible near the open mouth as a faint whish. This sound has no definite pitch because it has components over a wide range of frequencies. Sound of this kind is called white noise. When a healthy person lies supine, the breathing movements of the thorax are relatively slight. In contrast, the abdominal movements

---

* The clinically invisible parasternal muscles run from the sternum to the ribs. The scalene muscles run from the cervical vertebrae to the first two ribs. The internal and external intercostal muscles are no longer thought to play a major role in inspiration.

(which reflect diaphragmatic movements) are usually easy to see. In the sitting position, movements of the thorax become more prominent. These patterns are the same in both men and women.

During exercise and in certain diseases, extra work is required to breathe. The inspiratory contraction of the scalenes may become visible and, more obviously, the sternomastoids join in the inspiratory effort. Abdominal muscles assist in expiration. To see the inspiratory muscles, watch your own neck in a mirror as you inhale as deeply as possible.

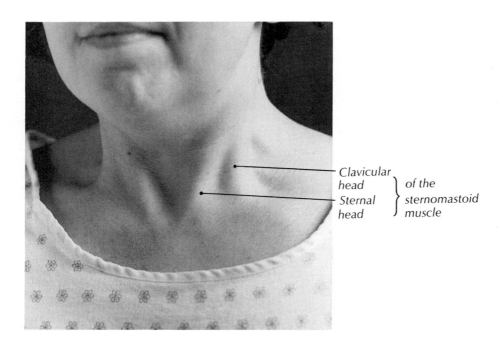

Clavicular head
Sternal head
} *of the sternomastoid muscle*

CHANGES WITH AGE

Throughout adult life, a person's vital capacity (the maximal volume of air that can be expired after a full inspiration) declines slowly. So does the maximal rate of expiration. These functional changes, along with others, may result from the aging process, from continued exposure to polluted air, or from disease. Skeletal changes associated with aging often accentuate the dorsal curve of the thoracic spine, producing kyphosis and an increased anteroposterior diameter of the chest. The resulting "barrel chest," however, does not by itself impair function.

Techniques of Examination

GENERAL APPROACH

1. The patient should undress to the waist and be examined with good lighting.
2. Proceed in an orderly fashion:
    a. Inspect, palpate, percuss, and auscultate.
    b. Compare one side with the other. Variations between patients are great; to some extent at least, comparison of one side with the other allows a patient to serve as his or her own control.
    c. Develop a pattern that assures relatively complete coverage, such as from the apices of the lungs to their bases.
3. Throughout your examination, try to visualize the underlying tissues, including the lobes of the lungs.
4. Examine the posterior thorax and lungs while the patient is still in the sitting position. The patient's arms should be folded across the chest with hands resting, if possible, on the opposite shoulders. This position moves the scapulae partly out of the way and increases your access to the lung fields.
5. Then ask the patient to lie down while you examine the anterior thorax and lungs. This supine position makes the examination of women easier because the breasts are less likely to get in the way. Furthermore, wheezes, if present, are more likely to be heard. (Some authorities, however, prefer to examine both the back and the front of the chest with the patient sitting. This technique is also satisfactory.)

When the patient cannot sit up without aid, try to get help so that you can examine the posterior chest in the sitting position. If this is impossible, roll the patient to one side and then the other. Percuss the upper lung and auscultate both lungs in each position. Because ventilation is relatively greater in the dependent lung, your chances of hearing wheezes or crackles are greater on the dependent side.

SURVEY OF THE THORAX AND RESPIRATION

During the examination of the skin, head, and neck, you have already made some preliminary observations relevant to the respiratory system. These include:

- The patient's color

  Cyanosis

- The shape of the fingernails

  Clubbing of the nails

- The position of the trachea

  May be displaced laterally by a pleural effusion, pneumothorax, or atelectasis

- Evidence of respiratory distress

Now carefully *observe the rate, rhythm, depth, and effort of breathing*. A normal adult breathes quietly and regularly about 14 to 20 times a minute. An occasional sigh is normal.

Inspect the neck for supraclavicular retraction and for contraction of the sternomastoid or other muscles during inspiration. Normally none is present.

Listen to the patient's breathing. Does the white noise of inspiration sound louder than usual? Are additional sounds such as wheezes audible? If so, where in the respiratory cycle do you hear them?

As you move around to the back of the patient, *observe the shape of the chest*. The anteroposterior diameter may increase with aging.

EXAMINATION OF THE POSTERIOR CHEST

Inspection

From a midline position behind the patient, note the *shape of the chest and the way in which it moves*, including:

● Deformities or asymmetry

● Abnormal retraction of the interspaces during inspiration. Retraction is most apparent in the lower interspaces. Supraclavicular retraction is often associated.

● Impairment in respiratory movement or a unilateral lag (or delay) in that movement

Palpation

Palpation of the chest has four potential uses:

1. *Identification of tender areas*. Carefully palpate any area where pain has been reported or where lesions are evident.
2. *Assessment of observed abnormalities* such as masses or sinus tracts (blind, inflammatory, tubelike structures opening onto the skin)

See Table 8-1, Abnormalities in Rate and Rhythm of Breathing (p. 256).

Inspiratory contraction of the sternomastoid muscles during rest suggests severe functional impairment.

In asthma and chronic bronchitis, the white noise of breathing becomes louder. Stridor, a wheeze that is solely or chiefly inspiratory, suggests airway obstruction in the neck.

The anteroposterior diameter of the chest may increase in chronic obstructive pulmonary disease.

See Table 8-2, Deformities of the Thorax (p. 257).

Retraction in severe asthma, chronic obstructive pulmonary disease, or upper airway obstruction

Unilateral impairment or lagging of respiratory movement suggests disease of the underlying lung or pleura.

Intercostal tenderness of an inflamed pleura. Although rare, sinus tracts usually indicate infection of the underlying pleura and lung (*e.g.*, tuberculosis, actinomycosis).

3. *Further assessment of respiratory expansion.* Place your thumbs about at the level of and parallel to the 10th ribs, your hands grasping the lateral rib cage. As you position your hands, slide them medially a bit in order to raise loose skin folds between thumbs and spine. Ask the patient to inhale deeply.

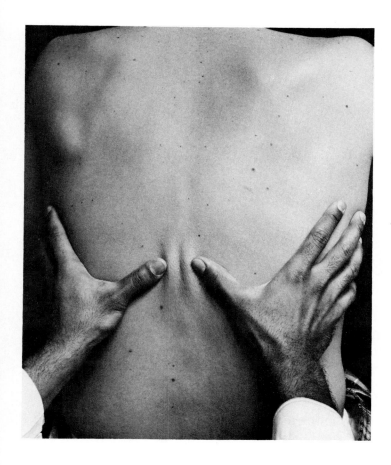

Watch the divergence of your thumbs during inspiration and feel for the range and symmetry of respiratory movement.

Causes of unilateral diminution of or delay in chest expansion include chronic fibrotic disease of the underlying lung or pleura, pleural effusion, lobar pneumonia, pleural pain with associated splinting, and unilateral bronchial obstruction.

4. *Assessment of tactile fremitus.* Fremitus refers to the palpable vibrations transmitted through the bronchopulmonary system to the chest wall when the patient speaks. Ask the patient to repeat the words "ninety-nine" or "one-one-one." If fremitus is faint, ask the patient to speak more loudly or in a lower voice.

Palpate and compare symmetrical areas of the lungs, using either the ball of your hand (the bony part of the palm at the base of the fingers) or the ulnar surface of your hand. In either case you are using the vibratory sensitivity of the bones in your hand to detect fremitus. Use one hand until you become thoroughly familiar with the feel of fre-

Fremitus is decreased or absent when the voice is soft or when the transmission of vibrations from the larynx to the surface of the chest is impeded. Causes include an obstructed bronchus; chronic obstructive pulmonary disease; separation of the pleural surfaces by fluid (pleural effusion), fibrosis (pleural thickening), air (pneu-

mitus. Some clinicians find this technique more accurate. The simultaneous use of both hands to compare sides, however, increases speed.

mothorax), or an infiltrating tumor; and also a very thick chest wall.

Fremitus is increased when transmission of sound is increased, as through the consolidated lung of lobar pneumonia.

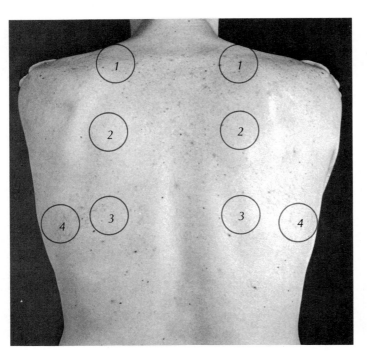

LOCATIONS FOR FEELING FREMITUS

Identify, describe, and localize any areas of increased or decreased fremitus. Fremitus is typically more prominent in the interscapular area than in the lower lung fields and is often more prominent on the right side than on the left. It disappears below the diaphragm.

Tactile fremitus is a relatively rough tool, but as a scouting maneuver it directs your attention to possible abnormalities. Later in the examination you will check any hypotheses that it raises by listening for breath sounds, voice sounds, and whispered voice sounds. All these attributes tend to increase or decrease together.

See Table 8-3, Normal and Altered Breath and Voice Sounds (p. 258).

Percussion

Percussion of the chest sets the chest wall and underlying tissues into motion, producing audible sounds and palpable vibrations. Percussion helps to determine whether the underlying tissues are air-filled, fluid-filled, or solid. It penetrates only about 5 cm to 7 cm into the chest, however, and will therefore not help you to detect deep-seated lesions.

The *technique of percussion* can be practiced on any surface. The key points, described for a right-handed person, follow.

Hyperextend the middle finger of your left hand (the pleximeter finger). Press its distal interphalangeal joint *firmly* on the surface to be percussed. Avoid contact by any other part of the hand, because this would damp the vibrations.

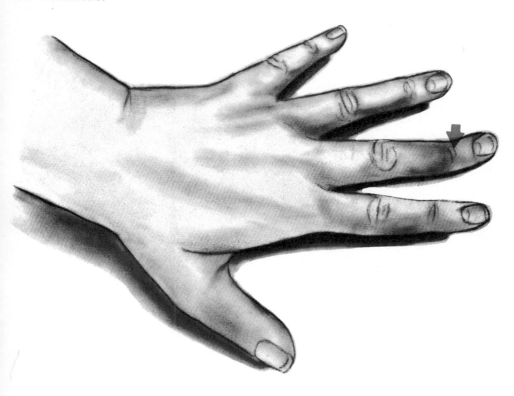

Position your right forearm quite close to the surface with the hand cocked upward. The right middle finger should be partially flexed, relaxed, and poised to strike.

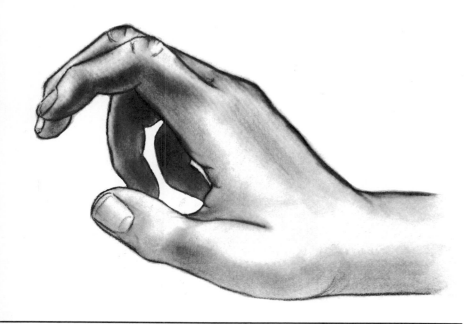

With a quick, sharp, but relaxed wrist motion, strike the pleximeter finger with the right middle finger (the plexor). Aim at your distal interphalangeal joint. You are trying to transmit vibrations through the bones of this joint to the underlying chest wall.

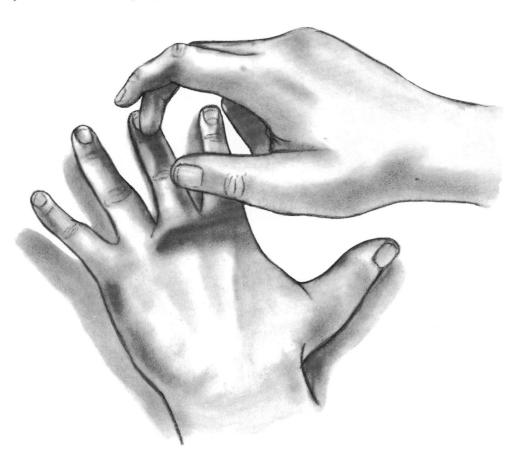

Use the tip of your plexor finger, not the finger pad. Your striking finger should be almost at right angles to the pleximeter. (A very short fingernail is required to avoid self-mutilation!)

Withdraw your striking finger quickly to avoid damping the vibrations that you have created.

In summary, the movement is at the wrist. It is direct, brisk yet relaxed, and a bit bouncy.

Use the lightest percussion that will produce a clear note. A thick chest wall requires heavier percussion than a thin one. In comparing two areas, however, keep your technique constant. Thump about twice in one location and then move on. You will perceive the sounds better by comparing one area with another than by repetitive thumping in one place. When percussing the lower posterior chest, stand somewhat to the side rather than directly behind the patient. Your hand position will feel more natural, and you will produce a clearer note.

Learn to identify five percussion notes, four of which you can reproduce on yourself. These notes can usually be distinguished by differences in their basic qualities of sound: intensity, pitch, and duration. Train your ear to detect these differences by concentrating on one quality at a time as you percuss first in one location, then in another.

Percussion Notes and Their Characteristics					PATHOLOGIC EXAMPLES
	RELATIVE INTENSITY	RELATIVE PITCH	RELATIVE DURATION	EXAMPLE LOCATION	
FLATNESS	Soft	High	Short	Thigh	Large pleural effusion
DULLNESS	Medium	Medium	Medium	Liver	Lobar pneumonia
RESONANCE	Loud	Low	Long	Normal lung	Bronchitis
HYPERRESONANCE	Very loud	Lower	Longer	None normally	Emphysema, pneumothorax
TYMPANY	Loud	High*	*	Gastric air bubble of puffed-out cheek	Large pneumothorax

* Distinguished mainly by its musical timbre

While the patient keeps both arms crossed in front of the chest, *percuss the thorax* in symmetrical locations from the apices to the lung bases. Percuss one side of the chest and then the other at each level, as shown by the numbers below.

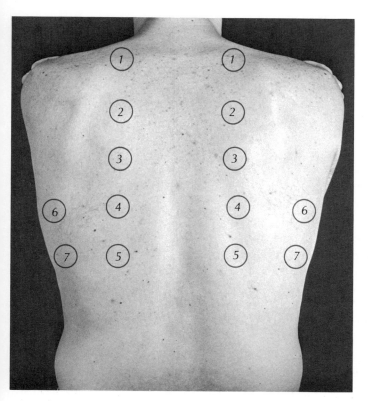

LOCATIONS FOR PERCUSSION AND AUSCULTATION

Dullness replaces resonance when fluid or solid tissue replaces air-containing lung or occupies the pleural space beneath your percussing fingers. Examples include: lobar pneumonia, in which the alveoli are filled with fluid and blood cells; and pleural accumulations of serous fluid (pleural effusion), blood (hemothorax), pus (empyema), fibrous tissue, or tumor.

Generalized hyperresonance may be heard over the hyperinflated lungs of emphysema or asthma, but it is not a reliable sign. Unilateral hyperresonance suggests a large pneumothorax or possibly a large air-filled bulla in the lung.

Omit the scapular areas; the thickness of musculoskeletal structures usually precludes worthwhile percussion there.

Identify, describe, and localize any area of abnormal percussion note.

Identify the level of diaphragmatic dullness during quiet respiration. With the pleximeter finger held parallel to the expected border of dullness, percuss in progressive steps downward until dullness clearly replaces resonance. Check the level of this change near the middle of the hemithorax and also more laterally.

An abnormally high level suggests pleural effusion or a high diaphragm, as from atelectasis or diaphragmatic paralysis.

A typical left pleural effusion of moderate size is represented below.

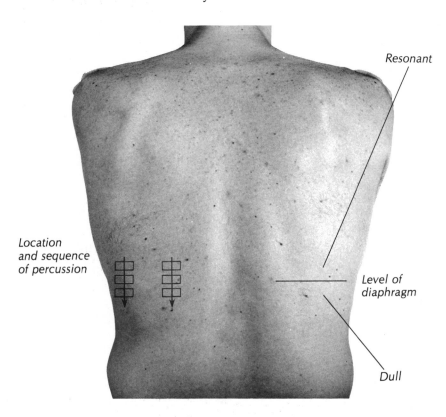

Location and sequence of percussion

Resonant

Level of diaphragm

Dull

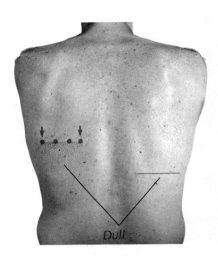

Dull

A paralyzed and therefore high left diaphragm causes similar dullness.

With this maneuver you are not percussing the diaphragm itself. If the boundary between the resonant lung tissue and the dull subdiaphragmatic tissue lies at a normal level, however, you can infer the probably normal location of the diaphragm.

Diaphragmatic excursion may be estimated by noting the distance between the levels of dullness on full expiration and on full inspiration, normally around 5 cm or 6 cm. This estimate, however, does not correlate well with radiologic assessment of diaphragmatic movement.

Auscultation

Auscultation of the lungs is useful in estimating air flow through the tracheobronchial tree and detecting obstruction to flow. Together with percussion, it also helps the clinician to assess the condition of the sur-

Sounds from bedclothes, paper gowns, and the chest itself can generate confusion in ausculta-

rounding lungs and pleural space. Auscultation involves (1) listening to the sounds generated by breathing, (2) listening for any adventitious (added) sounds, and (3) if abnormalities are suspected, listening to the sounds of the patient's spoken or whispered voice as they are transmitted through the chest wall.

BREATH SOUNDS (LUNG SOUNDS). Normal breath sounds have been classified into three categories according to their intensity, their pitch, and the relative duration of their inspiratory and expiratory phases. *Vesicular breath sounds* are soft and low-pitched. They are heard through inspiration, continue without pause into expiration, and then fade away about one third of the way through expiration. *Bronchial breath sounds* are louder and higher in pitch. There is a short silent period between the inspiratory and expiratory sounds, and the expiratory sounds last longer than the inspiratory ones. *Bronchovesicular sounds* are intermediate. Inspiratory and expiratory sounds are about equal in length, and a silent period between them may or may not be present. Differences in pitch and intensity are often more easily detected during expiration.

The characteristics of these three kinds of breath sounds are summarized in the table below. Also shown are the *tracheal breath sounds*—very loud, harsh sounds that are heard by listening over the trachea in the neck.

tion. Hair on the chest may cause crackling sounds. Either press harder or wet the hair. If the patient is cold or tense, you may hear muscle contraction sounds—muffled, low-pitched rumbling or roaring noises. A change in the patient's position may eliminate this noise. You can reproduce this sound on yourself by doing a Valsalva maneuver (straining down) as you listen to your own chest.

Characteristics of Breath Sounds

	DURATION OF SOUNDS	INTENSITY OF EXPIRATORY SOUND	PITCH OF EXPIRATORY SOUND	LOCATIONS WHERE HEARD NORMALLY
VESICULAR*	Inspiratory sounds last longer than expiratory ones.	Soft	Relatively low	Over most of both lungs
BRONCHO-VESICULAR	Inspiratory and expiratory sounds are about equal.	Intermediate	Intermediate	Often in the 1st and 2nd interspaces anteriorly and between the scapulae
BRONCHIAL	Expiratory sounds last longer than inspiratory ones.	Loud	Relatively high	Over the manubrium, if heard at all
TRACHEAL	Inspiratory and expiratory sounds are about equal.	Very loud	Relatively high	Over the trachea in the neck

* The thickness of the bars indicates intensity; the steeper their incline, the higher the pitch.

If bronchovesicular or bronchial breath sounds are heard in locations distant from those listed, suspect that air-filled lung has been replaced by fluid or solid lung tissue. See Table 8-3, Normal and Altered Breath and Voice Sounds (p. 258).

Listen to the breath sounds with the diaphragm of a stethoscope as the patient breathes somewhat more deeply than normal through an open mouth. Using locations similar to those recommended for percussion and moving from one side to the other, compare symmetrical areas of the lungs. Listen to at least one full breath in each location. Be alert for patient discomfort due to hyperventilation (*e.g.,* lightheadedness, faintness), and allow the patient to rest as needed.

Note the intensity of the breath sounds. Breath sounds are usually louder in the lower posterior lung fields and may also vary a bit from area to area. If the breath sounds seem faint, ask the patient to breathe more deeply. You may then hear them easily. When patients do not breathe deeply enough or when they have a thick chest wall, as in obesity, breath sounds may remain diminished.

Breath sounds may be decreased when air flow is decreased (as by obstructive lung disease or muscular weakness) or when the transmission of sound is poor (as in pleural effusion, pneumothorax, or emphysema).

Listen for the pitch, intensity, and duration of the expiratory and inspiratory sounds. Are vesicular breath sounds distributed normally over the chest wall? Or are there bronchovesicular or bronchial breath sounds in unexpected places? If so, where are they?

ADVENTITIOUS (ADDED) SOUNDS. Listen for any adventitious sounds, of which there are two basic types.*

See Table 8-4, Adventitious (Added) Lung Sounds (p. 259).

Discontinuous sounds, or *crackles,* are intermittent, nonmusical, and very brief, somewhat like dots in time. They can be simulated by rolling a lock of hair between your fingers close to your ear. Crackles are further divided into two subgroups according to their intensity, pitch, and duration.

See Table 8-5, Physical Signs in Selected Chest Disorders (pp. 260–261).

- *Fine crackles* (· · · · ·) are soft, high-pitched, and very brief (5–10 msec).
- *Coarse crackles* (• • • •) are somewhat louder, lower in pitch, and not quite so brief (20–30 msec).

If you hear crackles of either kind, note their number (few to many), their timing in relation to the respiratory cycle, and their location on the chest wall. It may also be helpful to note if they change with posture or after coughing. In some normal people, crackles that have no pathologic significance may be heard at the lung bases anteriorly after maximal expiration. Crackles in dependent portions of the lungs may also occur after prolonged recumbency.

---

* The nomenclature of lung sounds has been changing, and older terms often continue in use. For example, many clinicians still use "rales" instead of crackles. The term rales, however, has had several very different meanings, and authorities now discourage its use.

Continuous sounds last notably longer than crackles (>250 msec) but do not necessarily persist throughout the respiratory cycle. They may be likened to dashes in time. Their musical quality distinguishes them from breath sounds. Two subgroups are differentiated by pitch.

- *Wheezes* (〰) are relatively high-pitched (around 400 Hz or higher) and have a hissing or shrill quality.
- *Rhonchi* (〰) are relatively low-pitched (around 200 Hz or lower) and have a snoring quality.

This distinction is not useful in making diagnoses, however, and some authorities use the terms wheezes and rhonchi interchangeably.

If you hear such sounds,

> Are they inspiratory, expiratory, or both?
> Where on the chest wall do you hear them?
> Do they clear with deep breathing or coughing?

TRANSMITTED VOICE SOUNDS. If you note abnormally located bronchovesicular or bronchial breath sounds, continue on to assess transmitted voice sounds. With a stethoscope, listen in symmetrical areas over the chest wall as you—

- Ask the patient to say "ninety-nine." Normally the sounds transmitted through the chest wall are muffled and indistinct.

- Ask the patient to say "ee." You will normally hear a muffled long E sound.

- Ask the patient to whisper "ninety-nine" or "one-two-three." The whispered voice is normally heard faintly and indistinctly, if at all.

EXAMINATION OF THE ANTERIOR CHEST

The patient, when examined in the supine position, should lie comfortably with arms somewhat abducted. An orthopneic patient should be examined in the sitting position or with the bed elevated to a comfortable level.

Continuous sounds suggest that one or more airways are narrowed almost to the point of closure. This closure may be local (as from a tumor or foreign body) or generalized (as from bronchospasm, accumulated bronchial secretions, or edema of the bronchial mucosa).

Clearing suggests that secretions caused the sounds.

Increased transmission of voice sounds suggests that air-filled lung has become airless. See Table 8-3, Normal and Altered Breath and Voice Sounds (p. 258).

Louder, clearer voice sounds are called *bronchophony*.

When "ee" is heard as "ay," an *E-to-A change* (*egophony*) is present. The quality sounds nasal.

Louder, clearer whispered sounds are called *whispered pectoriloquy*.

Persons with severe chronic obstructive lung disease often prefer to sit leaning forward, with lips pursed during exhalation and arms supported on their knees or a table.

Inspection

Observe *the shape of the patient's chest* and *the way in which it moves.* Note:

● Deformities or asymmetry

See Table 8-2, Deformities of the Thorax (p. 257).

● Abnormal retraction of the lower interspaces during inspiration

Severe asthma, chronic obstructive pulmonary disease, or upper airway obstruction

● Local lag or impairment in respiratory movement

Underlying disease of lung or pleura

Palpation

Palpation has four potential uses:

1. *Identification of tender areas*

2. *Assessment of observed abnormalities*

Tender pectoral muscles or costal cartilages tend to corroborate, but do not prove, that chest pain has a musculoskeletal origin.

3. *Further assessment of respiratory expansion.* Place your thumbs along each costal margin, your hands along the lateral rib cage. As you position your hands, slide them medially a bit to raise a loose skin fold between your thumbs. Ask the patient to inhale deeply. Watch for divergence of your thumbs as the thorax expands, and feel for the range and symmetry of respiratory movement.

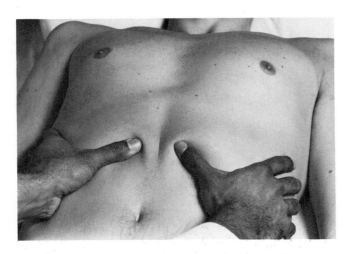

4. *Assessment of tactile fremitus.* Compare both sides of the chest, using the ball or ulnar surface of your hand. Fremitus is usually decreased or absent over the precordium. When examining a woman, gently displace the breasts as necessary.

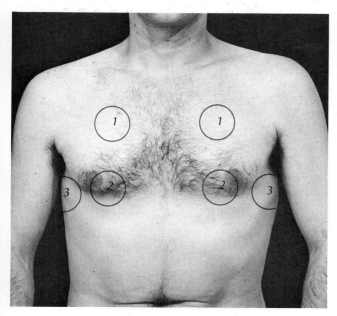

LOCATIONS FOR FEELING FREMITUS

Percussion

Percuss the anterior and lateral chest, again comparing both sides. The heart normally produces an area of dullness to the left of the sternum from the 3rd to the 5th interspaces. Percuss the left lung lateral to it.

Dullness replaces resonance when fluid or solid tissue replaces air-containing lung or occupies the pleural space. Because pleural fluid usually sinks to the lowest part of the pleural space (posteriorly in a supine patient), only a very large effusion can be detected anteriorly.

The hyperresonance of emphysema may totally replace cardiac dullness.

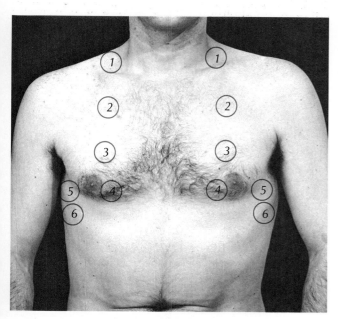

LOCATIONS FOR PERCUSSION AND AUSCULTATION

When a woman's breast interferes with percussion, gently displace it with your left hand while percussing with the right.

The dullness of right middle lobe pneumonia typically

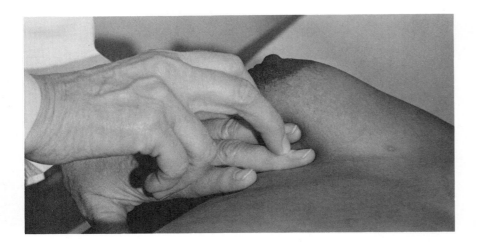

occurs behind the right breast. Unless you displace the breast, you may miss the abnormal percussion note.

Alternatively, you may ask the patient to move her breast for you.

Identify, describe, and localize any area of abnormal percussion note.

With your pleximeter finger parallel to the expected upper border of liver dullness, percuss in progressive steps downward in the right midclavicular line. Identify the upper border of liver dullness. Later, during the abdominal examination, you will use this method to estimate the size of the liver. As you percuss down the chest on the left, the resonance of normal lung usually changes to the tympany of the gastric air bubble.

An emphysematous lung often displaces this border downward. It also lowers the level of diaphragmatic dullness posteriorly.

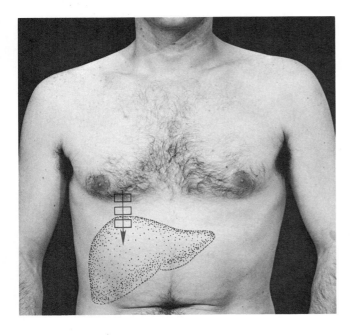

Auscultation

Listen to the chest, anteriorly and laterally, as the patient breathes with mouth open, somewhat more deeply than normal. Compare symmetrical areas of the lungs, using the pattern suggested for percussion.

Listen to the breath sounds, noting their intensity and identifying any variations from normal vesicular breathing. Breath sounds are usually louder in the upper anterior lung fields. Bronchovesicular breath sounds may be heard over the large airways, especially on the right.

Identify any adventitious sounds, time them in the respiratory cycle, and locate them on the chest wall. Do they clear with deep breathing?

See Table 8-4, Adventitious (Added) Lung Sounds (p. 259).

If indicated, *listen for transmitted voice sounds.*

See Table 8-5, Physical Signs in Selected Chest Disorders (pp. 260–261).

SPECIAL MANEUVERS

CLINICAL ASSESSMENT OF PULMONARY FUNCTION. A simple but informative way to assess the complaint of breathlessness in an ambulatory patient is to walk with the patient down the hall or climb one flight of stairs. Observe the rate, effort, and sound of the patient's breathing.

Obstructive pulmonary disease is characterized by a slowed expiratory phase. This can be quantitated clinically by measuring the *forced expiratory time.* Ask the patient to take a deep breath in and then breathe out as quickly and completely as possible, with mouth open. Listen over the trachea with the bell of a stethoscope and time the audible expiration. It should last less than 5 seconds. Try to get three consistent readings, allowing a short rest between efforts if necessary.

If the patient understands and cooperates in performing the test, a forced expiration time of more than 6 seconds strongly suggests obstructive pulmonary disease.

IDENTIFICATION OF A FRACTURED RIB. Local pain and tenderness of one or more ribs raise the question of fracture. By anteroposterior compression of the chest, you can help to distinguish a fracture from soft-tissue injury. With one hand on the sternum and the other on the thoracic spine, squeeze the chest. Is this painful, and where?

An increase in the local pain (distant from your hands) suggests rib fracture rather than just soft-tissue injury.

Table 8-1   Abnormalities in Rate and Rhythm of Breathing

When observing respiratory patterns, think in terms of *rate*, *depth*, and *regularity* of the patient's breathing. Describe what you see in these terms. Traditional terms, such as tachypnea, are given below so that you will understand them, but simple descriptions are recommended for use.

NORMAL

Inspiration   Expiration

Volume of air

Time

The respiratory rate is about 14–20 per min in normal adults and up to 44 per min in infants.

RAPID SHALLOW BREATHING
(Tachypnea)

Rapid shallow breathing has a number of causes, including restrictive lung disease, pleuritic chest pain, and an elevated diaphragm.

RAPID DEEP BREATHING
(Hyperpnea, Hyperventilation)

Rapid deep breathing also has a number of causes, including exercise, anxiety, and metabolic acidosis. In the comatose patient, infarction, hypoxia, or hypoglycemia affecting the midbrain or pons should be considered. *Kussmaul breathing* is deep breathing associated with metabolic acidosis. It may be fast, normal in rate, or slow.

SLOW BREATHING
(Bradypnea)

Slow breathing may be secondary to such causes as diabetic coma, drug-induced respiratory depression, and increased intracranial pressure.

CHEYNE-STOKES BREATHING

Hyperpnea   Apnea

Respiration waxes and wanes cyclically so that periods of deep breathing alternate with periods of apnea (no breathing). Children and aging people normally may show this pattern in sleep. Other causes include heart failure, uremia, drug-induced respiratory depression, and brain damage (typically on both sides of the cerebral hemispheres or diencephalon).

ATAXIC BREATHING
(Biot's Breathing)

Ataxic breathing is characterized by unpredictable irregularity. Breaths may be shallow or deep, and stop for short periods. Causes include respiratory depression and brain damage, typically at the medullary level.

SIGHING RESPIRATION

Sighs

Breathing punctuated by frequent sighs should alert you to the possibility of hyperventilation syndrome—a common cause of dyspnea and dizziness. Occasional sighs are normal.

OBSTRUCTIVE BREATHING

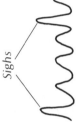

Prolonged expiration

Air trapping

In obstructive lung disease, expiration is prolonged because of increased airway resistance. If the respiratory rate increases, the patient lacks sufficient time for full expiration. The chest overexpands (air trapping) and breathing becomes more shallow.

Table 8-2 Deformities of the Thorax

Table 8-2 Deformities of the Thorax

NORMAL ADULT

CROSS SECTION OF THORAX

CLINICAL APPEARANCE

The thorax in the normal adult is wider than it is deep, i.e., its lateral diameter is larger than its anteroposterior diameter.

BARREL CHEST

CROSS SECTION OF THORAX

CLINICAL APPEARANCE

A barrel chest has an increased anteroposterior diameter. This shape is normal during infancy, and often accompanies normal aging and chronic obstructive pulmonary disease.

TRAUMATIC FLAIL CHEST

CROSS SECTION OF THORAX

Expiration

Inspiration

If multiple ribs are fractured, paradoxical movements of the thorax may be seen. As descent of the diaphragm decreases intrathoracic pressure on inspiration, the injured area caves inward; on expiration, it moves outward.

FUNNEL CHEST (*Pectus Excavatum*)

CROSS SECTION OF THE THORAX

CLINICAL APPEARANCE

A funnel chest is characterized by a depression in the lower portion of the sternum. Compression of the heart and great vessels may cause murmurs.

PIGEON CHEST (*Pectus Carinatum*)

CROSS SECTION OF THORAX

CLINICAL APPEARANCE

Depressed costal cartilages

Anteriorly displaced sternum

In a pigeon chest, the sternum is displaced anteriorly, increasing the anteroposterior diameter. The costal cartilages adjacent to the protruding sternum are depressed.

THORACIC KYPHOSCOLIOSIS

CLINICAL APPEARANCE

Spinal convexity to the right

Ribs widely separated

CROSS SECTION OF THORAX

Ribs close together

In thoracic kyphoscoliosis, abnormal spinal curvatures and vertebral rotation deform the chest. Distortion of the underlying lungs may make interpretation of lung findings very difficult.

Table 8-3   Normal and Altered Breath and Voice Sounds

The exact origins of breath sounds are still in dispute. It is thought that turbulent air flow in the central airways produces the tracheal and bronchial breath sounds, and that vesicular breath sounds arise somewhere distal to the trachea and proximal to the alveoli.

Tracheal and bronchial breath sounds are heard close to their anatomic origins but are not transmitted well through air-filled lung tissue. Over most of the chest wall, therefore, vesicular breath sounds predominate. When lung tissue loses its air, however, it transmits high-frequency sounds much better. The high-pitched bronchial breath sounds are then heard on the chest wall, where they replace the normal vesicular sounds. This change occurs typically in lobar pneumonia, in which the alveoli fill with fluid, red cells, and white cells—a process called consolidation.

The occurrence of bronchial breath sounds usually correlates with an increase in both tactile fremitus and transmitted voice sounds. These changes are summarized below.

	NORMALLY AIR-FILLED LUNG	AIRLESS LUNG, AS IN LOBAR PNEUMONIA
	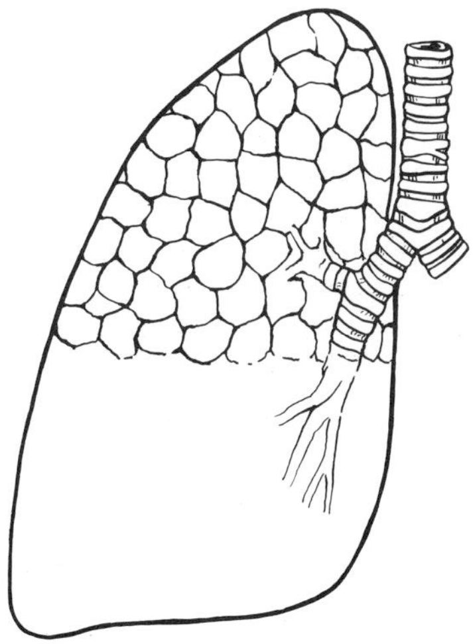	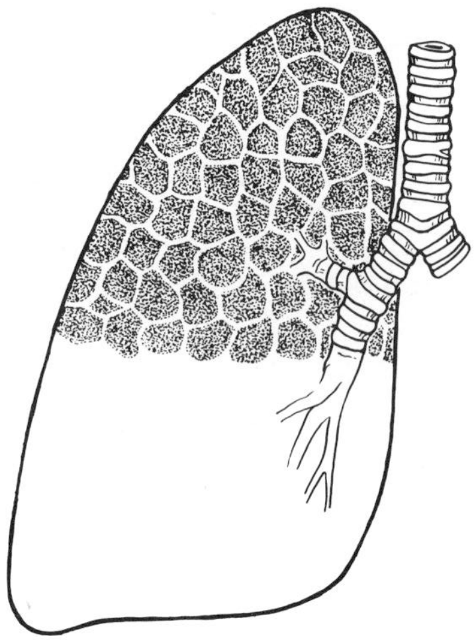
BREATH SOUNDS	Predominantly vesicular	Bronchial or bronchovesicular over the involved area
TRANSMITTED VOICE SOUNDS	Spoken words muffled and indistinct	Spoken words louder, clearer (bronchophony)
	Spoken "ee" heard as "ee"	Spoken "ee" heard as "ay" (egophony)
	Whispered words faint and indistinct, if heard at all	Whispered words louder, clearer (whispered pectoriloquy)
TACTILE FREMITUS	Normal	Increased

Table 8-4   Adventitious (Added) Lung Sounds

Table 8-4   Adventitious (Added) Lung Sounds

CRACKLES

Crackles have two leading explanations. (1) They result from a series of tiny explosions when small airways, deflated during expiration, pop open during inspiration. This mechanism probably explains the late inspiratory crackles of interstitial lung disease and early congestive heart failure. (2) Crackles result as air bubbles flow through secretions or lightly closed airways during respiration. This mechanism probably explains at least some coarse crackles.

Inspiration   Expiration

Late inspiratory crackles may begin in the first half of the inspiratory phase but must continue into late inspiration. They are usually fine, fairly profuse, and repeat themselves from breath to breath. They are not audible at the mouth. These crackles appear first at the bases of the lungs, spread upward as the condition worsens, and shift to dependent regions with changes in posture. Causes include interstitial lung disease (such as fibrosis) and early congestive heart failure.

Early inspiratory crackles appear soon after the start of inspiration and do not continue into late inspiration. They are often but not always coarse, are relatively few in number, and are commonly audible at the mouth as well as through the chest wall. Expiratory crackles are sometimes associated. Causes include chronic bronchitis and asthma.

Midinspiratory and expiratory crackles are heard in bronchiectasis but are not specific for this diagnosis. Wheezes and rhonchi may be associated.

WHEEZES AND RHONCHI

According to the leading theory, continuous lung sounds (wheezes and rhonchi) occur when air flows rapidly through bronchi that are narrowed nearly to the point of closure. They are often audible at the mouth as well as through the chest wall. Causes of continuous sounds that are generalized include bronchial asthma, chronic bronchitis, and congestive heart failure (cardiac asthma). In asthma, wheezes may be heard only in expiration or in both phases of the respiratory cycle. In chronic bronchitis, wheezes and rhonchi often clear with coughing.

Occasionally in severe obstructive pulmonary disease, the condition worsens to the point that the patient is no longer able to force enough air through the narrowed bronchi to produce wheezing. The disappearance of wheezing in such patients should signal concern and not be mistaken for improvement.

A persistent localized wheeze suggests a partial obstruction of a bronchus, as by a tumor or foreign body. It may be inspiratory, expiratory, or both.

STRIDOR

A wheeze that is entirely or predominantly inspiratory and that is also louder in the neck than over the chest wall is called stridor. It indicates a partial obstruction of the airway in the neck, *e.g.,* in the larynx or trachea.

PLEURAL RUB

Normal pleural surfaces move smoothly and noiselessly against each other during respiration. When pleural surfaces become inflamed, however, they move jerkily as they are momentarily and repeatedly delayed by increased friction. These movements, with their associated vibrations, produce creaking, grating sounds known as a pleural rub (or pleural friction rub).

Pleural rubs resemble crackles acoustically, although they are produced by different pathologic processes. The sounds may be heard as discrete, but sometimes are so numerous that they merge into an apparently continuous sound. A rub is usually confined to a relatively small area of the chest wall. It is often heard in both phases of respiration, but is sometimes confined to inspiration. When inflamed pleural surfaces are separated by fluid, the rub often disappears.

MEDIASTINAL CRUNCH
(*Hamman's Sign*)

A mediastinal crunch is a series of precordial crackles synchronous with the heart beat, not with respiration. Best heard in the left lateral position, it is due to mediastinal emphysema (pneumomediastinum).

259

Table 8-5   Physical Signs in Selected Chest Disorders

The changes described in this table vary importantly with the extent and severity of the disorder. Abnormalities deep in the chest, moreover, usually produce fewer signs than do superficial ones, and they may cause no signs at all. Use the table for the direction of typical changes rather than for fine distinctions.

The red boxes suggest a framework to guide clinical assessment. Start with the three clusters under Percussion Note, and move from there to other boxes.

CONDITION	TRACHEA	PERCUSSION NOTE	BREATH SOUNDS	TACTILE FREMITUS AND TRANSMITTED VOICE SOUNDS	ADVENTITIOUS SOUNDS
NORMAL The tracheobronchial tree and alveoli are clear; the pleurae are thin and close together; the mobility of the chest wall is unimpaired.	Midline	Resonant	Vesicular, except perhaps for bronchovesicular and bronchial sounds near the large bronchi and trachea respectively	Normal	None, except perhaps for a few transient inspiratory crackles at the bases of the lungs
CHRONIC BRONCHITIS The bronchi are chronically inflamed, and a productive cough is present. Airway obstruction may develop.	Midline	Resonant	Normal	Normal	None; or scattered coarse crackles in early inspiration and perhaps expiration; or wheezes or rhonchi
LEFT-SIDED HEART FAILURE (*Early*) Increased pressure in the pulmonary veins causes congestion and interstitial edema (around the alveoli). The bronchial mucosa may become edematous.	Midline	Resonant	Normal	Normal	Late inspiratory crackles in the dependent portions of the lungs; possibly wheezes
LOBAR PNEUMONIA Because of bacterial infection, the alveoli fill with fluid, red cells, and white cells in a process called consolidation.	Midline	Dull over the airless area	Bronchial over the involved area	Increased over the involved area with bronchophony, egophony, and whispered pectoriloquy	Late inspiratory crackles over the involved area

Table 8-5   Physical Signs in Selected Chest Disorders

Condition		Trachea	Percussion Note	Breath Sounds	(Transmitted Voice Sounds)	Adventitious Sounds
ATELECTASIS (Lobar Obstruction) When a plug in a mainstem bronchus (as from mucus or a foreign object) obstructs air flow, oxygen in the lobe is absorbed and the affected lung tissue collapses into an airless state.		May be shifted toward the involved side	Dull over the airless area	Usually absent when the bronchial plug persists. Exceptions include right upper lobe atelectasis, where adjacent tracheal sounds may be transmitted.	Usually absent when the bronchial plug persists. In exceptions, *e.g.*, right upper lobe atelectasis, may be increased	None
PLEURAL EFFUSION When fluid accumulates in the pleural space, it separates the air-filled lung from the chest wall and blocks the transmission of sound.		Toward the opposite side in a large effusion	Dull to flat over the fluid	Decreased to absent; but bronchial breath sounds may be heard near the top of a large effusion.	Decreased to absent; but may be increased toward the top of a large effusion	None, except for a possible pleural rub
PNEUMOTHORAX When air leaks into the pleural space, usually unilaterally, the lung recoils away from the chest wall. Pleural air blocks the transmission of sound.		Toward the opposite side if much air	Hyperresonant or tympanitic over the pleural air	Decreased to absent over the pleural air	Decreased to absent over the pleural air	None, except for a possible pleural rub
EMPHYSEMA This is a slowly progressive disorder in which the distal air spaces are enlarged and the lungs are hyperinflated. Chronic bronchitis is often associated.		Midline	Diffusely hyperresonant	Decreased to absent	Decreased	None, or the crackles, wheezes, and rhonchi of associated chronic bronchitis
BRONCHIAL ASTHMA Asthma occurs in episodes. The bronchi respond excessively to stimuli, causing restriction to air flow and hyperinflation.		Midline	Normal to diffusely hyperresonant	Often obscured by wheezes	Decreased	Wheezes, possibly crackles

Chapter 9
The Cardiovascular System

Anatomy and Physiology

SURFACE PROJECTIONS OF THE HEART AND GREAT VESSELS

The heart is assessed chiefly by examination through the anterior chest wall. Most of the anterior cardiac surface is made up of right ventricle. This chamber and the pulmonary artery may be visualized roughly as a wedge lying behind and to the left of the sternum.

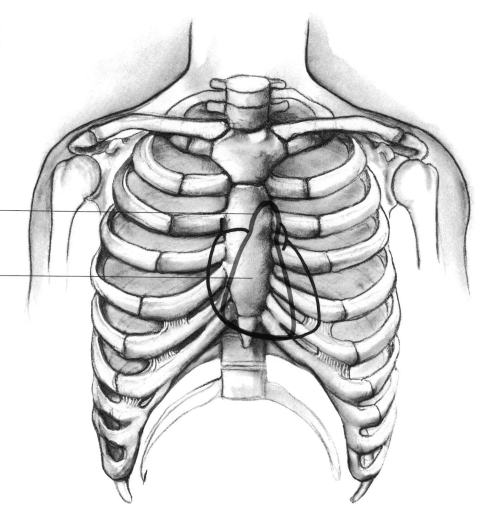

Pulmonary artery

Right ventricle

The inferior border of the right ventricle rests at a level somewhat below the junction of the sternum and the xiphoid process. The right ventricle narrows superiorly and meets the pulmonary artery at the level of the 3rd left costal cartilage close to the sternum.

The left ventricle, lying to the left of and behind the right ventricle, makes up only a small portion of the anterior cardiac surface. It is clinically important, however, forming the left border of the heart and producing the apical impulse.* This impulse is a brief systolic beat usually found in the 5th interspace, 7 cm to 9 cm from the midsternal line.

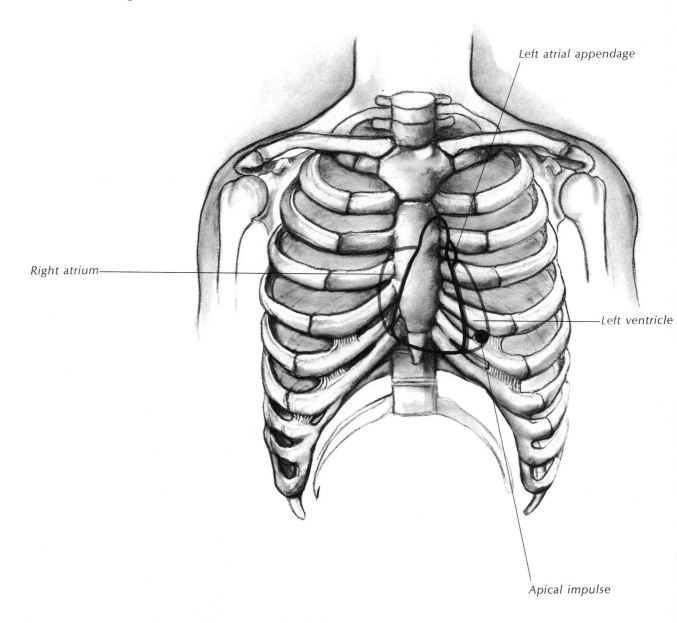

Left atrial appendage

Right atrium

Left ventricle

Apical impulse

The right border of the heart is formed by the right atrium, a chamber not usually identifiable on physical examination. The left atrium is mostly posterior and cannot be examined directly, although its small atrial appendage may make up a segment of the left cardiac border between the pulmonary artery and the left ventricle.

* The apical impulse is sometimes called the point of maximum impulse, or PMI. Because the most prominent cardiac impulse may not be apical, some authorities discourage use of this term.

Above the heart lie the great vessels. The pulmonary artery, already mentioned, bifurcates quickly into its left and right branches. The aorta curves upward from the left ventricle to the level of the sternal angle, where it arches backward and then down. On the right, the superior vena cava empties into the right atrium.

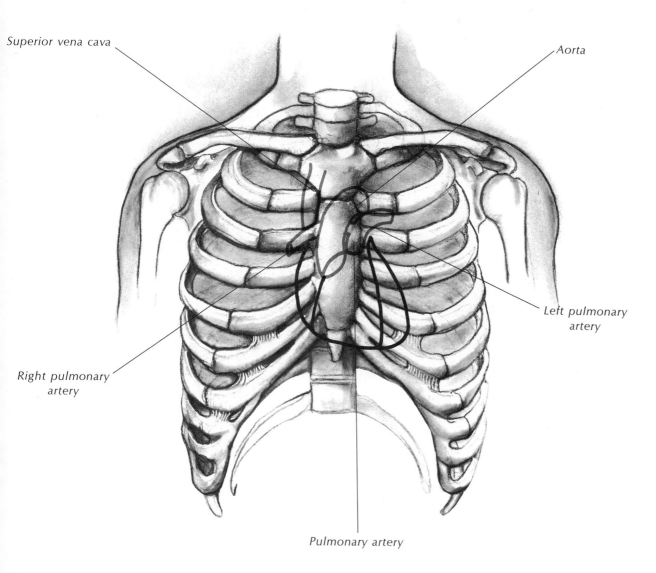

Superior vena cava

Aorta

Left pulmonary artery

Right pulmonary artery

Pulmonary artery

Although not illustrated above, the inferior vena cava also empties into the right atrium. The superior and inferior venae cavae carry venous blood from the upper and lower portions of the body, respectively.

CARDIAC CHAMBERS, VALVES, AND CIRCULATION

Circulation through the heart is illustrated in the following diagram, which identifies the cardiac chambers, valves, and direction of blood flow. Because of their positions, the tricuspid and mitral valves are often called atrioventricular valves. The aortic and pulmonic valves are called

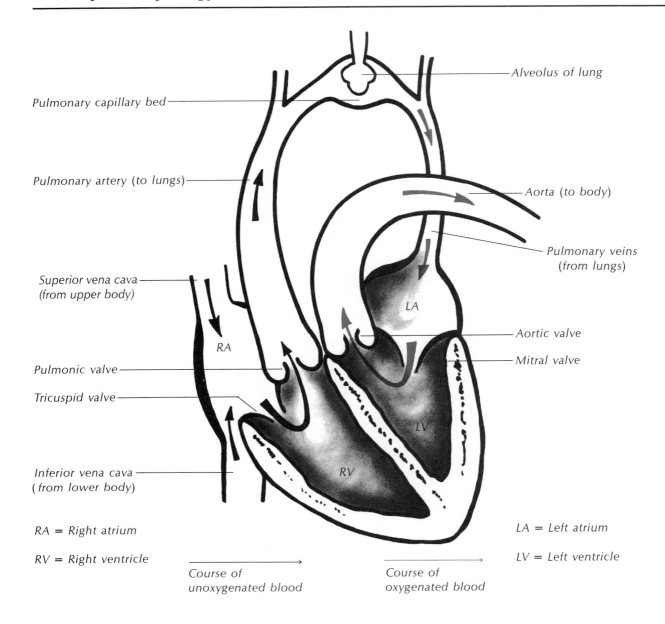

Pulmonary capillary bed

Alveolus of lung

Pulmonary artery (to lungs)

Aorta (to body)

Superior vena cava (from upper body)

Pulmonary veins (from lungs)

Pulmonic valve

Aortic valve

Tricuspid valve

Mitral valve

LA

RA

LV

RV

Inferior vena cava (from lower body)

RA = Right atrium

LA = Left atrium

RV = Right ventricle

LV = Left ventricle

Course of unoxygenated blood

Course of oxygenated blood

semilunar valves because each of their leaflets is shaped like a half moon. Although this diagram shows all valves in an open position, they are not all open simultaneously in the living heart.

When valves in the heart close, vibrations engendered in the leaflets, in adjacent cardiac structures, and in the blood produce normal heart sounds. The positions and movements of the valves must be understood in relation to events in the cardiac cycle.

EVENTS IN THE CARDIAC CYCLE

Measuring the pressure in the left ventricle throughout the cardiac cycle yields a pressure curve like the following:

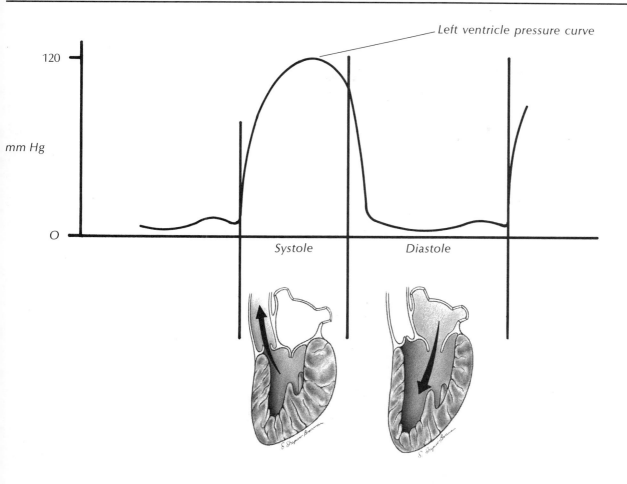

Left ventricle pressure curve

Systole is the period of ventricular contraction. Pressure in the left ventricle rises rapidly, then levels off, and starts to fall as most of its blood is ejected into the aorta. *Diastole* is the period of ventricular relaxation. Ventricular pressure falls almost to zero, and blood flows from atrium to ventricle. Late in diastole, ventricular pressure rises slightly during atrial contraction.

Note that during systole the aortic valve is open, allowing ejection of blood from the left ventricle into the aorta. The mitral valve is closed, preventing blood from regurgitating back into the left atrium. In contrast, during diastole the aortic valve is closed, preventing regurgitation of blood from the aorta back into the left ventricle. The mitral valve is open, allowing blood to flow from the left atrium into the relaxed left ventricle.

Understanding the interrelationships of the pressures in these three chambers—left atrium, left ventricle, and aorta—together with the position and movement of the valves is fundamental to the understanding of heart sounds. These changing pressures and the sounds that result will be traced here through one cardiac cycle.

During diastole, pressure in the blood-filled left atrium slightly exceeds that in the relaxed left ventricle, and blood flows from left atrium to left ventricle across the open mitral valve. Just before the onset of ventricular systole, atrial contraction produces a slight pressure rise in both chambers.

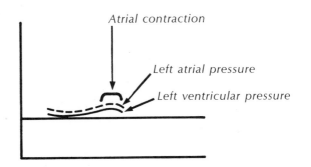

As the ventricle starts to contract, pressure within it rapidly exceeds left atrial pressure, thus shutting the mitral valve. Closure of the mitral valve produces the first heart sound (S_1).*

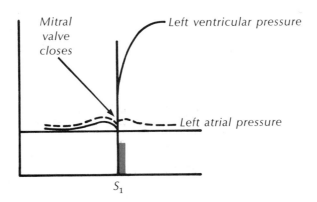

As the ventricular pressure continues to rise, it quickly exceeds the pressure in the aorta and forces the aortic valve open. Opening of the aortic valve is not usually heard, but in some pathologic conditions it is accompanied by an early systolic ejection sound (Ej).

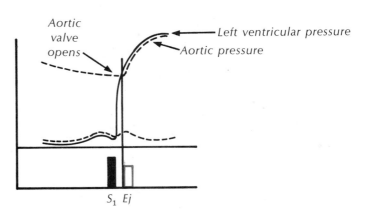

As the ventricle ejects most of its blood, its pressure begins to fall. When left ventricular pressure drops below the aortic pressure, the aortic valve shuts. Aortic valve closure causes the second heart sound (S_2).

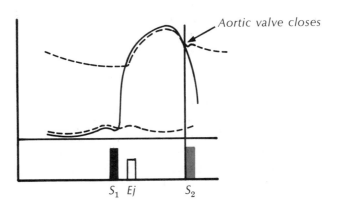

* An extensive literature deals with the exact causes of heart sounds (*e.g.*, actual closure of valve leaflets, tensing of related structures, and the impact of columns of blood). The explanations given here are oversimplified but retain clinical usefulness.

As the left ventricular pressure continues to drop during ventricular relaxation, it falls below left atrial pressure. The mitral valve opens. This is usually a silent event but may be audible as an opening snap (OS) in mitral stenosis.

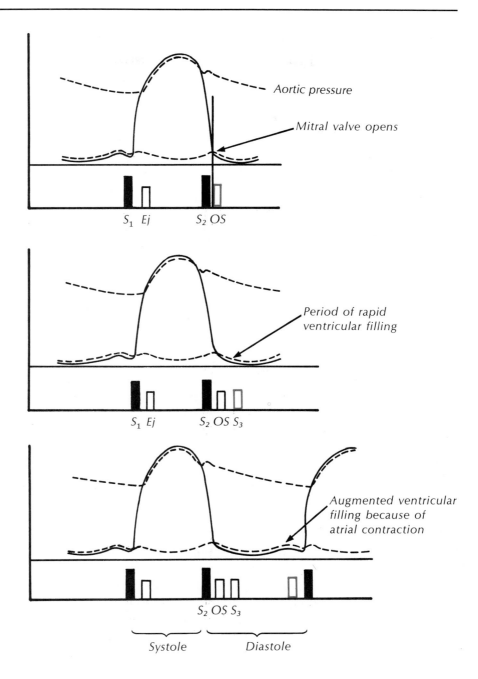

Aortic pressure

Mitral valve opens

S_1 Ej S_2 OS

Next occurs a period of rapid ventricular filling as blood flows early in diastole from left atrium to left ventricle. In children and young adults, this period may be marked by a third heart sound (S_3).

Period of rapid ventricular filling

S_1 Ej S_2 OS S_3

Finally, although not often heard in normal adults, a fourth heart sound (S_4) marks atrial contraction. It immediately precedes S_1 of the next beat.

During auscultation, S_1 and S_2 define the margins of systole and diastole.

Augmented ventricular filling because of atrial contraction

S_2 OS S_3

Systole   Diastole

THE SPLITTING OF HEART SOUNDS

While these events are occurring on the left side of the heart, similar changes are occurring on the right, involving the right atrium, right ventricle, tricuspid valve, pulmonic valve, and pulmonary artery. Right ventricular and pulmonary arterial pressures are significantly lower than corresponding levels on the left side. Furthermore, right-sided events usually occur slightly later than those on the left. Instead of a single heart sound, therefore, you may hear two discernible components, the first from left-sided valvular closure, the second from right-sided closure.

Consider the second heart sound and its two components, A_2 and P_2, which come from closure of the aortic and pulmonic valves, respectively. During expiration, these two components are fused into a single sound, S_2. During inspiration, however, A_2 and P_2 separate slightly, and S_2 splits into its two audible components.

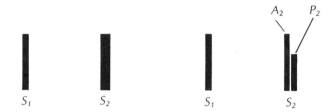

Current explanations of inspiratory splitting are technically complicated. In summary, inspiration prolongs ejection of blood from the right ventricle but shortens ejection from the left ventricle. P_2 is thus delayed, while A_2 comes slightly earlier.

Of the two components of the second heart sound, A_2 is normally the louder, reflecting the high pressure in the aorta. It is heard throughout the precordium. P_2, in contrast, is relatively soft, reflecting the lower pressure in the pulmonary artery. It is heard best in its own area—the 2nd and 3rd left interspaces close to the sternum. It is here that you should search for splitting of the second heart sound.

The first heart sound also has two components, an earlier mitral and a later tricuspid sound. The mitral sound, its principal component, is much louder, again reflecting the high pressures on the left side of the heart. It can be heard throughout the precordium and (like S_1 itself) is loudest at the cardiac apex. The softer tricuspid component is heard best at the lower left sternal border, and it is here that you should listen for a split S_1. The earlier, louder mitral component may mask the tricuspid sound, however, and splitting is not always detectable. Splitting of the first heart sound does not vary with respiration.

HEART MURMURS

Heart murmurs are distinguishable from heart sounds by their longer duration. They are attributed to turbulent blood flow. Heart murmurs often have no pathologic significance, but they may indicate serious heart disease. A stenotic (abnormally narrowed) valvular orifice that partially obstructs the flow of blood, for example, causes a murmur. So does a valve that fails to close fully and allows blood to regurgitate (leak) back in a retrograde direction. To interpret the meaning of murmurs, the clinician must be able to time them in the cardiac cycle and identify where they can be heard best. Further description of murmurs is given in Tables 9-11 through 9-15.

RELATION OF AUSCULTATORY FINDINGS TO THE CHEST WALL

The locations on the chest wall where heart sounds and murmurs are heard give important information as to their likely origins. Sounds and murmurs that originate in the mitral valve are usually heard best at and around the cardiac apex. Those that originate in the tricuspid valve are heard best at or near the lower left sternal border. Those originating in the pulmonic valve are usually heard best in the 2nd and 3rd left interspaces close to the sternum, but at times they may also be heard at higher or lower levels, and those originating in the aortic valve may be heard anywhere from the right 2nd interspace to the apex. These areas overlap, as illustrated below, and clinicians must often infer the origin of any single finding from other data.

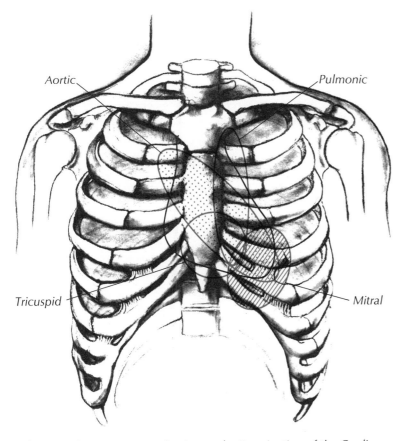

Redrawn from Leatham A: An Introduction to the Examination of the Cardiovascular System, 2nd ed, p 20. Oxford: Oxford University Press, 1979

The "base of the heart"—a term often used clinically—refers to the right and left 2nd interspaces close to the sternum.

THE CONDUCTION SYSTEM

An electrical conduction system stimulates and coordinates the contraction of cardiac muscle.

Each normal impulse is initiated in a group of cardiac cells known as the sinus node. Located in the right atrium, the *sinus node* acts as cardiac pacemaker and automatically discharges an impulse about 60 to 100 times a minute. This impulse travels through both atria to the *atrioventricular (or AV) node,* a specialized group of cells located low in the atrial septum. Here the impulse is delayed somewhat before its passage down the bundle of His and its branches and thence to the ventricular myocardium. Muscular contraction follows: first the atria, then the ventricles. The normal conduction pathway is diagrammed in simplified form at the right.

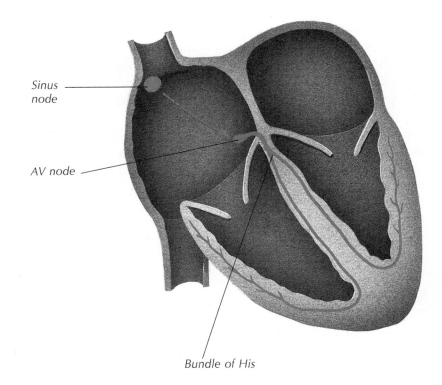

Sinus node

AV node

Bundle of His

The electrocardiogram records these events. Each normal impulse produces a series of waves:

1. A *small P wave* of atrial depolarization (electrical activation)

2. A *larger QRS complex* of ventricular depolarization. Each complex consists of one or more of the following:

   a. A *Q wave,* formed whenever the initial deflection is downward

   b. An *R wave,* the upward deflection

   c. An *S wave,* a downward deflection following an R wave

3. A *T wave* of ventricular repolarization (or recovery)

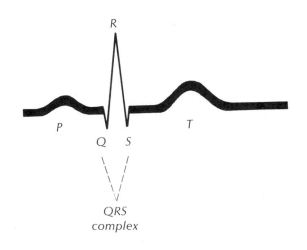

The electrical impulse slightly precedes the myocardial contraction that it stimulates. The relation of electrocardiographic waves to the cardiac cycle is shown below.

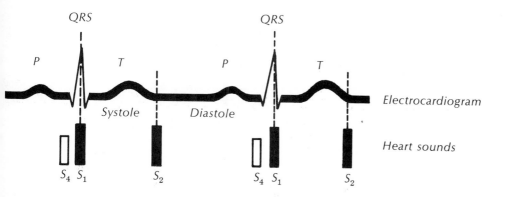

THE HEART AS A PUMP

The left and right ventricles pump blood into the systemic and pulmonary arterial trees, respectively. *Cardiac output*, the volume of blood ejected from each ventricle during one minute, is the product of *heart rate* and *stroke volume*. Stroke volume (the volume of blood ejected with each heartbeat) depends in turn on preload, myocardial contractility, and afterload.

Preload refers to the load that stretches the cardiac muscle prior to contraction. The volume of blood in the right ventricle at the end of diastole, then, constitutes its preload for the next beat. Right ventricular preload is increased by increasing venous return to the right heart. Physiologic causes include inspiration and the increased volume of blood that flows from exercising muscles. The increased volume of blood in a dilated ventricle of congestive heart failure also increases preload. Causes of decreased right ventricular preload include exhalation, decreased left ventricular output, and pooling of blood in the capillary bed or the venous system.

Myocardial contractility refers to the ability of the cardiac muscle, when given a load, to shorten. Contractility is increased by action of the sympathetic nervous system, and decreases when the myocardium is damaged.

Afterload refers to the resistance against which the ventricle must contract. Sources of resistance to left ventricular contraction include the walls of the aorta and the large arteries, the peripheral vascular tree (primarily the small arteries and arterioles), the volume of blood already in the aorta, and the viscosity of the blood.

Pathologic increases in preload and afterload, called *volume overload* and *pressure overload* respectively, produce different kinds of changes in the affected ventricles. These changes may be detectable by palpable differences in the ventricular impulses, by alterations in the heart sounds, and by the appearance of pathologic heart sounds and heart murmurs.

ARTERIAL PULSES AND BLOOD PRESSURE

With each contraction, the left ventricle ejects a volume of blood into the aorta and thence on into the arterial tree. A pressure wave moves rapidly through the arterial system, where it can be felt as the *arterial pulse.* Although the pressure wave travels quickly—many times faster than the blood itself—a palpable delay between ventricular contraction and peripheral pulses makes the pulses in the arms and legs unsuitable for timing cardiac events.

Blood pressure in the arterial system varies with the cardiac cycle, reaching a systolic peak and a diastolic trough, the levels of which are measured by sphygmomanometry. The difference between systolic and diastolic pressures is known as the *pulse pressure.*

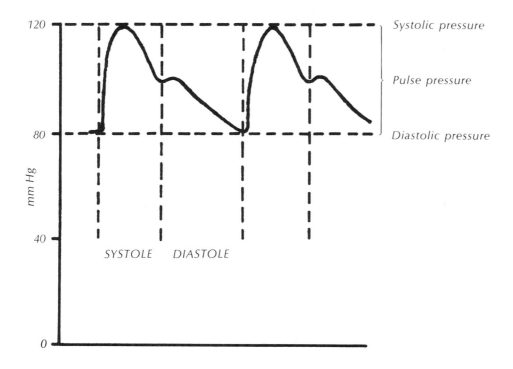

Several factors influence arterial pressure:

1. Left ventricular stroke volume
2. The distensibility of the aorta and the large arteries
3. The peripheral vascular resistance, principally at the arteriolar level. This is controlled by the autonomic nerve system.
4. The volume of blood in the arterial system
5. The viscosity of the blood

Changes in any of these five factors alter systolic pressure, diastolic pressure, or both. Blood pressure levels fluctuate strikingly through any 24-hour period, varying, for example, with physical activity, emotional state, pain, noise, environmental temperature, the use of coffee, tobacco, and other drugs, and even with the time of day.

JUGULAR VENOUS PRESSURE AND PULSES

Systemic venous pressure is much lower than the arterial pressure. It is ultimately dependent upon left ventricular contraction, but much of this force is dissipated as the blood passes through the arterial tree and the capillary bed. Other important determinants of systemic venous pressure include blood volume, venous tone, and the capacity of the right heart to receive blood and to eject it onward into the pulmonary arterial system. When any of these variables is altered pathologically, abnormalities in venous pressure result. For example, the venous pressure falls when left ventricular output or blood volume is significantly reduced; it rises when the right heart fails or when increased pressure in the pericardial sac impedes the return of blood to the right atrium.

The pressure in the jugular veins, which reflects right atrial pressure, can be estimated clinically. The best estimate is made from the internal jugular veins. If these are impossible to see, the external jugular veins can be used, but they are less reliable. The level of venous pressure is determined by finding the highest point of oscillation in the internal jugular veins or, if necessary, the point above which the external jugular veins appear collapsed.

The usual zero point for this estimate is the sternal angle, and the venous pressure is always measured in vertical distance from it. Regardless of the patient's position—supine, sitting upright, or at any angle between these positions—the sternal angle remains roughly 5 cm above the right atrium.

The observer arranges the patient's position in order to see the jugular veins and their pulsations in the lower half of the neck. Elevating the head of the bed to about 15° to 30° from horizontal is satisfactory for most normal people. In the illustrations on the next page, the pressure in the internal jugular vein is somewhat elevated. In *A*, the head of the bed is raised to about 30°. The venous pressure cannot be measured because the point that marks its level is above the jaw and therefore not visible. In *B*, the bed is raised to about 60°. The "top" of the jugular vein is now easily visible, and its vertical distance from the sternal angle can be measured. In *C*, the patient is upright and the veins are barely discernible above the clavicle. Note that the patient's venous pressure, measured from the sternal angle, is the same in all three positions, although the neck veins look much different.

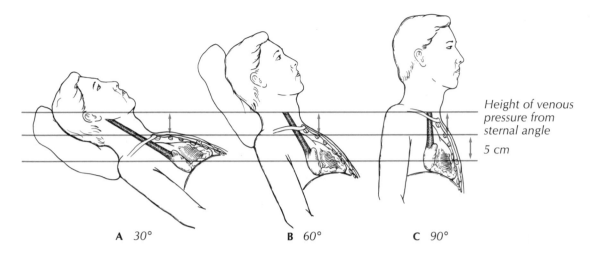

Height of venous
pressure from
sternal angle

5 cm

A 30°   B 60°   C 90°

Pressures measured as more than 3 cm or possibly 4 cm above the sternal angle are considered elevated.

The oscillations that you see in the internal jugular veins (and often in the externals as well) do not arise in the venous system itself. They reflect instead changing pressures within the right atrium. Of all the visible veins, the right internal jugular has the most direct channel to the right atrium and usually, therefore, reflects these pressure changes most satisfactorily.

Careful observation reveals that the undulating pulsations of the internal jugular veins (and sometimes the externals) are composed of two quick elevations and two troughs.

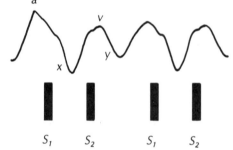

The first elevation, the *a wave*, reflects the slight rise in atrial pressure that accompanies atrial contraction. It occurs just before the first heart sound and before the carotid pulse. The following trough, the *x descent*, starts with atrial relaxation. It continues as the right ventricle, contracting during systole, pulls the floor of the atrium downward. During ventricular systole, blood continues to flow into the right atrium from the venae cavae. The tricuspid valve is closed, the chamber begins to fill, and right atrial pressure begins to rise again, creating the second elevation, the *v wave*. When the tricuspid valve opens early in diastole, blood in the right atrium flows passively into the right ventricle and right atrial pressure falls again, creating the second trough or *y descent*. To remember these four oscillations in a somewhat oversimplified way, think of the following sequence: atrial contraction, atrial relaxation, atrial filling, and atrial emptying.

To the naked eye, the two descents are the most obvious events in the normal jugular pulse. Of the two, the sudden collapse of the *x* descent late in systole is the more prominent, occurring just before the second heart sound. The *y* descent follows the second heart sound early in diastole.

CHANGES WITH AGE

Cardiovascular findings vary importantly with age. The *apical impulse* is usually felt easily in children and young adults but, as the chest deepens in its anteroposterior diameter, the impulse gets harder to find. For the same reason, *splitting of the second heart sound* may be harder to hear in older people as its pulmonic component becomes less audible. A physiologic *third heart sound*, commonly heard in children and young adults, may persist as late as the age of 40, especially in women. After approximately age 40, however, an S_3 strongly suggests either ventricular failure or volume overloading of the ventricle caused by valvular heart disease such as mitral regurgitation. In contrast, a *fourth heart sound* is seldom heard in young adults unless they are well conditioned athletes. An S_4 may be heard in apparently healthy older people, but is also frequently associated with heart disease. (See Table 9-9, Extra Heart Sounds in Diastole, p. 313.)

At some time over the life span, almost everyone has a *heart murmur.* Most murmurs occur without other evidence of cardiovascular abnormality, and may therefore be considered innocent normal variants. The nature of these common murmurs varies importantly with age, and familiarity with their patterns helps you to distinguish normal from abnormal.

Children, adolescents, and young adults frequently have an *innocent systolic murmur* that is usually heard best in the 2nd to 4th left interspaces (see p. 316).

Late in pregnancy and during lactation, many women have a so-called *mammary souffle** secondary to increased blood flow in their breasts. Although this murmur may be noted anywhere in the breasts, it is often heard most easily in the 2nd or 3rd interspace on either side of the sternum. A mammary souffle is typically both systolic and diastolic, but sometimes only the louder systolic component is audible.

Middle-aged and older adults commonly have an *aortic systolic murmur.* This has been heard in about a third of people near the age of 60, and in well over half of those reaching 85. Aging thickens the bases of the aortic cusps with fibrous tissue, calcification follows, and audible vibrations result. Turbulence produced by blood flow into a dilated aorta may contribute to this murmur. In most people, this process of fibrosis and calcification—known as aortic sclerosis—does not impede blood flow. In

---

* Souffle is pronounced soó-fl, not like cheese soufflé. Both words come from a French word meaning puff.

some, however, the valve cusps become progressively calcified and immobile, and true aortic stenosis, or obstruction of flow, develops. Clinical differentiation between benign aortic sclerosis and pathologic aortic stenosis may be difficult.

A similar aging process affects the mitral valve, usually about a decade later than aortic sclerosis. Here degenerative changes with calcification impair the ability of the mitral valve to close normally during systole, and cause the *systolic murmur of mitral regurgitation.* Because of the extra load placed on the heart by the leaking mitral valve, a murmur of mitral regurgitation cannot be considered innocent.

Murmurs may originate in large blood vessels as well as in the heart. The *jugular venous hum,* which is very common in children and may still be heard through young adulthood, illustrates this point (see p. 320). A second, more important example is the *cervical systolic murmur* or *bruit.* In older people, systolic bruits heard in the middle or upper portions of the carotid arteries suggest, but do not prove, a partial arterial obstruction secondary to atherosclerosis. In contrast, cervical bruits in younger people are usually innocent. In children and young adults, systolic murmurs (or bruits) are frequently heard just above the clavicle. One study has shown that, while cervical bruits can be heard in almost 9 out of 10 children under the age of 5, their prevalence falls steadily to about 1 out of 3 in adolescence and young adulthood and to less than 1 out of 10 in middle age. For further information on cardiovascular murmurs, see Tables 9-11 through 9-15, pages 315 to 320.

The aorta and large arteries stiffen with age as they become arteriosclerotic. As the aorta becomes less distensible, a given stroke volume causes a greater rise in systolic blood pressure; *systolic hypertension* with a *widened pulse pressure* often ensues. Peripheral arteries tend to lengthen, become tortuous, and feel harder and less resilient. These changes do not necessarily indicate atherosclerosis, however, and you can make no inferences from them as to disease in the coronary or cerebral vessels. Lengthening and tortuosity of the aorta and its branches occasionally result in kinking or buckling of the carotid artery low in the neck, especially on the right. The resulting pulsatile mass, which occurs chiefly in hypertensive women, may be mistaken for a carotid aneurysm—a true dilatation of the artery. A tortuous aorta occasionally raises the pressure in the jugular veins on the left side of the neck by impairing their drainage within the thorax.

In western societies, systolic blood pressure tends to rise from childhood through old age. Diastolic blood pressure stops rising, however, roughly around the sixth decade. On the other extreme, some elderly people develop an increased tendency toward *postural* (or *orthostatic*) *hypotension*—a sudden drop in blood pressure when they rise to a sitting or standing position. Elderly people are also more likely to have abnormal heart rhythms. These arrhythmias, like postural hypotension, may cause *syncope* (temporary loss of consciousness).

Techniques of Examination

The cardiovascular examination usually starts with measurements of the heart rate and blood pressure, although both may be taken along with other vital signs at the beginning of the physical examination. The clinician then examines the arterial pulsations, the jugular venous pulsations, and finally the heart itself. Position yourself on the patient's right side.

THE ARTERIAL PULSE

By examining arterial pulses you can count the rate of the heart, determine its rhythm, assess the amplitude and contour of the pulse wave, and sometimes detect obstructions to blood flow.

HEART RATE. The radial pulse is commonly used to assess the heart rate. With the pads of your index and middle fingers, compress the radial artery until a maximal pulsation is detected. If the rhythm is regular and the rate seems normal, count the rate for 15 seconds and multiply by 4. If the rate is unusually fast or slow, however, count it for 60 seconds.

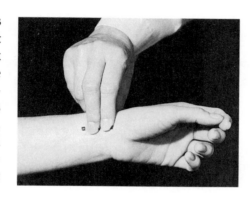

When the rhythm is irregular, the rate should be evaluated by cardiac auscultation, because beats that occur earlier than others may not be detected peripherally and the pulse rate can thus be seriously underestimated.

Irregular rhythms of this kind include atrial fibrillation and frequent premature contractions.

RHYTHM. Initial assessment of rhythm is also made by feeling the radial pulse. Abnormalities are assessed best, however, during cardiac auscultation. In either case, the questions are the same. Is the rhythm regular or irregular? If irregular, try to identify a pattern: (1) Do early beats appear in a basically regular rhythm? (2) Does the irregularity vary consistently with respiration? or (3), Is the rhythm totally irregular?

See Tables 9-1 to 9-3, Differentiation of Selected Heart Rates and Rhythms (pp. 304–307).

AMPLITUDE AND CONTOUR. These are best assessed in the carotid or brachial arteries. The carotid reflects the aortic pulsation more accurately, but in patients with carotid obstruction, kinking, or thrills it is unsuitable. Although either of these arteries can be felt with the fingers, the thumb is convenient and can be positioned more comfortably.* The patient should be lying down and the head of the bed elevated to about 30°.

When feeling the carotid artery, first inspect the neck for pulsations. Carotid pulsations may be visible just medial to the sternomastoid mus-

A tortuous and kinked carotid artery may produce a unilateral pulsatile bulge.

---

* Although there is a widespread prejudice against using thumbs to assess pulses, they are very useful for palpating large arteries.

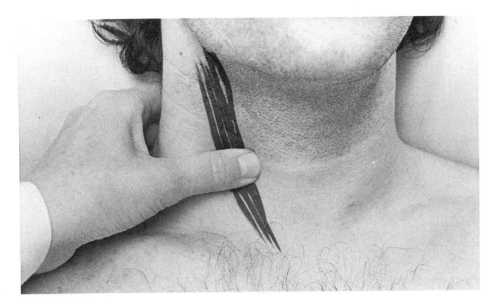

Decreased pulsations may be caused by decreased stroke volume, but may also be due to local factors in the artery such as atherosclerotic narrowing or occlusion.

cles. Then place your left thumb on the right carotid artery in the lower third of the neck, press posteriorly, and feel for the pulsations.

Your thumb should press just inside the medial border of a well relaxed sternomastoid muscle, roughly at the level of the cricoid cartilage. Avoid pressing on the carotid sinus, which lies at the level of the top of the thyroid cartilage. For the left carotid, use your right thumb. Do not press on both carotids at the same time because you might thereby decrease the blood supply to the brain in some patients.

Pressure on the carotid sinus may cause a reflex drop in pulse rate or blood pressure.

When feeling the brachial artery, use the thumb of your opposite hand. Cup your hand under the patient's elbow and feel for the pulse just

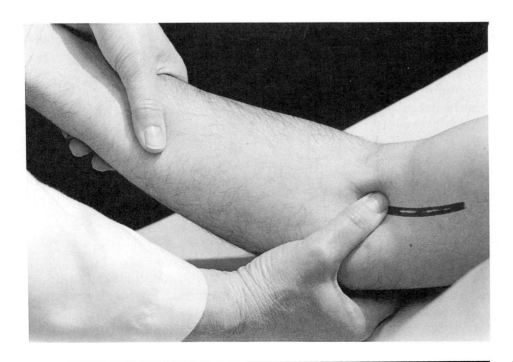

medial to the biceps tendon. The patient's arm should rest with the elbow extended, palm up. With your free hand, you may need to flex the elbow to a varying degree to get optimal muscular relaxation.

Whichever artery you use, slowly increase the pressure of your thumb until you feel a maximal pulsation, and then slowly decrease it until you can best sense the amplitude and contour. Try to assess:

See Table 9-4, Abnormalities of the Arterial Pulse (p. 308).

1. The amplitude of the pulse. This correlates reasonably well with the pulse pressure.
2. The contour of the pulse wave (*i.e.,* the speed of its upstroke, the duration of its summit, and the speed of its downstroke). The normal upstroke is smooth and rapid and follows the first heart sound almost immediately. The summit is smooth, rounded, and roughly midsystolic. The downstroke is less abrupt than the upstroke.
3. Any variations in amplitude
   a. From beat to beat

   b. With respiration

Small, weak pulses and large, bounding pulses (see p. 308).

Pulsus alternans, bigeminal pulse (see p. 308).

Paradoxical pulse (see p. 308).

BRUITS AND THRILLS. During palpation of the carotid artery, you may detect humming vibrations that feel like the throat of a purring cat. These are termed a *thrill*. If you feel them, listen over the area with the bell of a stethoscope for a *bruit*, a murmurlike sound of vascular rather than cardiac origin.

You should also listen over the carotid arteries if the patient is middle-aged or elderly or if you suspect cerebrovascular disease. Ask the patient to stop breathing for a moment so that breath sounds do not obscure the vascular sound. Heart sounds alone do not constitute a bruit.

A carotid bruit with or without a thrill in a middle-aged or older person suggests but does not prove arterial narrowing. An aortic murmur may radiate to the carotid artery and simulate a bruit.

Further examination of arterial pulses is described in Chapter 16, The Peripheral Vascular System.

BLOOD PRESSURE

CHOICE OF SPHYGMOMANOMETER. Blood pressure may be measured satisfactorily with a sphygmomanometer of either the aneroid or the mercury type. Because an aneroid instrument often becomes inaccurate with repeated use, it should be recalibrated periodically. Select a cuff with an inflatable bladder of appropriate size. Proper size depends on the circumference of the limb on which the cuff is to be used. The width of the bladder should be about 40% of this circumference—12 cm to 14 cm in an average adult. The length of the bladder should be about 80% of this circumference—almost long enough to encircle the arm.

Cuffs that are too short or too narrow may give falsely high readings. Using a regular-size cuff on an obese arm may lead to a false diagnosis of hypertension.

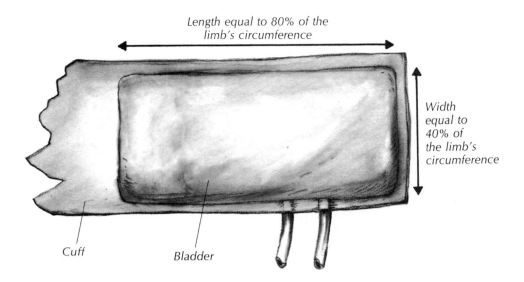

Length equal to 80% of the limb's circumference

Width equal to 40% of the limb's circumference

Cuff   Bladder

TECHNIQUE. The patient should have rested for at least 5 minutes and ideally should not have eaten or smoked for 30 minutes. The room should be quiet and comfortably warm. The patient's arm should be resting, free of clothing, and positioned so that the brachial artery (at the antecubital crease) is at heart level—roughly level with the 4th inter-space at its junction with the sternum. When the patient is seated, resting the arm on a table a little above the patient's waist is suitable. When taking a standing blood pressure, try to support the arm at a satisfactory level.

The patient's own effort to support the arm may raise the blood pressure.

If the brachial artery is much below heart level, blood pressure appears falsely high. To correct for this, subtract 0.8 mm Hg for each cm of vertical distance. Conversely, add an equivalent number if the arm is too high.

Find the brachial artery, which is usually just medial to the biceps tendon, and center the inflatable bladder over it. The lower border of the cuff should be about 2.5 cm above the antecubital crease. Secure the cuff snugly. Position the patient's arm so that it is slightly flexed at the elbow.

A loose cuff or a bladder that balloons outside the cuff leads to falsely high readings.

To determine how high to raise the cuff pressure, first estimate the systolic pressure by palpation. As you feel the radial artery with the fingers of one hand, rapidly inflate the cuff until the radial pulse disappears. Read this pressure on the manometer and add 30 mm Hg to it. Use of this sum as the target for subsequent inflations prevents discomfort from unnecessarily high cuff pressures. It also avoids the occasional error caused by an auscultatory gap—a silent interval that may be present between the systolic and the diastolic pressures.

An unrecognized auscultatory gap may lead to serious under-estimation of systolic pressure (*e.g.,* 150/98 in the example on p. 281) or overestimation of diastolic pressure.

Deflate the cuff promptly and completely and wait 15 to 30 seconds.

Now place the bell of a stethoscope lightly over the brachial artery, taking care to make an air seal with its full rim. Because the sounds to be heard (Korotkoff sounds) are relatively low in pitch, they are heard better with the bell.

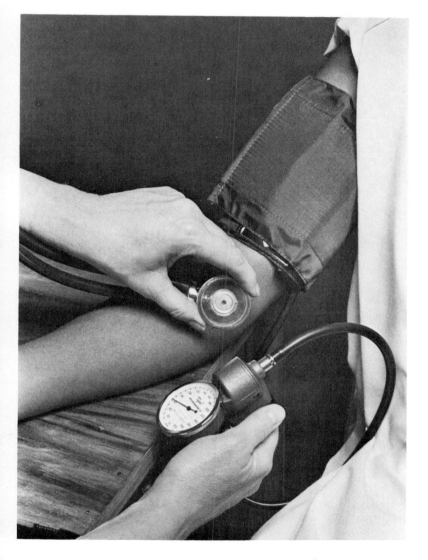

If you find an auscultatory gap, record your findings completely (*e.g.*, 200/98 with an auscultatory gap from 170 to 150).

Inflate the cuff rapidly again to the level just determined, then deflate it slowly at a rate of about 2 to 3 mm Hg per second. Note the level at which you hear the sounds of at least two consecutive beats. This is the systolic pressure.

Continue to lower the pressure slowly until the sounds become muffled and then disappear. To confirm the disappearance of sounds, listen as the pressure falls another 10 to 20 mm Hg. Then deflate the cuff rapidly to zero. The disappearance point, which is usually only a few mm Hg below the muffling point, gives the best estimate of true diastolic pressure in adults.

In some people, the muffling point and the disappearance point are farther apart. Occasionally, as in aortic regurgitation, the sounds never disappear. If there is more than 10 mm Hg difference, record both figures (*e.g.*, 154/80/68).

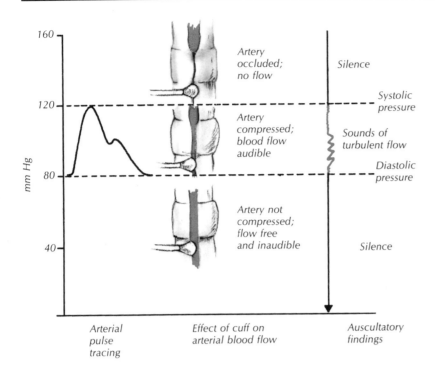

Read both the systolic and the diastolic levels to the nearest 2 mm Hg. Wait a minute or two and repeat. Average your readings.

When using a mercury sphygmomanometer, keep the manometer vertical (unless you are using a tilted floor model) and make all readings at eye level with the meniscus. When using an aneroid instrument, hold the dial so that it faces you directly. Avoid slow or repetitive inflations of the cuff, because the resulting venous congestion can cause false readings.

By making the sounds less audible, venous congestion may produce artifactually low systolic and high diastolic pressures.

Blood pressure should be taken in both arms at least once. Normally, there may be a difference in pressure of 5 mm Hg and sometimes up to 10 mm Hg. Subsequent readings should be made on the arm with the higher pressure.

Pressure difference of more than 10–15 mm Hg suggests arterial compression or obstruction on the side with the lower pressure.

When the patient is taking antihypertensive medications, when there is a history of fainting or postural dizziness, or when you suspect depletion of blood volume, take the blood pressure in three positions—supine, sitting, and standing (unless contraindicated). Normally, as the patient rises from the horizontal to a standing position systolic pressure drops slightly or remains unchanged while diastolic pressure rises slightly. Another measurement after 2 to 3 minutes of standing may identify orthostatic hypotension missed by the earlier readings. This repetition is especially useful in the elderly.

A fall in systolic pressure of 20 mm Hg or more, especially when accompanied by symptoms, indicates orthostatic (postural) hypotension. Causes include drugs, depletion of blood volume, prolonged bed rest, and diseases of the peripheral autonomic nervous system.

DEFINITIONS OF NORMAL AND ABNORMAL LEVELS. In 1988, the Joint National Committee on Detection, Evaluation, and Treatment of High Blood Pressure recommended that hypertension should be diagnosed only when a higher than normal level has been found on at least three visits. Either the diastolic blood pressure (DBP) or the systolic pressure (SBP) may be considered high. For adults (aged 18 or over) the Committee categorized the DBP in 5 levels:

Severe hypertension	≥115 mm Hg
Moderate hypertension	105–114
Mild hypertension	90–104
High normal blood pressure	85–89
Normal blood pressure	<85

When the DBP is less than 90, the Committee categorized blood pressure by its systolic level:

Isolated systolic hypertension	≥160 mm Hg
Borderline isolated systolic hypertension	140–159
Normal blood pressure	<140*

Relatively low levels of blood pressure should always be interpreted in the light of past readings and the patient's present clinical state.

Assessment of hypertension also includes its effects on target organs—the eyes, the heart, the brain, and the kidneys. Look for evidence of hypertensive retinopathy, left ventricular hypertrophy, and neurologic deficits suggesting a stroke. (Renal assessment requires urinalysis and blood tests.)

A pressure of 110/70 would usually be normal, for example, but could also indicate significant hypotension in a patient whose past pressures have been high.

SPECIAL PROBLEMS

The Apprehensive Patient. Anxiety is a frequent cause of high blood pressure, especially during an initial visit. Try to get the patient relaxed. Repeat your measurements later in the encounter.

The Obese Arm. Use a wide cuff (15 cm). If the arm circumference exceeds 41 cm, use a thigh cuff (18 cm wide).

Leg Pulses and Pressures. In order to rule out coarctation of the aorta, two observations should be made at least once with every hypertensive patient:

- Compare the volume and timing of the radial and femoral pulses.
- Compare blood pressures in the arm and leg.

A femoral pulse that is smaller and later than the radial pulse suggests coarctation of the aorta or occlusive aortic disease. Blood pressure is lower in the legs than in the arms in these conditions.

To determine blood pressure in the leg, use a wide, long cuff applied at the midthigh. Center the bladder over the posterior surface, wrap it securely, and listen over the popliteal artery. If possible, the patient should be prone. Alternatively, ask the supine patient to flex one leg slightly, with the heel resting on the bed. By sphygmomanometry, systolic pressure is usually found to be substantially higher in the legs than

---

* When the systolic and diastolic levels indicate different categories, isolated systolic hypertension of either kind takes precedence over high normal blood pressure (DBP 85–89), and high normal blood pressure takes precedence over normal blood pressure (SBP <140).

in the brachial artery. This does not reflect a true difference in intra-arterial pressures. A systolic pressure lower in the legs than in the arms is abnormal.

Weak or Inaudible Korotkoff Sounds. Consider technical problems such as erroneous placement of your stethoscope, failure to make full skin contact with the bell, and venous engorgement of the patient's arm from repeated inflations of the cuff. Consider also the possibility of shock.

When you cannot hear Korotkoff sounds at all, you may be able to estimate the systolic pressure by palpation. Alternative methods such as Doppler techniques or direct arterial puncture may be necessary.

To intensify Korotkoff sounds, one of the following methods may be helpful:

- Raise the patient's arm before and while you inflate the cuff. Then lower the arm and determine the blood pressure.
- Inflate the cuff. Ask the patient to make a fist several times, and then determine the blood pressure.

Arrhythmias. Irregular rhythms produce variations in pressure and therefore unreliable measurements. Ignore the effects of an occasional premature contraction. With frequent premature contractions or atrial fibrillation, determine the average of several observations and note that your measurements are approximate.

JUGULAR VENOUS PRESSURE AND PULSES

JUGULAR VENOUS PRESSURE (JVP). Examination of the jugular veins and their pulsations enables quite accurate estimation of the pressure in the right atrium (the central venous pressure). The internal jugular pulsations give a more accurate reading than the external pulsations. The jugular veins and pulses are difficult to see in children under 12 years of age, and are therefore of little use in evaluating the cardiovascular system in this age group.

Position the patient so as to promote comfort, with the head slightly elevated on a pillow and the sternomastoid muscles relaxed. Start with the head of the bed or table elevated about 30°; then adjust the angle so as to maximize the jugular venous pulsations and make them visible in the lower half of the neck. Turn the patient's head slightly away from the side you are inspecting.

Use tangential (oblique) lighting and *examine both sides of the neck.* Unilateral distention, especially of an external jugular vein, may be deceptive: it can be caused by local compression in the neck.

Identify the external jugular vein on each side. Then *find the pulsations of the internal jugular vein.* Because this vein lies deep to the sternomastoid

When the patient's venous pressure is increased, an elevation up to 60° or even 90° may be required. A hypovolemic patient, in contrast, may have to lie flat before you can see the veins. In all these positions the sternal angle remains roughly 5 cm above the right atrium, although individual variations do occur.

muscle, you will not see the vein itself. Watch instead for the pulsations transmitted through the surrounding soft tissues. Look for them in the suprasternal notch, between the attachments of the sternomastoid muscle on the sternum and clavicle, or just posterior to the sternomastoid muscle. Distinguish these pulsations from those of the adjacent carotid artery by the following points:

INTERNAL JUGULAR PULSATIONS	CAROTID PULSATIONS
Rarely palpable	Palpable
Soft, rapid, undulating quality, usually with two elevations and two troughs per heart beat	A more vigorous thrust with a single outward component
Pulsations eliminated by light pressure on the vein(s) just above the sternal end of the clavicle	Pulsations not eliminated by this pressure
Level of the pulsations changes with position, dropping as the patient becomes more upright.	Level of the pulsations unchanged by position
Level of the pulsations usually descends with inspiration.	Level of the pulsations not affected by inspiration

Identify the highest point at which pulsations of the internal jugular vein can be seen. With a centimeter ruler, measure the vertical distance between this point and the sternal angle. Establishing true vertical and horizontal lines is difficult—much like the problem of hanging a picture straight when you are close to it. Place your ruler on the sternal angle and line it up with something in the room that you know to be vertical. Then place a long rectangular object such as a packaged tongue blade at an exact right angle to the ruler. This object constitutes your horizontal line. Move it up or down—still horizontal—so that its lower edge rests at the top of the jugular pulsations, and read the vertical distance on the ruler. Round your measurement off to the nearest centimeter.

Increased pressure suggests right-sided heart failure or, less commonly, constrictive pericarditis, tricuspid stenosis, or superior vena cava obstruction.

In patients with obstructive lung disease, venous pressure may appear elevated on expiration only; the veins collapse on inspiration. This finding does not indicate congestive heart failure.

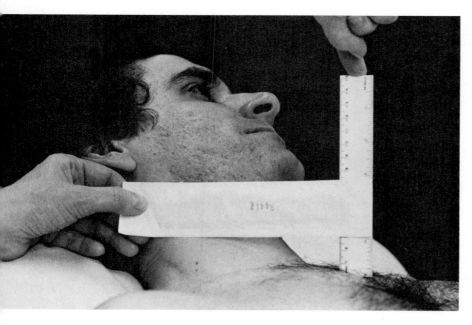

The highest point of venous pulsations may lie below the level of the sternal angle. Under these circumstances, venous pressure is not elevated and seldom needs to be measured.

If you are unable to visualize pulsations in the internal jugular veins, look for them in the external jugulars, although they may not be visible here. If you see none, use *the point above which the external jugular veins appear to be collapsed.* Make this observation on each side of the neck. Measure the vertical distance of this point from the sternal angle.

Venous pressure measured as greater than 3 cm or possibly 4 cm above the sternal angle is considered elevated.

*THE ABDOMINOJUGULAR TEST.** This test may show evidence of congestive heart failure even when the jugular venous pressure is normal. After measuring the JVP, put the bladder of a blood-pressure cuff flat on the patient's midabdomen, and partially inflate the bladder with six full squeezes of the bulb. Place one hand (palm and slightly spread fingers) on this bladder, and compress the patient's abdomen for 10 seconds at a pressure level of about 20 mm Hg. The patient should breathe easily throughout this period. Note any change in the JVP during the abdominal pressure and at the time of release. A transient rise or no rise in the JVP constitutes a normal response.

JUGULAR VENOUS PULSATIONS. Observe the amplitude and timing of the jugular venous pulsations. In order to time these pulsations, feel the left carotid artery with your right thumb or listen to the heart simultaneously. The *a* wave just precedes S_1 and the carotid pulse, the *x* descent can be seen as a systolic collapse, the *v* wave almost coincides with S_2, and the *y* descent follows early in diastole. Look for absent or unusually prominent waves.

Considerable practice and experience are required to master jugular venous pulsations. A beginner is probably well advised to concentrate primarily on jugular venous pressure.

Unilateral distention of the external jugular vein is usually due to local kinking or obstruction. Occasionally, even bilateral distention has a local cause.

A rise in the JVP followed by an abrupt fall of at least 4 cm at the time of release constitutes a positive test. It may be due to isolated right-sided heart failure, but it has been found more commonly in left-sided heart failure. If the patient guards against the pressure, thus performing a Valsalva maneuver, a falsely positive response may occur.

Prominent *a* waves indicate increased resistance to right atrial contraction. Causes include tricuspid stenosis or, more commonly, the decreased compliance of a hypertrophied right ventricle. The *a* waves disappear in atrial fibrillation. Large *v* waves characterize tricuspid regurgitation.

THE HEART

General Approach

For most of the cardiac examination, the patient should be supine with the upper body raised by elevating the head of the bed or table to about

---

* This is a modification of the older abdominojugular (hepatojugular) reflux and has a new interpretation.

30°. When examining a woman with large breasts, gently displace the left breast upward or laterally as necessary. Alternatively, ask her to do this for you. The room must be quiet.

You should inspect and palpate the anterior chest for impulses, listen to the first and second heart sounds, and listen for additional heart sounds and for heart murmurs. In order to interpret these observations, you will need to identify their location both anatomically and chronologically.

Note the anatomic location of sounds in terms of interspaces and their distance from the midsternal, midclavicular, or axillary lines. The midsternal line offers the most reliable zero point for measurement, but the midclavicular line accommodates to the different sizes and shapes of patients.

Identify the timing of impulses or sounds in relation to the cardiac cycle. Timing of sounds is often possible through auscultation alone. In most people with normal or slow heart rates, it is easy to identify the paired heart sounds by listening through a stethoscope. S_1 is the first of these sounds, S_2 is the second, and the relatively long diastolic interval separates one pair from the next.

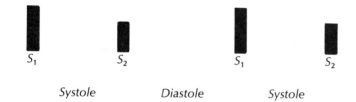

S_1 S_2 S_1 S_2

     Systole   *Diastole*   *Systole*

The relative intensity of these sounds may also be helpful. S_1 is usually louder than S_2 at the apex and, more reliably, S_2 is usually louder than S_1 at the base. Precordial impulses or murmurs may be timed by these sounds.

Even experienced clinicians sometimes become confused in timing what they hear, especially when they encounter extra heart sounds and murmurs. "Inching" can then be helpful. Return to a place on the chest—most often the base—where it is easy to identify S_1 and S_2. Get their rhythm clearly in mind. Then inch your stethoscope down the chest in steps until you hear the new sound.

Auscultation alone, however, can be a misleading tool for timing. The intensities of S_1 and S_2, for example, may be abnormal. At rapid heart rates, moreover, diastole shortens, and at about a rate of 120 the durations of systole and diastole become indistinguishable. Palpation of either the carotid artery or the apical impulse must then guide the timing of observations. Both occur in early systole, right after the first heart sound.

For example, S_1 is decreased in first-degree heart block, and S_2 is decreased in aortic stenosis.

Inspection and Palpation

Careful inspection of the anterior chest may reveal the location of the apical impulse or, less commonly, the ventricular movements of a left-sided S_3 or S_4.

Palpation yields further information. The characteristics of the apical impulse help you to determine the size of the left ventricle, and a left parasternal impulse may suggest enlargement of the right ventricle. An S_3 or an S_4 may be palpable, as may accentuated first and second heart sounds and exaggerated pulsations of the aorta or pulmonary artery. In addition, a loud heart murmur may be palpable as a thrill.

The proper techniques facilitate these observations. Tangential light much improves your changes of seeing impulses. For feeling impulses, use your fingerpads, held flat or obliquely on the body surface: light pressure for the low-pitched S_3 and S_4 and firmer pressure for the relatively high-pitched S_1 and S_2. Thrills, like tactile fremitus, are felt best through bone—the ball of your hand pressed firmly on the chest. It is probably more efficient to feel for thrills only after auscultation has revealed a loud murmur, although detecting one prior to auscultation may reward you for your skill in palpation.

From the patient's right side, systematically examine the anterior chest, paying special attention to each of the five areas illustrated below.

Thrills most often accompany loud, harsh or rumbling murmurs such as those of aortic stenosis, patent ductus arteriosus, ventricular septal defect, and mitral stenosis. They are felt most easily in patient positions that accentuate the murmur.

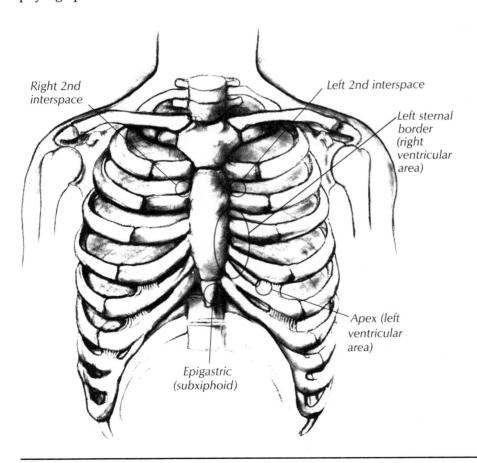

Right 2nd interspace

Left 2nd interspace

Left sternal border (right ventricular area)

Apex (left ventricular area)

Epigastric (subxiphoid)

THE CARDIAC APEX (LEFT VENTRICULAR AREA). This is normally at or medial to the midclavicular line in the 5th or possibly the 4th interspace. Here you can often see the apical impulse, the brief early systolic pulsation of the left ventricle as it rotates to the right and upward and touches the chest wall.

The apical impulse may not be visible in the supine patient, and often is most easily felt in the partial left lateral decubitus position. Ask the patient to roll partly onto the left side and look again. Then feel for the impulse. If inspection does not reveal its location, search for it first with the palmar surfaces of several fingers. If you cannot find it, ask the patient to exhale fully and stop breathing for a few seconds.

Cardiac impulses lateral to the midclavicular line suggest cardiac enlargement or displacement.

Occasionally, a patient has dextrocardia—a heart situated on the right side. The apical impulse will then be found on the right. If you cannot find an apical impulse, percuss for the dullness of heart and liver and for the tympany of the stomach. In situs inversus, all three of these structures are on opposite sides from normal. A right-sided heart (dextrocardia) with a normally placed liver and stomach is usually associated with congenital heart disease.

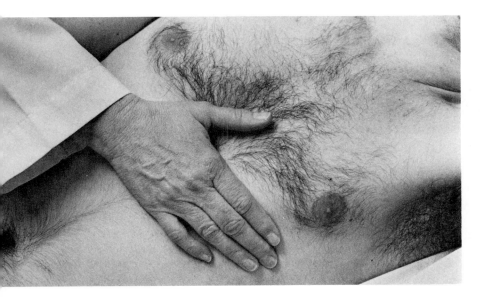

Once you have found the apical impulse, make finer assessments with your fingertips, and then with one finger.

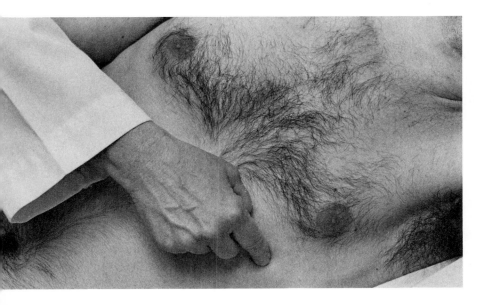

With experience, you will learn to feel the apical impulse in a high percentage of patients, but obesity, a very muscular chest wall, or an increased anteroposterior diameter of the chest may make it undetectable. Some apical impulses hide behind the rib cage, despite positioning.

Assess the location, diameter, amplitude, and duration of the apical impulse. Having the patient breathe out and briefly stop breathing is helpful.

Location. If possible, assess the location of the apical impulse when the patient is supine. The left lateral decubitus position displaces this impulse to the left, though not normally beyond the midclavicular line. Note the interspace(s) that the impulse occupies, and measure its distance in centimeters from the midsternal or the midclavicular line.

See Table 9-5, Variations and Abnormalities of the Ventricular Impulses (p. 309).

The apical impulse may be displaced upward and to the left by pregnancy or a high left diaphragm. It may also be displaced by deformities of the thorax, by a mediastinal shift, or by enlargement of the heart.

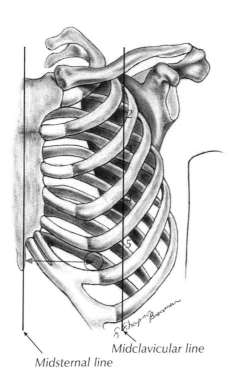

Midclavicular line

Midsternal line

Diameter. Note the diameter of the apical impulse. In the supine patient, it usually measures less than 2.5 cm and occupies only one interspace. It may be larger in the left lateral decubitus position.

In the left lateral decubitus position, a diameter greater than 3 cm indicates left ventricular enlargement.

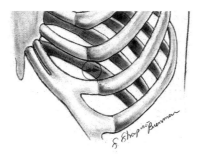

Amplitude. Estimate the amplitude of the impulse. It is usually small and feels like a gentle tap. An increased amplitude (hyperkinetic impulse) may be felt in some young persons, especially with excitement or after exercise. Duration, however, is normal.

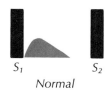 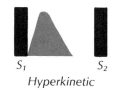

Normal   Hyperkinetic

Amplitude is increased in hyperkinetic states (*e.g.,* hyperthyroidism, severe anemia), in pressure overload of the left ventricle (*e.g.,* aortic stenosis), and in volume overload of the left ventricle (*e.g.,* mitral regurgitation).

Duration. Of all the characteristics of the apical impulse, duration is the most useful in identifying hypertrophy of the left ventricle. To assess duration, listen to the heart sounds while you are feeling the apical impulse, or watch the movement of your stethoscope as you listen at the apex. Estimate the proportion of systole occupied by the apical impulse. The normal impulse may be sustained during the first two thirds of systole, and often less, but does not continue to the second heart sound.

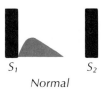

Normal

Sustained contraction that approaches the second heart sound indicates left ventricular enlargement.

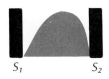

A sustained, high-amplitude impulse that is normally located suggests left ventricular hypertrophy without dilatation (from pressure overload). If such an impulse is displaced laterally, volume overload is suggested.

A sustained but hypokinetic impulse (decreased amplitude) is noted in the dilated heart of cardiomyopathy.

S_3 and S_4. By inspection and palpation you may also be able to detect the ventricular movements that are synchronous with pathologic third and fourth heart sounds. For the left ventricular impulses, feel the apical beat gently with one finger. The patient should lie partly on the left side, breathe out, and briefly stop breathing. A brief middiastolic impulse indicates an S_3; an impulse just before the systolic apical beat itself indicates an S_4. By inking an X on the apex you may be able to see these movements.

For the significance of these movements and their associated sounds, see Table 9-9, Extra Heart Sounds in Diastole (p. 313).

THE LEFT STERNAL BORDER IN THE 3RD, 4TH, AND 5TH INTERSPACES (RIGHT VENTRICULAR AREA). The patient should rest supine at 30°. Place the tips of your curved fingers in the 3rd, 4th, and 5th interspaces and try to feel the systolic impulse of the right ventricle.

Again, asking the patient to breathe out and hold the breath out improves your observation.

If an impulse is palpable, assess it according to location, amplitude, and duration. A brief systolic tap of low or slightly increased amplitude is sometimes felt in thin or shallow-chested persons, especially when stroke volume is increased, as by anxiety.

A marked increase in amplitude with little or no change in duration occurs in chronic volume overload of the right ventricle, as from an atrial septal defect.

An impulse with increased amplitude and duration occurs with pressure overload of the right ventricle, as in pulmonic stenosis or pulmonary hypertension.

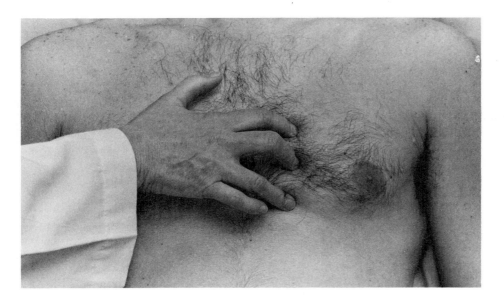

The diastolic movements of right-sided third and fourth heart sounds may be felt occasionally. Feel for them in the 4th and 5th left interspaces. Time them by auscultation or carotid palpation.

See Table 9-9, Extra Heart Sounds in Diastole (p. 313).

THE EPIGASTRIC (SUBXIPHOID) AREA. This location is especially useful when you are examining a person with an increased anteroposterior

In pulmonary emphysema, hyperinflated lung may prevent palpation of an enlarged right ventricle in the left parasternal area. The impulse is easily felt, however, high in the epigastrium. In such patients, heart sounds are also often heard best here.

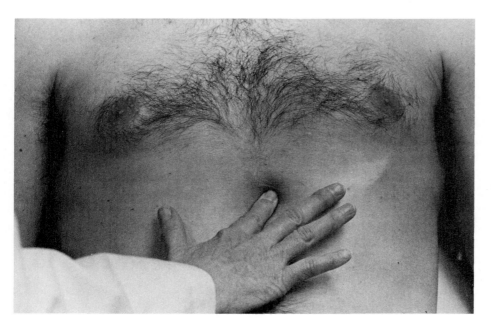

diameter of the chest. With your hand flattened, press your index finger just under the rib cage and up toward the left shoulder and try to feel right ventricular pulsations.

Asking the patient to inhale and hold the breath is helpful. The inspiratory position moves your hand well away from the pulsations of the abdominal aorta, which might otherwise be confusing.

The diastolic movements of S_3 and S_4, if present, may also be felt here.

THE LEFT 2ND INTERSPACE, which overlies the *pulmonary artery.* During held expiration, look and feel for an impulse and feel for possible heart sounds. Firmer pressure is needed for the heart sounds. In thin or shallow-chested people, the pulsation of a pulmonary artery may sometimes be felt here, especially after exercise or with excitement.

A prominent pulsation here often accompanies dilatation or increased flow in the pulmonary artery. A palpable second heart sound suggests increased pressure in the pulmonary artery (pulmonary hypertension).

THE RIGHT 2ND INTERSPACE. Again, search for pulsations and palpable heart sounds.

A palpable second heart sound suggests systemic hypertension. A pulsation here suggests a dilated or aneurysmal aorta.

Percussion

In most cases, palpation has replaced percussion in the estimation of cardiac size. When you cannot feel the apical impulse, however, percussion may suggest where to search for it. Occasionally, percussion may be your only tool. Under these circumstances, cardiac dullness often occupies a large area. Starting well to the left on the chest, percuss from resonance toward cardiac dullness in the 3rd, 4th, 5th, and possibly 6th interspaces.

A markedly dilated failing heart may have a hypokinetic apical impulse that is displaced far to the left. A large pericardial effusion may make the impulse undetectable.

Auscultation

LOCATIONS. You should listen to the heart with your stethoscope in the right 2nd interspace close to the sternum, along the left sternal border in each interspace from the 2nd through the 5th, and at the apex.

In the past, most of these areas have had auscultatory names (shown in parentheses on p. 296 because they are still commonly used). Because murmurs of more than one origin may occur in a given area these names may be misleading, and some authorities now discourage their use.

The areas designated on page 296 should not limit your auscultation. If the heart is enlarged or displaced, you should alter your pattern accordingly. You should also listen in any area where you have observed an abnormality, and you should listen in areas adjacent to murmurs in order to determine where they are loudest and to trace their radiation.

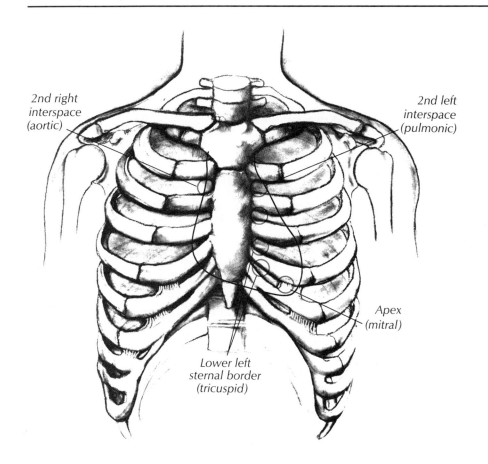

Heart sounds and murmurs that originate in the four valves are illustrated in the diagram below. Pulmonic sounds are usually heard best in the 2nd and 3rd left interspaces, but may extend further.

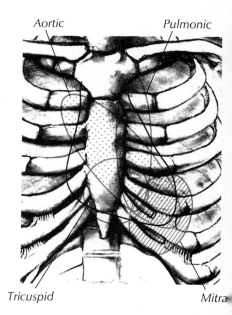

(Redrawn from Leatham A: Introduction to the Examination of the Cardiovascular System, 2nd ed, p 20. Oxford: Oxford University Press, 1979)

SEQUENCE. Clinicians vary in their sequence of auscultation, some preferring to start at the apex, others preferring to start at the base. Either pattern is satisfactory.

USE OF THE STETHOSCOPE. You should listen throughout the precordium with the diaphragm of your stethoscope, pressing it firmly on the chest. The diaphragm is better for picking up relatively high-pitched sounds such as S_1, S_2, the murmurs of aortic and mitral regurgitation, and pericardial friction rubs. The bell is more sensitive to low-pitched sounds such as S_3, S_4, and the murmur of mitral stenosis. Use the bell at the apex and more medially along the lower sternal border. Apply it lightly, with just enough pressure to produce an air seal with its full rim. Resting the heel of your hand on the chest, like a fulcrum, helps to maintain this light pressure.

Pressing the bell firmly on the chest stretches the underlying skin and makes the bell function more like a diaphragm. Low-pitched sounds such as S_3 and S_4 may disappear with this maneuver—an observation that helps to identify them. High-pitched sounds such as a midsystolic click, an ejection sound, or an opening snap, in contrast, persist or get louder.

PATIENT POSITIONS. Listen to the entire precordium with the patient supine, as described on pp. 288–289. In addition, use two other positions:

1. Ask the patient to *roll partly onto the left side*, thus bringing the left ventricle closer to the chest wall. Place the bell of your stethoscope lightly on the apical impulse.

This position accentuates or brings out a left-sided S_3 and S_4 and mitral murmurs, especially the murmur of mitral stenosis. You may otherwise miss these important findings.

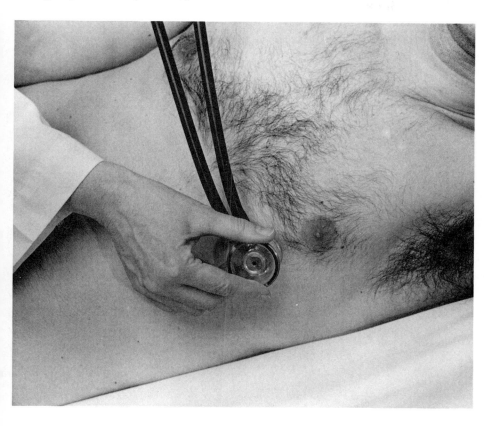

2. Ask the patient to *sit up, lean forward, exhale completely, and stop breathing* in expiration. With the diaphragm of your stethoscope pressed on the chest, listen along the left sternal border and at the apex, pausing periodically so the patient may breathe.

This position accentuates or brings out aortic murmurs. You may easily miss the murmur of aortic regurgitation unless you use this position.

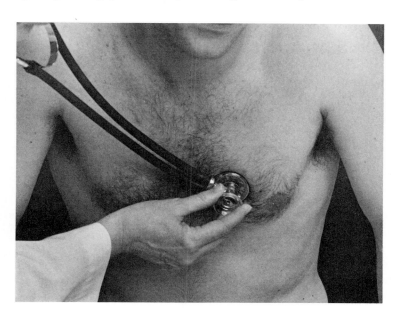

WHAT TO LISTEN FOR. Throughout your examination, take your time at each auscultatory area, concentrating in turn on each of the following places in the cardiac cycle:

- *The first heart sound.* Note its intensity and any apparent splitting. Normal splitting is often detectable along the lower left sternal border.

See Table 9-6, Variations in the First Heart Sound (p. 310).

- *The second heart sound.* Note its intensity.

Listen for splitting of this sound in the left 2nd and 3rd interspaces. Ask the patient to breathe quietly, and then slightly more deeply than normal. Does S_2 split into its two components, as it usually does? If not, ask the patient to (1) breathe a little more deeply, or (2) sit up. Listen again. A thick chest wall or an increased anteroposterior diameter of the chest may make the pulmonic component of S_2 inaudible.

See Table 9-7, Variations in the Second Heart Sound (p. 311).

When either A_2 or P_2 is absent, as in disease of the respective valves, S_2 is persistently single.

How wide is the split? It is normally quite narrow.

When in the respiratory cycle do you hear the split? It is normally heard late in inspiration.

Expiratory splitting suggests an abnormality (see p. 311).

Does the split disappear, as it should, during exhalation? If not, listen again with the patient sitting up.

Persistent splitting results from delayed closure of the pulmonic valve or early closure of the aortic valve.

Compare the intensity of the two components, A_2 and P_2. A_2 is usually louder.

A loud P_2 suggests pulmonary hypertension.

- *Extra sounds in systole,* such as ejection sounds or systolic clicks. Note their location, timing, intensity, and pitch, and the effects of respiration on the sounds.

The systolic click of mitral valve prolapse is the most common of these sounds. See Table 9-8, Extra Heart Sounds in Systole (p. 312).

- *Extra sounds in diastole,* such as S_3, S_4, or an opening snap. Note their location, timing, intensity, and pitch, and the effects of respiration on the sounds. Most well conditioned athletes have an audible S_3 and many have an audible S_4.

See Table 9-9, Extra Heart Sounds in Diastole (p. 313).

See Table 9-10, Causes of an Apparently Split First Heart Sound (p. 314).

- *Systolic murmurs.* Murmurs are differentiated from heart sounds by their longer duration.

See Table 9-11, Mechanisms of Heart Murmurs (p. 315).

- *Diastolic murmurs*

ATTRIBUTES OF HEART MURMURS. Any murmur should be described in terms of its timing, shape, location of maximal intensity, radiation or transmission from this location, intensity, pitch, and quality.

Timing. You must first be sure whether you are hearing a *systolic murmur*, which occurs somewhere between S_1 and S_2, or a *diastolic murmur*, which occurs somewhere between S_2 and S_1.

Diastolic murmurs usually indicate heart disease. Systolic murmurs may indicate heart disease but often occur when the heart is entirely normal.

Systolic murmurs are further divided into two principal categories:

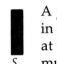

A midsystolic murmur begins after S_1 and stops before S_2. Brief gaps are audible between the murmur and the heart sounds.* Listen carefully for the gap just before S_2. It is more easily heard and, if present, usually confirms the murmur as midsystolic, not pansystolic.

Midsystolic murmurs most often are related to blood flow across the semilunar valves. See Table 9-12, Midsystolic Murmurs (pp. 316–317).

A pansystolic (holosystolic) murmur, in contrast, starts with S_1 and stops at S_2, without a gap between murmur and heart sounds.*

Pansystolic murmurs often occur with regurgitant (backward) flow across the atrioventricular valves. See Table 9-13, Pansystolic Murmurs (p. 318).

In addition, a *late systolic murmur* may be heard. It usually starts in mid- or late systole and persists up to S_2.

This is the murmur of mitral valve prolapse and is often, but not always, preceded by a systolic click (see p. 312).

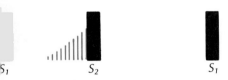

Diastolic murmurs are divided into 3 categories:

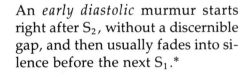

An *early diastolic* murmur starts right after S_2, without a discernible gap, and then usually fades into silence before the next S_1.*

Early diastolic murmurs typically accompany regurgitant flow across incompetent semilunar valves.

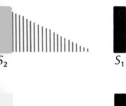

A *mid-diastolic murmur* starts a short time after S_2. It may fade away, as illustrated, or merge into a late diastolic murmur.

Mid-diastolic and presystolic murmurs are related to turbulent flow across the atrioventricular valves. See Table 9-14, Diastolic Murmurs (p. 319).

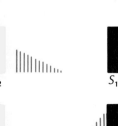 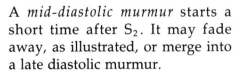

A *late diastolic (presystolic)* murmur starts late in diastole and typically continues up to S_1.

* To be more precise, systolic and early diastolic murmurs should be timed in relation to A_2 or P_2, depending on whether the murmur is aortic or pulmonic, respectively. This subtle difference, however, is difficult to discern, especially for beginning students.

An occasional murmur, such as that caused by a patent ductus arteriosus, starts in systole and continues without pause through S_2 into but not necessarily throughout diastole. It is then called a *continuous* murmur. Like continuous murmurs, some other cardiovascular sounds, such as pericardial friction rubs or venous hums, have *both systolic and diastolic components.* Observe and describe these sounds according to the characteristics used for systolic and diastolic murmurs.

The combination of two murmurs—one systolic and the other diastolic, each with its own characteristics—is not a continuous murmur, although it might have similar timing. See Table 9-15, Differentiation of Cardiovascular Sounds With Both Systolic and Diastolic Components (p. 320).

Shape. The shape or configuration of a murmur is determined by its intensity over time.

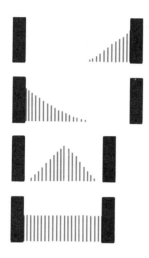

A *crescendo murmur* grows louder.

The presystolic murmur of mitral stenosis in normal sinus rhythm

A *decrescendo murmur* grows softer.

The early diastolic murmur of aortic regurgitation

A *crescendo–decrescendo murmur* first rises in intensity, then falls.

The midsystolic murmur of aortic stenosis

A *plateau murmur* has the same intensity throughout.

The pansystolic murmur of mitral regurgitation

Location of Maximal Intensity. This is determined by the site where the murmur originates. Find the location by exploring the area in which you can hear the murmur, and describe where you hear it best in terms of the interspace and its relation to the sternum, the apex, or the midsternal, the midclavicular, or one of the axillary lines.

For example, a murmur best heard in the 2nd right interspace usually originates at or near the aortic valve.

Radiation or Transmission from the Point of Maximal Intensity. This is determined not only by the site of origin but also by the intensity of the murmur and the direction of blood flow. Explore the area around a murmur and determine where else you can hear it.

A loud murmur of aortic stenosis often radiates into the neck (in the direction of arterial flow).

Intensity. This is usually graded on a 6-point scale and expressed as a fraction. The numerator describes the intensity of the murmur wherever it is loudest, and the denominator indicates the scale you are using. (There is also a 4-point scale.)

The 6 categories are defined as follows:

  Grade 1—very faint, heard only after the listener has "tuned in"; may not be heard in all positions

Intensity is influenced by the thickness of the chest wall and the presence of intervening tissue. For example, an identical degree of turbulence would cause a louder murmur in a thin person than in a very muscular or obese one. Emphysematous lungs may diminish the intensity of murmurs.

Grade 2—quiet but heard immediately upon placing the stethoscope on the chest

Grade 3—moderately loud

Grade 4—loud

Grade 5—very loud, may be heard with a stethoscope partly off the chest

Grade 6—may be heard with the stethoscope entirely off the chest

Pitch. This is categorized as high, medium, and low.

Quality. This is described in terms such as blowing, harsh, rumbling, and musical.

Other useful characteristics of murmurs—and heart sounds too—include their variations, if any, with respiration, with the position of the patient, or with other special maneuvers.

Thrills are usually associated with murmurs of grades 4 through 6.

A fully descriptive example might be: a harsh, medium-pitched, grade 3/6, midsystolic crescendo–decrescendo murmur, heard best in the 2nd right interspace, with radiation to the neck.

Murmurs originating in the right side of the heart tend to change more with respiration than do left-sided murmurs.

A Note on Cardiovascular Assessment

A good cardiovascular examination requires more than observation. You need to think about the possible meanings of your individual observations, fit them together in a logical pattern, and correlate your cardiac findings with the patient's blood pressure, arterial pulses, venous pulsations, and venous pressure, and with the remainder of your history and physical examination.

Evaluating the common systolic murmur illustrates this point. In examining an asymptomatic teenager, for example, you might hear a Grade 2 midsystolic murmur localized in the 2nd and 3rd left interspaces. Since this suggests a murmur of pulmonic origin, you should pay special attention to the size of the right ventricle by carefully palpating the left parasternal area. Because pulmonic stenosis and atrial septal defects can occasionally cause such murmurs, listen carefully to the splitting of the second heart sound and try to hear any ejection sounds. Listen to the murmur after the patient sits up. Look for evidence of anemia, hyperthyroidism, or pregnancy that could produce such a murmur by increasing the flow across the aortic or the pulmonic valve. If all your findings are normal, your patient probably has an *innocent murmur*—one with no pathologic significance.

In a 60-year-old person with anginal pains, you might hear a Grade 3 harsh midsystolic murmur maximal in the right 2nd interspace and radiating to the neck vessels. You cannot feel a thrill. These findings suggest aortic stenosis, but could be related to a sclerotic valve without stenosis, to a dilated aorta, or to increased flow across a normal valve. Evaluate the apical impulse for evidence of left ventricular enlargement. Listen for the murmur of aortic regurgitation as the patient leans forward and exhales. Assess the carotid pulse contour and the blood pressure for evidence of aortic stenosis. Put all this information together and make a tentative hypothesis as to the nature of the murmur.

SPECIAL MANEUVERS

AUSCULTATORY AIDS. Elsewhere in this chapter, you have already read how to improve your auscultation of the heart by positioning the patient in different ways. Two additional maneuvers extend these methods.

Squatting and Standing. When a person squats, venous return to the heart increases and so does peripheral vascular resistance. Arterial blood pressure, stroke volume, and the volume of blood in the left ventricle all rise. On standing, changes occur in opposite directions. These changes help (1) to identify a prolapsed mitral valve, and (2) to distinguish hypertrophic cardiomyopathy from aortic stenosis.

The temporary increase in left ventricular volume decreases the prolapse of a mitral valve, delays the click and murmur, and may decrease the intensity of the murmur. Standing reverses these changes (p. 312).

Secure the patient's gown so that it will not interfere with your examination, and ready yourself for prompt auscultation. Instruct the patient in how to squat next to the examining table and how to hold on to it for balance. Listen to the heart with the patient in the squatting position and again in the standing position.

The increased stroke volume increases the intensity of the murmur of aortic stenosis. In contrast, the increase in left ventricular volume decreases the outflow obstruction in hypertrophic cardiomyopathy and decreases the intensity of its murmur. Standing reverses both changes.

Valsalva Maneuver. When a person strains down against a closed glottis, venous return to the right heart is decreased and after a few seconds left ventricular volume and arterial blood pressure both fall. Release of the effort has the opposite effects. These changes, like those of squatting, help to identify prolapse of the mitral valve and hypertrophic cardiomyopathy.

The decreased left ventricular volume increases the tendency of the mitral valve to prolapse, moves the click earlier in systole, and lengthens the murmur

The patient should be lying down. Place one hand on the midabdomen and instruct the patient to strain against it. By adjusting your pressure you can alter the patient's effort to the desired level. Use your other hand to place your stethoscope on the patient's chest.

The decreased left ventricular volume increases the obstruction of hypertrophic cardiomyopathy and often increases the intensity of the murmur. The murmur of aortic stenosis, in contrast, decreases.

PULSUS ALTERNANS. If you suspect left-sided heart failure, feel the pulse specifically for alternating amplitudes. These are usually felt best in

Alternately loud and soft Korotkoff sounds or a sudden dou-

the radial or the femoral arteries. A blood-pressure cuff gives you a more sensitive method. After raising the cuff pressure, lower it slowly to the systolic level and then below it. While you do this, the patient should breathe quietly or stop breathing in the respiratory midposition. If dyspnea prevents this, help the patient to sit up and dangle both legs over the side of the bed.

PARADOXICAL PULSE. If you have noted that the pulse varies in amplitude with respiration or if you suspect pericardial tamponade (because of increased jugular venous pressure, a rapid and diminished pulse, and dyspnea, for example), use a blood-pressure cuff to check for a paradoxical pulse. This is a greater than normal drop in systolic pressure during inspiration. As the patient breathes, quietly if possible, lower the cuff pressure slowly to the systolic level. Note the pressure level at which the first sounds can be heard. Then drop the pressure very slowly until sounds can be heard throughout the respiratory cycle. Again note the pressure level. The difference between these two levels is normally no greater than 3 or 4 mm Hg.

bling of the apparent heart rate as the cuff pressure declines indicates a pulsus alternans (see p. 308).

The upright position may accentuate the alternation.

The level identified by first hearing Korotkoff sounds is the highest systolic pressure during the respiratory cycle. The level identified by hearing sounds throughout the cycle is the lowest systolic pressure. A difference between these levels of more than 10 mm Hg indicates a paradoxical pulse and suggests pericardial tamponade, possibly constrictive pericarditis, but, most commonly, obstructive airway disease (see p. 308).

Table 9-1 Approach to the Differentiation of Selected Heart Rates and Rhythms

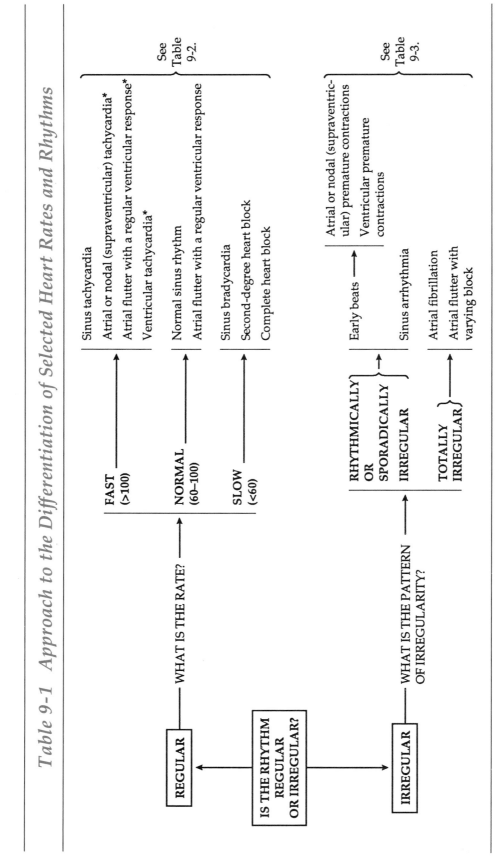

IS THE RHYTHM REGULAR OR IRREGULAR?		
REGULAR → WHAT IS THE RATE? →	**FAST (>100)** →	Sinus tachycardia / Atrial or nodal (supraventricular) tachycardia* / Atrial flutter with a regular ventricular response* / Ventricular tachycardia* } See Table 9-2.
	NORMAL (60–100) →	Normal sinus rhythm / Atrial flutter with a regular ventricular response
	SLOW (<60) →	Sinus bradycardia / Second-degree heart block / Complete heart block
IRREGULAR → WHAT IS THE PATTERN OF IRREGULARITY? →	**RHYTHMICALLY OR SPORADICALLY IRREGULAR** →	Early beats → Atrial or nodal (supraventricular) premature contractions / Ventricular premature contractions } See Table 9-3. / Sinus arrhythmia
	TOTALLY IRREGULAR →	Atrial fibrillation / Atrial flutter with varying block

* Less commonly, these arrhythmias may occur with slower ventricular rates.

Table 9-2 Differentiation of Selected Regular Rhythms

Table 9-2 Differentiation of Selected Regular Rhythms

DESCRIPTION	CLINICAL MANIFESTATIONS			FIRST AND SECOND HEART SOUNDS
	VENTRICULAR RATE			
	USUAL RESTING RATE	RESPONSE TO EXERCISE	RESPONSE TO VAGAL STIMULATION*	
RHYTHMS WITH FAST VENTRICULAR RATES				
SINUS TACHYCARDIA — A fast rhythm originating normally in the sinus node and conducted over normal pathways through the heart. Causes include exercise, anxiety, fever, hyperthyroidism, and blood loss.	100–150		Smooth slowing	Normal
ATRIAL OR NODAL (*Supraventricular*) TACHYCARDIA — A fast rhythm typically occurring in episodes or paroxysms. Young adults with no other evidence of heart disease are often affected. Conduction within the atria is abnormal, but the ventricles usually respond to each impulse.	160–200		Abrupt slowing or no change	Normal
ATRIAL FLUTTER WITH A REGULAR VENTRICULAR RESPONSE — A very fast atrial rhythm, often around 300–320 per min. There is usually a partial conduction block at the AV node. In a 2:1 block, for example, every second atrial beat is followed by a ventricular response.	150–160		Abrupt slowing or no change	Normal
VENTRICULAR TACHYCARDIA — A fast rhythm originating in the ventricles. This is an ominous arrhythmia, usually associated with organic heart disease, and may herald ventricular fibrillation and sudden death.	150–200		No change	Split S_1, S_2; varying intensity of S_1

Continued

Table 9-2 *Differentiation of Selected Regular Rhythms*

Table 9-2 (Cont'd.)

DESCRIPTION		CLINICAL MANIFESTATIONS			
		VENTRICULAR RATE			FIRST AND SECOND HEART SOUNDS
		USUAL RESTING RATE	RESPONSE TO EXERCISE	RESPONSE TO VAGAL STIMULATION*	
RHYTHMS WITH NORMAL VENTRICULAR RATES					
NORMAL SINUS RHYTHM	A rhythm of normal origin and conduction through the heart. Note, however, that a regular rhythm with a normal rate is not necessarily a normal sinus rhythm.	60–100	Smooth increase	Smooth slowing	Normal
ATRIAL FLUTTER WITH A REGULAR VENTRICULAR RESPONSE	A very fast atrial rhythm, as described above, but with a greater degree of AV block, *e.g.,* a 4:1 block, in which every fourth atrial impulse is followed by a ventricular response.	60–100	Abrupt increase or no change	Abrupt slowing or no change	Normal
RHYTHMS WITH SLOW VENTRICULAR RATES					
SINUS BRADYCARDIA	A slow rhythm with normal sinus origin and normal conduction. A very common rhythm, it may indicate excellent physical fitness. Other causes include hypothyroidism, hypothermia, acute myocardial infarction, and sick sinus syndrome (a condition associated with additional arrhythmias), and drugs such as digitalis and propranolol.	50–60, may be down to 40	Smooth increase		Normal
SECOND-DEGREE HEART BLOCK	A slow rhythm produced by impaired conduction through the AV node or the bundle of His. Some of the atrial impulses fail to get through to the ventricles. Causes include heart disease and drugs such as digitalis.	35–60	Smooth increase		Normal S₁, S₂; atrial sounds may also be heard
COMPLETE HEART BLOCK	A very slow rhythm produced by a complete block of conduction through the AV node or the bundle of His or its branches. Ventricular beats originate in the ventricles themselves. The most common cause is an acute myocardial infarction.	25–45, may be up to 60	No change		Varying intensity of S_1

* Vagal stimulation may be produced by holding a deep breath, by the induction of gagging or retching, and by carotid sinus massage. Careful monitoring is required.

Table 9-3   Differentiation of Selected Irregular Rhythms

Table 9-3   Differentiation of Selected Irregular Rhythms

TYPE OF RHYTHM	DIAGRAMMATIC REPRESENTATION	RHYTHM	HEART SOUNDS
ATRIAL OR NODAL (*Supraventricular*) **PREMATURE CONTRACTIONS**	QRS Aberrant P wave Normal QRS and T P T S_1 S_2 Early beat Pause	A beat of atrial or nodal origin comes earlier than the next expected normal beat. A pause follows and then the rhythm resumes.	S_1 may differ in intensity from the S_1 of normal beats, and S_2 may be decreased. Both sounds are otherwise similar to those of normal beats.
VENTRICULAR PREMATURE CONTRACTIONS	No P wave Aberrant QRS and T S_1 S_2 Early beat with split sounds Pause	A beat of ventricular origin comes earlier than the next expected normal beat. A pause follows and the rhythm resumes.	S_1 may differ in intensity from the S_1 of the normal beats, and S_2 may be decreased. Both sounds are likely to be split.
SINUS ARRHYTHMIA	S_1 S_2 S_1 S_2 S_1 S_2 S_1 S_2 S_1 S_2 INSPIRATION EXPIRATION	The heart varies cyclically, usually speeding up with inspiration and slowing down with expiration.	Normal, though S_1 may vary with the heart rate
ATRIAL FIBRILLATION AND ATRIAL FLUTTER WITH VARYING AV BLOCK	No P waves Fibrillation waves S_1 S_2 S_1 S_2 S_1 S_2 S_1 S_2 S_1 S_2	The ventricular rhythm is totally irregular, although short runs of the irregular ventricular rhythm may seem regular.	S_1 varies in intensity.

Table 9-4   Abnormalities of the Arterial Pulse

NORMAL

$mm\ Hg$

The pulse pressure is about 30–40 mm Hg. The pulse contour is smooth and rounded. (The notch on the descending slope of the pulse wave is not palpable.)

SMALL, WEAK PULSES

The pulse pressure is diminished, and the pulse feels weak and small. The upstroke may feel slowed, the peak prolonged. Causes include (1) decreased stroke volume, as in heart failure, hypovolemia, and severe aortic stenosis; and (2) increased peripheral resistance, as in exposure to cold and severe congestive heart failure.

LARGE, BOUNDING PULSES

The pulse pressure is increased and the pulse feels strong and bounding. The rise and fall may feel rapid, the peak brief. Causes include (1) an increased stroke volume, a decreased peripheral resistance, or both, as in fever, anemia, hyperthyroidism, aortic regurgitation, arteriovenous fistulas, and patent ductus arteriosus; (2) an increased stroke volume due to slow heart rates, as in bradycardia and complete heart block; and (3) decreased compliance (increased stiffness) of the aortic walls, as in aging or atherosclerosis.

BISFERIENS PULSE

A bisferiens pulse is an increased arterial pulse with a double systolic peak. Causes include pure aortic regurgitation, combined aortic stenosis and regurgitation, and, though less commonly palpable, hypertrophic cardiomyopathy.

PULSUS ALTERNANS

The pulse alternates in amplitude from beat to beat even though the rhythm is basically regular (and must be for you to make this judgment). When the difference between stronger and weaker beats is slight, it can be detected only by sphygmomanometry. Pulsus alternans indicates left ventricular failure and is usually accompanied by a left-sided S_3.

BIGEMINAL PULSE

Premature contractions

This is a disorder of rhythm that may masquerade as pulsus alternans. A bigeminal pulse is caused by a normal beat alternating with a premature contraction. The stroke volume of the premature beat is diminished in relation to that of the normal beats, and the pulse varies in amplitude accordingly.

PARADOXICAL PULSE

Inspiration

Expiration

A paradoxical pulse may be detected by a palpable decrease in the pulse's amplitude on quiet inspiration. If the sign is less pronounced, a blood-pressure cuff is needed. Systolic pressure decreases by more than 10 mm Hg during inspiration. A paradoxical pulse is found in pericardial tamponade, constrictive pericarditis (though less commonly), and obstructive lung disease.

Table 9-5 Variations and Abnormalities of the Ventricular Impulses

Table 9-5 Variations and Abnormalities of the Ventricular Impulses

When a ventricle works under conditions of chronic pressure overload (increased afterload), its walls gradually thicken (hypertrophy). Volume overload (increased preload), in contrast, produces dilatation of the ventricle as well as thickening of its walls. A hyperkinetic impulse results from an increased stroke volume and does not necessarily signify heart disease. An impulse may feel hyperkinetic when the chest wall is unusually thin.

	LEFT VENTRICLE				RIGHT VENTRICLE			
THE IMPULSE	NORMAL	HYPERKINETIC	PRESSURE OVERLOAD	VOLUME OVERLOAD	NORMAL	HYPERKINETIC	PRESSURE OVERLOAD	VOLUME OVERLOAD
LOCATION	5th or possibly 4th left interspace, medial to the midclavicular line	Normal	Normal	Displaced to the left and possibly downward	Indeterminate	3rd, 4th, or 5th left interspaces	3rd, 4th or 5th left interspaces, also subxiphoid	Left sternal border, extending toward the left cardiac border, also subxiphoid
DIAMETER	Little more than 2 cm in adults (1 cm in children); 3 cm or less in left-sided position	Normal, though increased amplitude may make it seem larger	Increased	Increased	Indeterminate	Not useful	Not useful	Not useful
AMPLITUDE	Small, gentle	Increased	Increased	Increased	Not palpable beyond infancy	Slightly increased	Increased	Slightly to markedly increased
DURATION	Usually less than two thirds of systole; the impulse stops before S_2	Normal	Prolonged, may be sustained up to S_2	Often slightly prolonged	Indeterminate	Normal	Prolonged	Normal to slightly prolonged
EXAMPLES OF CAUSES		Anxiety, hyperthyroidism, severe anemia	Aortic stenosis, systemic hypertension	Aortic or mitral regurgitation		Anxiety, hyperthyroidism, severe anemia	Pulmonic stenosis, pulmonary hypertension	Atrial septal defect

Table 9-6 Variations in the First Heart Sound

Category	Diagram	Description
NORMAL VARIATIONS	S_1 S_2 (at base)	S_1 is softer than S_2 at the *base* (right and left 2nd interspaces).
	S_1 S_2 (at apex)	S_1 is often but not always louder than S_2 at the *apex*.
ACCENTUATED S_1	S_1 S_2	S_1 is accentuated (1) by tachycardia and by high cardiac output states (*e.g.*, exercise, anemia, hyperthyroidism), and (2) in mitral stenosis. In these conditions, the mitral valve is still open wide at the onset of ventricular systole and then closes quickly.
DIMINISHED S_1	S_1 S_2	S_1 is diminished in first-degree heart block (delayed conduction from atria to ventricles). Here the mitral valve has had time after atrial contraction to float back into an almost closed position before ventricular contraction shuts it. It closes less loudly. S_1 is also diminished (1) when the mitral valve is calcified and relatively immobile, as in mitral regurgitation, and (2) when left ventricular contractility is markedly reduced, as in congestive heart failure or coronary heart disease.
VARYING S_1	S_1 S_2	S_1 varies in intensity (1) in complete heart block, where atria and ventricles are beating independently of each other, and (2) in any totally irregular rhythm (*e.g.*, atrial fibrillation). In these situations, the mitral valve is in varying positions before being shut by ventricular contraction. Its closure sound, therefore, varies in loudness.
SPLIT S_1	S_1 S_2	S_1 may be split normally along the lower left sternal border where the tricuspid component, often too faint to be heard, becomes audible. This split may sometimes be heard at the apex, but other explanations for it must then be considered (see Table 9-10). Abnormal splitting of both heart sounds may be heard in right bundle branch block and in beats of ventricular origin such as premature ventricular contractions.

Table 9-7 Variations in the Second Heart Sound

Table 9-7 Variations in the Second Heart Sound

	EXPIRATION	INSPIRATION	
PHYSIOLOGIC SPLITTING	S_1 ... S_2	S_1 ... A_2 P_2 (S_2)	*Physiologic splitting* of the second heart sound can usually be detected in the 2nd or 3rd left interspace. The pulmonic component of S_2 is usually too faint to be heard at the apex or aortic area, where S_2 is single and derived from aortic valve closure alone. Normal splitting is accentuated by inspiration and usually disappears on expiration. In some patients, however, especially younger ones, S_2 may not become completely single on expiration. It may do so when the patient sits up.
PATHOLOGIC SPLITTING (*All of these involve splitting during expiration and all suggest heart disease.*)	S_1 ... S_2	S_1 ... S_2	*Wide splitting* of S_2 refers to an increase in the usual splitting that persists throughout the respiratory cycle. Wide splitting can be caused by delayed closure of the pulmonic valve (*e.g.,* by pulmonic stenosis or right bundle branch block). As illustrated here, right bundle branch block also causes splitting of S_1 into its mitral and tricuspid components. Wide splitting can also be caused by early closure of the aortic valve, as in mitral regurgitation.
	S_1 ... S_2	S_1 ... S_2	*Fixed splitting* refers to wide splitting that does not vary with respiration. It occurs in atrial septal defect and right ventricular failure.
	S_1 ... P_2 A_2 (S_2)	S_1 ... S_2	*Paradoxical* or *reversed splitting* refers to splitting that appears on expiration and disappears on inspiration. Closure of the aortic valve is abnormally delayed so that A_2 follows P_2 in expiration. Normal inspiratory delay of P_2 makes the split disappear. The most common cause of paradoxical splitting is left bundle branch block

INCREASED INTENSITY OF S_2 IN THE RIGHT SECOND INTERSPACE (where only A_2 can usually be heard) occurs in systemic hypertension because of the increased pressure. It also occurs when the aortic root is dilated, probably because the aortic valve is then closer to the chest wall.

A DECREASED OR ABSENT S_2 IN THE RIGHT SECOND INTERSPACE is noted in calcific aortic stenosis because of immobility of the valve. If A_2 is inaudible, no splitting is heard.

INCREASED INTENSITY OF THE PULMONIC COMPONENT OF S_2. When P_2 is equal to or louder than A_2, pulmonary hypertension may be suspected. Other causes include a dilated pulmonary artery and an atrial septal defect. Splitting of the second heart sound that is heard widely, even at the apex and the right base, indicates an accentuated P_2.

A DECREASED OR ABSENT P_2 is most commonly due to the increased anteroposterior diameter of the chest associated with aging. It can also result from pulmonic stenosis. If P_2 is inaudible, no splitting is heard.

Table 9-8 Extra Heart Sounds in Systole

Extra heart sounds in systole are of two kinds: (1) early ejection sounds, and (2) clicks, most commonly heard in mid- and late systole.

EARLY SYSTOLIC EJECTION SOUNDS

Early systolic ejection sounds occur shortly after the first heart sound, coincident with the opening of the aortic and pulmonic valves. They are relatively high in pitch, have a sharp, clicking quality, and are heard better with the diaphragm of the stethoscope. An ejection sound indicates cardiovascular disease.

An *aortic ejection sound* is heard at both base and apex and may be louder at the apex. It does not usually vary with respiration. An aortic ejection sound may accompany a dilated aorta or aortic valve disease, such as congenital stenosis or a bicuspid valve.

A *pulmonic ejection sound* is heard best in the 2nd and 3rd left interspaces. When the first heart sound, usually relatively soft in this area, appears to be loud, you may instead be hearing a pulmonic ejection sound. Its intensity often decreases with inspiration. Causes include dilatation of the pulmonary artery, pulmonary hypertension, and pulmonic stenosis.

S_1 E_j S_2

SYSTOLIC CLICKS

Systolic clicks are usually due to *mitral valve prolapse*—an abnormal systolic ballooning of part of the mitral valve into the left atrium. The clicks are usually mid- or late systolic, but occasionally they are early systolic. Prolapse of the mitral valve is a common cardiac condition, affecting about 5% of young adults. It is more common in women. The click is usually single, but more than one may be heard. A click is heard best at or medial to the apex but may also be heard at the lower left sternal border. It is high-pitched and clicking in quality and is heard better with the diaphragm. The click is often followed by a late systolic murmur, which indicates a usually mild mitral regurgitation—a flow of blood from left ventricle to left atrium. The murmur usually crescendos up to S_2.

Auscultatory findings are notably variable. Most patients have only a click, some have only a murmur, and some have both. Findings vary from time to time and often change with body position. Several positions are recommended to identify the syndrome: supine, seated, squatting, and standing. Squatting delays the click and murmur; standing moves them closer to S_1.

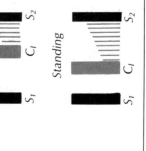

S_1 C_1 S_2

Squatting

S_1 C_1 S_2

Standing

S_1 C_1 S_2

Table 9-9   Extra Heart Sounds in Diastole

Table 9-9   Extra Heart Sounds in Diastole

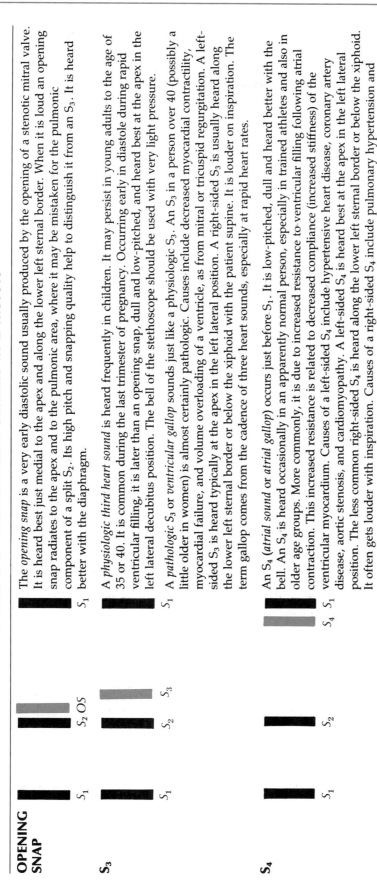

OPENING SNAP	The *opening snap* is a very early diastolic sound usually produced by the opening of a stenotic mitral valve. It is heard best just medial to the apex and along the lower left sternal border. When it is loud an opening snap radiates to the apex and to the pulmonic area, where it may be mistaken for the pulmonic component of a split S_2. Its high pitch and snapping quality help to distinguish it from an S_3. It is heard better with the diaphragm.
S_3	A *physiologic third heart sound* is heard frequently in children. It may persist in young adults to the age of 35 or 40. It is common during the last trimester of pregnancy. Occurring early in diastole during rapid ventricular filling, it is later than an opening snap, dull and low-pitched, and heard best at the apex in the left lateral decubitus position. The bell of the stethoscope should be used with very light pressure.
	A *pathologic S_3 or ventricular gallop* sounds just like a physiologic S_3. An S_3 in a person over 40 (possibly a little older in women) is almost certainly pathologic. Causes include decreased myocardial contractility, myocardial failure, and volume overloading of a ventricle, as from mitral or tricuspid regurgitation. A left-sided S_3 is heard typically at the apex in the left lateral position. A right-sided S_3 is usually heard along the lower left sternal border or below the xiphoid with the patient supine. It is louder on inspiration. The term gallop comes from the cadence of three heart sounds, especially at rapid heart rates.
S_4	An S_4 (*atrial sound or atrial gallop*) occurs just before S_1. It is low-pitched, dull and heard better with the bell. An S_4 is heard occasionally in an apparently normal person, especially in trained athletes and also in older age groups. More commonly, it is due to increased resistance to ventricular filling following atrial contraction. This increased resistance is related to decreased compliance (increased stiffness) of the ventricular myocardium. Causes of a left-sided S_4 include hypertensive heart disease, coronary artery disease, aortic stenosis, and cardiomyopathy. A left-sided S_4 is heard best at the apex in the left lateral position. The less common right-sided S_4 is heard along the lower left sternal border or below the xiphoid. It often gets louder with inspiration. Causes of a right-sided S_4 include pulmonary hypertension and pulmonic stenosis.
	An S_4 may also be associated with delayed conduction between atria and ventricles. This delay separates the normally faint atrial sound from the louder S_1 and makes it audible. An S_4 is never heard in the absence of atrial contraction, as occurs with atrial fibrillation.
	Occasionally, a patient has both an S_3 and an S_4, producing a *quadruple rhythm* of four heart sounds. At rapid heart rates, the S_3 and S_4 may merge into one loud extra heart sound called a *summation gallop*.

Table 9-10   Causes of An Apparently Split First Heart Sound

Normal splitting of the first heart sound occurs when the soft second tricuspid component is audible. Additional causes of an apparently split S₁ are compared below. A pulmonic ejection sound is not included in this table because its location in the 2nd and 3rd left interspaces should alone make the differentiation. An early systolic click has the same significance as a midsystolic or late systolic click—mitral valve prolapse.

	LEFT-SIDED S₄	RIGHT-SIDED S₄	SPLIT S₁	AORTIC EJECTION SOUND	EARLY SYSTOLIC CLICK
LOCATION OF MAXIMAL INTENSITY	Apex	Lower left sternal border or subxiphoid	Lower left sternal border, but may be heard at the apex too	Aortic area, apex, or both	At or medial to the apex or at the lower left sternal border
PITCH AND QUALITY	Low-pitched, dull	Low-pitched, dull	High-pitched; both components of similar quality	High-pitched, clicking	High-pitched, clicking
BETTER HEARD WITH	Bell	Bell	Diaphragm	Diaphragm	Diaphragm
PALPABLE SPLIT	May be present as a double impulse at the apex	May be present as a double impulse at the left sternal border or in the subxiphoid area	Absent	Absent	Absent
SPECIAL AUSCULTATORY AIDS	The left lateral decubitus position accentuates this S₄.	Inspiration often accentuates this S₄.	None	None	The squatting position delays the click and widens the split.

Table 9-11   Mechanisms of Heart Murmurs

Table 9-11   Mechanisms of Heart Murmurs

Heart murmurs are of longer duration than heart sounds. They originate within the heart itself or in its great vessels, and are usually caused by one of the following mechanisms:

1. Flow across a partial obstruction (*e.g.,* aortic stenosis)

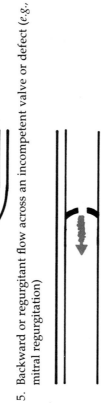

2. Flow across a valvular or intravascular irregularity without obstruction (*e.g.,* a biscuspid aortic valve without true stenosis)

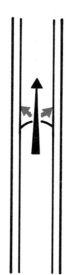

3. Increased flow through normal structures (*e.g.,* aortic systolic murmur associated with anemia)

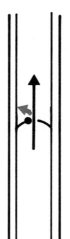

4. Flow into a dilated chamber (*e.g.,* aortic systolic murmur associated with aneurysmal dilatation of the ascending aorta)

5. Backward or regurgitant flow across an incompetent valve or defect (*e.g.,* mitral regurgitation)

6. Shunting of blood out of a high-pressure chamber or artery through an abnormal passage (*e.g.,* ventricular septal defect, patent ductus arteriosus)

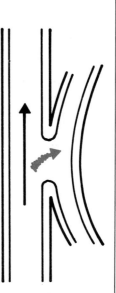

Table 9-12   Midsystolic Murmurs

Table 9-12   Midsystolic Murmurs

Midsystolic (ejection) murmurs—the most common kind of heart murmur—may be (1) *pathologic* (secondary to structural cardiovascular abnormality), (2) *physiologic* (secondary to physiologic alteration in the body), and (3) *innocent* (not associated with any detectable physiologic or structural abnormality). Midsystolic murmurs tend to peak near midsystole, and usually stop before S_2. The crescendo–decrescendo shape is not always obvious to the ear, but the gap between the murmur and S_2 helps to distinguish midsystolic from pansystolic murmurs.

	MECHANISM	THE MURMUR	ASSOCIATED FINDINGS
INNOCENT MURMURS S_1 S_2	Innocent murmurs result from turbulent blood flow probably generated by left ventricular ejection of blood into the aorta. Occasionally, turbulence from right ventricular ejection may also cause them. There is no evidence of cardiovascular disease. Innocent murmurs—very common in children and young adults—may also be heard in older people.	*Location.* 2nd to 4th left interspaces between the left sternal border and the apex *Radiation.* Little *Intensity.* Grade 1 to 2, possibly 3 *Pitch.* Medium *Quality.* Variable *Aids.* Usually decreases or disappears on sitting	None: normal splitting, no ejection sounds, no diastolic murmurs, and no palpable evidence of ventricular enlargement. Occasionally, a patient has both an innocent murmur and another kind of murmur.
PHYSIOLOGIC MURMURS S_1 S_2	Turbulence due to a temporary increase in blood flow causes this murmur. Predisposing conditions include anemia, pregnancy, fever, and hyperthyroidism.	Similar to innocent murmurs	Possible signs of a likely cause

Table 9-12 Midsystolic Murmurs

PATHOLOGIC MURMURS

AORTIC STENOSIS

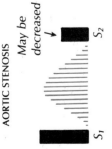

Significant stenosis of the aortic valve impairs blood flow across the valve, causing turbulence, and increases the afterload on the left ventricle. Causes are congenital, rheumatic, and degenerative, and findings may differ with each cause.

Other conditions may mimic the murmur of aortic stenosis without obstructing flow:

- *Aortic sclerosis,* a stiffening of aortic valve leaflets associated with aging
- A *bicuspid aortic valve,* a congenital condition, which may not be recognized until adulthood
- A *dilated aorta,* as from arteriosclerosis, syphilis, or Marfan's syndrome
- *A pathologically increased flow across the aortic valve during systole,* as in aortic regurgitation

Location. Right 2nd interspace

Radiation. Often to the neck and down the left sternal border, even to the apex

Intensity. Sometimes soft but often loud, with a thrill

Pitch. Medium; at the apex, it may be higher

Quality. Often harsh; at the apex it may be more musical

Aids. Heard best with the patient sitting and leaning forward

A_2 decreases as the stenosis worsens. A_2 may be delayed, merging with P_2 to form a single sound or causing paradoxical splitting. An S_4, reflecting the decreased compliance of the hypertrophied left ventricle, may be present at the apex. An aortic ejection sound, if present, suggests a congenital cause. A sustained apical impulse often reveals left ventricular hypertrophy. The carotid artery impulse may rise slowly and feel small in amplitude.

HYPERTROPHIC CARDIOMYOPATHY

Massive hypertrophy of ventricular muscle is associated with unusually rapid systolic ejection of blood from the left ventricle during systole. Obstruction to flow may coexist. Accompanying distortion of the mitral valve may cause mitral regurgitation.

Location. 3rd and 4th left interspaces

Radiation. Down the left sternal border to the apex, possibly to the base, but not to the neck

Intensity. Variable

Pitch. Medium

Quality. Harsh

Aids. Decreases with squatting, increases with straining down

As S_3 may be present.

An S_4 is often present at the apex (unlike in mitral regurgitation).

The apical impulse may be sustained and have two palpable components.

The carotid pulse rises quickly (unlike the pulse in aortic stenosis).

PULMONIC STENOSIS

Stenosis of the pulmonic valve impairs flow across the valve, and increases the afterload on the right ventricle. It is congenital and most often found in children.

Pathologically increased flow across the pulmonic valve may mimic the murmur of pulmonic stenosis. The systolic murmur associated with an atrial septal defect originates from this flow, not from the defect itself.

Location. 2nd and 3rd left interspaces

Radiation. If loud, toward the left shoulder and neck, especially on the left

Intensity. Soft to loud; if loud, associated with a thrill

Pitch. Medium

Quality. Often harsh

In severe stenosis, S_2 is widely split and P_2 is diminished. When P_2 is inaudible, no splitting is heard.

An early pulmonic ejection sound is common.

A right-sided S_4 may be present. The right ventricular impulse is often increased in amplitude and may be prolonged.

Table 9-13 Pansystolic (Holosystolic) Murmurs

Table 9-13 Pansystolic (Holosystolic) Murmurs

Pansystolic (holosystolic) murmurs are pathologic. They are heard when blood flows from a chamber of high pressure to one of lower pressure through a valve or other structure that should be closed. The murmur begins immediately with S_1 and continues up to S_2.

	MECHANISM	THE MURMUR	ASSOCIATED FINDINGS
MITRAL REGURGITATION	When the mitral valve fails to close fully in systole, blood regurgitates from left ventricle to left atrium, causing a murmur. This leakage creates a volume overload on the left ventricle, with subsequent dilatation and hypertrophy. Several structural abnormalities cause this condition, and findings may vary accordingly.	*Location.* Apex *Radiation.* To the left axilla, less often to the left sternal border *Intensity.* Soft to loud; if loud, associated with an apical thrill *Pitch.* Medium to high *Quality.* Blowing *Aids.* Unlike the murmur of tricuspid regurgitation, it does not become louder in inspiration.	S_1 is often decreased. An apical S_3 reflects the volume overload on the left ventricle. The apical impulse is increased in amplitude and may be prolonged.
TRICUSPID REGURGITATION	When the tricuspid valve fails to close fully in systole, blood regurgitates from right ventricle to right atrium, producing a murmur. The most common cause is right ventricular failure and dilatation, with resulting enlargement of the tricuspid orifice. Either pulmonary hypertension or left ventricular failure is the usual initiating cause.	*Location.* Lower left sternal border *Radiation.* To the right of the sternum, to the xiphoid area, and perhaps to the midclavicular line, but not into the axilla *Intensity.* Variable *Pitch.* Medium *Quality.* Blowing *Aids.* Unlike in the murmur of mitral regurgitation, the intensity may increase slightly with inspiration.	The right ventricular impulse is increased in amplitude and may be prolonged. An S_3 may be audible along the lower left sternal border. The jugular venous pressure is often elevated, and large v waves may be seen in the jugular veins.
VENTRICULAR SEPTAL DEFECT	A ventricular septal defect is a congenital abnormality in which blood flows from the relatively high-pressure left ventricle into the low-pressure right ventricle through a hole. The defect may be accompanied by other abnormalities, but an uncomplicated lesion is described here.	*Location.* 3rd, 4th, and 5th left interspaces *Radiation.* Often wide *Intensity.* Often very loud, with a thrill *Pitch.* High *Quality.* Often harsh	A_2 may be obscured by the loud murmur. Findings vary with the severity of the defect and with associated lesions.

Table 9-14   Diastolic Murmurs

Diastolic murmurs almost always indicate heart disease. There are two basic types. *Early decrescendo diastolic murmurs* signify regurgitant flow through an incompetent semilunar valve, more commonly the aortic. *Rumbling diastolic murmurs in mid- or late diastole* suggest stenosis of an atrioventricular valve, more often the mitral.

	MECHANISM	THE MURMUR	ASSOCIATED FINDINGS
AORTIC REGURGITATION	The leaflets of the aortic valve fail to close completely during diastole, and blood regurgitates from the aorta back into the left ventricle. A volume overload on the left ventricle results. Two other murmurs may be associated: (1) a midsystolic murmur from the resulting increased forward flow across the aortic valve, and (2) a mitral diastolic (or Austin Flint) murmur. The latter is attributed to diastolic impingement of the regurgitant flow on the anterior leaflet of the mitral valve.	*Location.* 2nd to 4th left interspaces	An ejection sound may be present.
		Radiation. If loud, to the apex, perhaps to the right sternal border	An S_3 or S_4, if present, suggest severe regurgitation.
		Intensity. Grade 1 to 3	Progressive changes in the apical impulse include increased amplitude, displacement laterally and downward, widened diameter, and increased duration.
		Pitch. High. Use a diaphragm.	
		Quality. Blowing; may be mistaken for breath sounds	
		Aids. The murmur is heard best with the patient sitting, leaning forward, with breath held in exhalation.	The pulse pressure increases, and arterial pulses are often large and bounding.
			Either a midsystolic flow murmur or an Austin Flint murmur suggests a large regurgitant flow.
MITRAL STENOSIS	When the leaflets of the mitral valve thicken, stiffen, and become distorted from the effects of rheumatic fever, it fails to open sufficiently in diastole. The resulting murmur has two components: (1) middiastolic (during rapid ventricular filling), and (2) presystolic (during atrial contraction). The latter disappears if atrial fibrillation develops, leaving only a middiastolic rumble.	*Location.* Usually limited to the apex	S_1 is accentuated and may be palpable at the apex.
		Radiation. Little or none	An opening snap (OS) often follows S_2 and initiates the murmur.
		Intensity. Grade 1 to 4	If pulmonary hypertension develops, P_2 is accentuated and the right ventricular impulse becomes palpable.
		Pitch. Low. Use a bell.	
		Aids. Placing the bell exactly on the apical impulse, turning the patient into a left lateral position, and mild exercise all help to make the murmur audible. It is heard better in exhalation.	Mitral regurgitation and aortic valve disease may be associated with mitral stenosis.

Table 9-15 Cardiovascular Sounds With Both Systolic and Diastolic Components

Some cardiovascular sounds are not confined to one portion of the cardiac cycle. Three examples are (1) a pericardial friction rub, produced by inflammation of the pericardial sac; (2) patent ductus arteriosus, a congenital abnormality in which an open channel persists between aorta and pulmonary artery; and (3) a venous hum, a benign sound produced by turbulence of blood in the jugular veins (common in children). Their characteristics are contrasted below. The term *continuous murmur* is defined as one that begins in systole and continues through the second sound into all or part of diastole. It need not continue through diastole. The murmur of patent ductus arteriosus, therefore, may be classified as continuous.

	PERICARDIAL FRICTION RUB	PATENT DUCTUS ARTERIOSUS	VENOUS HUM
TIMING	May have three short components, each associated with cardiac movement: (1) atrial systole, (2) ventricular systole, and (3) ventricular diastole. Usually the first two components are present; all three make diagnosis easy; only one (usually the systolic) invites confusion with a murmur.	Continuous murmur in both systole and diastole, often with a silent interval late in diastole. Is loudest in late systole, obscures S_2, and fades in diastole	Continuous murmur without a silent interval. Loudest in diastole
LOCATION	Variable, but usually heard best in the 3rd interspace to the left of the sternum	Left 2nd interspace	Above the medial third of the clavicles, especially on the right
RADIATION	Little	Toward the left clavicle	1st and 2nd interspaces
INTENSITY	Variable. May increase when the patient leans forward and exhales	Usually loud, sometimes associated with a thrill	Soft to moderate. Can be obliterated by pressure on the jugular veins
QUALITY	Scratchy, scraping	Harsh, machinerylike	Humming, roaring
PITCH	High (heard better with a diaphragm)	Medium	Low (heard better with a bell)

Chapter 10
The Breasts and Axillae

Anatomy and Physiology

The female breast lies between the 2nd and 6th ribs, between the sternal edge and the midaxillary line. About two thirds of it is superficial to the pectoralis major, about one third to the serratus anterior. The nipple and the areola that surrounds it are somewhat lateral to the midline of the breast.

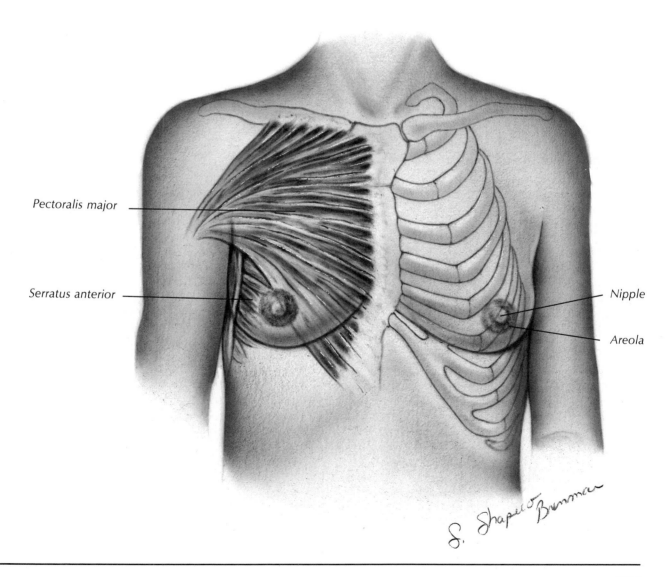

Pectoralis major

Serratus anterior

Nipple

Areola

For purposes of description, the breast may be divided into four quadrants by horizontal and vertical lines crossing at the nipple. In addition, a tail of breast tissue frequently extends toward or into the axilla. An alternative method of localizing findings visualizes the breast as the face of a clock. A lesion may be located by the "time" (*e.g.*, 4 o'clock) and by the distance in centimeters from the nipple.

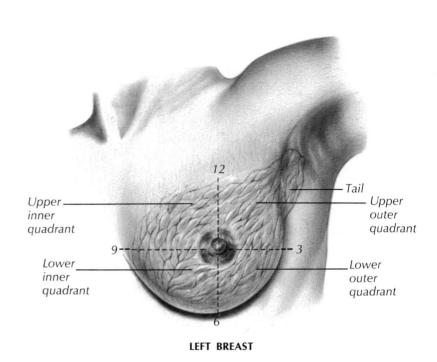

LEFT BREAST

Breast tissue has three principal components. (1) The *glandular tissue* produces milk after the delivery of an infant. This tissue is organized into 15 to 20 lobes that radiate around the nipple. Each lobe is drained by a duct that opens onto the nipple surface. Deep to the areola, each duct has a dilated portion that accumulates milk during lactation. (2) The glandular tissue is supported by *fibrous tissue*, including suspensory ligaments that are connected both to the skin and to fascia underlying the breast. (3) *Fat* surrounds the breast and predominates both superficially and peripherally. The proportions of these components vary with age, the general state of nutrition, pregnancy, and other factors.

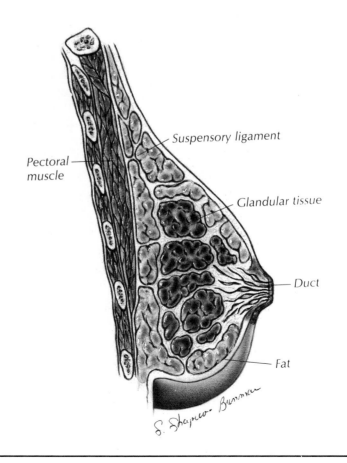

The surface of the areola has small, rounded elevations that mark the locations of sebaceous glands (glands of Montgomery). Both the nipple and the areola are well supplied with smooth muscle that helps to empty the ductal system of milk when a woman is nursing an infant. Tactile stimulation of the area, including that associated with breast examination, makes the nipple smaller, firmer, and more erect, while the areola puckers and wrinkles. These normal smooth muscle reflexes should not be mistaken for signs of breast disease.

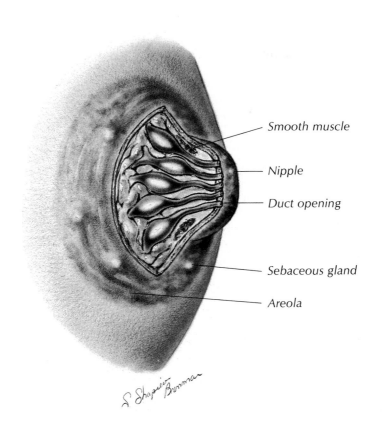

Occasionally, one or more extra (supernumerary) breasts are located along the "milk line," illustrated on the right. They are found most commonly in the axilla or just below the normal breast. Only a small nipple and areola are usually present, then often mistaken for a common mole. Glandular tissue may be present. An extra breast has no pathologic significance.

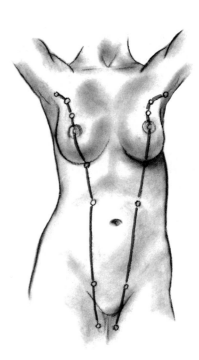

The male breast consists chiefly of a small nipple and areola. These overlie a thin disc of undeveloped breast tissue that may not be distinguishable clinically from the surrounding tissues. A firm button of breast tissue 2 cm or more in diameter has been described in roughly one out of three adult men. The limits of normal have not yet been clearly established.

CHANGES WITH AGE

Adolescence. Development of a woman's breasts begins during puberty. The preadolescent breast consists of a small elevated nipple with no elevation of underlying breast tissue. Between the ages of 8 and 13 (average around 11), secondary sex characteristics become apparent. Breast buds appear, and further enlargement of breasts and areolae follows. The five stages of breast development as defined by Tanner's sex maturity ratings (SMR) are shown below.

Sex Maturity Ratings in Girls: Breasts

STAGE 1

Preadolescent. Elevation of nipple only

STAGE 2 | **STAGE 3**

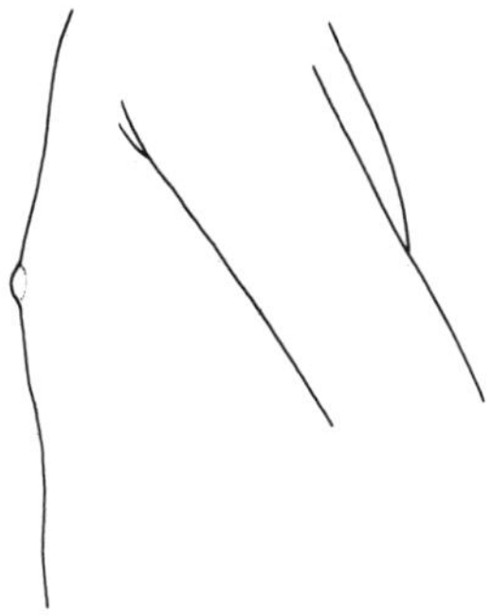

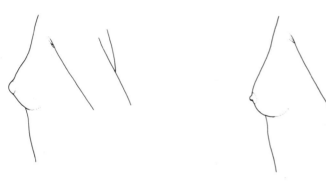

Breast bud stage. Elevation of breast and nipple as a small mound; enlargement of areolar diameter

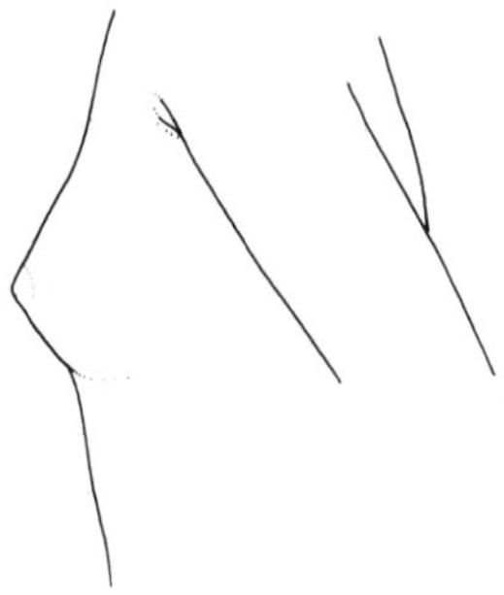

Further enlargement and elevation of breast and areola, with no separation of their contours

STAGE 4 | **STAGE 5**

Projection of areola and nipple to form a secondary mound above the level of breast

Mature stage; projection of nipple only. Areola has receded to general contour of the breast (although in some normal individuals the areola continues to form a secondary mound).

(Illustrations through the courtesy of W.A. Daniel, Jr., Division of Adolescent Medicine, University of Alabama, Birmingham)

Concomitantly, pubic hair appears and spreads, as illustrated on page 388. These two developmental changes—in breasts and pubic hair—are useful in assessing growth and maturation, although they do not necessarily proceed synchronously in any given person. The sequence from SMR 2 to SMR 5 takes about 3 years on the average, with a range of 1.5 to 6 years. Axillary hair usually appears about 2 years after pubic hair.

Menarche ordinarily occurs when a girl is in breast stage 3 or 4. By the time of menarche a girl has characteristically reached the peak of her adolescent growth spurt. Although she may continue to grow somewhat, her rate of growth has begun to taper off. The relationships of menarche to breast development and to the growth spurt are useful in counseling a girl who is worried that she may grow too tall or that her menarche is too late. The usual sequence of these changes is summarized in the diagram below.

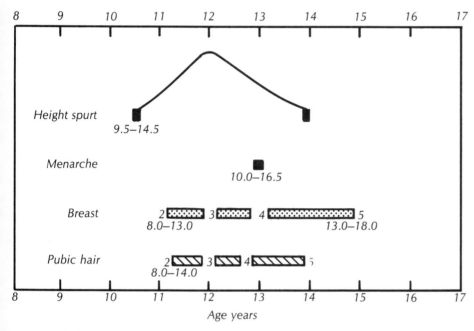

Numbers below the bars indicate the ranges in age within which certain changes occur. (Redrawn from Marshall WA, Tanner JM: Variations in the pattern of pubertal changes in boys. Arch Dis Child 45:22, 1970)

Tanner's figures are based on studies of white English girls. An American survey indicates that black girls tend to be more advanced in their secondary sex characteristics than are whites of the same age. Black girls, too, develop axillary hair earlier than their white counterparts, sometimes before their pubic hair appears. These differences, together with the relatively fine, sparse pubic hair described in Oriental women, illustrate the caution required in applying group norms.

Breasts vary normally in several ways. In about 1 out of 12 girls, breasts develop at different rates, and considerable asymmetry may result. This is usually a temporary phenomenon; unless the difference is unusually marked, reassurance is indicated.

Adulthood. The normal adult breast may be soft but may also feel diffusely granular, nodular, or lumpy. This texture, termed physiologic nodularity, is often bilateral. It may be evident throughout the breast or only in parts of it. The nodularity may increase premenstrually—a time that breasts often enlarge and become tender or even painful. For breast changes during pregnancy, see pp. 409–410.

Aging. The breasts of an aging woman tend to diminish in size as glandular tissue atrophies and is replaced by fat. Although the proportion of fat increases, its total amount may also decrease. The breasts often get flabby and hang lower on the chest, as shown on page 131. The ducts surrounding the nipple may become more easily palpable as firm stringy strands. Axillary hair diminishes.

The Adolescent Male. Approximately 2 out of 3 adolescent boys develop *gynecomastia*—breast enlargement on one or both sides. This is usually a slight change, but obvious enlargement may cause considerable embarrassment. Pubertal gynecomastia usually resolves spontaneously within a year or two.

LYMPHATICS

Because the lymphatics of much of the breast drain toward the axilla, an understanding of the axillary lymph nodes will help you in assessing the breasts. Of these, the central axillary nodes are most frequently palpable. They are located along the chest wall, usually high in the axilla and midway between the anterior and posterior axillary folds. Into them drain channels from three other groups of lymph nodes:

1. The pectoral (or anterior) group of nodes is located along the lower border of the pectoralis major inside the anterior axillary fold. These nodes drain the anterior chest wall and most of the breast.
2. The subscapular (or posterior) group is located along the lateral border of the scapula and is felt deep in the posterior axillary fold. These nodes drain the posterior chest wall and a portion of the arm.
3. The lateral group is felt along the upper humerus. These nodes drain most of the arm.

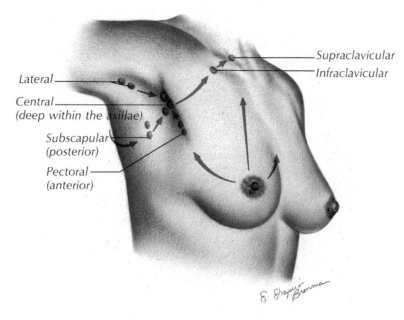

ARROWS INDICATE DIRECTION OF LYMPH FLOW

Lymph drains from the central axillary nodes to the infraclavicular and supraclavicular nodes.

Note that the lymphatics of the breast do not all drain into the axilla. Depending upon the location of a lesion in the breast, malignant cells or infection may spread directly to the infraclavicular nodes or into deep channels within the chest.

Techniques of Examination

THE FEMALE BREAST

General Approach

Women and girls may feel embarrassed about having their breasts examined, and they may be fearful about what the clinician may discover. Be alert to such feelings, and use courtesy, gentleness, and a matter-of-fact approach. An adequate inspection requires full exposure of the chest, but later in the examination you may find it helpful to cover one breast while you are palpating the other.

Tell the patient that you are going to examine her breasts. This may be a good time to ask if she has noted any lumps or other problems or whether she does monthly self-examinations. If she is unfamiliar with self-examination, you have a good opportunity to explain what you are doing and help her to repeat maneuvers after you.

Risk factors for breast cancer include increasing age, prior cancer in the opposite breast, a mother or sister who has had it, early menarche, late or no pregnancies, late menopause, and exposure to ionizing radiation.

Because breasts tend to swell and become more nodular premenstrually, the best time to examine them is a week or two after a menstrual period. If you find suspicious nodules during the premenstrual phase, arrange to reevaluate them later.

Inspection

With the patient in the sitting position, disrobed to the waist and with her arms at her sides—

Inspect the breasts. Note:

- The appearance of the skin, including

    Color

    Thickening of the skin and unusually prominent pores, which may accompany lymphatic obstruction

Redness in infection or inflammatory carcinoma

Thickening and prominent pores suggest a breast cancer.

- The size and symmetry of the breasts. Some difference in the size of the breasts, including the areolae, is common and is usually normal, as shown in the photograph on p. 329.

- The contour of the breasts. Look for changes such as masses, dimpling, or flattening. Compare one side with the other.

See Table 10-1, Visible Signs of Breast Cancer (p. 336).

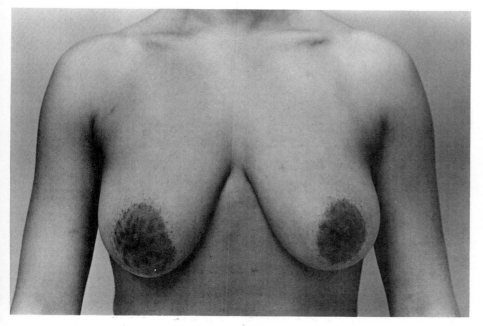

ARMS AT SIDES

Flattening of the normally convex breast, shown below, suggests cancer.

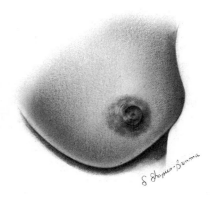

Inspect the nipples. Note:

- Their size and shape. Occasionally, a nipple is inverted—depressed below the areolar surface and sometimes enveloped by folds of areolar skin. Long-standing inversion is usually a normal variant and, except for possible difficulty in nursing an infant, is of no clinical conse-quence.

Recent or fixed flattening or depression of the nipple suggests
nipple retraction. A retracted
nipple may also be broadened
and thickened. It suggests an
underlying cancer.

- The direction in which they point (normally outward and often downward)

Asymmetry of the directions in
which nipples point suggests an
underlying cancer.

- Any rashes or ulcerations

Paget's disease of the breast
(see p. 336).

- Any discharge

When examining an adolescent girl, assess her breast development ac-cording to Tanner's sex maturity ratings (SMR) described on page 324. Because an adolescent girl is often concerned about her breasts, it may be helpful to tell her that she is developing normally (if she is) and, using the diagrams, to review with her the usual developmental sequence. You will rate pubic hair development separately, later in the examination.

In order to bring out dimpling or retraction that may otherwise be invisi-ble, ask the patient (1) to raise her arms over her head, and (2) to press her hands against her hips. Again inspect the breast contour carefully.

Dimpling or retraction of the
breasts with either of these maneuvers suggests an underlying

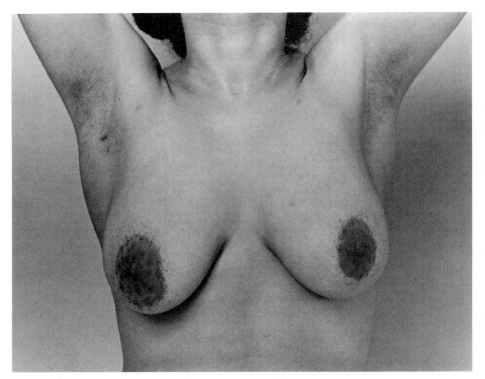

ARMS OVER HEAD

cancer. Occasionally, these signs may be associated with benign lesions such as post-traumatic fat necrosis or mammary duct ectasia, but they must always be evaluated with great care.

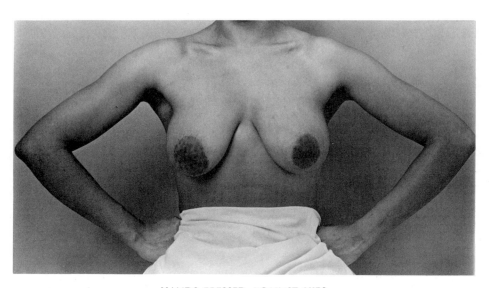

HANDS PRESSED AGAINST HIPS

Pressing against the hips contracts the pectoral muscles. When a cancer or its associated fibrous strands are attached to both the skin and the fascia overlying these muscles, pectoral contraction can draw the skin inward, causing dimpling.

Occasionally, other maneuvers may be useful:

If the breasts are large or pendulous, ask the patient to stand and lean forward, supported by the back of a chair or the examiner's hands.

This position may reveal an asymmetry of the breast or nipple not otherwise visible, and may thus help you to identify a cancer.

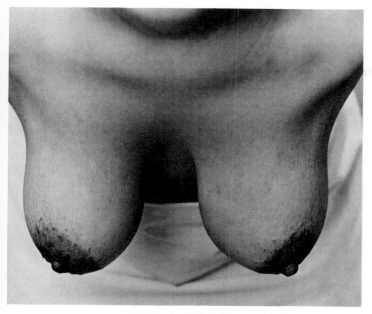

LEANING FORWARD

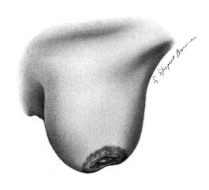

If you suspect a mass, gently move or compress the breast and watch for dimpling.

Dimpling suggests an underlying cancer.

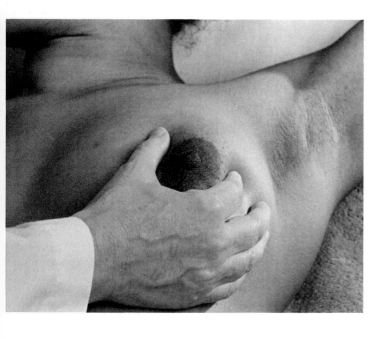

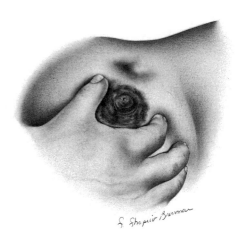

Palpation

Ask the patient to lie down. Unless the breasts are small, place a small pillow under the patient's shoulder on the side you are examining and ask her to rest her arm over her head. These maneuvers help to spread the breast more evenly across the chest and make it easier to find nodules.

With your fingers flat on the breast, compress the tissues gently in a rotary motion against the chest wall. Proceed systematically, examining the entire breast including the periphery, tail, and areola.

Nodules in the tail of the breast are sometimes mistaken for enlarged axillary lymph nodes (and *vice versa*).

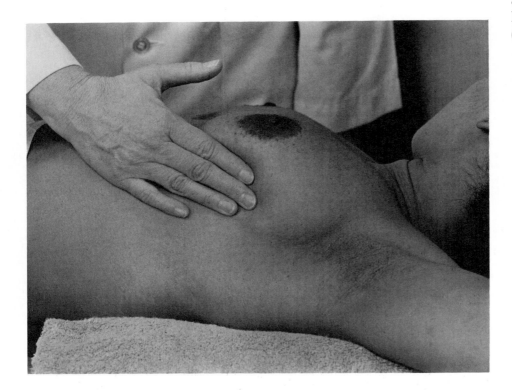

Use a uniform pattern of palpation to assure that you examine the entire breast from the clavicle to below the inframammary fold, from the midsternal line to the posterior axillary line, and well into the axilla for the tail of the breast. Possible patterns include concentric circles and a series of parallel lines.

Note:

> The *consistency of the tissues.* Normal consistency varies widely, depending in part on the relative proportions of soft fat and firmer glandular tissue. Physiologic nodularity may be present and may increase premenstrually. Especially in large breasts, a firm transverse ridge of compressed tissue may be present along the lower edge of the breast. This is the normal inframammary ridge and should not be confused with a tumor.

Tender cords suggest *mammary duct ectasia*, a benign but sometimes painful condition with dilatation of the ducts and inflammation around them. Masses may be associated.

> *Tenderness*

Premenstrual fullness, cysts, inflamed areas, and sometimes cancer may be tender.

> *Nodules.* Feel for any lump or mass that is larger or qualitatively different from the rest of the breast tissue. This is sometimes called a dominant mass and suggests a pathologic rather than a physiologic change. If one or more nodules are present, describe:

See Table 10-2, Differentiation of Common Breast Nodules (p. 337).

- Their location, by quadrant or the clock method, with centimeters from the nipple
- Size in centimeters
- Shape (*e.g.*, round or discoid, regular or irregular)
- Consistency (*e.g.*, soft, firm, or hard)
- Delimitation in relationship to surrounding tissues (*e.g.*, well circumscribed or not)
- Tenderness
- Mobility, with special reference to the skin, the pectoral fascia, and the underlying chest wall. Try to move the skin over the mass. Next, try to move the mass itself while the patient relaxes her arm and then while she presses her hand against her hip.

Hard, irregular, poorly circumscribed nodules, fixed to the skin or underlying tissues, strongly suggest cancer.

If a mobile mass becomes fixed when the patient presses her hand against her hip, the mass is attached to the pectoral fascia. If it is immobile with the patient relaxed, it is attached to the ribs and intercostal muscles.

Palpate each nipple, noting its elasticity.

Thickening of the nipple and loss of elasticity suggest an underlying cancer.

Compress the nipple and adjacent areola gently between your thumb and index finger, trying to strip them of any discharge. Note the color, consistency, and quantity of discharge and the exact location where it appears. Small amounts of milky discharge may persist for long periods after normal lactation.

Milky discharge unrelated to a prior pregnancy and lactation is called *nonpuerperal galactorrhea*. Leading causes are hormonal and drug-related.

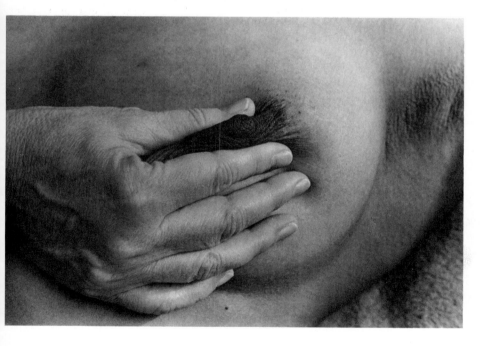

If you see any discharge, or if there is a history of nipple discharge, try to determine its origin by compressing the areola with your index finger placed in radial positions around the nipple. Watch for discharge appearing through one of the duct openings on the nipple's surface.

A nonmilky discharge suggests local breast disease. Causes include both benign and malignant processes, and there is no

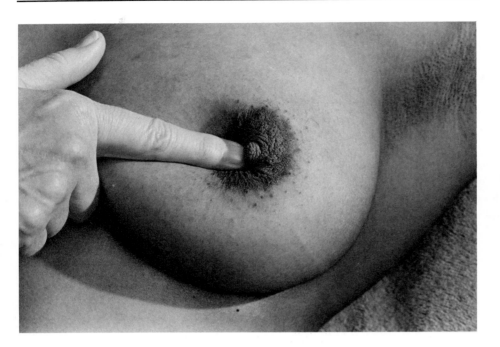

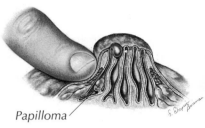

reliable way to distinguish them by the appearance of the discharge alone. One cause is an intraductal papilloma, shown below in its usual subareolar location.

Papilloma

THE MALE BREAST

Examination of the male breast may be brief but is sometimes important.

Inspect the nipple and areola for nodules, swelling, or ulceration.

Palpate the areola for nodules. If the breast appears enlarged, distinguish between the soft fatty enlargement that may accompany obesity and the firm disc of glandular enlargement, called gynecomastia.

Gynecomastia is attributed to an imbalance of estrogens and androgens, sometimes drug-related. A hard, irregular, eccentric, or ulcerating nodule is not gynecomastia and suggests breast cancer.

THE AXILLAE

Although the axillae may be examined with the patient lying down, a sitting position is preferable.

Inspection

Inspect the skin of each axilla, noting evidence of:

● Rash

Deodorant and other rashes

● Infection

Sweat gland infections (hidradenitis suppurativa)

● Unusual pigmentation

Deeply pigmented, velvety axillary skin suggests acanthosis nigricans, one form of which is associated with internal malignancy.

Palpation

To examine the left axilla, ask the patient to relax with the left arm down. Help by supporting the left wrist or hand with your left hand. Cup together the fingers of your right hand and reach as high as you can toward the apex of the axilla. Your fingers should lie directly behind the pectoral muscles, pointing toward the midclavicle. Now press your fingers in toward the chest wall and slide them downward, trying to feel the central nodes against the chest wall. Of the axillary nodes, these are the most often palpable. One or more soft, small, nontender nodes are frequently felt.

Enlarged axillary nodes are most commonly due to infection of the hand or arm, but a search for them is an important part of the evaluation for breast cancer.

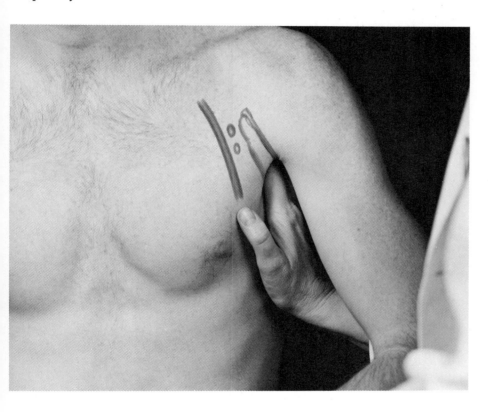

Use your left hand to examine the right axilla.

If the central nodes feel large, hard, or tender, or if there is a suspicious lesion in the drainage areas for the axillary nodes, feel for the other groups of lymph nodes:

- Pectoral nodes: grasp the anterior axillary fold between your thumb and fingers, and with your fingers palpate inside the border of the pectoral muscle.
- Lateral nodes: from high in the axilla feel along the upper humerus.
- Subscapular nodes: step behind the patient and with your fingers feel inside the muscle of the posterior axillary fold.

If you detect enlarged or tender axillary nodes, feel for infraclavicular nodes and reexamine the supraclavicular nodes.

Table 10-1   Visible Signs of Breast Cancer

Table 10-1   Visible Signs of Breast Cancer

RETRACTION SIGNS

MECHANISM

As breast cancer advances, it causes fibrosis (scar tissue). Shortening of this fibrotic tissue produces retraction signs, including dimpling, changes in contour, and retraction or deviation of the nipple. Illustrated is a cancer with fibrotic strands that have caused skin dimpling and a retracted nipple. Other causes of retraction signs include fat necrosis and mammary duct ectasia.

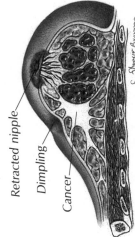

Retracted nipple

Dimpling

Cancer

SKIN DIMPLING

Look for this sign with the patient's arm at rest, during special positioning, and on moving or compressing the breast, as illustrated here.

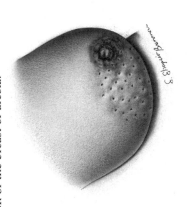

EDEMA OF THE SKIN

Edema of the skin is produced by lymphatic blockade. It appears as thickened skin with enlarged pores—the so-called peau d'orange (orange peel) sign. It is often seen first in the lower portion of the breast or areola.

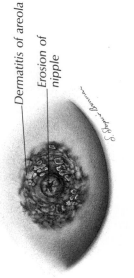

NIPPLE RETRACTION AND DEVIATION

A retracted nipple is flattened or pulled inward, as illustrated here. It may also be broadened, and feels thickened. When involvement is radially asymmetrical, the nipple may deviate, *i.e.,* point in a different direction from its normal counterpart, typically toward the underlying cancer.

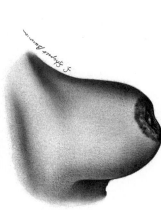

ABNORMAL CONTOURS

Look for any variation in the normal convexity of each breast, and compare one side with the other. Special positioning may again be useful. Shown here is marked flattening of the lower outer quadrant of the left breast.

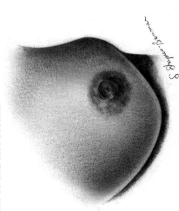

PAGET'S DISEASE OF THE NIPPLE

This is an uncommon form of breast cancer that usually starts as a scaly, eczemalike lesion. The skin may also weep, crust, or erode. A breast mass may be present. Suspect Paget's disease in any persisting dermatitis of the nipple and areola.

Dermatitis of areola

Erosion of nipple

Table 10-2 Differentiation of Common Breast Nodules

Table 10-2 Differentiation of Common Breast Nodules

The three most common kinds of breast nodules are gross cysts, fibroadenoma (a benign tumor), and breast cancer. The classic clinical characteristics of these three conditions, outlined below, are not always predictive of the final diagnosis. The nodules illustrated are rather large for illustrative purposes. Identification of a breast cancer is made ideally when it is small.

	GROSS CYSTS	FIBROADENOMA	CANCER
USUAL AGE	30–60, regresses after menopause	Puberty and young adulthood, up to age 55	30–90, most common in middle-aged and elderly women
NUMBER	Single or multiple	Usually single, may be multiple	Usually single, although may coexist with other nodular lesions
SHAPE	Round	Round, discoid, or lobular	Irregular or stellate
CONSISTENCY	Soft to firm, usually elastic	May be soft, usually firm	Firm or hard
DELIMITATION	Well delineated	Well delineated	Not clearly delineated from surrounding tissues
MOBILITY	Mobile	Very mobile	May be fixed to skin or underlying tissues
TENDERNESS	Often tender	Usually nontender	Usually nontender
RETRACTION SIGNS	Absent	Absent	Often present

Chapter 11
The Abdomen

Anatomy and Physiology

Review the anatomy of the abdominal wall, identifying the landmarks illustrated. The rectus abdominis muscles can be identified when a person raises head and shoulders from the supine position.

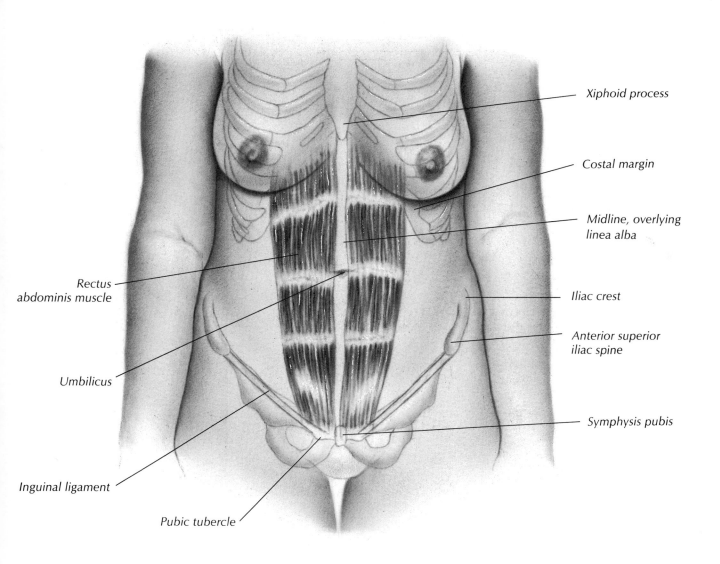

Xiphoid process

Costal margin

Midline, overlying linea alba

Iliac crest

Anterior superior iliac spine

Symphysis pubis

Rectus abdominis muscle

Umbilicus

Inguinal ligament

Pubic tubercle

For descriptive purposes, the abdomen is often divided into four quadrants by imaginary lines crossing at the umbilicus: right upper, right lower, left upper, and left lower quadrants. Another system divides the abdomen into nine sections. Terms for three of them are commonly used: epigastric, umbilical, and hypogastric or suprapubic.

When examining the abdomen, you may be able to feel several normal structures. The sigmoid colon is frequently palpable as a firm, narrow tube in the left lower quadrant, while the cecum and part of the ascending colon form a softer, wider tube in the right lower quadrant. Portions of the transverse and descending colon may also be palpable. None of these structures should be mistaken for a tumor. Although the normal liver often extends down just below the right costal margin, its soft consistency makes it difficult to feel through the abdominal wall. Occasionally, however, it may be palpable. Also in the right upper quadrant, but usually on a deeper level, lies the lower pole of the right kidney. It may be palpable, especially in thin women with relaxed abdominal muscles. Pulsations of the abdominal aorta are frequently visible and usually palpable in the upper abdomen, while the pulsations of the iliac arteries may sometimes be felt in the lower quadrants.

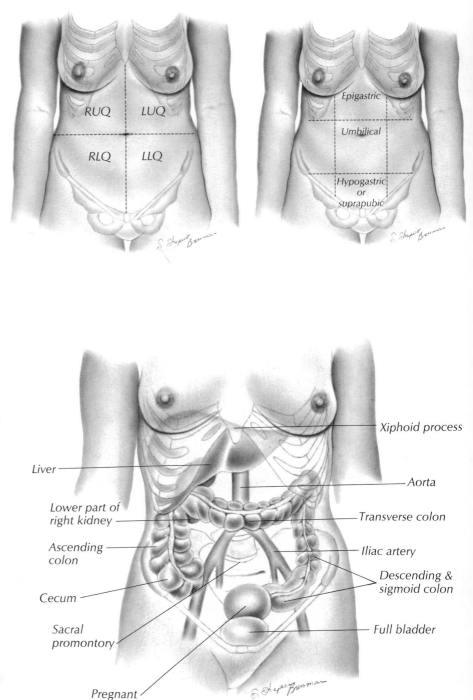

A distended bladder and a pregnant uterus each may rise above the symphysis pubis. With deep palpation several centimeters below the umbilicus in thin relaxed persons you can sometimes feel the sacral promontory, the anterior edge of the first sacral vertebra. Until you are familiar with this normal structure, you may mistake its stony hard outlines for a tumor. Another stony hard lump that can sometimes mislead you, and occasionally also alarms a patient who discovers it first, is a normal xiphoid process.

The abdominal cavity extends up under the rib cage to the dome of the diaphragm. In this protected location, beyond the reach of the palpating hand, are much of the liver and stomach and all of the usual normal spleen. Percussion may help you to assess these organs. The tip of a normal spleen is palpable in a small percentage of adults.

Most of the normal gallbladder lies deep to the liver, from which it cannot be clinically distinguished. The duodenum and pancreas lie deep in the upper abdomen, where they are not normally palpable.

The kidneys are posterior organs, the upper portions of which are protected by the ribs. The costovertebral angle—the angle formed by the lower border of the 12th rib and the transverse processes of the upper lumbar vertebrae—defines the region to assess for kidney tenderness.

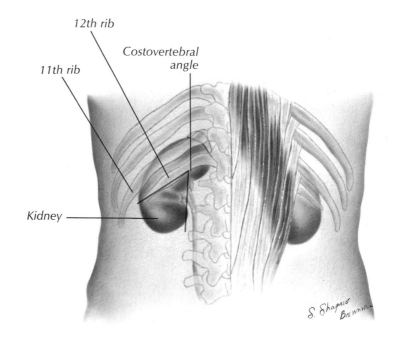

CHANGES WITH AGE

During the middle and later years, fat tends to accumulate in the lower abdomen and near the hips, even when total body weight is stable. This accumulation, together with weakening of the abdominal muscles, often produces a potbelly. Occasionally a person notes this change with alarm and interprets it as fluid or evidence of disease.

Old age may blunt the manifestations of acute abdominal disease. Pain may be less severe, fever is often less pronounced, and signs of peritoneal inflammation, such as muscular guarding and rebound tenderness (pp. 350–351), may be diminished or even absent.

Techniques of Examination

GENERAL APPROACH

Essential conditions for a good abdominal examination include (1) good light, (2) a relaxed patient, and (3) full exposure of the abdomen from above the xiphoid process to the symphysis pubis. The groins should be visible, although the genitalia should be kept draped. To encourage relaxation:

- The patient should *not* have a full bladder.

- Make the patient comfortable in a supine position, with a pillow for the head and perhaps another under the knees. You can ascertain whether or not the patient is relaxed flat on the table by trying to insert your hand underneath the low back.

An arched back thrusts the abdomen forward, thus tightening the abdominal muscles.

- The patient should keep arms at the sides or folded across the chest. Although patients commonly put their arms over their heads, this move should be discouraged because it stretches and tightens the abdominal wall and makes palpation difficult.

- Before palpation, ask the patient to point to any areas of pain, and examine painful or tender areas last.

- Have warm hands, a warm stethoscope, and short fingernails. Rubbing your hands together or running hot water over them may help to warm them. If necessary, you may start your palpation through the patient's gown. This contact with the patient's body usually warms your hand, and you can then expose the abdomen properly. Anxious examiners, unfortunately, often have cold hands. This problem decreases over time.

- Approach slowly and avoid quick, unexpected movements.

- Distract the patient if necessary with conversation or questions.

- If the patient is very frightened or very ticklish, begin palpation with his or her own hand beneath yours. In a few moments you can slip your hand underneath to palpate directly.

- Monitor your examination by watching the patient's face for signs of discomfort.

Make a habit of visualizing each organ in the region you are examining. From the patient's right side, proceed in an orderly fashion: inspection, auscultation, percussion, palpation.

INSPECTION

Starting from your usual standing position at the right side of the bed, inspect the abdomen. When looking at the contour of the abdomen and watching for peristalsis, it is helpful to sit or bend down so that you can view the abdomen tangentially.

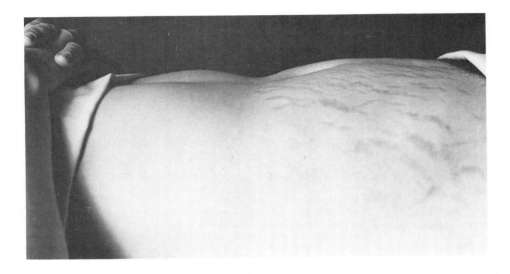

Note:

● *The skin*, including:

    Scars. Describe or diagram their location.

    Striae. Old silver striae or stretch marks, as illustrated above, are normal.

      Pink purple striae of Cushing's syndrome

    Dilated veins. A few small veins may be visible normally.

      Dilated veins of hepatic cirrhosis or of inferior vena cava obstruction

    Rashes and lesions

● *The umbilicus*—its contour and location, and any signs of inflammation or hernia

      See Table 11-1, Localized Bulges in the Abdominal Wall (p. 362).

● *The contour of the abdomen.*

    Is it flat, rounded, protuberant, or scaphoid (markedly concave or hollowed)?

      See Table 11-2, Protuberant Abdomens (p. 363).

    Do the flanks bulge or are there any local bulges? Include in this survey the inguinal and femoral areas.

      Bulging flanks of ascites

      Suprapubic bulge of distended bladder or pregnant uterus

Is the abdomen symmetrical?

Asymmetry of an enlarged organ or mass

Are there visible organs or masses? Look for an enlarged liver or spleen that has descended below the rib cage.

Lower abdominal mass of an ovarian or a uterine tumor

- *Peristalsis.* Observe for several minutes if you suspect intestinal obstruction. Peristalsis may be visible normally in very thin people.

Increased peristaltic waves of intestinal obstruction

- *Pulsations.* The normal aortic pulsation is frequently visible in the epigastrium.

Increased pulsation of aortic aneurysm or of increased pulse pressure

AUSCULTATION

bowel = intestine (small & large)
↳ duodenum, jejunum, ileon
caecum, colon, rectum

Auscultation of the abdomen is useful in assessing bowel motility and abdominal complaints, in searching for renal artery stenosis as a cause of hypertension, and in exploring for other vascular obstructions. You should practice the technique until you become thoroughly familiar with normal variations and can listen intelligently when you need to. In most other situations, however, auscultation may safely be omitted.

Listen to the abdomen before percussing and feeling it, because the latter maneuvers may alter the frequency of bowel sounds. Place the diaphragm of your stethoscope gently on the abdomen.

Listen for *bowel sounds* and note their frequency and character. Normal sounds consist of clicks and gurgles, the frequency of which has been estimated at from 5 to 34 per minute. Occasionally you may hear borborygmi—loud prolonged gurgles of hyperperistalsis—the familiar "stomach growling." Because bowel sounds are widely transmitted through the abdomen, listening in one spot, such as the right lower quadrant, is usually sufficient.

Bowel sounds may be altered in diarrhea, intestinal obstruction, paralytic ileus, and peritonitis. See Table 11-3, Sounds in the Abdomen (p. 364).

If the patient has high blood pressure, listen in the epigastrium and in each upper quadrant for *bruits*—vascular sounds resembling heart murmurs. Later in the examination, when the patient sits up, listen also in the costovertebral angles. Epigastric bruits confined to systole may be heard in normal persons.

In a hypertensive patient, a bruit in the upper abdomen with both systolic and diastolic components strongly suggests renal artery stenosis.

If you suspect arterial insufficiency in the legs, listen for bruits over the aorta, the iliac arteries, and the femoral arteries. Bruits confined to systole are relatively common, however, and do not necessarily signify occlusive disease.

Bruits with both systolic and diastolic components suggest the turbulent blood flow of partial arterial occlusion.

Listening points for bruits in these vessels are illustrated on p. 346.

See Table 11-3, Sounds in the Abdomen (p. 364).

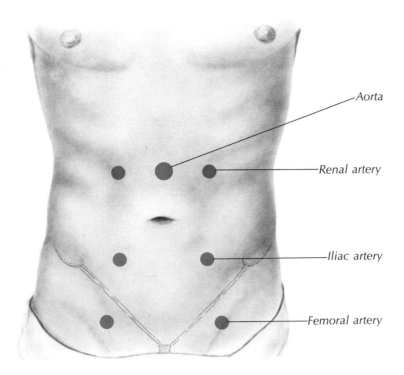

Aorta

Renal artery

Iliac artery

Femoral artery

If you suspect a liver tumor, gonococcal infection around the liver, or splenic infarction, listen over the liver and spleen for *friction* rubs.

See Table 11-3, Sounds in the Abdomen (p. 364).

PERCUSSION

Percussion is useful for orientation to the abdomen, for measuring the liver and sometimes the spleen, and for identifying ascitic fluid, solid or fluid-filled masses, and air in the stomach and bowel. Although percussion for all these purposes is described in this section, some practitioners prefer to alternate percussion with palpation as they examine liver, spleen, and other areas of the abdomen. Either approach is satisfactory.

ORIENTATION. Percuss the abdomen lightly in all four quadrants to assess the distribution of tympany and dullness. Tympany usually predominates because of gas in the gastrointestinal tract, but normal fluid and feces here may also produce a duller sound. On each side, note where abdominal tympany changes to the dullness of solid posterior structures. Check the suprapubic area for the dullness of a distended bladder or an enlarged uterus.

See Table 11-2, Protuberant Abdomens (p. 363).

Dullness in both flanks indicates further assessment for ascites (see pp. 358–359).

Lightly percuss the lower anterior chest, between lungs above and costal margins below. You will usually find on the right the dullness of liver and on the left the tympany that overlies the gastric air bubble and the splenic flexure of the colon.

Dullness above the left costal margin indicates need for a careful search for an enlarged spleen.

THE LIVER. Measure the vertical span, or height, of liver dullness in the right midclavicular line. Starting at a level below the umbilicus (in an area of tympany, not dullness), lightly percuss upward toward the liver. Ascertain the lower border of liver dullness in the midclavicular line.

Next, identify the upper border of liver dullness in the midclavicular line. Lightly percuss from lung resonance down toward liver dullness. Gently displace a woman's breast as necessary to be sure that you start in a resonant area. The course of percussion is shown below.

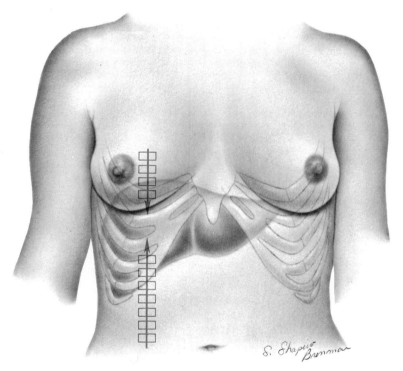

PERCUSSING LIVER SPAN

The span of liver dullness is increased when the liver is enlarged.

The span of liver dullness is decreased when the liver is small. It may also be decreased when free air is present below the diaphragm, as from a perforated hollow viscus. Serial observations may show a decreasing span of dullness as a liver, enlarged due to hepatitis or congestive heart failure, improves or, less commonly, as fulminant hepatitis progresses.

Liver dullness may be displaced downward by the low diaphragm of chronic obstructive lung disease. Span, however, remains normal.

Now measure in centimeters the vertical span, or height, of liver dullness. Normal liver spans are shown at the top of page 348. They are generally greater in men than in women, in tall people than in short. If the liver seems to be enlarged, outline the lower edge by percussing in other areas.

Although percussion is probably the most accurate clinical method for estimating liver size, it typically results in underestimation of the true vertical span of the liver.

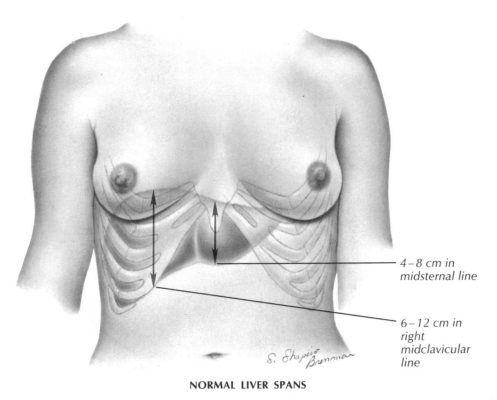

4–8 cm in
midsternal line

6–12 cm in
right
midclavicular
line

NORMAL LIVER SPANS

Dullness of a right pleural effusion or consolidated lung, if adjacent to liver dullness, may
falsely increase the estimated
liver size.

Gas in the colon may produce
tympany in the right upper
quadrant, obscure liver dullness, and falsely decrease the
estimated liver size.

THE SPLEEN. The normal spleen lies in the curve of the diaphragm just
posterior to the midaxillary line. A small oval area of splenic dullness can
sometimes be found between pulmonary resonance above and abdominal tympany anteriorly, but searching for it is seldom worthwhile.

Percussion may give you a clue, however, to *splenomegaly,* an enlarged
spleen. When a spleen enlarges, it does so anteriorly, downward, and
medially, replacing the tympany of stomach and colon with the dullness
of a solid organ. If you suspect splenomegaly, try two further maneuvers:

1. Percuss the lowest interspace in the left anterior axillary line as illustrated on p. 349. This area is usually tympanitic. Then ask the patient
   to take a deep breath, and percuss again. When spleen size is normal,
   the percussion note usually remains tympanitic.

A change in percussion note
from tympany to dullness on
inspiration suggests splenic enlargement. This is a positive
splenic percussion sign. Dullness,
however, may appear during
inspiration even when spleen
size is normal, thus giving a
falsely positive sign.

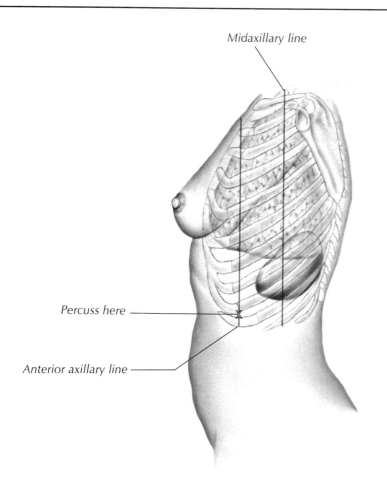

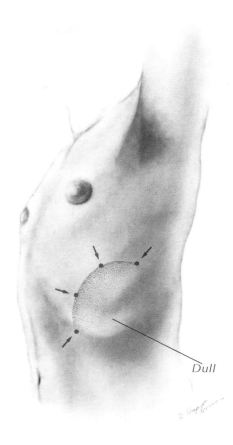

A large dull area, shown above, suggests splenic enlargement.

2. Percuss in several directions from resonance or tympany toward the estimated area of splenic dullness so that you can outline its edges. You cannot, of course, distinguish between the dullness of the posterior flank and that of the spleen.

Percussion as a method for estimating splenic size is impaired by the varying contents of stomach and colon, but it may suggest splenomegaly even before the organ becomes palpable. Further, it may help you to position your hands properly to feel for the splenic edge.

PALPATION

Light palpation is especially helpful in identifying muscular resistance, abdominal tenderness, and some superficial organs and masses. Its gentleness helps also to reassure and relax the patient.

Keeping your hand and forearm on a horizontal plane, with fingers together and flat on the abdominal surface, palpate the abdomen with a

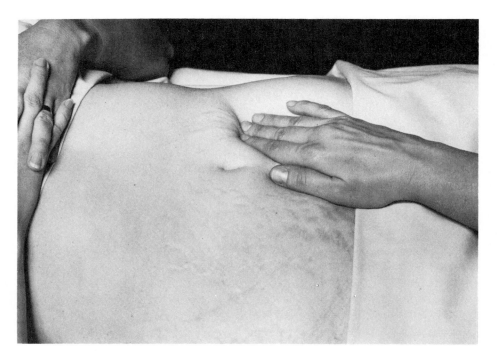

light, gentle, dipping motion. When moving your hand from place to place, raise it just off the skin. Moving smoothly, feel in all quadrants.

Identify any superficial organs or masses, any area of tenderness or increased resistance to palpation. If resistance is present, try to determine whether it is voluntary resistance or involuntary muscular spasm. (1) Try all the maneuvers to relax the patient (see p. 343) and ask the patient to mouth-breathe with the jaw dropped open. (2) Feel for the relaxation of the rectus muscles that normally accompanies expiration. If the rigidity remains unaltered by all these maneuvers, it is probably involuntary.

Involuntary rigidity or spasm of the abdominal muscles indicates peritoneal inflammation.

Deep palpation is usually required to delineate abdominal masses. Again using the palmar surfaces of your fingers, feel in all four quadrants. Identify any masses and note their location, size, shape, consistency, tenderness, pulsations, and mobility (*e.g.,* with respiration or with the examining hand).

Abdominal masses may be categorized in several ways: physiologic (pregnant uterus), inflammatory (diverticulitis of the colon or a pseudocyst of the pancreas), vascular (an aneurysm of the abdominal aorta), neoplastic (a myomatous uterus or a carcinoma of the colon or ovary), or obstructive (a distended bladder or a dilated loop of bowel).

When deep palpation is difficult—because of obesity, for example, or muscular resistance—use two hands, one on top of the other, as shown on the next page. Exert pressure with the outside hand while concentrating on feeling with the inside hand.

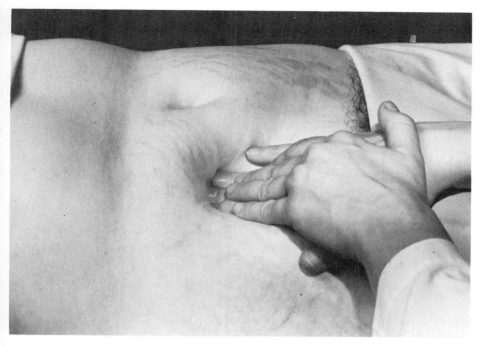

TWO-HANDED DEEP PALPATION

ASSESSMENT FOR PERITONEAL IRRITATION. Abdominal pain and tenderness, especially when associated with muscular spasm, suggest inflammation of the parietal peritoneum. Localize it as accurately as possible. First, even before palpation, *ask the patient to cough* and determine where the cough produced pain. Thus guided, *palpate gently with one finger* to map the tender area. Pain produced by light percussion has similar localizing value. These gentle maneuvers may be all you need to establish an area of peritoneal inflammation.

Abdominal pain on coughing or with light percussion suggests peritoneal inflammation. See Table 11-4, Tender Abdomens (pp. 365–366).

If not, *look for rebound tenderness.* Press your fingers in firmly and slowly, and then quickly withdraw them. Watch and listen to the patient for signs of pain. Ask the patient (1) to compare which hurt more, the pressing or the letting go, and (2) to show you exactly where it hurt. Pain induced or increased by quick withdrawal constitutes rebound tenderness. It results from the rapid movement of inflamed peritoneum. If tenderness is felt elsewhere than where you were trying to elicit rebound, that area may be the real source of the problem.

Rebound tenderness suggests peritoneal inflammation.

THE LIVER. Place your left hand behind the patient, parallel to and supporting the right 11th and 12th ribs. Remind the patient to relax on your hand if necessary. By pressing your left hand forward, the patient's liver is felt in front more easily.

Place your right hand on the patient's right abdomen lateral to the rectus muscle, with your fingertips well below the lower border of liver dullness.

Some examiners like to point their fingers up toward the patient's head, while others prefer a somewhat more oblique position, as shown in the two photos below. In either case, press gently in and up.

The liver below is palpable about 4 cm below the right costal margin in the midclavicular line.

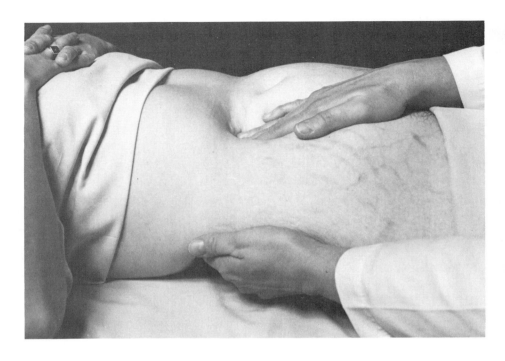

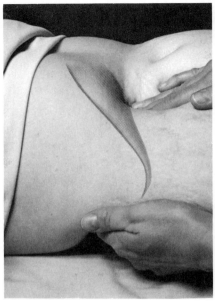

The edge of an enlarged liver may be missed by starting palpation too high in the abdomen.

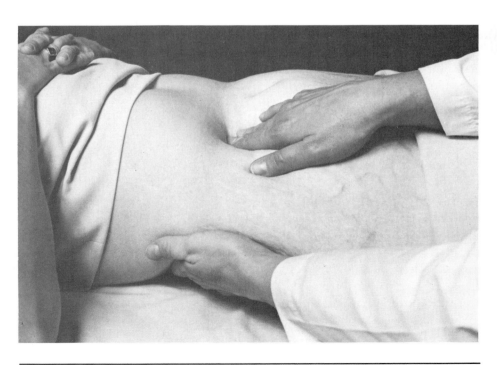

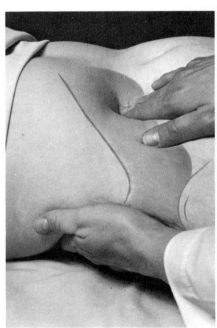

Ask the patient to take a deep breath. Try to feel the liver as it comes down to meet your fingertips. If you feel it, release the pressure of your palpating hand slightly so that the liver can slip under your finger pads and you can feel its anterior surface. Note any tenderness. If palpable at all, the edge of a normal liver is soft, sharp, and regular, its surface smooth. The normal liver may be slightly tender.

Try to trace the liver edge both laterally and medially. Palpation through the rectus muscles, however, is especially difficult. Describe or sketch the liver edge, and measure its distance from the right costal margin in the midclavicular line.

In order to feel the liver, you may have to alter your pressure according to the thickness and resistance of the abdominal wall. If you cannot feel it, move your palpating hand closer to the costal margin and try again.

The liver may also be felt by the "hooking technique." Stand to the right of the patient's chest. Place both hands, side by side, on the right abdomen below the border of liver dullness. Press in with your fingers and up toward the costal margin. Ask the patient to take a deep breath.

Firmness or hardness of the liver, bluntness or rounding of its edge, and irregularity of its contour suggest an abnormality of the liver. See Table 11-5, Liver Enlargement: Apparent and Real (pp. 367–368).

An obstructed, distended gallbladder may form an oval mass below the edge of the liver and merging with it. It is dull to percussion.

The liver edge shown below is palpable with the fingerpads of both hands.

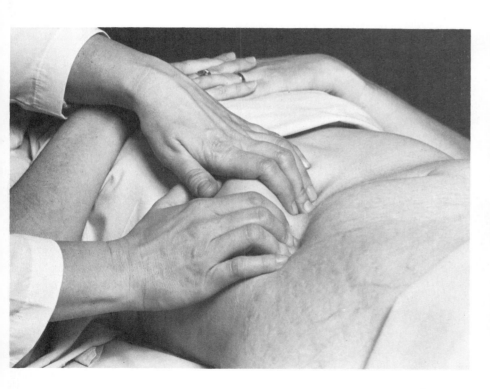

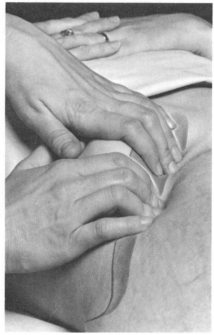

Some people breathe more with their chests than with their diaphragms. It may be helpful to train such a patient to "breathe with the abdomen," thus bringing the liver, as well as the spleen and kidneys, into a palpable position during inspiration.

To check for liver tenderness when the organ is not palpable, place your left hand flat on the lower right rib cage and then gently strike your hand with the ulnar surface of your right fist. Ask the patient to compare the sensation with that produced by a similar maneuver on the left side.

Tenderness suggests inflammation, as in hepatitis.

THE SPLEEN. With your left hand, reach over and around the patient to support and press forward the lower left rib cage. With your right hand below the left costal margin, press in toward the spleen. Begin palpation low enough to be sure that you are below a possibly enlarged spleen. (If your hand is too close to the costal margin, furthermore, it is not sufficiently mobile to reach up under the rib cage.) Ask the patient to take a deep breath. Try to feel the tip or edge of the spleen as it comes down to meet your fingertips. Note any tenderness, assess the splenic contour, and measure the distance between the spleen's lowest point and the left costal margin. In a small percentage of normal adults, the tip of the spleen is palpable. Likely causes include a low, flat diaphragm, as in chronic obstructive pulmonary disease, and a deep inspiratory descent of the diaphragm.

An enlarged spleen may be missed if the examiner starts too high in the abdomen to feel the lower edge.

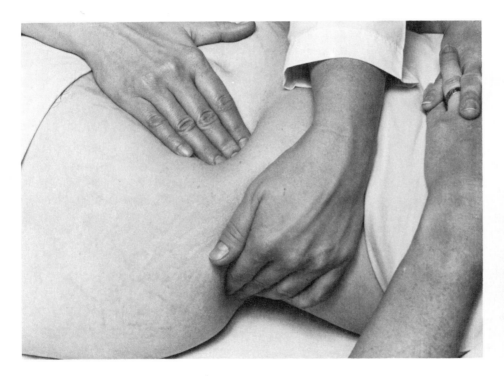

A palpable spleen tip, though not necessarily abnormal, may indicate splenic enlargement. The spleen tip below is just palpable deep to the left costal margin.

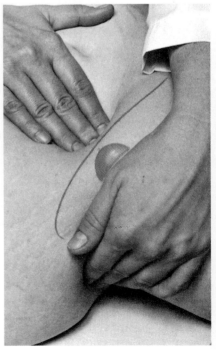

Repeat with the patient lying on the right side with legs somewhat flexed at hips and knees. In this position, gravity may bring the spleen forward and to the right into a palpable location.

The enlarged spleen below is palpable about 2 cm below the left costal margin on deep inspiration.

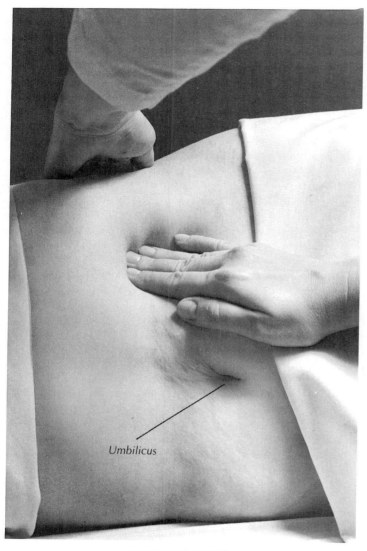

Umbilicus

PALPATING SPLEEN—
ANTERIOR VIEW WITH PATIENT LYING ON RIGHT SIDE

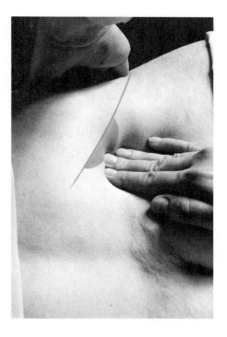

Marked and massive splenomegaly are shown below.

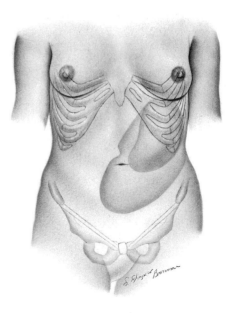

In assessment of a mass in the left flank, attributes that favor an enlarged spleen over an en-

THE KIDNEYS

The Right Kidney. Place your left hand behind the patient just below and parallel to the 12th rib, with your fingertips just reaching the costovertebral angle. Lift, trying to displace the kidney anteriorly. Place your right hand gently in the right upper quadrant, lateral and parallel to the rectus muscle. Ask the patient to take a deep breath. At the peak of inspiration, press your right hand firmly and deeply into the right upper quadrant, just below the costal margin, and try to "capture" the kidney between your two hands. Ask the patient to breathe out and then to stop breathing briefly. Slowly release the pressure of your right hand, feeling at the same time for the kidney to slide back into its expiratory position. If the kidney is palpable, describe its size, contour, and tenderness.

larged left kidney are a notch on the medial border, extension beyond the midline, dullness to percussion, and the ability to get your fingers deep to its medial and lower borders but not between the mass and the costal margin. Definitive differentiation, however, cannot usually be made on clinical criteria alone.

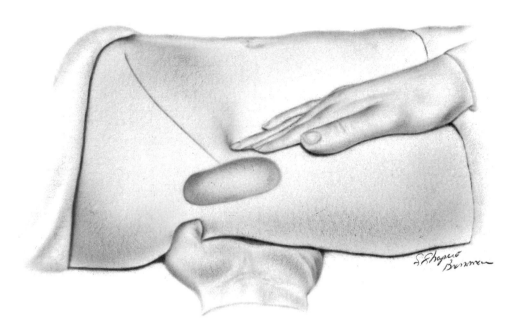

A normal right kidney may be palpable, especially in thin, well relaxed women. It may or may not be slightly tender. The patient is usually aware of a capture and release. Occasionally, a right kidney is located more anteriorly than usual and then must be distinguished from the liver. The edge of the liver, if palpable, tends to be sharper and to extend farther medially and laterally. It cannot be captured. The lower pole of the kidney is rounded.

Causes of kidney enlargement include hydronephrosis, cysts, and tumors. Bilateral enlargement suggests polycystic disease.

The Left Kidney. To capture the left kidney, move to the patient's left side. Use your right hand to lift from in back, and your left hand to feel deep in the left upper quadrant. Proceed as before.

Alternatively, try to feel for the left kidney by a method somewhat similar to feeling for the spleen. With your left hand, reach over and

In assessment of a mass in the left flank, attributes that favor an enlarged kidney over an enlarged spleen are the preservation of normal tympany in the left upper quadrant, and the

around the patient to lift the left loin, and with your right hand feel deep in the left upper quadrant. Ask the patient to take a deep breath, and feel for a mass.

A normal left kidney is rarely palpable.

Kidney Tenderness. Tenderness may be noted during abdominal palpation, but search for it also in each costovertebral angle. Pressure from your fingertips may be enough to reveal tenderness here; if not, use fist percussion. Place the ball of one hand in the costovertebral angle and strike it with the ulnar surface of your fist. Use force sufficient to cause a perceptible but painless jar or thud in a normal person.

ability to get your fingers between the mass and the costal margin but not deep to its medial and lower borders.

Pain with pressure or with fist percussion in the costovertebral angle suggests kidney infection, but it may also have a musculoskeletal cause.

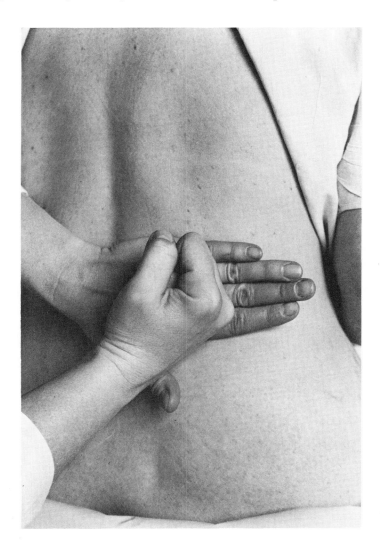

To save the patient needless exertion, integrate this maneuver with your examination of the back (see p. 123).

THE AORTA. Press firmly deep in the upper abdomen, slightly to the left of the midline, and identify the aortic pulsations. In persons over age 50, try to assess the width of the aorta by pressing deeply in the upper

In an older person, a periumbilical or upper abdominal mass

abdomen with one hand on each side of the aorta, as illustrated. A normal adult aorta is not more than 2.5 cm wide. This measurement does not include the thickness of the abdominal wall. The ease with which you can feel aortic pulsations varies greatly with the thickness of the abdominal wall and with the anteroposterior diameter of the abdomen.

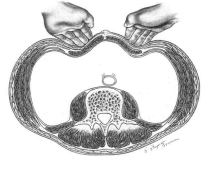

with expansile pulsations suggests an aortic aneurysm.

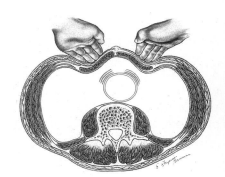

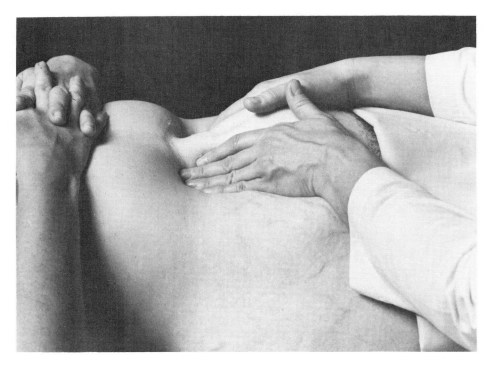

This is a pathologic dilatation of the aorta, usually due to arteriosclerosis. A merely tortuous abdominal aorta, however, may be difficult to distinguish from an aneurysm on clinical grounds.

Although an aneurysm is usually painless, pain may herald its most dreaded and frequent complication—rupture of the aorta.

SPECIAL MANEUVERS

TO ASSESS POSSIBLE ASCITES. A protuberant abdomen with bulging flanks suggests the possibility of ascitic fluid. Because ascitic fluid characteristically sinks with gravity while gas-filled loops of bowel float to the top, percussion gives a dull note in dependent areas of the abdomen. Look for such a pattern by percussing outward in several directions from the central area of tympany. Map the border between tympany and dullness.

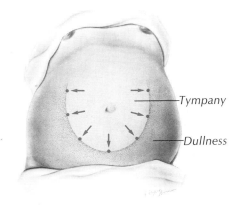

Tympany

Dullness

Two further maneuvers help to confirm the presence of ascites, although both signs may be misleading.

1. *Test for shifting dullness.* After mapping the borders of tympany and dullness, ask the patient to turn onto one side. Percuss and mark the borders again. In a person without ascites, the borders between tympany and dullness usually stay relatively constant.

In ascites, dullness shifts to the more dependent side, while tympany shifts to the top.

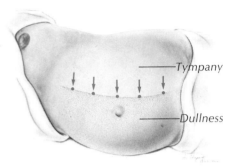

2. *Test for a fluid wave.* Ask the patient or an assistant to press the edges of both hands firmly down the midline of the abdomen. This pressure helps to stop the transmission of a wave through fat. While you tap one flank sharply with your fingertips, feel on the opposite flank for an impulse transmitted through the fluid. Unfortunately, this sign is often negative until ascites is obvious, and it is sometimes positive in people without ascites.

An easily palpable impulse suggest ascites.

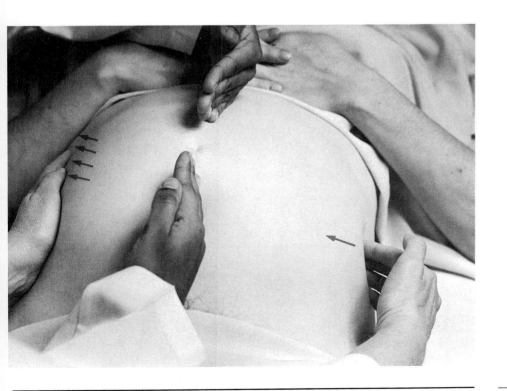

TO IDENTIFY AN ORGAN OR A MASS IN AN ASCITIC ABDOMEN.
Try to *ballotte* the organ or mass, exemplified here by an enlarged liver. Straighten and stiffen the fingers of one hand together, place them on the abdominal surface, and make a brief jabbing movement directly toward the anticipated structure.

This quick movement often displaces the fluid so that your fingertips can briefly touch the surface of the structure through the abdominal wall.

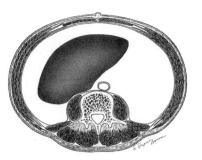
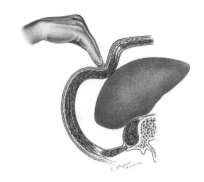

TO ASSESS POSSIBLE APPENDICITIS

● Ask the patient to point to where the pain began and where it is now. Ask the patient to cough. Determine whether and where pain results.

The pain of appendicitis classically begins near the umbilicus and then shifts to the right lower quadrant, where coughing increases it. Elderly patients report this pattern less frequently than younger ones.

● Search carefully for an area of local tenderness.

Localized tenderness anywhere in the right lower quadrant, even in the right flank, may indicate appendicitis.

● Feel for muscular rigidity.

Early voluntary guarding may be replaced by involuntary muscular rigidity.

● Perform a rectal examination and, in women, a pelvic examination. These maneuvers may not help you to discriminate well between a normal and an inflamed appendix, but they may help to identify an inflamed appendix atypically located within the pelvic cavity. They may also suggest other causes of the abdominal pain.

Right-sided rectal tenderness may be caused by, for example, inflamed adnexa or an inflamed seminal vesicle, as well as by an inflamed appendix.

Some additional maneuvers are sometimes helpful.

● Check the tender area for rebound tenderness. (If other signs are typically positive, you can save the patient unnecessary pain by omitting this test.)

Rebound tenderness suggests peritoneal inflammation, as from appendicitis.

● Check for Rovsing's sign and for referred rebound tenderness. Press deeply and evenly in the *left* lower quadrant. Then quickly withdraw your fingers.	Pain in the *right* lower quadrant during *left*-sided pressure suggests appendicitis (a positive Rovsing's sign). So does right lower quadrant pain on quick withdrawal (referred rebound tenderness).
● Look for a psoas sign. Place your hand just above the patient's right knee and ask the patient to raise the thigh against your hand. Alternatively, ask the patient to turn onto the left side. Then extend the patient's right leg at the hip. Flexion of the leg at the hip makes the psoas muscle contract; extension stretches it.	Increased abdominal pain on either maneuver constitutes a positive psoas sign, suggesting irritation of the psoas muscle by an inflamed appendix.
● Look for an obturator sign. Flex the patient's right thigh at the hip, with the knee bent, and rotate the leg internally at the hip. This maneuver stretches the internal obturator muscle. (Internal rotation of the hip is illustrated on p. 470, lower right.)	Right hypogastric pain constitutes a positive obturator sign, suggesting irritation of the obturator muscle by an inflamed appendix.
● Test for cutaneous hyperesthesia. At a series of points down the abdominal wall, gently pick up a fold of skin between your thumb and index finger, without pinching it. This maneuver should not normally be painful.	Localized pain with this maneuver, in all or part of the right lower quadrant, may accompany appendicitis.

TO ASSESS POSSIBLE ACUTE CHOLECYSTITIS. When right upper quadrant pain and tenderness suggest acute cholecystitis, look for Murphy's sign. Hook your left thumb or the fingers of your right hand under the costal margin at the point where the lateral border of the rectus muscle intersects with the costal margin. Alternatively, if the liver is enlarged, hook your thumb or fingers under the liver edge at a comparable point below. Ask the patient to take a deep breath. Watch the patient's breathing and note the degree of tenderness.

A sharp increase in tenderness with a sudden stop in inspiratory effort constitutes a positive Murphy's sign of acute cholecystitis. Hepatic tenderness may also increase with this maneuver, but is usually less well localized.

TO ASSESS VENTRAL HERNIAS (hernias in the abdominal wall exclusive of groin hernias). If you suspect but do not see an umbilical or incisional hernia, ask the patient to raise both head and shoulders off the table.

The bulge of a hernia will usually appear with this action (see p. 362).

Inguinal and femoral hernias are discussed in the next chapter. They can give rise to important abdominal problems and must not be overlooked.

The cause of intestinal obstruction or peritonitis may be missed by overlooking a strangulated femoral hernia.

TO DISTINGUISH AN ABDOMINAL MASS FROM A MASS IN THE ABDOMINAL WALL. An occasional mass is in the abdominal wall rather than inside the abdominal cavity. Ask the patient either to raise the head and shoulders or to strain down, thus tightening the abdominal muscles. Feel for the mass again.

A mass in the abdominal wall remains palpable; an intra-abdominal mass is obscured by muscular contraction.

Table 11-1   Localized Bulges in the Abdominal Wall

Localized bulges in the abdominal wall include ventral hernias (defects in the wall through which tissue protrudes) and subcutaneous tumors such as lipomas. The more common ventral hernias are umbilical, incisional, and epigastric. Rectus diastasis is also sometimes so classified. Hernias and a rectus diastasis usually become more evident when the patient raises head and shoulders from a supine position.

UMBILICAL HERNIA

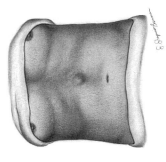

INFANT

Umbilical hernias protrude through a defective umbilical ring. They are most common in infants but also occur in adults. In infants, but not in adults, they usually close spontaneously within a year or two.

INCISIONAL HERNIA

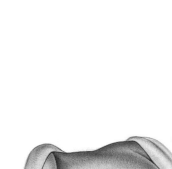

An incisional hernia protrudes through an operative scar. By palpation, note the length and width of the defect in the abdominal wall. A small defect, through which a large hernia has passed, has a greater risk of complications than a large defect.

DIASTASIS RECTI

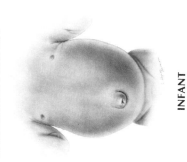

Ridge

A rectus diastasis is a separation of the two rectus abdominis muscles, through which abdominal contents bulge to form a midline ridge when the patient raises head and shoulders. Repeated pregnancies, obesity, and chronic lung disease may predispose to it. It has no clinical consequences.

EPIGASTRIC HERNIA

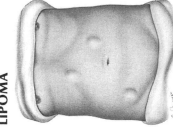

An epigastric hernia is a small midline protrusion through a defect in the linea alba, somewhere between the xiphoid process and the umbilicus. With the patient's head and shoulders raised (or with the patient standing), look for it, and run your fingerpad down the linea alba to feel it.

LIPOMA

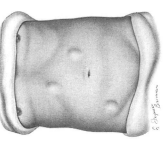

Lipomas are common, benign, fatty tumors usually located in the subcutaneous tissues almost anywhere in the body, including the abdominal wall. Small or large, they are usually soft and often lobulated. When your finger presses down on the edge of a lipoma, the tumor typically slips out from under it.

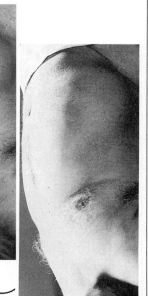

Table 11-2   Protuberant Abdomens

Table 11-2   Protuberant Abdomens

FAT

Fat is the most common cause of a protuberant abdomen and is associated with generalized obesity. The abdominal wall is thick. Fat in the mesentery and omentum also contributes to abdominal size. The umbilicus may appear sunken. The percussion note is normal. An apron of fatty tissue may extend below the inguinal ligaments. Lift it to look for inflammation in the skin fold or even for a hidden hernia.

GAS

Gaseous distention may be localized, as shown, or generalized. It causes a tympanitic percussion note. Increased intestinal gas production due to certain foods may cause mild distention. More serious are intestinal obstruction and adynamic (paralytic) ileus. Note the location of the distention. Distention becomes more marked in colonic than in small bowel obstruction.

TUMOR

Tympany

Dullness

A large, solid tumor, usually rising out of the pelvis, is dull to percussion. Air-filled bowel is displaced to the periphery. Causes include ovarian tumors and uterine myomata. Occasionally, a markedly distended bladder may be mistaken for such a tumor.

PREGNANCY

Tympany

Dullness

Pregnancy is a common cause of a pelvic "tumor." Listen for the fetal heart (see p. 419).

ASCITIC FLUID

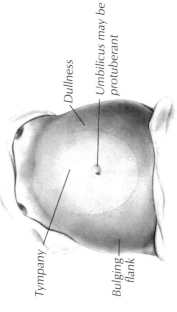

Dullness

Umbilicus may be protuberant

Tympany

Bulging flank

Tympany

Dullness

Ascitic fluid seeks the lowest point in the abdomen, producing bulging flanks that are dull to percussion. The umbilicus may protrude. Turn the patient onto one side to detect the shift in position of the fluid level (shifting dullness). (See pp. 358–359 for the assessment of ascites.)

Table 11-3   Sounds in the Abdomen

Table 11-3   Sounds in the Abdomen

BOWEL SOUNDS

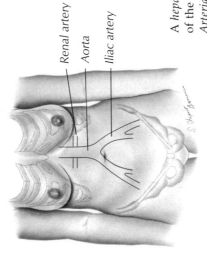

Bowel sounds may be:

- Increased, as from diarrhea or early intestinal obstruction
- Decreased, then absent, as in adynamic ileus and peritonitis. Before deciding that bowel sounds are absent, sit down and listen where shown for 2 min or even longer.

High-pitched tinkling sounds suggest intestinal fluid and air under tension in a dilated bowel. Rushes of high-pitched sounds coinciding with an abdominal cramp indicate intestinal obstruction.

BRUITS

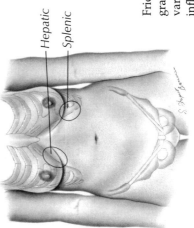

Renal artery
Aorta
Iliac artery

A *hepatic bruit* suggests carcinoma of the liver or alcoholic hepatitis. *Arterial bruits* with both systolic and diastolic components suggest partial occlusion of the aorta or large arteries.

VENOUS HUM

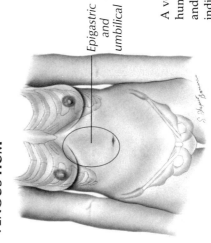

Epigastric and umbilical

A venous hum is rare. It is a soft humming noise with both systolic and diastolic components. It indicates increased collateral circulation between portal and systemic venous systems, as in hepatic cirrhosis.

FRICTION RUBS

Hepatic
Splenic

Friction rubs are rare. They are grating sounds with respiratory variation. They indicate inflammation of the peritoneal surface of an organ, as from a liver tumor, chlamydial or gonococcal perihepatitis, recent liver biopsy, or splenic infarct. When a systolic bruit accompanies a hepatic friction rub, suspect carcinoma of the liver.

Table 11-4   Tender Abdomens

Table 11-4   Tender Abdomens

ABDOMINAL WALL TENDERNESS

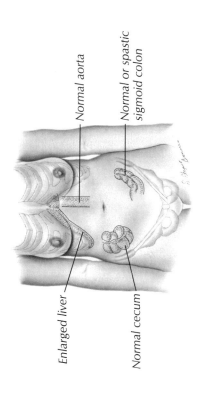

Superficial tender area

Deep tender areas

Tenderness may originate in the abdominal wall. When the patient raises head and shoulders, this tenderness persists, whereas tenderness from a deeper lesion (protected by the tightened muscles) decreases.

ACUTE PLEURISY

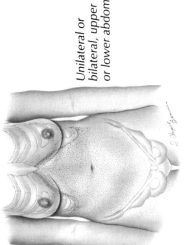

Unilateral or bilateral, upper or lower abdomen

Abdominal pain and tenderness may be due to acute pleural inflammation. When unilateral, it may mimic acute cholecystitis or appendicitis. Rebound tenderness and rigidity are less common; chest signs are usually present.

VISCERAL TENDERNESS

Normal aorta

Normal or spastic sigmoid colon

Enlarged liver

Normal cecum

The structures shown may be tender to deep palpation. Usually the discomfort is dull and there is no muscular rigidity or rebound tenderness. A reassuring explanation to the patient may prove quite helpful.

TENDERNESS FROM DISEASE IN THE CHEST AND PELVIS

ACUTE SALPINGITIS

Frequently bilateral, the tenderness of acute salpingitis is usually maximal just above the inguinal ligaments. Rebound tenderness and rigidity may be present. On pelvic examination, motion of the uterus causes pain.

Continued

Table 11-4   *Tender Abdomens*

Table 11-4 (Cont'd.)

TENDERNESS OF PERITONEAL INFLAMMATION

Tenderness associated with peritoneal inflammation is usually more severe than visceral tenderness. Muscular rigidity and rebound tenderness are frequently but not necessarily present. Generalized peritonitis causes exquisite tenderness throughout the abdomen, together with boardlike muscular rigidity. Local causes of peritoneal inflammation include:

ACUTE CHOLECYSTITIS

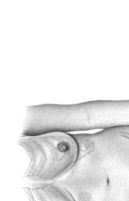

Signs are maximal in the right upper quadrant. Check for Murphy's sign (see p. 361).

ACUTE APPENDICITIS

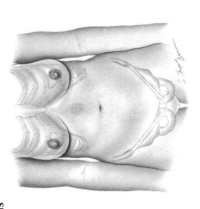

Right rectal tenderness

Just below the middle of a line joining the umbilicus and the anterior superior iliac spine

Right lower quadrant signs are typical of acute appendicitis, but may be absent early in the course. The typical area of tenderness is illustrated. Explore other portions of the right lower quadrant as well as the right flank.

ACUTE PANCREATITIS

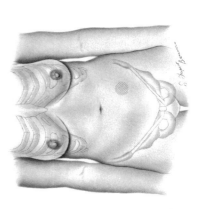

In acute pancreatitis, epigastric tenderness and rebound tenderness are usually present but the abdominal wall may be soft.

ACUTE DIVERTICULITIS

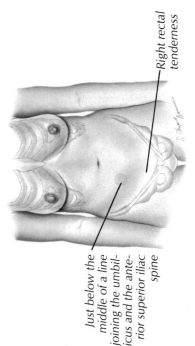

Acute diverticulitis most often involves the sigmoid colon and then resembles a left-sided appendicitis.

Table 11-5   Liver Enlargement: Apparent and Real

Table 11-5   Liver Enlargement: Apparent and Real

A palpable liver does not necessarily indicate hepatomegaly (an enlarged liver), but more often results from a change in consistency—from the normal softness to an abnormal firmness or hardness, as in cirrhosis. Clinical estimates of liver size should be based on both percussion and palpation, although even then they are far from perfect.

DOWNWARD DISPLACEMENT OF THE LIVER BY A LOW DIAPHRAGM

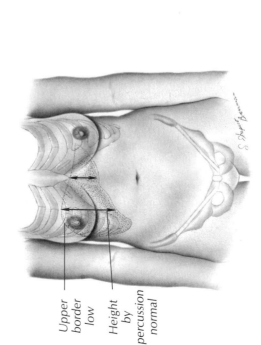

Upper border low

Height by percussion normal

This is a common finding (*e.g.,* in emphysema) when the diaphragm is low. The liver edge may be readily palpable well below the costal margin. Percussion, however, reveals a low upper edge also, and the total span or height is normal.

NORMAL VARIATIONS IN LIVER SHAPE

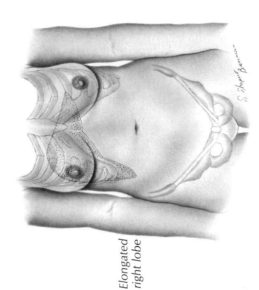

Elongated right lobe

In some persons, especially those with a lanky build, the liver tends to be somewhat elongated so that its right lobe is easily palpable as it projects downward toward the iliac crest. Such an elongation, sometimes called Riedel's lobe, represents a variation in shape, not an increase in liver volume or size. This variant illustrates the basic limitations of assessing liver size. We can only estimate the upper and lower borders of an organ that has three dimensions and differing shapes. Some error is unavoidable.

▶ *Continued*

Table 11-5   Liver Enlargement: Apparent and Real

Table 11-5 (Cont'd.)

SMOOTH LARGE NONTENDER LIVER

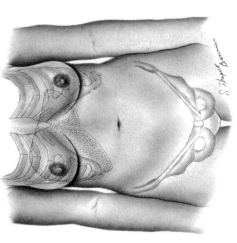

Cirrhosis may produce an enlarged liver with a firm nontender edge. The liver is not always enlarged in this condition, however, and many other diseases may produce similar findings.

SMOOTH LARGE TENDER LIVER

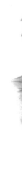
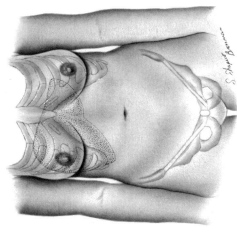

An enlarged liver with a smooth tender edge suggests inflammation, as in hepatitis, or venous congestion, as in right-sided heart failure.

LARGE IRREGULAR LIVER

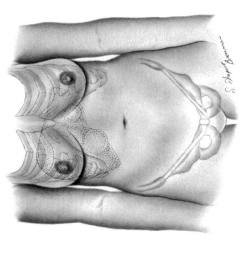

An enlarged liver that is firm or hard and has an irregular edge or surface suggests malignancy. There may be one or more nodules. The liver may or may not be tender.

Chapter 12
Male Genitalia and Hernias

Anatomy and Physiology

Review the anatomy of the male genitalia.

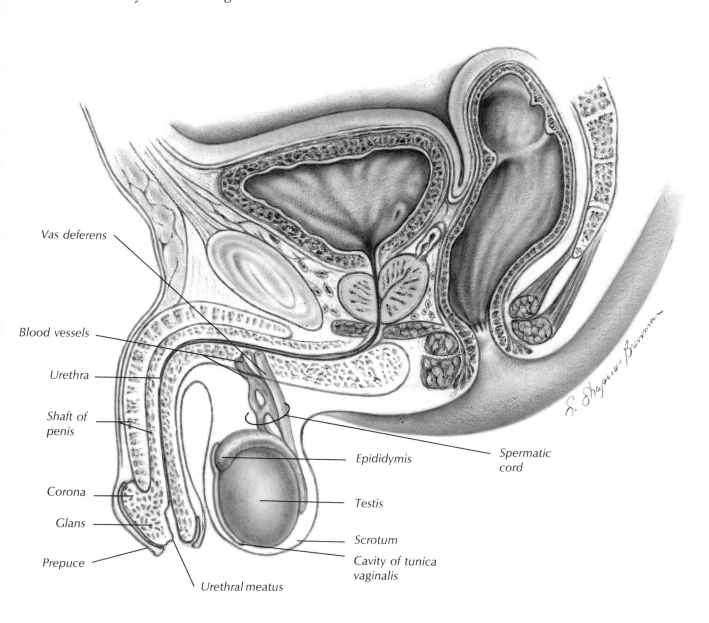

Vas deferens

Blood vessels

Urethra

Shaft of penis

Corona

Glans

Prepuce

Urethral meatus

Epididymis

Spermatic cord

Testis

Scrotum

Cavity of tunica vaginalis

The shaft of the penis is formed by three columns of vascular erectile tissue bound together by fibrous tissue. At the end of the penis is the cone-shaped glans with its expanded base, or corona. Unless the person has been circumcised, the glans is covered by a loose, hoodlike fold of skin called the prepuce, or foreskin. The urethra is located ventrally in the shaft of the penis, within one of the vascular columns, and urethral abnormalities may sometimes be felt here. The urethra opens into the vertical, slitlike urethral meatus, located somewhat ventrally at the tip of the glans.

The scrotum is a loose, wrinkled pouch divided into two compartments, each of which contains a testicle. The testes are ovoid, somewhat rubbery structures, about 4.5 cm long in the adult, with a range from 3.5 cm to 5.5 cm. The left usually lies somewhat lower than the right. On the postero-lateral surface of each testis is the softer, comma-shaped epididymis. It is most prominent along the superior margin of the testis. (The epididymis may be located anteriorly in 6% to 7% of males.) Surrounding the testis, except posteriorly, is the tunica vaginalis, a serous membrane enclosing a potential cavity.

The testes produce spermatozoa and testosterone. Testosterone stimulates the pubertal growth of the male genitalia, prostate, and seminal vesicles. It also stimulates the development of masculine secondary sex characteristics, including the beard, body hair, musculoskeletal development, and the enlarged larynx with its male voice.

The vas deferens, a cordlike structure, begins at the tail of the epididymis, ascends within the scrotal sac, and passes through the external inguinal ring on its way to the abdomen and pelvis. Behind the bladder it is joined by the duct from the seminal vesicle and enters the urethra within the prostate gland. Sperm thus pass from the testis and the epididymis through the vas deferens into the urethra. Secretions from the vasa deferentia, the seminal vesicles, and the prostate all contribute to the semen. Within the scrotum each vas is closely associated with blood vessels, nerves, and muscle fibers, with which it makes up the spermatic cord.

Lymphatics from the penile and scrotal surfaces drain into the inguinal nodes. When you find an inflammatory or possibly malignant lesion on these surfaces, assess the inguinal nodes especially carefully for enlargement or tenderness. The lymphatics of the testes, however, drain into the abdomen, where enlarged nodes are clinically undetectable. See page 439 for further discussion of the inguinal nodes.

Because hernias are relatively common, it is important to understand the anatomy of the groin. The basic landmarks are the anterior superior iliac spine, the pubic tubercle, and the inguinal ligament which runs between them. Find these on yourself or a colleague.

The inguinal canal, which lies above and approximately parallel to the inguinal ligament, forms a tunnel for the vas deferens as it passes through the abdominal muscles. The exterior opening of the tunnel—the external inguinal ring—is a triangular slitlike structure palpable just above and lateral to the pubic tubercle. The internal opening of the canal—or internal inguinal ring—is about 1 cm above the midpoint of the inguinal ligament. Neither canal nor internal ring is palpable through the abdominal wall. When loops of bowel force their way through weak areas of the inguinal canal they produce inguinal hernias, as illustrated on page 382.

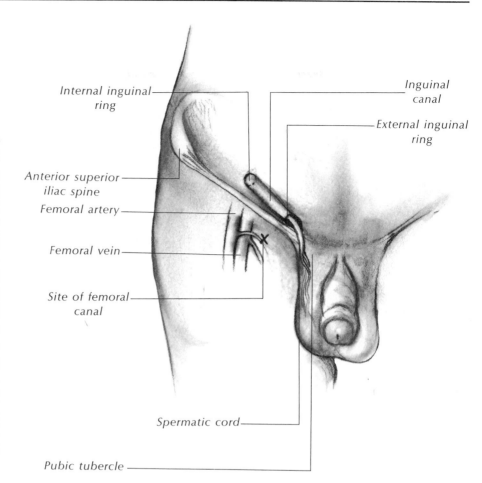

Another potential route for a herniating mass is the femoral canal. This lies below the inguinal ligament. Although you cannot see it, you can estimate its location by placing your right index finger, from below, on the right femoral artery. Your middle finger will then overlie the femoral vein; your ring finger, the femoral canal. Femoral hernias protrude here.

CHANGES WITH AGE

Adolescence. Important anatomic changes in the male genitalia accompany puberty and help to define its progress. A noticeable increase in the size of the testes constitutes the first reliable sign and usually begins between the ages of 9.5 years and 13.5 years. Next, pubic hair appears and the penis begins to grow. The complete change from preadolescent to adult form requires about 3 years, with a range from less than 2 years to almost 5 years.

By observing the pubic hair and the development of the penis, testes, and scrotum, you can assess sexual development according to the five stages described by Tanner. These are outlined and illustrated on page 372.

Sex Maturity Ratings in Boys

In assigning SMRs in boys, observe each of the three characteristics separately because they may develop at different rates. Record two separate ratings: pubic hair and genital. If the penis and testes differ in their stages, average the two into a single figure for the genital rating.

| | **PUBIC HAIR** | GENITAL | |
		PENIS	TESTES AND SCROTUM
STAGE 1	Preadolescent—no pubic hair except for the fine body hair (vellus hair) similar to that on the abdomen	Preadolescent—same size and proportions as in childhood	Preadolescent—same size and proportions as in childhood
STAGE 2 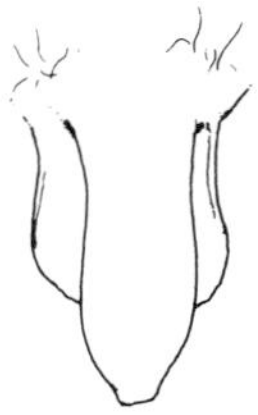	Sparse growth of long, slightly pigmented, downy hair, straight or only slightly curled, chiefly at the base of the penis	Slight or no enlargement	Testes larger; scrotum larger, somewhat reddened, and altered in texture
STAGE 3 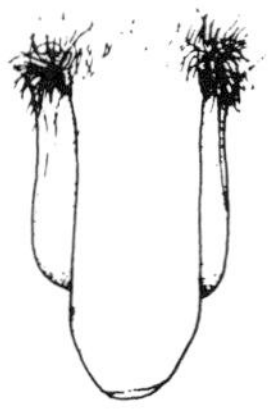	Darker, coarser, curlier hair spreading sparsely over the pubic symphysis	Larger, especially in length	Further enlarged
STAGE 4 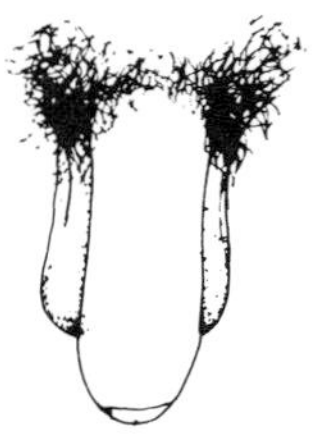	Coarse and curly hair, as in the adult; area covered greater than in stage 3 but not as great as in the adult and not yet including the thighs	Further enlarged in length and breadth, with development of the glans	Further enlarged; scrotal skin darkened
STAGE 5 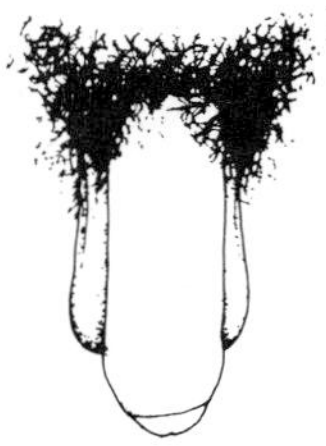	Hair adult in quantity and quality, spread to the medial surfaces of the thighs but not up over the abdomen	Adult in size and shape	Adult in size and shape

(Illustrations through the courtesy of W.A. Daniel, Jr, Division of Adolescent Medicine, University of Alabama, Birmingham)

In about 80% of men, pubic hair spreads further up the abdomen in a triangular pattern pointing toward the umbilicus. Because this kind of spread, known as stage 6, is not completed until the mid-20s or later, it is not considered a pubertal change.

An average developmental sequence is diagrammed below. Note the rather wide age ranges for the start and completion of pubertal changes. Some normal boys may have completed their genital development while others of the same age have not yet begun. Boys often begin to experience ejaculation as they approach SMR 3, and sometimes mistake nocturnal emissions for the discharge of venereal disease. Discussion and explanation are indicated.

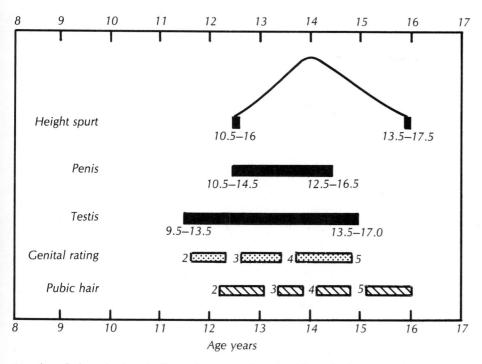

Numbers below the bars indicate the ranges in age within which certain changes occur. (Redrawn from Marshall WA, Tanner JM: Variations in the pattern of pubertal changes in boys. Arch Dis Child 45:22, 1970)

Aging. In elderly patients, pubic hair may decrease and become gray. The penis decreases in size and the testicles hang lower in the scrotum. Although the testes often decrease in size with protracted, debilitating illnesses, they do not necessarily decrease with aging *per se.*

Techniques of Examination

GENERAL APPROACH

Many students—especially women but also men—feel anxious about examining a man's genitalia. "How will the patient react?" "Will he have an erection?" "Will he let me examine him?" In fact, a male patient, regardless of who examines him, does occasionally have an erection, though rarely, and is probably more embarrassed about it than you are. You should explain to him that this is a normal response, finish your examination, and proceed on with an unruffled demeanor. Occasionally, too, a man may refuse to be examined by a woman just as a woman sometimes refuses to allow a man to do a pelvic examination. Your own comfort with the procedures will minimize these difficulties, but you should respect the patient's wishes and rights.

A good genital examination can be done with the patient either standing or supine. To check for hernias or varicoceles, however, the patient should stand, and you should sit comfortably on a chair or stool. A gown conveniently covers the patient's chest and abdomen. If there is any chance of an infectious process, wear gloves. Expose the genitalia and inguinal areas.

ASSESSMENT OF SEXUAL DEVELOPMENT

Assess sexual maturation by noting the size and shape of the penis and testes, the color and texture of the scrotal skin, and the character and distribution of the pubic hair. Assessment of testicular size requires palpation (see p. 376).

In adolescents, make two separate sex maturity ratings according to Tanner's stages: one for pubic hair, the other for genital development. If a boy's testes have increased in size to 2.5 cm or more, or if his pubic hair has reached stage 2, you can tell him that his sexual development has started. You may also use Tanner's diagrams to show your patient how he is developing, to review the wide range of normals for his age, and to answer any questions he may have.

Delayed puberty is often familial or related to chronic illness. It may also be due to abnormalities in the hypothalamus, anterior pituitary gland, or testes.

THE PENIS

Inspection

Inspect the penis, including:

See Table 12-1, Abnormalities of the Penis (p. 379).

● The skin

- The prepuce (foreskin). If it is present, retract it or ask the patient to retract it. This step is essential for the detection of many chancres and carcinomas. A cheesy, whitish material called smegma may accumulate normally under the foreskin.

Phimosis is a tight prepuce that cannot be retracted over the glans. Paraphimosis is a tight prepuce that, once retracted, gets caught behind the glans and cannot be returned. Edema ensues.

- The glans. Look for any ulcers, scars, nodules, or signs of inflammation.

Balanitis (inflammation of the glans); balanoposthitis (inflammation of the glans and prepuce)

Check the skin around the base of the penis for excoriations or inflammation. Look for nits or lice at the bases of the pubic hairs.

Pubic or genital excoriations suggest the possibility of lice (crabs) or sometimes scabies.

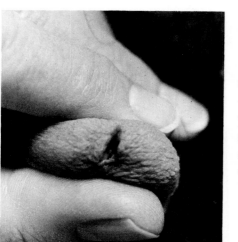

Note the location of the urethral meatus.

Hypospadias is a congenital, ventral displacement of the meatus on the penis (p. 379).

Compress the glans gently between your index finger above and your thumb below. This maneuver should open the urethral meatus and allow you to inspect it for discharge. Normally there is none.

The discharge of gonococcal urethritis tends to be profuse and yellow, while that of nongonococcal urethritis tends to be scanty and white or clear. Definitive diagnosis, however, requires a Gram stain and culture.

If the patient has reported a discharge but you do not see any, ask him to strip, or milk, the shaft of the penis from its base to the glans. Alternatively, do it yourself. This maneuver may bring some discharge out of the urethral meatus for appropriate examination. Have a glass slide and culture materials ready.

Palpation

Palpate any abnormality of the penis, noting any tenderness or induration. Palpate the shaft of the penis between your thumb and first two fingers, noting any induration. Palpation of the shaft may be omitted in a young asymptomatic male patient.

Induration along the ventral surface of the penis suggests a urethral stricture or possibly a carcinoma. Tenderness of such an indurated area suggests periurethral inflammation secondary to a urethral stricture.

If you retracted the foreskin, replace it before proceeding on to examine the scrotum.

THE SCROTUM AND ITS CONTENTS

Inspection

Inspect the scrotum, including

See Table 12-2, Abnormalities in the Scrotum (pp. 380–381).

- The skin. Lift up the scrotum so that you can see its posterior surface.

Rashes, sebaceous cysts, rarely skin cancer

- The scrotal contours. Note any swelling, lumps, or veins.

A poorly developed scrotum on one or both sides suggests cryptorchidism. Common scrotal swellings include indirect inguinal hernias, hydroceles, and scrotal edema. A tender, painful scrotal swelling occurs in acute epididymitis, acute orchitis, torsion of the spermatic cord, and a strangulated inguinal hernia.

Palpation

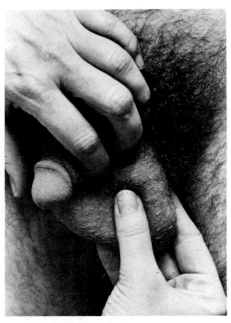

Between your thumb and first two fingers, palpate each testis and epididymis.

Note their size, shape, consistency, and tenderness; feel for any nodules. Pressure on the testis normally produces a deep visceral pain.

Any painless nodule in the testis must raise the possibility of testicular cancer, a potentially curable cancer with a peak incidence between the ages of 20 and 35 years.

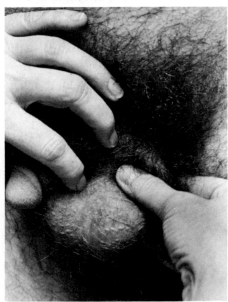

Identify each spermatic cord with its vas deferens, and palpate it between your thumb and fingers along its course from epididymis to superficial inguinal ring.

Multiple tortuous veins in this area, usually on the left, may be palpable and even visible. They indicate a varicocele (p. 380).

Note any nodules or swellings.

The vas deferens, if chronically infected, may feel thickened or beaded. A cystic structure in the spermatic cord suggests a hydrocele of the cord.

Any swelling in the scrotum other than the testicles should be evaluated by transillumination. After darkening the room, shine the beam of a strong flashlight from behind the scrotum through the mass. Look for transmission of the light as a red glow.

Swellings that contain serous fluid, such as a hydrocele, transilluminate: they light up with a red glow. Those that contain blood or tissue, such as a normal testis, a tumor, and most hernias, do not.

HERNIAS

Inspection

Inspect the inguinal and femoral areas carefully for bulges. While you continue your observation, ask the patient to strain down.

A bulge that appears on straining suggests a hernia.

Palpation

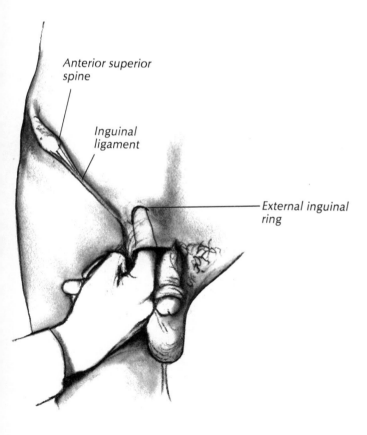

Anterior superior spine

Inguinal ligament

External inguinal ring

Using in turn your right hand for the patient's right side and your left hand for the patient's left side, invaginate loose scrotal skin with your index finger. Start at a point low enough to be sure that your finger will have enough mobility to reach as far as the internal inguinal ring if this proves possible. Follow the spermatic cord upward to above the inguinal ligament and find the triangular slitlike opening of the external inguinal ring. This is just above and lateral to the pubic tubercle. If the ring is somewhat enlarged, it may admit your index finger. If possible, gently follow the inguinal canal laterally in its oblique course. With your finger

See Table 12-3, Course and Presentation of Hernias in the Groin (p. 382).

See Table 12-4, Differentiation of Hernias in the Groin (p. 383).

located either at the external ring or within the canal, ask the patient to strain down or cough. Note any palpable herniating mass as it touches your finger.

Palpate the anterior thigh in the region of the femoral canal. Ask the patient to strain down again or cough. Note any swelling or tenderness.

If you find a large scrotal mass and suspect that it may be a hernia, ask the patient to lie down. The mass may return to the abdomen by itself. If so, it is a hernia. If not—

- Can you get your fingers above the mass in the scrotum?

- Listen to the mass with a stethoscope for bowel sounds.

If the findings suggest a hernia, gently try to reduce it (return it to the abdominal cavity) by sustained pressure with your fingers. Do not attempt this maneuver if the mass is tender or the patient reports nausea and vomiting.

History may be helpful here. The patient can usually tell you what happens to his swelling on lying down and may be able to demonstrate how he reduces it himself. Remember to ask him.

If you can, suspect a hydrocele.

Bowel sounds may be heard over a hernia, but not over a hydrocele.

A hernia is *incarcerated* when its contents cannot be returned to the abdominal cavity. A hernia is *strangulated* when the blood supply to the entrapped contents is compromised. Suspect strangulation in the presence of tenderness, nausea, and vomiting.

Table 12-1 Abnormalities of the Penis

Table 12-1   Abnormalities of the Penis

HYPOSPADIAS

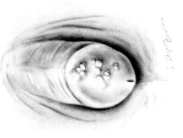

Hypospadias is a congenital displacement of the urethral meatus to the inferior surface of the penis. A groove extends from the actual urethral meatus to its normal location on the tip of the glans.

SYPHILITIC CHANCRE

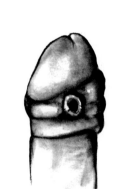

A syphilitic chancre usually appears as an oval or round, dark red, painless erosion or ulcer with an indurated base. Nontender enlarged inguinal lymph nodes are typically associated. Chancres may be multiple and when secondarily infected may be painful. They may then be mistaken for the lesions of herpes. Chancres are infectious.

GENITAL HERPES

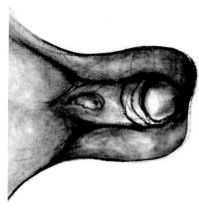

A cluster of small vesicles, followed by shallow, painful, nonindurated ulcers on red bases, suggests a herpes simplex infection. The lesions may occur anywhere on the penis. Usually there are fewer lesions when the infection recurs.

VENEREAL WART (*Condyloma acuminatum*)

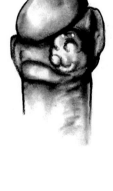

Venereal warts are rapidly growing excrescences that are moist and often malodorous. They result from infection by human papillomavirus.

CARCINOMA OF THE PENIS

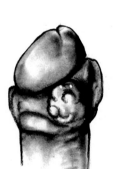

Carcinoma may appear as an indurated nodule or ulcer that is usually nontender. Limited almost completely to men who are not circumcised in childhood, it may be masked by the prepuce. Any persistent penile sore must be considered suspicious.

PEYRONIE'S DISEASE

In Peyronie's disease there are palpable nontender hard plaques just beneath the skin, usually along the dorsum of the penis. The patient complains of crooked, painful erections.

Table 12-2   Abnormalities in the Scrotum

Table 12-2   Abnormalities in the Scrotum

TUMOR OF THE TESTIS

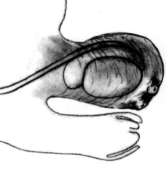

LATE

As a testicular neoplasm grows and spreads, it may seem to replace the entire organ. The testicle characteristically feels heavier than normal.

EARLY

A tumor of the testis usually appears as a painless nodule. It does not transilluminate. Any nodule within the testis must raise the suspicion of malignancy.

SCROTAL HERNIA

Fingers cannot get above mass

A hernia located within the scrotum is usually an indirect inguinal hernia. Since it comes through the external inguinal ring, the examining fingers cannot get above it in the scrotum.

HYDROCELE

Fingers can get above mass

A hydrocele is a nontender, fluid-filled mass that occupies the space within the tunica vaginalis. The examining fingers can get above the mass within the scrotum. The mass transilluminates.

SEBACEOUS CYSTS

These are firm, yellowish, nontender, cutaneous cysts up to about 1 cm in diameter. They are common and frequently multiple.

TUBERCULOUS EPIDIDYMITIS

The chronic inflammation of tuberculosis produces a firm enlargement of the epididymis, sometimes tender, with thickening or beading of the vas deferens.

VARICOCELE

Varicocele refers to varicose veins of the spermatic cord, usually found on the left. It feels like a soft "bag of worms" separate from the testis and slowly collapses when the scrotum is elevated in the supine patient. Infertility may be associated.

SPERMATOCELE AND CYST OF THE EPIDIDYMIS

A painless, movable cystic mass just above the testis suggests a spermatocele or an epididymal cyst. Both transilluminate. The former contains sperm, the latter does not, but they are clinically indistinguishable.

Table 12-2   Abnormalities in the Scrotum

Table 12-2   (Cont'd.)

ACUTE ORCHITIS

An acutely inflamed testis is painful, tender, and swollen. The testis may be difficult to distinguish from the epididymis. The scrotum may be reddened. Look for evidence of postpubertal mumps, such as parotid swelling, or other less common infectious causes.

ACUTE EPIDIDYMITIS

An acutely inflamed epididymis is tender and swollen and may be difficult to distinguish from the testis. The scrotum may be reddened, and the vas deferens may also be inflamed. Epididymitis occurs chiefly in adults. Coexisting urinary tract infection or prostatitis supports the diagnosis.

TORSION OF THE SPERMATIC CORD

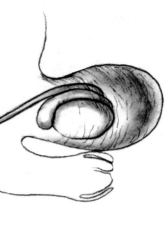

Torsion, or twisting, of the testicle on its spermatic cord produces an acutely painful, tender, and swollen organ that is retracted upward in the scrotum. The scrotum becomes red and edematous. There is no associated urinary infection. Torsion, most common in adolescents, is a surgical emergency because of obstructed circulation.

SMALL TESTIS

Adult testes are considered small when they are less than 3.5 cm long. Small firm testes (usually less than 2 cm long) suggest Klinefelter's syndrome. Small soft testes suggest atrophy, associated with several conditions (*e.g.*, cirrhosis, myotonia dystrophica, administration of estrogens, and hypopituitarism). Atrophy may also follow orchitis (*e.g.*, from mumps).

CRYPTORCHIDISM

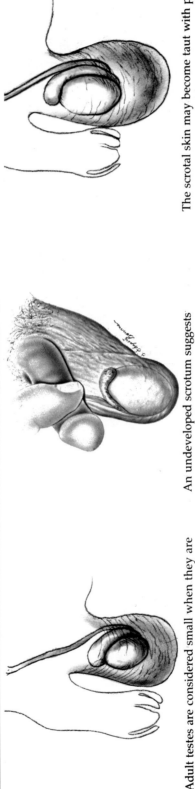

An undeveloped scrotum suggests cryptorchidism (an undescended testicle), as shown here on the patient's left. No left testis or epididymis is palpable in this scrotal sac. They may lie in the inguinal canal or abdomen. Cryptorchidism eventually leads to testicular atrophy on the involved side(s) and increases the risk of testicular cancer.

SCROTAL EDEMA

The scrotal skin may become taut with pitting edema. Scrotal edema is usually associated with generalized edema, as in chronic congestive heart failure or the nephrotic syndrome.

Table 12-3   Course and Presentation of Hernias in the Groin

Table 12-3   Course and Presentation of Hernias in the Groin

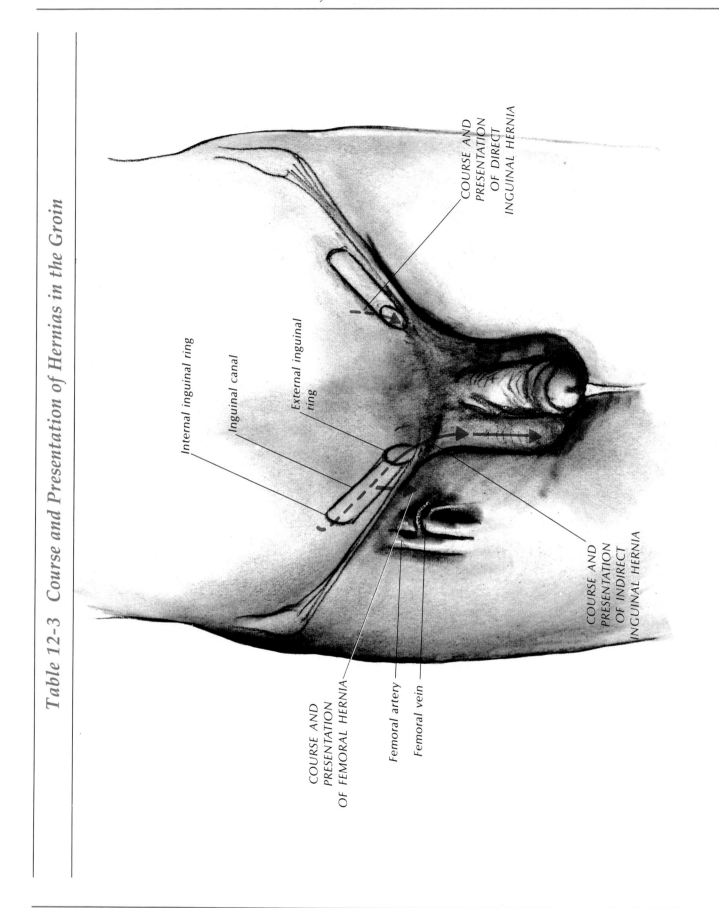

Internal inguinal ring

Inguinal canal

External inguinal ring

COURSE AND PRESENTATION OF DIRECT INGUINAL HERNIA

COURSE AND PRESENTATION OF INDIRECT INGUINAL HERNIA

COURSE AND PRESENTATION OF FEMORAL HERNIA

Femoral artery

Femoral vein

Table 12-4   Differentiation of Hernias in the Groin

Table 12-4   Differentiation of Hernias in the Groin

Differentiation among these hernias is not always clinically possible. Understanding their features, however, improves your observation.

| | INGUINAL | | FEMORAL |
	INDIRECT	DIRECT	
FREQUENCY	Most common, all ages, both sexes	Less common	Least common
AGE AND SEX	Often in children, may be in adults	Usually men over age 40, rare in women	More common in women than in men
POINT OF ORIGIN	Above inguinal ligament, near its midpoint (the internal inguinal ring)	Above inguinal ligament, close to the pubic tubercle (near the external inguinal ring)	Below the inguinal ligament; appears more lateral than an inguinal hernia and may be hard to differentiate from lymph nodes
COURSE	Often into the scrotum	Rarely into the scrotum	Never into the scrotum
	The hernia comes down the inguinal canal and touches the fingertip.	The hernia bulges anteriorly and pushes the side of the finger forward.	The inguinal canal is empty.
With the examining finger in the inguinal canal during straining or cough			

Chapter 13
Female Genitalia

Anatomy and Physiology

Review the anatomy of the external female genitalia, or vulva, including the mons pubis, a hair-covered fat pad overlying the symphysis pubis; the labia majora, rounded folds of adipose tissue; the labia minora, thinner pinkish red folds that extend anteriorly to form the prepuce; and the clitoris. The vestibule is the boat-shaped fossa between the labia minora. In its posterior portion lies the vaginal opening or introitus, which in virgins may be hidden by the hymen. The term perineum, as commonly used clinically, refers to the tissues between the introitus and the anus.

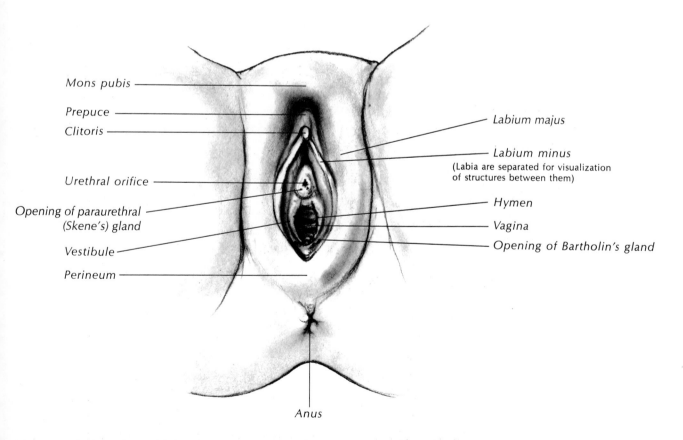

Mons pubis

Prepuce

Clitoris

Labium majus

Labium minus
(Labia are separated for visualization of structures between them)

Urethral orifice

Opening of paraurethral (Skene's) gland

Hymen

Vagina

Opening of Bartholin's gland

Vestibule

Perineum

Anus

The urethral orifice (urethral meatus) opens into the vestibule between the clitoris and the vagina. Just posterior to it on either side can sometimes be discerned the openings of the paraurethral or Skene's glands.

The openings of Bartholin's glands are located posteriorly on either side of the vaginal opening, but are not usually visible. Bartholin's glands themselves are situated more deeply.

The vagina is a hollow tube extending between urethra and rectum upward and posteriorly. It terminates in the cup-shaped fornix. The vaginal mucosa lies in transverse folds, or rugae.

At almost right angles to the vagina sits the uterus, a flattened fibromuscular structure shaped like an inverted pear. The uterus has two parts: the body (or corpus) and the cervix, which are joined together by the isthmus. The convex upper surface of the body is called the fundus of the uterus. The lower part of the uterus, the cervix, protrudes into the vagina, dividing the fornix into anterior, posterior, and lateral fornices.

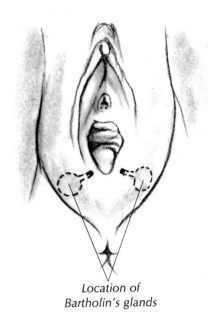

Location of
Bartholin's glands

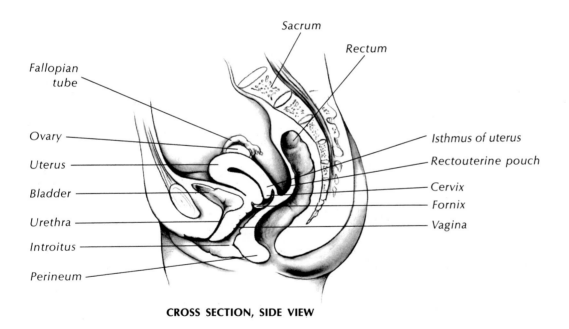

CROSS SECTION, SIDE VIEW

The vaginal surface of the cervix, the ectocervix, is easily seen with the help of a speculum. At its center is a round, oval, or slitlike depression, the external os of the cervix, that marks the opening into the endocervical canal. The ectocervix is covered by epithelium of two possible types: a shiny pink squamous epithelium, contiguous with the vaginal lining, and a deep red columnar epithelium similar to that which lines the endocervical canal. The latter is often visible around the os. The squamocolumnar junction marks the boundary between the two types of epithelium.

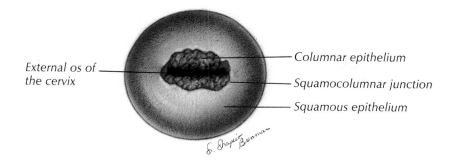

External os of the cervix

Columnar epithelium

Squamocolumnar junction

Squamous epithelium

From each side of the uterine fundus extends a fallopian tube, the fringed, funnel-shaped end of which curves toward the ovary. An ovary is an almond-shaped structure that varies considerably in size but averages about $3.5 \times 2 \times 1.5$ cm from adulthood through menopause. The ovaries are often palpable on pelvic examination during a woman's reproductive years, but normal fallopian tubes cannot be felt. The term adnexa (a plural Latin word meaning appendages) refers to the ovaries, tubes, and supporting tissues.

The ovaries have two primary functions: the production of ova and the secretion of hormones, including estrogen, progesterone, and testosterone. Increased hormonal secretions during puberty stimulate the growth of the uterus and its endometrial lining. They enlarge the vagina and thicken its epithelium. They also stimulate the development of secondary sex characteristics, including the breasts and pubic hair.

The parietal peritoneum extends downward behind the uterus into a cul de sac called the rectouterine pouch (or pouch of Douglas). You can just reach this area on rectal examination.

The pelvic organs are supported by a sling of tissues composed of muscle, ligaments, and fascia, through which the urethra, vagina, and rectum all pass.

Lymph from the vulva and the lower vagina drains to the inguinal nodes, but that from the internal genitalia, including the upper vagina, flows into pelvic and abdominal lymph nodes which are not palpable clinically.

CHANGES WITH AGE

Adolescence. During the pubertal years, the vulva and the internal genitalia grow and change to their adult proportions. Assessment of sexual maturity in girls, as classified by Tanner, depends not on internal examination, however, but on the growth of pubic hair and the development of breasts. Tanner's stages, or sex maturity ratings, as they relate to pubic hair are shown below; those relating to breasts are shown on page 324.

Sex Maturity Ratings in Girls: Pubic Hair

STAGE 1
Preadolescent—no pubic hair except for the fine body hair (vellus hair) similar to that on the abdomen

STAGE 2

STAGE 3

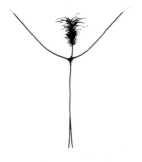

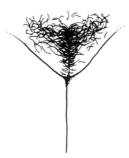

Sparse growth of long, slightly pigmented, downy hair, straight or only slightly curled, chiefly along the labia

Darker, coarser, curlier hair, spreading sparsely over the pubic symphysis

STAGE 4

STAGE 5

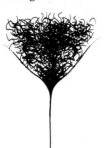

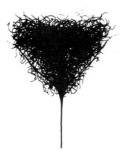

Coarse and curly hair as in adults; area covered greater than in stage 3 but not as great as in the adult and not yet including the thighs

Hair adult in quantity and quality, spread on the medial surfaces of the thighs but not up over the abdomen

(Illustrations through the courtesy of W.A. Daniel, Jr., Division of Adolescent Medicine, University of Alabama, Birmingham)

A girl's first sign of puberty is usually the appearance of breast buds. Sometimes, however, pubic hair appears first. On the average, these changes start at around 11 years of age, with a range from 8 to 13 years for breast buds, 8 to 14 years for pubic hair. The transformation from preadolescent to adult form takes about 3 years, with a range of 1.5 to 6 years. Menarche tends to occur during breast stage 3 or 4, at ages ranging from 10 to 16.5 years according to Tanner's studies, which are summarized graphically on p. 389. The age of menarche in the United States is a little earlier, roughly from 9 to 16 years.

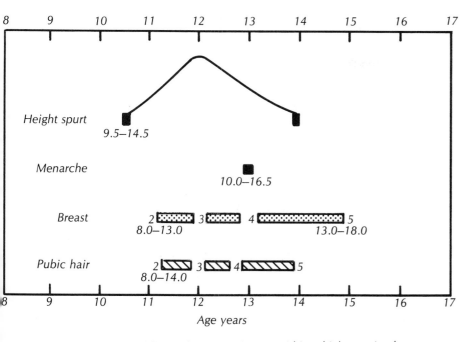

Numbers below the bars indicate the ranges in age within which certain changes occur. (Redrawn from Marshall WA, Tanner JM: Variations in the pattern of pubertal changes in boys. Arch Dis Child 45:22, 1970)

As in boys, there is a wide range of normal in pubertal development. Some girls may have completed the development of their secondary sex characteristics while others of the same age have not yet begun.

In 10% or more of women, pubic hair spreads further up the abdomen in a triangular pattern, pointing toward the umbilicus. This spread can be classified as stage 6 but, because it is usually not completed until the mid-20s or later, it is not considered a pubertal change.

Just before menarche there is a physiologic increase in vaginal secretion —a normal change that sometimes worries a girl or her mother. As menses become established, increased secretions, or leukorrhea, coincide with ovulation. They also accompany sexual arousal. These normal kinds of discharges must be differentiated from those of infectious processes.

Aging. Ovarian function usually starts to diminish during a woman's 40s, and menstrual periods cease on the average between the ages of 45 and 52, sometimes earlier and sometimes later. Pubic hair becomes sparse as well as gray. With the decline of estrogenic stimulus, the labia and the clitoris become smaller. The vagina narrows and shortens and its mucosa becomes thin, pale, and dry. The uterus and ovaries diminish in size.

Techniques of Examination

GENERAL APPROACH

Most students feel anxious, embarrassed, or uncomfortable when first examining the genitalia of another person. At the same time, patients have their own concerns. Some women have had painful, embarrassing, or even demeaning experiences during previous pelvic examinations, while others may be facing their first examination. Fear of what the clinician may find and what this may mean in the patient's life adds to potential tensions.

A patient's reactions and behavior may give you important clues to such feelings and to her attitudes toward sexuality. If she adducts her thighs, pulls away, or expresses negative feelings during the examination, you can gently confront her as you would during the interview. "I notice you are having some trouble relaxing . . . or seem disgusted. . . . Is it just being here or is it the same way at home? . . . or during intercourse?" Behavior that seems to present an annoying obstacle to your examination may become the key to understanding your patient's problem.

A patient who has never had a pelvic examination is often fearful of it, embarrassed, and ignorant of what to expect. Try to make the experience one in which she learns about both her body and the examination itself and becomes more comfortable with them. Before she undresses, explain the relevant anatomy with the help of three-dimensional models. Show her the speculum and other equipment and encourage her to handle them. During the examination, then, she can better understand your explanations and procedures. It is especially important not to hurt the patient during her first encounter.

Indications for a pelvic examination during adolescence include menstrual abnormalities such as amenorrhea, excessive bleeding, or dysmenorrhea, unexplained abdominal pain, vaginal discharge, the prescription of contraceptives, bacteriological and cytological studies in a sexually active girl, and the patient's own desire for assessment. Rape requires special evaluation for which specialty references should be consulted.

At any age, getting the patient to relax is essential for an adequate examination. Sensitivity to her feelings may help here. In addition—

1. Ask the patient to empty her bladder before the examination.
2. Position and drape her appropriately. Elevating her head and shoulders slightly helps the patient to relax her abdominal muscles and to see what is going on. The drape should cover her thighs and knees. Depressing it in the midline enables both patient and examiner to see each other's face. A girl or woman may wish to use a mirror to see her genitalia during the examination. When possible, offer her this opportunity.

3. The patient's arms should be at her sides or folded across her chest—not over her head, since this last position tends to tighten the abdominal muscles.

4. Explain in advance each step of the examination and tell the patient what she may feel. Avoid any sudden or unexpected movements. When beginning palpation or using a speculum, it may be helpful to make initial contact not on the genitalia themselves but on the upper inner thigh.

5. Your hands and the speculum should be warm.

6. Monitor your examination when possible by watching the patient's face.

7. Finally, of course, be as gentle as possible.

Wear gloves throughout the examination and afterward when handling equipment used.

EQUIPMENT. You should have within reach a good light, a vaginal speculum of appropriate size, water-soluble lubricant, and equipment for taking Papanicolaou smears, bacteriologic cultures, or other diagnostic tests. Review the supplies and procedures of your own facility before taking cultures and other samples.

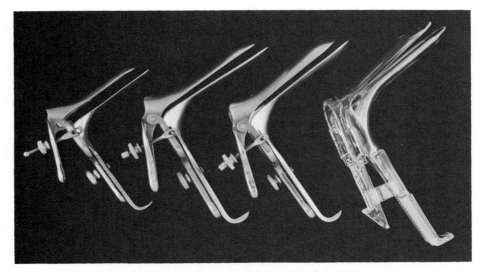

Specula are made of metal or plastic and come in two basic shapes. Graves specula are usually best for sexually active women. They are available in small, medium, and large sizes. The narrow-bladed Pedersen speculum is useful for a patient with a relatively small introitus, such as a virgin or an elderly woman, and is often more comfortable for other patients as well.

Before using a speculum, become thoroughly familiar with how to open and close its blades, lock the blades in an open position, and release them again. Although the instructions in this chapter refer to a metal speculum, you can easily adapt them to a plastic one by handling the speculum before using it. Plastic specula typically make a

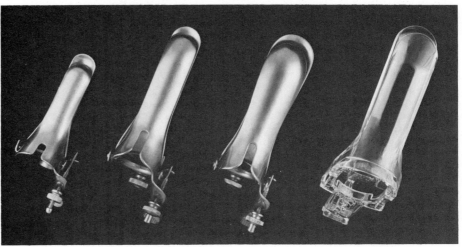

Specula, from left to right: small metal Pedersen, medium metal Pedersen, medium metal Graves, and large plastic Pedersen

loud click when locked or released. Forewarning the patient about this click helps to avoid unnecessary surprise.

Male examiners are customarily attended by female assistants. Female examiners may or may not prefer to work alone but should also be assisted if the patient is physically disabled or emotionally disturbed.

POSITION. Drape the patient appropriately and then assist her into the lithotomy position. Help her to place first one heel and then the other into the stirrups. She may be more comfortable with shoes on than with bare feet. Then ask her to move toward the end of the examining table until her buttocks extend slightly beyond the edge. Her thighs should be flexed and abducted. A pillow should support her head.

EXTERNAL EXAMINATION

ASSESS THE SEXUAL MATURITY OF AN ADOLESCENT PATIENT. You can assess pubic hair during either the abdominal or the pelvic examination. Note its character and distribution, and rate it according to Tanner's stages described on page 388.

Delayed puberty is often familial or related to chronic illness. It may also be due to abnormalities in the hypothalamus, anterior pituitary gland, or ovaries.

INSPECT THE PATIENT'S EXTERNAL GENITALIA. Seat yourself comfortably and inspect the mons pubis, labia, and perineum. Separate the labia and inspect:

Excoriations or itchy, small, red maculopapules suggest pediculosis pubis (lice or "crabs"). Look for nits or lice at the bases of the pubic hairs.

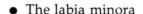

- The labia minora

- The clitoris

Enlarged clitoris in masculinizing conditions

- The urethral orifice

Urethral caruncle, prolapse of the urethral mucosa (p. 402)

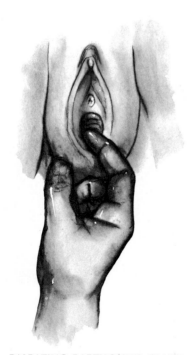

- The vaginal opening or introitus

See Table 13-1, Lesions of the Vulva (p. 401).

Note any inflammation, ulceration, discharge, swelling, or nodules. If there are any lesions, palpate them.

Syphilitic chancre, sebaceous cyst

If there is a history or an appearance of labial swelling, check Bartholin's glands. Insert your index finger into the vagina near the posterior end of the introitus. Place your thumb outside the posterior part of the labium majus. On

A Bartholin's gland may become acutely or chronically infected and then produces a swelling. See Table 13-2, Bulges and Swellings of Vulva, Vagina, and Urethra (p. 402).

PALPATING BARTHOLIN'S GLAND

each side in turn, palpate between your finger and thumb for swelling or tenderness. Note any discharge exuding from the duct opening of the gland. If any is present, culture it.

If you suspect urethritis or inflammation of the paraurethral glands, insert your index finger into the vagina and milk the urethra gently from inside outward. Note any discharge from or about the urethral orifice. If any is present, culture it.

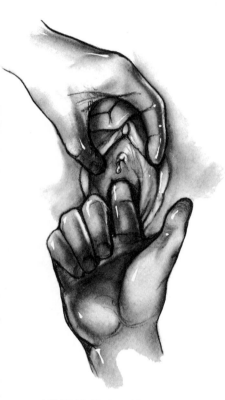

MILKING THE URETHRA

INTERNAL EXAMINATION

LOCATE THE CERVIX. Insert your index finger into the vagina and identify the firm, rounded surface of the cervix. Locating the cervix manually will help you to find it more easily with a speculum. This maneuver also helps you to assess the size of the introitus and guides your choice of speculum. You may need to lubricate your finger with water, but do not use other lubricants.

ASSESS THE SUPPORT OF THE VAGINAL OUTLET. With the labia separated by your middle and index fingers, ask the patient to strain down. Note any bulging of the vaginal walls.

Cystocele and rectocele. See Table 13-2, Bulges and Swellings of Vulva, Vagina, and Urethra (p. 402).

INSERT THE SPECULUM. Select a speculum of appropriate size and shape, and lubricate and warm it with warm water. (Other lubricants may interfere with cytological or other studies but may be used if no such tests are planned.) If you have your speculum ready during assessment of the vaginal outlet, you can ease speculum insertion and increase your efficiency by proceeding to this next maneuver while the patient is still straining down.

Place two fingers at the introitus and gently press down on the perineal body. With your other hand, introduce the closed speculum past your fingers at a somewhat downward angle. Be careful not to pull on the pubic hair or pinch the labia with the speculum.

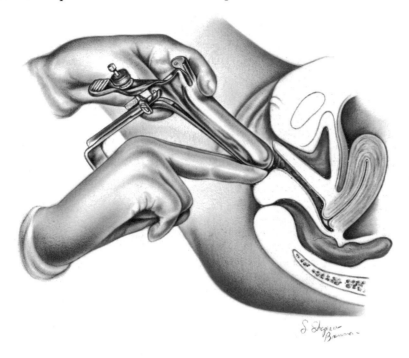

Two methods avoid the discomfort caused by pressure on the sensitive urethra. (1) When inserting the speculum, hold the blades obliquely, and then (2) slide the speculum inward along the posterior wall of the vagina.

After the speculum has entered the vagina, remove your fingers from the introitus. Rotate the blades of the speculum into a horizontal position, maintaining the pressure posteriorly, and insert the speculum to its full length.

ENTRY ANGLE

ANGLE AT FULL INSERTION

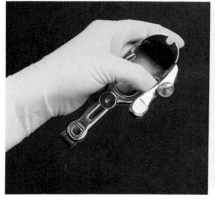
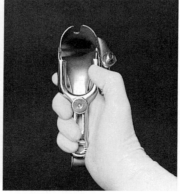

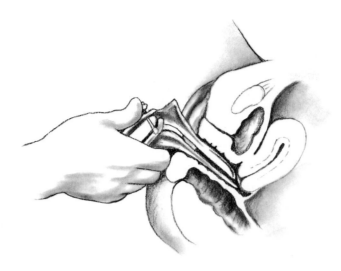

INSPECT THE CERVIX. Open the blades and maneuver the speculum, if necessary, so that the cervix comes into full view. Adjust the light for good visualization. When the uterus is retroverted, the cervix points more anteriorly than illustrated. If you have difficulty finding such a cervix, withdraw the speculum slightly and position it more anteriorly (*i.e.,* more horizontally). If discharge obscures your view, wipe it away gently with a large cotton swab.

See retroversion of the uterus, page 407.

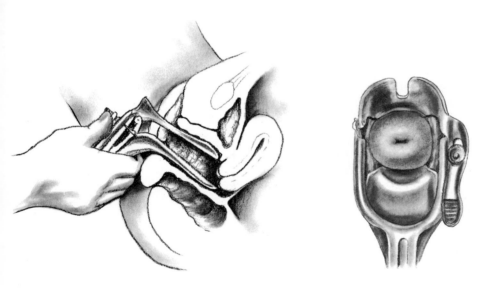

Inspect the cervix and its os. Note the color of the cervix, its position, the characteristics of its surface, and any ulcerations, nodules, masses, bleeding, or discharge.

See Table 13-3, Variations in the Cervix (p. 403), and Table 13-4, Abnormalities of the Cervix (p. 404).

Secure the speculum with the blades open by tightening the thumb screw.

OBTAIN TWO SPECIMENS FOR CERVICAL CYTOLOGY (PAPANICO-LAOU SMEARS), one from the endocervical canal and the other from the ectocervix.

Endocervical Swab. Moisten the end of a cotton applicator stick with saline and insert it into the cervical os. Roll it between your thumb and index finger, clockwise and counterclockwise. Remove it. Smear a glass slide with the cotton swab, gently, in a painting motion. (Rubbing hard on the slide will destroy the cells.) Either place the slide into an ether-alcohol fixative at once, or spray it promptly with a special fixative. Special brushes may also be used to collect the endocervical sample.

A yellowish discharge on the endocervical swab suggests a mucopurulent cervicitis, which is commonly caused by *Chlamydia trachomatis.*

Cervical Scrape. Place the longer end of the scraper into the os of the cervix. Press, turn, and scrape in a full circle, making sure to include the squamocolumnar junction. Prepare a second slide as before.

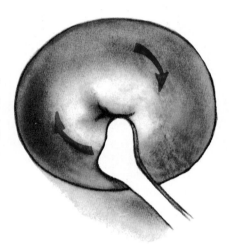

INSPECT THE VAGINA. Withdraw the speculum slowly while observing the vagina. As the speculum clears the cervix, release the thumb screw and maintain the open position of the speculum with your thumb. Close the blades as the speculum emerges from the introitus, avoiding both excessive stretching and pinching of the mucosa. During withdrawal inspect the vaginal mucosa, noting its color and any inflammation, discharge, ulcers, or masses.

See Table 13-5, Vaginitis (p. 405).

Cancer of the vagina

PERFORM A BIMANUAL EXAMINATION. Lubricate the index and middle fingers of one of your gloved hands, and from a *standing position* insert them into the vagina, again exerting pressure primarily posteriorly. Your thumb should be abducted, your ring and little fingers flexed into your palm. Pressing inward on the perineum with your flexed fingers causes little if any discomfort and allows you to position your palpating fingers correctly. Note any nodularity or tenderness in the vaginal wall, including the region of the urethra and the bladder anteriorly.

Stool in the rectum may simulate a rectovaginal mass, but unlike a tumor mass can usually be dented by digital pressure. Rectovaginal examination confirms the distinction.

Palpate the cervix, noting its position, shape, consistency, regularity, mobility, and tenderness. Normally the cervix can be moved somewhat without pain. Feel the fornix around the cervix.

Pain on movement of the cervix, together with adnexal tenderness, suggests pelvic inflammatory disease.

Place your other hand on the abdomen about midway between the umbilicus and the symphysis pubis. While you elevate the cervix and uterus with your pelvic hand, press your abdominal hand in and down, trying to grasp the uterus between your two hands. Note its size, shape, consistency, and mobility, and identify any tenderness or masses.

See Table 13-6, Abnormalities and Positions of the Uterus (pp. 406–407).

Uterine enlargement suggests pregnancy or benign or malignant tumors.

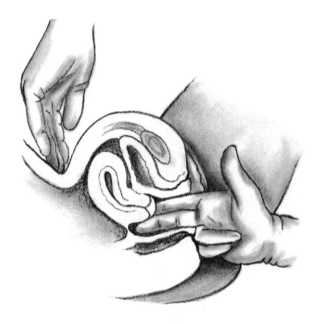

Now slide both fingers of your pelvic hand into the anterior fornix and palpate the body of the uterus between your hands. In this position your pelvic hand can feel the anterior surface of the uterus, and your abdominal hand can feel part of the posterior surface.

Nodules on the uterine surfaces suggest myomas (see p. 406).

If you cannot feel the uterus with either of these maneuvers, it may be tipped posteriorly (retrodisplaced). In this case, slide your pelvic fingers into the posterior fornix and feel for the uterus butting against your fingertips. An obese or poorly relaxed abdominal wall may also prevent you from feeling the uterus even when it is located anteriorly.

See retroversion and retroflexion of the uterus (p. 407).

Next, place your abdominal hand on the right lower quadrant, your pelvic hand in the right lateral fornix. Press your abdominal hand in and down, trying to push the adnexal structures toward your pelvic hand. Try to identify the right ovary or any adjacent adnexal masses. By moving

Three to five years after menopause, the ovaries have usually atrophied and are no longer palpable. If you can feel an

your hands slightly, slide the adnexal structures between your fingers, if possible, and note their size, shape, consistency, mobility, and tenderness. Repeat the procedure on the left side.

ovary in a postmenopausal woman, consider an abnormality such as a cyst or a tumor.

Adnexal masses include ovarian cysts and tumors, the swollen fallopian tube(s) of pelvic inflammatory disease, and a tubal pregnancy. A uterine myoma may simulate an adnexal mass. See Table 13-7, Adnexal Masses (p. 408).

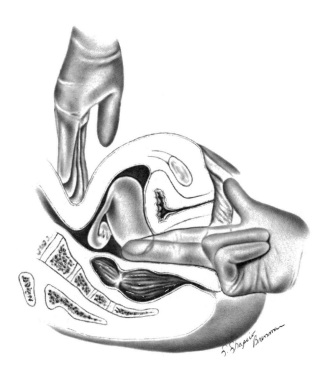

Normal ovaries are somewhat tender. They are usually palpable in slender, relaxed women but are difficult or impossible to feel in others who are obese or poorly relaxed.

ASSESS THE STRENGTH OF THE PELVIC MUSCLES. Withdraw your two fingers slightly, just clear of the cervix, and spread them to touch the sides of the vaginal walls. Ask the patient to squeeze her muscles around them as hard and long as she can. A squeeze that compresses your fingers snugly, moves them upward and inward, and lasts 3 seconds or more is full strength.

Impaired strength may be due to age, vaginal deliveries, or neurologic deficits. Weakness may be associated with urinary stress incontinence.

DO A RECTOVAGINAL EXAMINATION. Withdraw your fingers. Lubricate your gloves again if necessary. (See note on using lubricant, p. 399.) Then slowly reintroduce your index finger into the vagina, your middle finger into the rectum. Ask the patient to strain down as you do this so that her anal sphincter will relax. Tell her that this examination may make her feel as if she has to move her bowels but that she will not do so. Repeat the maneuvers of the bimanual examination, giving special attention to the region behind the cervix that may be accessible only to the rectal finger. Rectovaginal palpation is especially valuable in assessing a retrodisplaced uterus, as illustrated.

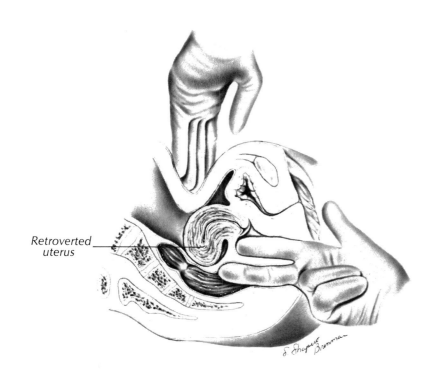

Retroverted uterus

Proceed to the rectal examination (see Chap. 15). After your examination, wipe off the external genitalia and anus or offer the patient some tissue with which to do it herself.

A NOTE ON THE SMALL INTROITUS. Many virginal vaginal orifices will readily admit a single examining finger. Modify your technique so as to use your index finger only. A small Pedersen speculum may make inspection possible. When the vaginal orifice is even smaller, a fairly good bimanual examination can be performed by placing one finger in the rectum rather than in the vagina.

An imperforate hymen occasionally delays menarche. Be sure to check for this possibility when menarche seems unduly late in relation to the development of a girl's breasts and pubic hair.

Similar techniques may be indicated in elderly women in whom the introitus has become atrophied and tight.

A NOTE ON USING LUBRICANT. If you use a large tube of lubricant during a pelvic or rectal examination, you may inadvertently contaminate it by touching the tube with your gloved fingers after touching the patient. To avoid this problem, let the lubricant drop onto your gloved fingers without allowing contact between the tube and the gloves. If you or your assistant should inadvertently contaminate the tube, discard it. Small disposable tubes for use with one patient circumvent this problem.

HERNIAS

Hernias of the groin occur in women as well as in men, but they are much less common. Search for one if symptoms suggest the possibility. The examination techniques (see pp. 377–378) are basically the same as for men, and a woman too should stand up to be examined. To feel an indirect inguinal hernia, however, palpate in the labia majora and upward to just lateral to the pubic tubercles.

An indirect inguinal hernia is the most common hernia that occurs in the female groin. A femoral hernia ranks next in frequency.

Table 13-1 Lesions of the Vulva

Table 13-1 Lesions of the Vulva

SEBACEOUS CYST

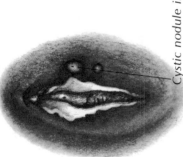

Cystic nodule in skin

Small, firm, round cystic nodules in the labia suggest sebaceous cysts. They are sometimes yellowish in color. Look for the dark punctum marking the blocked opening of the gland.

VENEREAL WART (Condyloma Acuminatum)

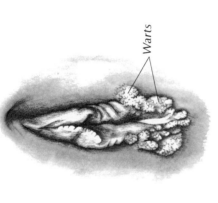

Warts

Warty lesions on the labia and within the vestibule suggest condylomata acuminata. They are due to infection with human papillomavirus.

SECONDARY SYPHILIS (Condyloma Latum)

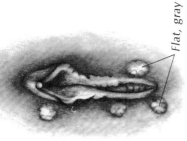

Flat, gray papules

Slightly raised, flat, round or oval papules covered by a gray exudate suggest condylomata lata. These constitute one manifestation of secondary syphilis and are contagious.

SYPHILITIC CHANCRE

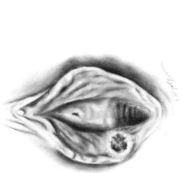

A firm, painless ulcer suggests the chancre of primary syphilis. Since most chancres in women develop internally, they often go undetected.

GENITAL HERPES

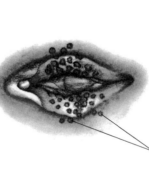

Shallow ulcers on red bases

Shallow, small, painful ulcers on red bases suggest a herpes infection. Initial infection may be extensive, as illustrated here. Recurrent infections are usually confined to a small local patch.

CARCINOMA OF THE VULVA

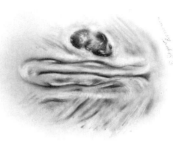

An ulcerated or raised red vulvar lesion in an elderly woman may indicate vulvar carcinoma.

Table 13-2 Bulges and Swelling of Vulva, Vagina, and Urethra

Table 13-2 Bulges and Swelling of Vulva, Vagina, and Urethra

CYSTOCELE

A cystocele is a bulge of the anterior vaginal wall, together with the bladder above it, that results from weakened supporting tissues. The upper two thirds of the vaginal wall are involved.

CYSTOURETHROCELE

Urethrocele

Cystocele

When the entire anterior vaginal wall, together with the bladder and the urethra, is involved in the bulge, a cystourethrocele is present. A groove sometimes defines the border between urethrocele and cystocele but is not always present.

RECTOCELE

Bulge

A rectocele is a bulging of the posterior wall of the vagina, together with the rectal wall behind it. Weakened supporting structures are the cause.

BARTHOLIN'S GLAND INFECTION

Labial swelling

Causes of a Bartholin's gland infection include gonococci, *Chlamydia trachomatis*, and other organisms. Acutely, it appears as a tense, hot, very tender abscess. Look for pus coming out of the duct or erythema around the duct opening. Chronically, a nontender cyst is felt. It may be large or small.

URETHRAL CARUNCLE

Caruncle

A urethral caruncle is a small, red, benign tumor, visible at the posterior part of the urethral meatus. It occurs chiefly in postmenopausal women and usually causes no symptoms. Occasionally, a carcinoma of the urethra is mistaken for a caruncle. To check for this, palpate the urethra through the vagina for thickening, nodularity, or tenderness, and feel for inguinal lymphadenopathy.

PROLAPSE OF THE URETHRAL MUCOSA

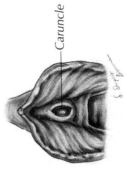

Prolapsed urethral mucosa

Prolapsed urethral mucosa forms a swollen red ring around the urethral meatus. It usually occurs before menarche or after menopause. Identify the urethral meatus at the center of the swelling to make this diagnosis.

Table 13-3   Variations in the Cervix

SHAPES OF THE CERVICAL OS

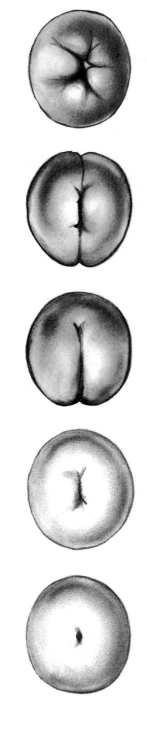

The normal cervical os may be round, oval, or slitlike. The trauma of one or more vaginal deliveries may tear the cervix, producing lacerations. Illustrated here, from left to right, are an oval os, a slitlike os, and lacerations described as unilateral transverse, bilateral transverse, and stellate.

VARIATIONS IN THE CERVICAL SURFACE

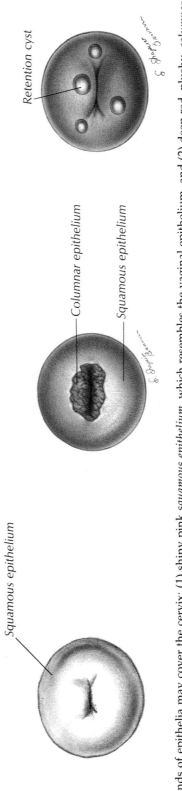

Two kinds of epithelia may cover the cervix: (1) shiny pink *squamous epithelium*, which resembles the vaginal epithelium, and (2) deep red, plushy, *columnar epithelium*, which is continuous with the endocervical lining. These two meet at the squamocolumnar junction. When this junction is at or inside the cervical os, only squamous epithelium is seen. A ring of columnar epithelium is often visible to a varying extent around the os—the result of a normal process that accompanies fetal development, menarche, and the first pregnancy.*

By another process termed metaplasia, all or part of this columnar epithelium is transformed into squamous epithelium again. This change may block the secretions of columnar epithelium and thus cause retention cysts (nabothian cysts). These appear as one or more translucent nodules on the cervical surface and have no pathologic significance.

* Terminology is in flux. Other terms for the columnar epithelium that is visible on the ectocervix are ectropion, ectopy, and eversion.

Table 13-4   Abnormalities of the Cervix

Table 13-4   Abnormalities of the Cervix

CARCINOMA OF THE CERVIX

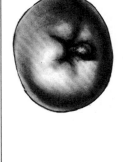

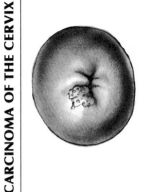

Carcinoma of the cervix begins in an area of metaplasia. In its earliest stages, it cannot be distinguished from a normal cervix. In a late stage, an extensive, irregular, cauliflowerlike growth may develop. Early, frequent intercourse and multiple partners increase the risk for cervical cancer.

MUCOPURULENT CERVICITIS

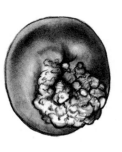

Mucopurulent cervicitis is usually due to infection from *Chlamydia trachomatis*. Gonorrhea (from *Neisseria gonorrhoeae*) may coexist or may itself be the cause. Both infections are sexually transmitted. A yellowish, mucopurulent discharge coming from the os suggests this diagnosis. Both infections may occur without symptoms or signs.

CERVICAL POLYP

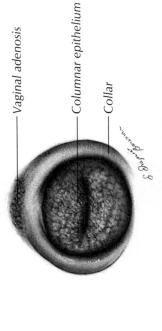

A cervical polyp usually arises from the endocervical canal, becoming visible when it protrudes through the cervical os. It is bright red, soft, and rather fragile. When only the tip is seen, it cannot be differentiated clinically from a polyp originating in the endometrium. Polyps are benign but may bleed.

FETAL EXPOSURE TO DIETHYLSTILBESTROL (DES)*

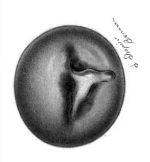

Vaginal adenosis

Columnar epithelium

Collar

Daughters of women who took diethylstilbestrol during pregnancy are at much higher risk for a number of abnormalities, including (1) columnar epithelium that covers most or all of the cervix, (2) vaginal adenosis, *i.e.,* extension of this epithelium to the vaginal wall, and (3) a circular collar or ridge of tissue, of varying shapes, between cervix and vagina. Much less common is an otherwise rare carcinoma of the upper vagina.

*In the United States, exposure to DES diminished in the late 1960s and stopped in 1971 when the drug was banned.

Table 13-5   Vaginitis

Table 13-5   Vaginitis

The vaginal discharge that often accompanies vaginitis must be distinguished from a physiologic discharge. The latter is clear or white and may contain white clumps of epithelial cells; it is not malodorous. Mucopurulent cervicitis (p. 404) may also cause a discharge.

	TRICHOMONAS VAGINITIS	CANDIDA VAGINITIS (MONILIA)	BACTERIAL VAGINOSIS*	ATROPHIC VAGINITIS
CAUSE	*Trichomonas vaginalis*, a protozoa. Often but not always acquired sexually	*Candida albicans*, a yeast (a normal vaginal inhabitant). Many factors predispose.	*Gardnerella vaginalis*, together with anaerobic bacteria. May be transmitted sexually.	Decreased estrogen production after menopause
DISCHARGE	Yellowish green or gray, possibly frothy; often profuse and pooled in the vaginal fornix; may be malodorous	White and curdy; may be thin but typically thick; not as profuse as in *Trichomonas* infection; not malodorous	Gray or white, thin, homogeneous, malodorous; coats the vaginal walls. Usually not profuse, may be minimal	Variable in color, consistency, and amount; may be blood-tinged; rarely profuse
OTHER SYMPTOMS	Pruritus, though not usually as severe as with *Candida* infection; pain on urination (from skin inflammation or possibly urethritis); and dyspareunia	Pruritus, vaginal soreness, pain on urination (from skin inflammation), and dyspareunia	Unpleasant fishy or musty genital odor	Pruritus, vaginal soreness or burning, and dyspareunia
VULVA	The vestibule and labia minora may be reddened.	The vulva and even the surrounding skin are often inflamed and sometimes swollen to a variable extent.	Usually normal	Atrophic
VAGINAL MUCOSA	May be diffusely reddened, with small red granular spots or petechiae in the posterior fornix. In mild cases, the mucosa looks normal.	Often reddened, with white, often tenacious patches of discharge. The mucosa may bleed when these patches are scraped off. In mild cases, the mucosa looks normal.	Usually normal	Atrophic, dry, pale; may be red, petechial, or ecchymotic; bleeds easily; may show erosions or filmy adhesions

* Previously termed Gardnerella vaginitis.

Table 13-6   Abnormalities and Positions of the Uterus

Table 13-6   Abnormalities and Positions of the Uterus

MYOMAS OF THE UTERUS (*Fibroids*)

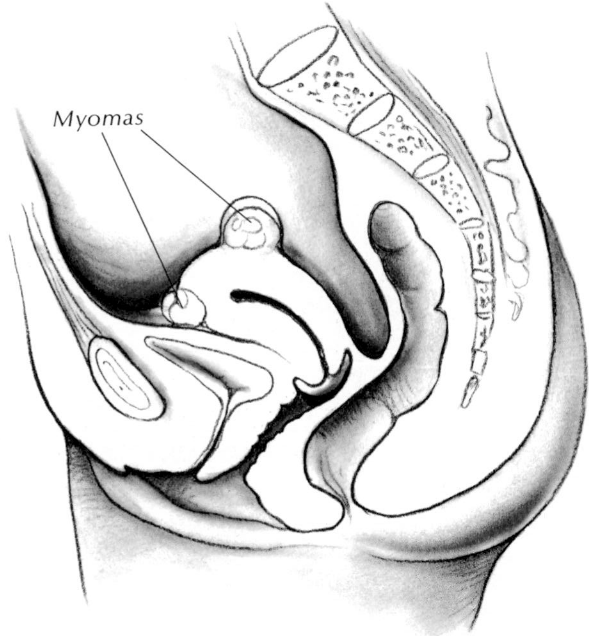

PROLAPSE OF THE UTERUS

Normal position

Myomas

Myomas are very common benign uterine tumors. They may be single or multiple and vary greatly in size, occasionally reaching massive proportions. They feel like firm, irregular nodules in continuity with the uterine surface. Occasionally, a myoma projecting laterally can be confused with an ovarian mass; a nodule projecting posteriorly can be mistaken for a retroflexed uterus. Submucous myomas project toward the endometrial cavity and are not themselves palpable, although they may be suspected because of an enlarged uterus.

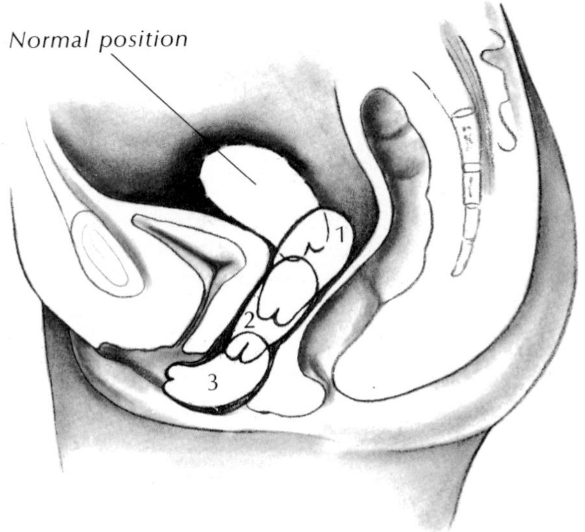

Prolapse of the uterus results from weakness of the supporting structures of the pelvic floor and is often associated with a cystocele and rectocele. In progressive stages, the uterus becomes retroverted and descends down the vaginal canal to the outside. In first-degree prolapse, the cervix is still well within the vagina. In second-degree prolapse, it is at the introitus. In third-degree prolapse, also called procidentia uteri, the cervix and vagina are outside the introitus.

Table 13-6   Abnormalities and Positions of the Uterus

RETROVERSION OF THE UTERUS

MODERATE

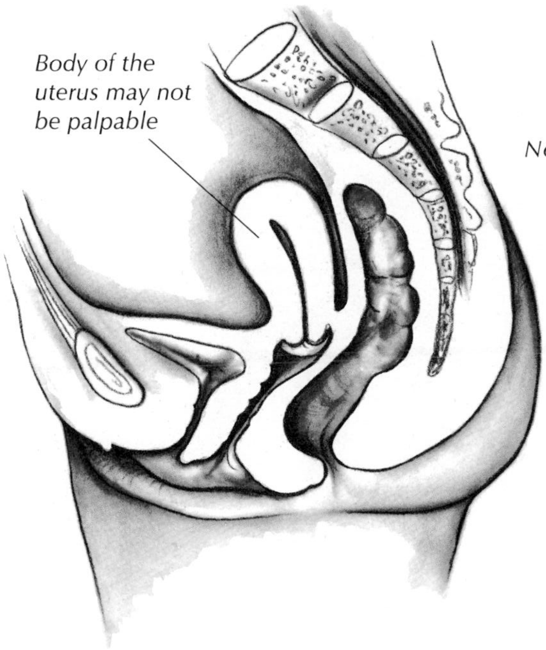

Body of the uterus may not be palpable

MARKED

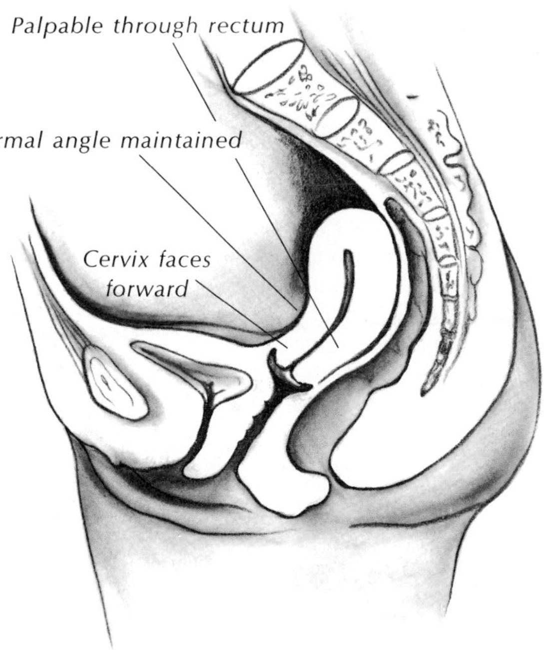

Palpable through rectum

Normal angle maintained

Cervix faces forward

RETROFLEXION OF THE UTERUS

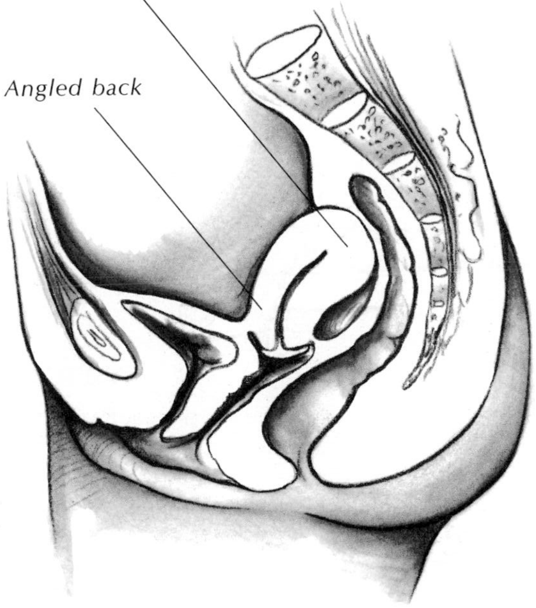

May be palpable through rectum

Angled back

Retroversion of the uterus refers to a tilting backward of the entire uterus, including both body and cervix. It is a common variant occurring in about 1 out of 5 women. Early clues on pelvic examination are a cervix that faces forward and a uterine body that cannot be felt by the abdominal hand. In moderate retroversion, shown on the left, the body may not be palpable with either hand. In marked retroversion, shown on the right, the body can be felt posteriorly, either through the posterior fornix or through the rectum. A retroverted uterus is usually both mobile and asymptomatic. Occasionally, such a uterus is fixed and immobile, held in place by conditions such as endometriosis or pelvic inflammatory disease.

Retroflexion of the uterus refers to a backward angulation of the body of the uterus in relationship to the cervix. The cervix maintains its usual position. The body of the uterus is often palpable through the posterior fornix or through the rectum. Both retroversion and retroflexion are usually normal variants.

Table 13-7   Adnexal Masses

Table 13-7   Adnexal Masses

Adnexal masses most commonly result from disorders of the fallopian tubes or ovaries. Three examples—often hard to differentiate—are described. In addition, inflammatory disease of the bowel (such as diverticulitis), carcinoma of the colon, and a pedunculated myoma of the uterus may simulate an adnexal mass.

OVARIAN CYSTS AND TUMORS

Ovarian cysts and tumors may be detected as adnexal masses on one or both sides. Later, they may grow up out of the pelvis. Cysts tend to be smooth and compressible, tumors more solid and often nodular. Uncomplicated cysts and tumors are not usually tender.

Small (≤ 6cm in diameter), mobile, cystic masses in a young woman are usually benign and often disappear after the next menstrual period.

RUPTURED TUBAL PREGNANCY

A ruptured tubal pregnancy spills blood into the peritoneal cavity, causing severe abdominal pain and tenderness. Guarding and rebound tenderness are sometimes associated. A unilateral adnexal mass may be palpable, but tenderness often prevents its detection. Faintness, syncope, nausea, vomiting, tachycardia, and shock may be present, reflecting the hemorrhage. There may be a prior history of amenorrhea or other symptoms of a pregnancy.

PELVIC INFLAMMATORY DISEASE

Pelvic inflammatory disease (PID) is a result of sexually transmitted infection of the fallopian tubes (salpingitis) or of the tubes and ovaries (salpingo-oophoritis). It is caused by *Neisseria gonorrhoeae*, *Chlamydia trachomatis*, and other organisms. *Acute* disease is associated with very tender, bilateral adnexal masses, although pain and muscle spasm usually make it impossible to delineate them. Movement of the cervix produces pain. *Chronic* disease is manifested by bilateral, tender, usually irregular, and fairly fixed adnexal masses.

Infection of the fallopian tubes and ovaries may also follow delivery of a baby or gynecologic surgery.

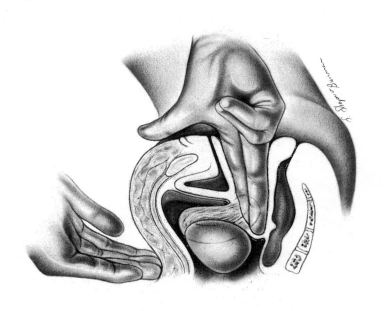

Chapter 14
The Pregnant Woman

Joyce E. (Beebe) Thompson

Assessment of the pregnant woman is similar to that of other women. Changes in anatomy and physiology during pregnancy, however, result in symptoms and physical signs that are important to recognize as pregnancy-related rather than abnormal. This chapter focuses on the evaluation of healthy adult women who are pregnant, and the ways in which this differs from evaluation of healthy nonpregnant women. Common variations of normal findings are presented, and easily identified problems or danger signs are discussed briefly.

The chapter concentrates on the initial assessment of the pregnant woman by any primary provider, including the history and physical examination used to diagnose or confirm pregnancy. This assessment ideally takes place within 6 to 8 weeks of conception, although some women do not come for their first pregnancy visit until much later. If a woman appears late in pregnancy for her first visit, additional techniques such as modified Leopold's maneuvers for abdominal palpation are needed. Because normal pregnancy lasts 38 to 42 weeks and changes in the organs of reproduction that begin with conception continue throughout, these changes will be outlined briefly. The text does not, however, present the detail needed to provide care throughout pregnancy.

Anatomy and Physiology

In preparation for physical examination of the pregnant woman, you may wish to review the anatomy in Chapter 10, Breasts and Axillae, and Chapter 13, Female Genitalia. The major anatomical changes related to pregnancy occur in the thyroid gland, breasts, abdomen, and pelvis. Minor skin changes, including the mask of pregnancy and abdominal striae, may be noted in some women.

During pregnancy, the thyroid gland enlarges moderately due to hyperplasia of the glandular tissue and increased vascularity. The breasts also enlarge for the same reasons, and become nodular by the third month of gestation as the mammary tissue hypertrophies. The nipples enlarge, darken, and become more erectile. From mid- to late pregnancy a normal thick, yellowish discharge called colostrum may be expressed from the nipple. The areolae darken, and Montgomery's glands appear prominent around the nipples. The venous pattern over the breasts becomes increasingly visible as pregnancy progresses.

The abdomen's most notable anatomical change is distention, primarily related to the increasing size of the growing uterus and fetus. Early distention from fluid retention and from the relaxation of abdominal muscles may be noted before the uterus becomes an abdominal organ (12–14 weeks of gestation). The expected growth patterns of the normal uterus and fetus are illustrated on the right, and the standing contours of the primigravid abdomen in each trimester of pregnancy are illustrated below.

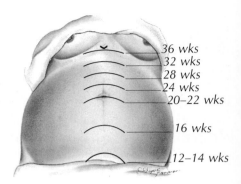

36 wks
32 wks
28 wks
24 wks
20–22 wks
16 wks
12–14 wks

EXPECTED HEIGHT OF THE UTERINE FUNDUS BY MONTH OF PREGNANCY

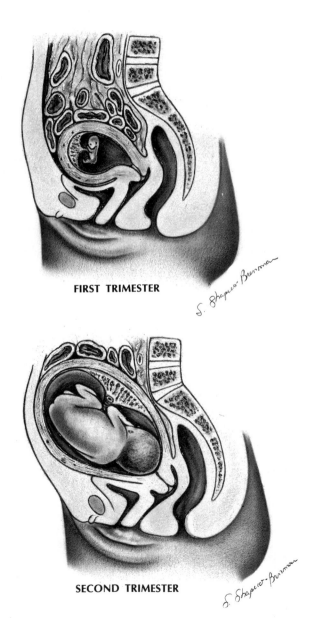

FIRST TRIMESTER

SECOND TRIMESTER

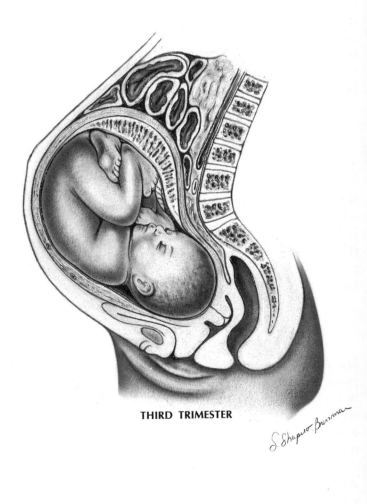

THIRD TRIMESTER

CHANGING CONTOURS OF THE PRIMIGRAVID ABDOMEN

As the skin stretches to accommodate the growth of the fetus, purplish striae may appear. Linea nigra, a brownish black pigmented line following the midline of the abdomen, may become evident. Muscle tone is diminished as pregnancy advances, and diastasis recti (separation of the rectus muscles at the midline of the abdomen) may be noticeable in the latter trimesters of pregnancy. If diastasis is severe (as it may be in multiparous women), only a layer of skin, fascia, and peritoneum covers most of the anterior uterine wall. The fetus is felt easily through this muscular gap.

Many anatomical changes take place in the pelvis through the course of pregnancy. The early diagnosis of pregnancy is based in part on the changes in the vagina and the uterus. With the increased vascularity throughout the pelvic region, the vagina takes on a bluish or violet color. The vaginal walls appear thicker and deeply rugated because of an increased thickness of the mucosa, loosening of the connective tissue, and hypertrophy of smooth muscle cells. Vaginal secretions are considerably increased, thick, and white. The pH becomes more acidic as a result of increased lactic acid from the action of *Lactobacillus acidophilus* on the increased levels of glycogen stored in the vaginal epithelium. This changing pH protects the pregnant woman from some vaginal infections, but the increased glycogen may contribute to higher rates of *Candida* (yeast) infection during pregnancy (see Table 13-5).

The uterus is clearly the organ most affected. Early in pregnancy, it loses the firmness and resistance of the nonpregnant organ. The palpable softening at the isthmus (Hegar's sign) is an early diagnostic sign of pregnancy, and is illustrated on the right.

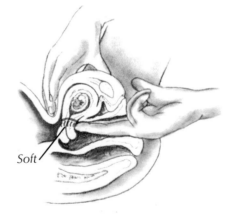

Soft

HEGAR'S SIGN

Over 9 months, the uterus increases in weight from 2 ounces to 2 pounds, largely because of increased size of muscle cells, an accumulation of fibrous tissue, a considerable increase in elastic tissue, and a great increase in the size and number of blood vessels and lymphatics. There is a 500- to 1,000-fold increase in size, so that by the end of pregnancy the uterus has a capacity of approximately 10 liters.

As the uterus grows, it changes shape and position. Prior to 12 weeks of gestation, it is a pelvic organ. As it enlarges, the anteverted uterus quickly takes up space normally occupied by the bladder, thus creating a need for frequent voiding. Irrespective of uterine position (anteverted, retroverted, or retroflexed), the uterus straightens and rises out of the pelvis by the end of 12 weeks' gestation, then becoming palpable abdominally. As it grows, it displaces the intestinal contents laterally and superiorly and also stretches the ligaments that support it, sometimes resulting in lower quadrant pain. The usually pear-shaped organ is altered by fetal growth and positions, and as the uterus grows it tends to rotate to the right to accommodate the rectosigmoid in the left side of the pelvis.

The cervix also looks and feels quite different during pregnancy than in a nonpregnant state. Pronounced softening and cyanosis appear very early after conception and continue throughout pregnancy (Chadwick's sign). The cervical canal is filled with a tenacious mucus (mucous plug) that protects the developing fetus from infection. Red, velvety mucosa around the os is common on the cervix during pregnancy and is considered normal.

COMMON COMPLAINTS OF PREGNANCY AND THEIR EXPLANATION

COMMON COMPLAINT	TIME IN PREGNANCY	EXPLANATION AND EFFECTS ON WOMAN'S BODY
No menses (amenorrhea)	Throughout	Continued high levels of estrogen, progesterone, and human chorionic gonadotropin following fertilization of the ovum allow the uterine endometrium to build up and support the developing pregnancy rather than to slough as menses.
Nausea with or without vomiting	First trimester	Possible causes include hormonal changes of pregnancy leading to slowed peristalsis throughout the GI tract, changes in taste and smell, the growing uterus, or emotional factors. Women may have a modest (2–5 lb) weight loss in the first trimester.
Breast tenderness, tingling	First trimester	The hormones of pregnancy stimulate the growth of breast tissue. As the breasts enlarge throughout pregnancy, women may experience upper backache from their increased weight. There is also increased blood flow throughout the breasts, increasing pressure on the tissue.
Urinary frequency (nonpathological)	First/third trimesters	There is increased blood volume and increased filtration rate in the kidneys with increased urine production. Due to less space for the bladder from pressure from the growing uterus (1st trimester) or from the descent of the fetal head (3rd trimester), the woman needs to empty her bladder more frequently.
Fatigue	First trimester	Mechanism(s) not clearly understood.
Heartburn Constipation	Throughout	Relaxation of the lower esophageal sphincter allows stomach contents to back up into the lower esophagus. The decreased GI motility caused by pregnancy hormones slows peristalsis and causes constipation. Constipation may cause or aggravate existing hemorrhoids.
Leukorrhea	Throughout	Increased secretions from the cervix and the vaginal epithelium, due to the hormones and vasocongestion of pregnancy, result in an asymptomatic milky white vaginal discharge.
Weight loss	First trimester	If a woman experiences nausea and vomiting, she may not be eating normally in early pregnancy. (See nausea above.)
Backache (nonpathological)	Throughout	Hormonally induced relaxation of joints and ligaments and the minor lordosis required to balance the growing uterus sometimes result in a lower backache. Pathological causes must be ruled out.

The ovaries and fallopian tubes undergo changes as well, but few are noticeable during physical examination. Early in pregnancy, the corpus luteum (the ovarian follicle that has discharged its ovum) may be sufficiently prominent to be felt on the affected ovary as a small nodule, but it disappears by midpregnancy. The major reason for thorough examination of the fallopian tubes is the need to rule out a tubal pregnancy (see p. 408).

Reproductive physiology is reviewed briefly in the table on p. 412. Physiological alterations during pregnancy affect anatomical changes that explain many of the normal symptoms and physical findings. One example is what happens to a woman's breasts in early pregnancy. Hormonal influences (estrogen, progesterone, and prolactin) lead to vasodilation and growth and proliferation of ducts and glands. These changes, in turn, result in tenderness, fullness, and tingling of the breasts and can make breast examination difficult as well as uncomfortable for the newly pregnant woman. Care needs to be taken during palpation to avoid undue discomfort while distinguishing between normal nodular changes of pregnancy and other breast masses.

THE PREGNANCY HISTORY

Accurate historical details are essential for directing both the order and the content of the physical examination. This examination is usually done to confirm the woman's suspicion of pregnancy, and the woman is most interested in pregnancy-related information and symptoms. The examiner, however, should also ascertain the general health of the woman. Details of the medical and psychosocial history related to pregnancy can be found in texts of nurse-midwifery and obstetrics noted in the bibliography.

In large measure, the history is directed toward risk factors known or suspected to diminish the health of either the woman or her developing fetus. The sociodemographic history includes age, income, adequacy of the social support network, and the woman's attitude toward this pregnancy, including whether she plans to keep it. Personal and family history of chronic diseases such as hypertension, diabetes, and cardiac conditions are important to know, along with family history of genetic disease. Past obstetrical history is particularly significant when the woman has had any major complication of pregnancy, labor, or birth or has given birth to a premature or growth-retarded infant. These conditions tend to repeat in subsequent pregnancies.

Exposure to teratogenic drugs, toxic substances in the workplace, or high levels of stress need to be known early in pregnancy, though prevention is done better before the woman conceives. Personal behaviors known to have adverse effects on the health of the pregnant woman and/or her fetus include over- or undernutrition, cigarette smoking, and use of alcohol and illicit drugs. Knowledge of these behaviors can lead to appropriate counseling during this first pregnancy assessment.

In addition, the clinician should get the history necessary to calculate the *expected weeks of gestation by dates.* This is currently counted in weeks from either (1) the first day of the last menstrual period (LMP), known as menstrual age, or (2) the date of conception, if this is known (conception age). Menstrual age is used most frequently to express the weeks of gestation calculated by dates. The first day of the last menstrual period (LMP) is also used to calculate the *expected date of confinement* (EDC) or projected time of term labor and birth for women with regular 28- to 30-day cycles. The EDC can be determined by adding 7 days to the first day of the last menstrual period, subtracting 3 months, and adding one year (Naegele's rule). This information is often one of the first questions the pregnant woman asks when seeking confirmation of pregnancy.

The weeks of gestation at the time of examination tell you what size the uterus should be if the LMP was normal, the dates were remembered accurately, and conception actually occurred. You should ascertain this size before examining the woman. You can then compare the expected size by dates with what you actually palpate during the bimanual examination (or abdominally, if pregnancy is beyond 14 weeks of gestation). Uterine size is measured by the palpable size of the uterus if still within the pelvic cavity, or by the height of the fundus if above the symphysis pubis. If there is a discrepancy, you need to look for the causes. Accurately dating the pregnancy is best done early, and contributes to good decision making later in pregnancy if the fetus is not growing well, if preterm labor is suspected, or if the pregnancy goes beyond 42 weeks of gestation. If the woman does not remember her LMP or has irregular menstrual cycles, dating the pregnancy is done by palpation and subsequent monitoring of the growth curve (see p. 410) along with the time of first fetal movements. In some cases, ultrasound is an appropriate adjunct in dating an early pregnancy.

The other historical data needed prior to examination include the symptoms of pregnancy such as breast tenderness, nausea or vomiting, urinary frequency, change in bowel habits, and fatigue (see table on p. 412). It is also important to find out whether the woman has ever had a complete pelvic examination before. If not, time will be needed to explain its details and seek her cooperation throughout. Explaining what you do and what you find are important if you are to maintain that cooperation and educate the woman about her body and what is happening to it in response to pregnancy.

Techniques of Examination

GENERAL APPROACH

The general approach to examining a pregnant woman is much the same as used with other patients. Equipment needs to be ready, the room prepared for privacy, the temperature comfortable, and the examiner aware of individual needs and sensitivities of the woman about to be examined. The dressing gown is put on most efficiently with the opening in the front. This allows for ease of examining both the breasts and the pregnant abdomen. Draping for the abdominal and pelvic examinations is similar to that discussed in earlier chapters.

POSITIONING

Positioning is important when examining the abdomen of a pregnant woman because of the added time and attention needed to palpate the uterus and listen to the fetal heart. The position affording the greatest comfort as well as protection from the negative effects of the weight of the gravid uterus on abdominal organs and vessels is semi-sitting with knees slightly bent, as shown below. This position is especially important

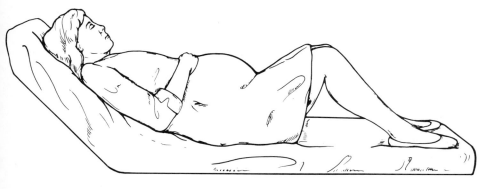

when examining a woman with an advanced pregnancy. In this case, prolonged periods of lying on the back should be avoided because the uterus then lies directly on the woman's vertebral column and may compress the descending aorta and inferior vena cava, thus interfering with the return of venous blood from the lower extremities and the pelvic vessels. Supine hypotension is a severe form of this diminished circulation in which the woman may experience dizziness and faint, especially when lying down. Therefore, abdominal palpation should be efficient in time and results. It is also recommended that the woman be allowed to sit again briefly before proceeding to the pelvic evaluation. This is a good time to allow the woman to empty her bladder again. Make sure, however, that she is acclimated to sitting before allowing her to stand up. The pelvic examination should likewise be relatively quick. All other examination procedures should be done in sitting or left-side-lying positions.

EQUIPMENT

The examiner's hands are the primary equipment for examination of the pregnant woman; they should be warm, and firm yet gentle in palpation. Whenever possible, the fingers should be together and flat against the abdominal or pelvic tissue, thus causing minimal discomfort. Likewise, all touching and palpation should be done with smooth, continuous movement in contact with the skin rather than kneading or abrupt contacts. The more sensitive palmar surfaces of the ends of the fingers will attain the greatest amount of information. Tender areas on the woman's body should be avoided until the end of the examination.

The gynecologic speculum is used for inspecting the cervix and the vagina and for taking specimens for cytologic or bacteriologic study. Because the vaginal walls are relaxed during pregnancy and may fall medially, obscuring your view, a speculum of larger than expected size may be needed. The relaxation of perineal and vulvar structures allows its use with minimal discomfort for the woman. Because of the increased vascularity of the vaginal and cervical structures, insert and open the speculum gently. You will thus avoid tissue trauma and bleeding. (Bleeding interferes with the interpretation of Pap smears.)

The cervical brush is not recommended for Pap smears in pregnant women because it often causes bleeding. The Ayre wooden spatula and/or cotton-tipped applicator are appropriate. (Review Chapter 13 for instruments and techniques used to take cervical smears).

GENERAL INSPECTION

Inspection for overall health, nutritional status, neuromuscular coordination, and emotional state can be made as the woman is walking into the exam room and climbing onto the examination table. Conversation related to the woman's priorities for the examination, her responses to pregnancy, and her general health provide the examiner with needed information and help to put the woman at ease.

VITAL SIGNS AND WEIGHT

Take the blood pressure. A baseline reading helps to determine the woman's usual range. In early and midpregnancy, blood pressure is normally lower than in the nonpregnant state.

High blood pressure prior to 24 weeks indicates chronic hypertension. After 24 weeks, it requires further evaluation to diagnose and treat pregnancy-induced hypertension (PIH).

Weigh the woman. First trimester weight loss related to nausea and vomiting is common, but should not exceed 5 pounds.

Weight loss of more than 5 pounds during the first trimester may be due to excessive vomiting (hyperemesis).

HEAD AND NECK

Stand facing the seated woman and observe the head and neck, including:

The face. The mask of pregnancy (chloasma) is normal. It consists of irregular brownish patches around the eyes or across the bridge of the nose.

Facial edema after 24 weeks of gestation suggests PIH.

Hair, including texture, moisture, and distribution. Dryness, oiliness, and sometimes minor generalized hair loss may be noted.

Localized patches of hair loss should not be attributed to pregnancy.

Eyes. Note the conjunctival color.

Anemia of pregnancy may cause pallor.

Nose, including the mucous membranes and the septum. Nasal congestion is common during pregnancy.

Nosebleeds are more common during pregnancy. Signs of cocaine use may be present.

Mouth, especially the gums and teeth

Gingival enlargement with bleeding (p. 225) is common during pregnancy.

Thyroid gland. Inspect and palpate the gland. Symmetrical enlargement is expected.

Marked or asymmetrical enlargement is not due to pregnancy.

THORAX AND LUNGS

Inspect the thorax for the pattern of breathing. Although women late in pregnancy sometimes report difficulty in breathing, there are usually no abnormal physical signs.

If signs of respiratory distress are noted, examine the lungs thoroughly.

HEART

Palpate for the apical impulse (PMI). In advanced pregnancy, it may be slightly higher than normal because of dextrorotation of the heart due to the higher diaphragm.

Auscultate the heart. Soft, blowing murmurs are common during pregnancy, reflecting increased blood flow in normal vessels.

These murmurs may also accompany anemia.

BREASTS

Inspect the breasts and nipples for symmetry and color. The venous pattern may be marked, the nipples and areolae are dark, and Montgomery's glands are prominent.

An inverted nipple needs attention if breast-feeding is planned.

Palpate for masses. During pregnancy, breasts are tender and nodular.

A pathologic mass may be difficult to isolate.

Compress each nipple between your index finger and thumb. This maneuver may express colostrum from the nipples.

A bloody or purulent discharge should not be attributed to pregnancy.

ABDOMEN

Position the pregnant woman in a semi-sitting position with her knees flexed (see p. 415).

Inspect for scars, striae, the shape and contour of the abdomen, and the fundal height. Purplish striae and linea nigra are normal in pregnancy. The shape and contour may indicate pregnancy size (see figures on p. 410).

Scars may confirm the type of prior surgery, especially cesarean section.

Palpate the abdomen for:

- *Organs or masses.* The mass of pregnancy is expected.

- *Fetal movements.* These can usually be felt by the examiner after 24 weeks (and by the mother at 18–20 weeks).

If movements cannot be felt after 24 weeks, consider error in calculating gestation, fetal death or morbidity, or false pregnancy.

- *Uterine contractility.* The uterus contracts irregularly after 12 weeks and often in response to palpation during the third trimester. The abdomen then feels tense or firm to the examiner, and it is difficult to feel fetal parts. If the hand is left resting on the fundal portion of the uterus, the fingers will sense the relaxation of the uterine muscle.

Prior to 37 weeks, regular uterine contractions with or without pain or bleeding are abnormal, suggesting preterm labor.

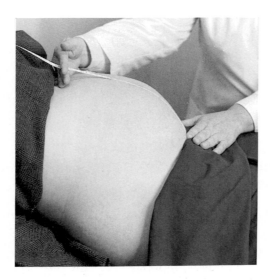

Measure the fundal height with a tape measure if the woman is more than 20 weeks pregnant. Holding the tape as illustrated and following the

If fundal height is more than 2 cm higher than expected, con-

midline of the abdomen, measure from the top of the symphysis pubis to the top of the uterine fundus. After 20 weeks, measurement in centimeters should roughly equal the weeks of gestation. For estimating fetal height between 12 and 20 weeks, see page 410.

Auscultate the fetal heart, noting its rate (FHR), location, and rhythm. Use either:

● Doptone, with which the FHR is audible after 12 weeks, or

● A fetoscope, with which it is audible after 18 wks.

sider multiple gestation, a big baby, extra amniotic fluid, or uterine myomata. If it is lower than expected by more than 2 cm, consider missed abortion, transverse lie, growth retardation, or false pregnancy.

Lack of an audible fetal heart may indicate pregnancy of fewer weeks than expected, fetal demise, or false pregnancy. An FHR that near term drops noticeably with movement could indicate poor placental circulation.

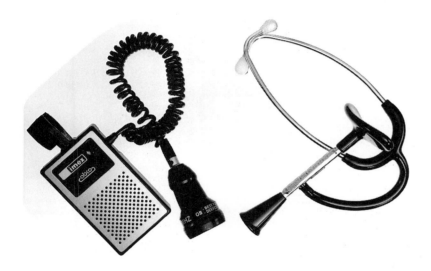

DOPTONE (LEFT) AND FETOSCOPE (RIGHT)

The *rate* is usually in the 160s during early pregnancy, then slows to the 120s to 140s near term. After 32 to 34 weeks, the FHR should increase with fetal movement.

The *location* of the audible FHR is in the midline of the lower abdomen from 12 to 18 weeks. After 28 weeks of gestation, the fetal heart is heard best over the fetal back or chest. The location of the FHR then depends on how the fetus is positioned. Palpating the fetal head and back helps you to know where to listen for it. (See Leopold's Maneuvers, pp. 422–424.) If the fetus is head down with the back on the woman's left side, the FHR is heard best in the lower left quadrant. If the fetal head is under the xiphoid process (breech presentation) with the back on the right, the FHR is heard in the upper right quadrant.

After 24 weeks, auscultation of more than one FHR in different locations on the maternal abdomen suggests more than one fetus.

Rhythm becomes important in the third trimester. Expect a variance of 10 to 15 beats per minute (BPM) over 1 to 2 minutes.

Lack of beat-to-beat variability late in pregnancy suggests fetal compromise.

FEMALE GENITALIA, ANUS, AND RECTUM

Inspect the *external genitalia,* noting the hair distribution, the color, and any scars. Parous relaxation of the introitus and noticeable enlargement of the labia and clitoris are normal. Scars from an episiotomy (a perineal incision to facilitate delivery of an infant) or from perineal lacerations may be present in multiparous women.

Some women have labial varicosities that become tortuous and painful.

Inspect the *anus* for varicosities (hemorrhoids). If these are present, note their size and location.

Varicosities often engorge later in pregnancy. They may be painful and bleed.

Palpate *Bartholin's and Skene's glands.* No discharge or tenderness should be present.

Check for a *cystocele* or *rectocele.*

May be pronounced due to the muscle relaxation of pregnancy

Speculum Examination. Take *Pap smears* and, if indicated, other vaginal or cervical specimens. The cervix may bleed more easily when touched due to the vasocongestion of pregnancy.

Vaginal infections are more common during pregnancy, and specimens may be needed for diagnosis.

Inspect the *vaginal walls* for color, discharge, rugae, and relaxation. A bluish or violet color, deep rugae, and an increased milky white discharge (leukorrhea) are normal.

A pink vagina suggests a non-pregnant state. Vaginal irritation and itching with discharge suggest infection.

Inspect the *cervix* for color, shape, and healed lacerations. A parous cervix may look irregular because of lacerations (see p. 403).

A pink cervix suggests a non-pregnant state.

Bimanual Examination. Insert two lubricated fingers into the introitus, palmar side down, with slight pressure downward on the perineum. Slide the fingers into the posterior vaginal vault. Maintaining downward pressure, gently turn the fingers palmar side up. Avoid the sensitive urethral structures at all times. With the relaxation of pregnancy, the bimanual examination is usually accomplished more easily. Tissues are soft and the vaginal walls usually close in on the examining fingers, giving the sensation of being immersed in a bowl of oatmeal. It may be difficult to distinguish the cervix at first because of its softer texture.

Place your finger gently in the os, then sweep it around the *surface of the cervix.* A nulliparous cervix should be closed, while a multiparous cervix may admit a fingertip through the external os. The internal os—the narrow passage between the endocervical canal and the uterine cavity—

should be closed in both situations. The surface of a normal multiparous cervix may feel irregular due to the healed lacerations from a previous birth.

Estimate the *length of the cervix* by palpating the lateral surface of the cervix from the cervical tip to the lateral fornix. Prior to 34 to 36 weeks, the cervix should retain its normal length of about 1.5 to 2 cm.

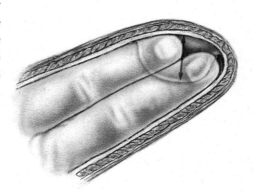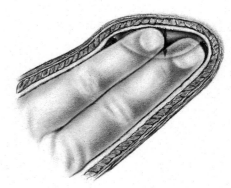

A shortened (effaced) cervix prior to 32 weeks may indicate preterm labor.

Palpate the *uterus* for size, shape, consistency, and position. These depend on the weeks of gestation. Early softening of the isthmus (Hegar's sign) is characteristic of pregnancy. The uterus is shaped like an inverted pear until 8 weeks, with slight enlargement in the fundal portion. The uterus becomes globular by 10 to 12 weeks. Anteflexion or retroflexion is lost by 12 weeks, with the fundal portion measuring about 8 cm in diameter.

With your internal fingers placed at either side of the cervix, palmar surfaces upward, gently lift the uterus toward the abdominal hand. Capture the fundal portion of the uterus between your two hands and gently estimate uterine size.

An irregularly shaped uterus suggests uterine myomata or a bicornuate uterus (two distinct uterine cavities separated by a septum).

Palpate the *left and right adnexa*. The corpus luteum may feel like a small nodule on the affected ovary during the first few weeks after conception. Late in pregnancy, adnexal masses may be difficult to feel.

Early in pregnancy, it is important to rule out a tubal (ectopic) pregnancy. See Table 13-7, Adnexal Masses, p. 408.

Palpate for *pelvic muscle strength* as you withdraw your examining fingers.

A *rectovaginal examination* may be done if you need to confirm uterine size or the integrity of the rectovaginal septum. A pregnancy of less than 10 weeks in a retroverted and retroflexed uterus lies totally in the posterior pelvis. Its size can be confirmed only by this examination.

EXTREMITIES

General inspection may be done with the woman seated or lying on her left side.

Inspect the legs for *varicose veins.*

Inspect the hands and legs for *edema.* Palpate for pretibial, ankle, and pedal edema. Edema is rated on a 0 to 4+ scale. Physiologic edema is more common in advanced pregnancy, during hot weather, and in women who stand a lot.

Obtain knee and ankle *reflexes.*

SPECIAL MANEUVERS

MODIFIED LEOPOLD'S MANEUVERS. These maneuvers are important adjuncts to palpation of the pregnant abdomen from 28 weeks of gestation onward. The information gained is translated into where the fetus is lying in relation to the woman's back (longitudinal or transverse), what end of the fetus is presenting at the pelvic inlet (head or buttocks), where the fetal back is located, how far the presenting part of the fetus has descended into the maternal pelvis, and the estimated weight of the fetus. This information is necessary to assess the adequacy of fetal growth and the probability of successful vaginal birth.

First Maneuver (Upper Pole). Stand at the woman's side facing her head. Keeping the fingers of both examining hands together, palpate gently with the fingertips to determine what part of the fetus is in the upper pole of the uterine fundus.

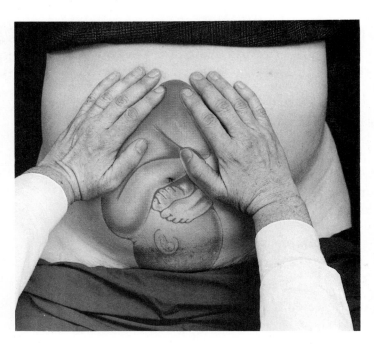

Varicose veins may begin or worsen during pregnancy.

Pathologic edema associated with PIH is often 3+ or more pretibially; it also affects the hands and face.

After 24 weeks, reflexes greater than 2+ may indicate PIH.

Interpretation

Common deviations include breech presentation (the fetal buttocks presenting at the outlet of the maternal pelvis) and absence of the presenting part well down into the maternal pelvis at term. Neither situation necessarily precludes vaginal birth. The most serious findings are a transverse lie close to term and slowed fetal growth that could represent intrauterine growth retardation (IUGR).

Most commonly, the fetal buttocks are at the upper pole. They feel firm but irregular, and less globular than the head. The fetal head feels firm, round, and smooth.

Second Maneuver (Sides of the Maternal Abdomen). Place one hand on each side of the woman's abdomen, aiming to capture the body of the fetus between them. Use one hand to steady the uterus and the other to palpate the fetus.

The hand on the fetal back feels a smooth, firm surface the length of the hand (or longer) by 32 weeks of gestation. The hand on the fetal arms and legs feels irregular bumps, and also perhaps kicking, if the fetus is awake and active.

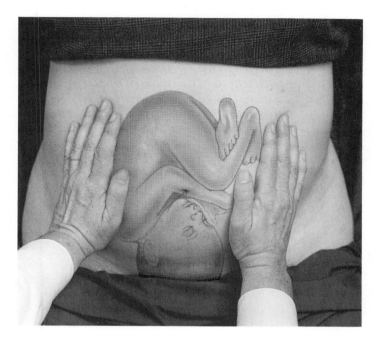

Third Maneuver (Lower Pole). Turn and face the woman's feet. Using the flat palmar surfaces of the fingers of both hands and, at the start, touching the fingertips together, palpate the area just above the symphysis pubis. Note whether the hands diverge with downward pressure or stay together. This tells you whether or not the presenting part of the fetus (head or buttocks) is descending into the pelvic inlet.

If the fetal head is presenting, the fingers feel a smooth, firm, rounded surface on both sides.

If the hands diverge, the presenting part is descending into the pelvic inlet, as illustrated. If the hands stay together and you can gently depress the tissue over the bladder without touching the fetus, the presenting part is above your hands.

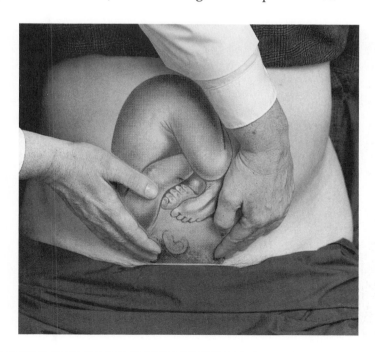

If the presenting fetal part is descending, palpate its texture and firmness. If not, gently move your hands up the lower abdomen and capture the presenting part between your hands.

Fourth Maneuver (Confirmation of the Presenting Part). With your dominant hand grasp the part of the fetus in the lower pole, and with your nondominant hand the part of the fetus in the upper pole. With this maneuver, you may be able to distinguish between the head and the buttocks.

The fetal head feels smooth, firm, and rounded; the buttocks, firm but irregular.

Most commonly, the head is in the lower pole and the fetal buttocks are in the upper pole. If the head is above the pelvic inlet, it moves somewhat independently of the rest of the fetal body.

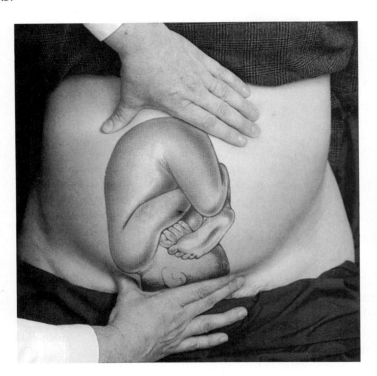

CONCLUDING THE VISIT

Once the examination is completed and the woman is dressed, review the findings with her. If further data are necessary to confirm pregnancy, discuss how these may be obtained. Reinforce the woman's need to continue with prenatal supervision. Record all the findings on the prenatal record.

Chapter 15
The Anus, Rectum, and Prostate

Anatomy and Physiology

The gastrointestinal tract terminates in a short segment, the anal canal. Its external margin is poorly demarcated, but generally the skin of the anal canal can be distinguished from the surrounding perianal skin by its moist, hairless appearance. The anal canal is normally held in a closed position by action of the voluntary external muscular sphincter and the involuntary internal sphincter, the latter an extension of the muscular coat of the rectal wall.

The direction of the anal canal on a line roughly between anus and umbilicus should be noted carefully. Unlike the rectum above it, the canal is liberally supplied by somatic sensory nerves, and a poorly directed finger or instrument will produce pain.

The anal canal is demarcated from the rectum superiorly by a serrated line marking the change from skin to mucous membrane. This anorectal

CROSS SECTION, SIDE VIEW

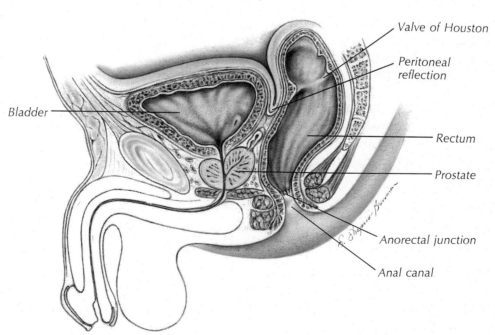

Valve of Houston

Peritoneal reflection

Bladder

Rectum

Prostate

Anorectal junction

Anal canal

junction (often called the pectinate or dentate line) also denotes the boundary between somatic and visceral nerve supplies. It is readily visible on proctoscopic examination, but is not palpable.

Above the anorectal junction, the rectum balloons out and turns posteriorly into the hollow of the coccyx and the sacrum. In the male, the prostate gland is palpable anteriorly as a rounded, heart-shaped structure about 2.5 cm in length. Its two lateral lobes are separated by a shallow median sulcus or groove. The seminal vesicles, shaped like rabbit ears above the prostate, are not normally palpable.

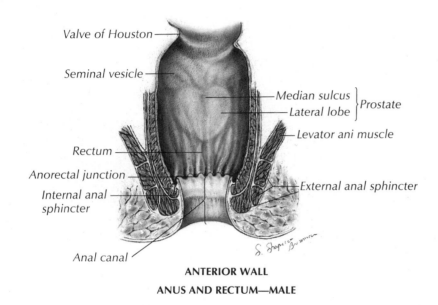

ANTERIOR WALL

ANUS AND RECTUM—MALE

Through the anterior wall of the female rectum, the uterine cervix can usually be felt.

The rectal wall contains three inward foldings, called valves of Houston. The lowest of these can sometimes be felt, usually on the patient's left.

Most of the rectum that is accessible to digital examination does not have a peritoneal surface. The anterior rectum usually does, however, and you may reach it with the tip of your examining finger. You may thus be able to identify the tenderness of peritoneal inflammation or the nodularity of peritoneal metastases.

CHANGES WITH AGE

The prostate gland is small during boyhood, but between puberty and the age of about 20 years it increases roughly five-fold in size. Starting in about the fifth decade, further enlargement is increasingly common as the gland becomes hyperplastic (see p. 433).

Techniques of Examination

For most patients, the rectal examination is probably the least popular segment of the entire physical examination. It may cause discomfort for the patient, perhaps embarrassment, but, if skillfully done, should not be truly painful in most circumstances. Although you may choose to omit a rectal examination in adolescents who have no relevant complaints, you should do one in adult patients. In middle-aged and older persons, omission risks missing an asymptomatic carcinoma. A successful examination requires gentleness, slow movement of your finger, a calm demeanor, and an explanation to the patient of what he or she may feel.

MALE

The anus and rectum may be examined with the patient in one of several positions. For most purposes, the side-lying position is satisfactory and allows good visualization of the perianal and sacrococcygeal areas. This is the position described below. The lithotomy position may help you to reach a cancer high in the rectum. It also permits a bimanual examination, enabling you to delineate a pelvic mass. Some clinicians prefer to examine a patient while he stands with his hips flexed and his upper body resting across the examining table.

No matter how you position the patient, your examining finger cannot reach the full length of the rectum. If a rectosigmoid cancer is suspected, direct visualization by proctosigmoidoscopy is necessary.

Ask the patient to lie on his left side with his buttocks close to the edge of the examining table near you. Flexing the patient's hips and knees, especially in the top leg, stabilizes his position and improves visibility. Drape the patient appropriately and adjust the lighting for good visualization of the anus and surrounding area. Glove one or both of your hands and spread the buttocks apart.

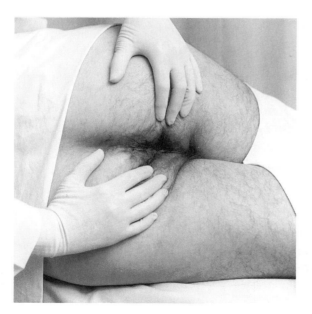

Inspect the sacrococcygeal and perianal areas for lumps, ulcers, inflammation, rashes, or excoriations. Adult perianal skin is normally more pigmented and somewhat coarser than the skin over the buttocks. Palpate any abnormal areas, noting lumps or tenderness.

Examine the anus and rectum. Lubricate your gloved index finger, explain to the patient what you are going to do, and tell him that the examination may make him feel as if he were moving his bowels but that he will not do so. Ask him to strain down. Inspect the anus, noting any lesions.

As the patient strains, place the pad of your lubricated and gloved index finger over the anus. As the sphincter relaxes, gently insert your fingertip into the anal canal, in a direction pointing toward the umbilicus.

Anal and perianal lesions include hemorrhoids, venereal warts, herpes, syphilitic chancre, and carcinoma. A perianal abscess produces a painful, tender, indurated, and reddened mass. Pruritus ani causes swollen, thickened, fissured skin with excoriations.

Soft, pliable tags of redundant skin at the anal margin are common. Though sometimes due to past anal surgery or previously thrombosed hemorrhoids, they are often unexplained.

See Table 15-1, Abnormalities of the Anus, Surrounding Skin, and Rectum (pp. 431–432).

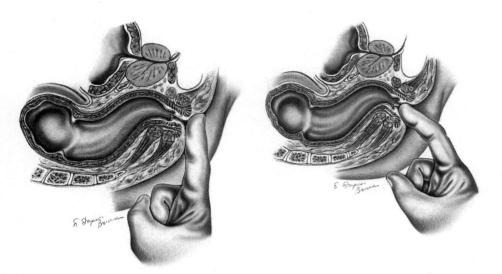

If you feel the sphincter tighten, pause and reassure the patient. When in a moment the sphincter relaxes, proceed. Occasionally, severe tenderness prevents you from examining the anus. Do not try to force it. Instead, place your fingers on both sides of the anus, gently spread the orifice, and ask the patient to strain down. Look for a lesion such as an anal fissure.

Note:

● The sphincter tone of the anus. Normally, the muscles of the anal sphincter close snugly around your finger.

Sphincter tightness in anxiety, inflammation, or scarring; laxity in some neurologic diseases

● Tenderness

- Induration

Induration may be due to inflammation, scarring, or malignancy.

- Irregularities or nodules

Insert your finger into the rectum as far as possible. Rotate your hand clockwise, then counterclockwise, to palpate as much of the rectal surface as you can reach—first toward the patient's right side, then posteriorly, and then toward the patient's left. Note any nodules, irregularities, or induration. To bring a possible lesion into reach, take your finger off the rectal surface, ask the patient to strain down, and palpate again.

The irregular border of a rectal cancer is shown below.

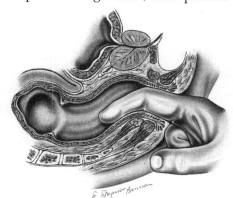

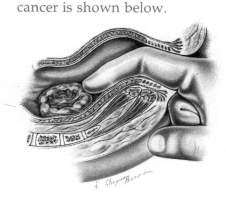

Then rotate your hand further counterclockwise so that your finger can *examine the posterior surface of the prostate gland.* By turning your body somewhat away from the patient, you can feel this area more easily. Tell the patient that you are going to feel his prostate gland, and that it may make him want to urinate but he will not do so.

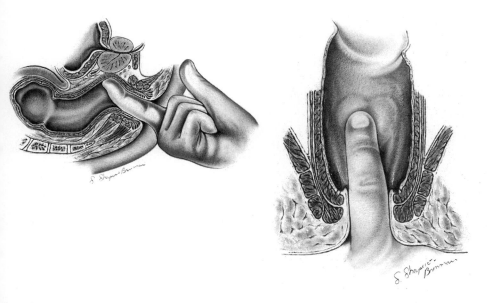

Sweep your finger carefully over the prostate gland, identifying its lateral lobes and the median sulcus between them. Note the size, shape, and consistency of the prostate, and identify any nodules or tenderness. The normal prostate is rubbery and nontender.

See Table 15-2, Abnormalities of the Prostate (p. 433).

If possible, *extend your finger above the prostate* to the region of the seminal vesicles and the peritoneal cavity. Note nodules or tenderness.

Gently withdraw your finger, and wipe the patient's anus or give him tissues to do it himself. Note the color of any fecal matter on your glove, and test it for occult blood.

A rectal "shelf" of peritoneal metastases (see p. 432) or the tenderness of peritoneal inflammation.

FEMALE

The rectum is usually examined after the female genitalia, while the patient is in the lithotomy position. If a rectal examination alone is indicated, the lateral position offers a satisfactory alternative. It affords much better visualization of the perianal and sacrococcygeal areas.

The technique is basically similar to that described for males. The cervix is usually felt readily through the anterior rectal wall. Sometimes, a retroverted uterus is also palpable. Neither of these, nor a vaginal tampon, should be mistaken for a tumor.

Table 15-1   Abnormalities of the Anus, Surrounding Skin, and Rectum

Table 15-1   Abnormalities of the Anus, Surrounding Skin, and Rectum

PILONIDAL CYST AND SINUS

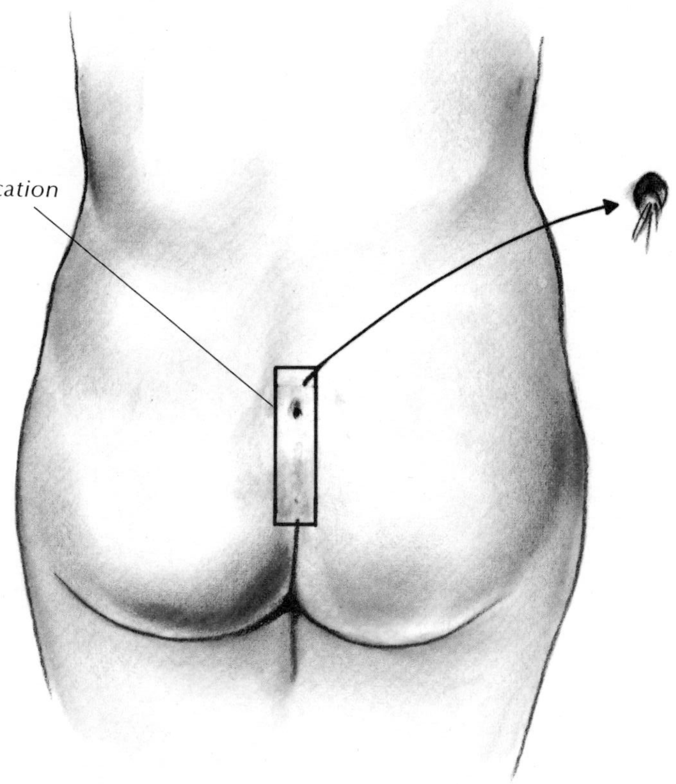

Location

A pilonidal cyst is a fairly frequent, probably congenital abnormality located in the midline superficial to the coccyx or the lower sacrum. It is clinically identified by the opening of a sinus tract. This opening may exhibit a small tuft of hair and be surrounded by a halo of erythema. Although pilonidal cysts are generally asymptomatic, except perhaps for slight drainage, abscess formation and secondary sinus tracts may complicate the picture.

ANORECTAL FISTULA

Opening

Fistula

Fissure

Sentinel tag

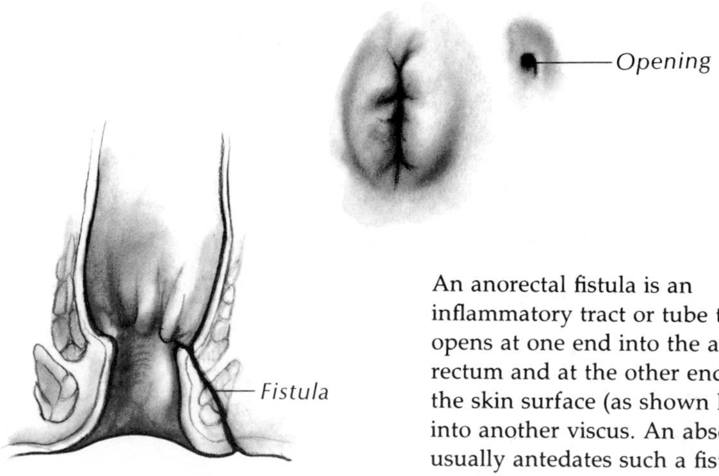

An anorectal fistula is an inflammatory tract or tube that opens at one end into the anus or rectum and at the other end onto the skin surface (as shown here) or into another viscus. An abscess usually antedates such a fistula. Look for the fistulous opening or openings anywhere in the skin around the anus.

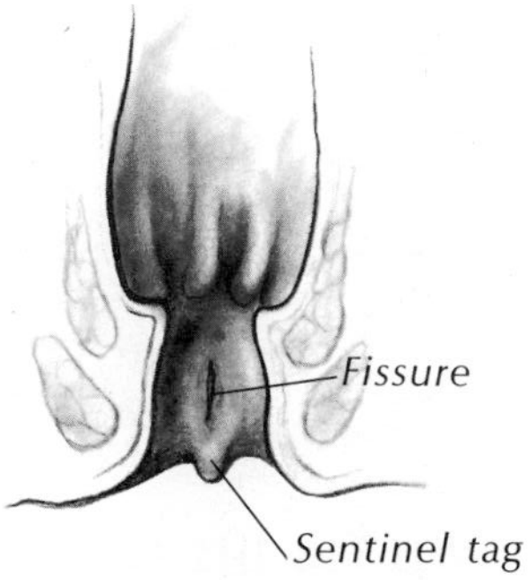

An anal fissure is a very painful oval ulceration of the anal canal, found most commonly in the midline posteriorly, less commonly in the midline anteriorly. Its long axis lies longitudinally. Inspection may show a swollen "sentinel" skin tag just below it, and gentle separation of the anal margins may reveal the lower edge of the fissure. The sphincter is spastic; the examination painful. Local anesthesia may be required.

▶ *Continued*

Table 15-1 Abnormalities of the Anus, Surrounding Skin, and Rectum

Table 15-1 (Cont'd.)

EXTERNAL HEMORRHOIDS

External hemorrhoids are dilated hemorrhoidal veins that originate below the pectinate line and are covered with skin. They seldom produce symptoms unless thrombosis occurs. This causes acute local pain that is increased by defecation and by sitting. A tender, swollen, bluish, ovoid mass is visible at the anal margin.

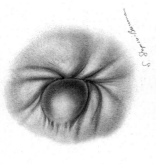

INTERNAL HEMORRHOIDS

ANTERIOR

Internal hemorrhoids are an enlargement of the normal vascular cushions that are located above the pectinate line. Here they are not usually palpable. Sometimes, especially during defecation, internal hemorrhoids may cause bright red bleeding. They may also prolapse through the anal canal and appear as reddish, moist, protruding masses, typically located in one or more of the positions illustrated.

POSTERIOR

PROLAPSED HEMORRHOIDS

PROLAPSE OF THE RECTUM

On straining for a bowel movement the rectal mucosa, with or without its muscular wall, may prolapse through the anus, appearing as a doughnut or rosette of red tissue. A prolapse involving only mucosa is relatively small and shows radiating folds, as illustrated. When the entire bowel wall is involved, the prolapse is larger and covered by concentrically circular folds.

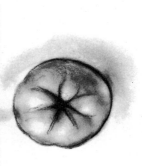

POLYPS OF THE RECTUM

Polyps of the rectum are fairly common. Variable in size and number, they can develop on a stalk (pedunculated) or lie close to the mucosal surface (sessile). They are soft and may be difficult or impossible to feel even when in reach of the examining finger. Proctoscopy is usually required for diagnosis, as is biopsy for the differentiation of benign from malignant lesions.

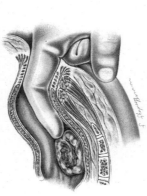

CANCER OF THE RECTUM

Asymptomatic carcinoma of the rectum makes routine rectal examination important for adults. Illustrated here is the firm, nodular, rolled edge of an ulcerated cancer. Polyps, as noted above, may also be malignant.

RECTAL SHELF

Widespread peritoneal metastases from any source may develop in the area of the peritoneal reflection anterior to the rectum. A firm to hard nodular rectal "shelf" may be just palpable with the tip of the examining finger. In a woman, this shelf of metastatic tissue develops in the rectouterine pouch, behind the cervix and the uterus.

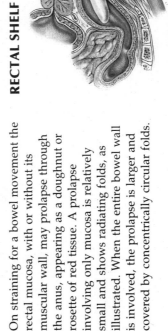

Table 15-2   Abnormalities of the Prostate

Table 15-2 Abnormalities of the Prostate

THE NORMAL PROSTATE GLAND

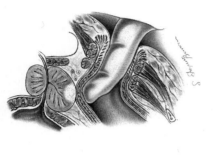

As palpated through the anterior rectal wall, the normal prostate is a rounded, heart-shaped structure about 2.5 cm in length. The median sulcus can be felt between the two lateral lobes. Only the posterior surface of the prostate is palpable. Anterior lesions, including those that may obstruct the urethra, may not be detectable by physical examination.

CANCER OF THE PROSTATE

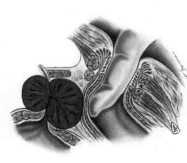

Cancer of the prostate is suggested by an area of hardness in the gland. A distinct hard nodule that alters the contour of the gland may or may not be palpable. As the cancer enlarges, it feels irregular and may extend beyond the confines of the gland. The median sulcus may be obscured.

Hard areas in the prostate are not always malignant. They may also result from prostatic stones, chronic inflammation, and other conditions.

BENIGN PROSTATIC HYPERPLASIA *(HYPERTROPHY)*

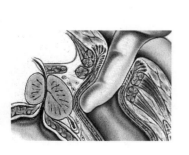

Starting in the fifth decade of life, benign prostatic hyperplasia becomes increasingly prevalent. The affected gland usually feels symmetrically enlarged, smooth, and firm though slightly elastic. It seems to protrude more into the rectal lumen. The median sulcus may be obliterated. Finding a normal-sized gland by palpation, however, does not rule out this diagnosis. Prostatic hyperplasia may obstruct urinary flow, causing symptoms, yet not be palpable.

PROSTATITIS

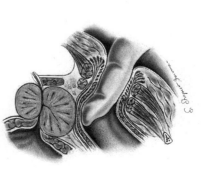

Acute prostatitis (illustrated here) is an acute, febrile condition caused by bacterial infection. The gland is very tender, swollen, firm, and warm. Examine it gently.

Chronic prostatitis does not produce consistent physical findings and must be evaluated by other methods.

433

Chapter 16
The Peripheral Vascular System

Anatomy and Physiology

This chapter focuses on the circulatory supply to the arms and legs. It includes the arteries, the veins, the capillary bed that connects them, and the lymphatic system with its lymph nodes.

ARTERIES

Arterial pulses are palpable when an artery lies close to the body surface. In the arms, there or two or sometimes three such locations. Pulsations of the *brachial artery* can be felt in and above the bend of the elbow, just medial to the biceps tendon and muscle. The brachial artery divides into the radial and ulnar arteries. *Radial artery* pulsations can be felt on the flexor surface of the wrist laterally. Medially, pulsations of the *ulnar artery* may be palpable, but overlying tissues frequently obscure them.

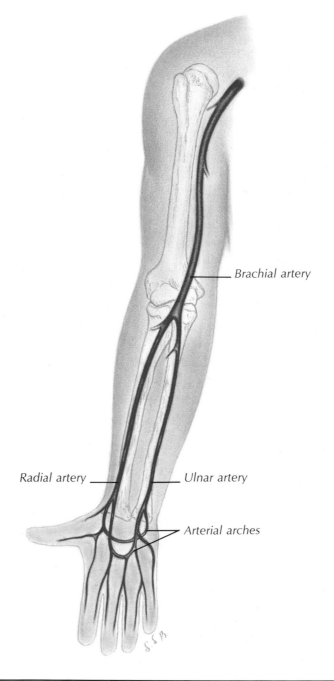

Brachial artery

Radial artery   *Ulnar artery*

Arterial arches

The radial and ulnar arteries are interconnected by two vascular arches within the hand. Circulation to the hand and fingers is thereby doubly protected against possible arterial occlusion.

In the legs, arterial pulsations can usually be felt in four places. Those of the *femoral artery* are palpable below the inguinal ligament, midway between the anterior superior iliac spine and the symphysis pubis. The femoral artery travels downward deep within the thigh, passes medially behind the femur, and becomes the *popliteal artery*. Popliteal pulsations can be felt in the tissues behind the knee. Below the knee, the popliteal artery divides into two branches, both of which continue to the foot. There the anterior branch becomes the *dorsalis pedis artery*. Its pulsations are palpable on the dorsum of the foot just lateral to the extensor tendon of the big toe. The posterior branch, the *posterior tibial artery*, can be felt as it passes behind the medial malleolus of the ankle.

Like the hand, the foot is protected by an interconnecting arch between the two chief arterial branches that supply it.

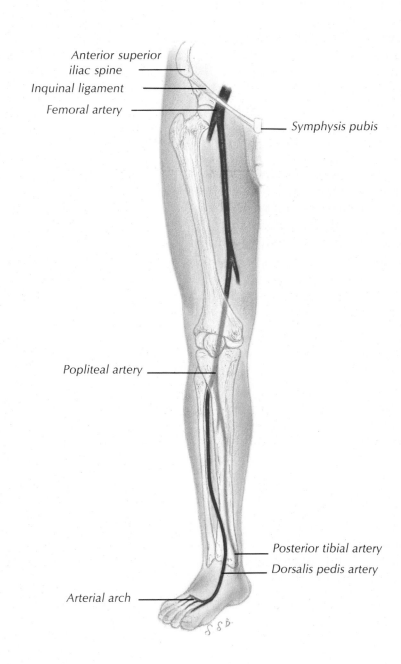

Anterior superior iliac spine

Inquinal ligament

Femoral artery

Symphysis pubis

Popliteal artery

Posterior tibial artery

Dorsalis pedis artery

Arterial arch

VEINS

The veins from the arms, together with those from the upper trunk and the head and neck, drain into the superior vena cava and on into the right atrium. Veins from the legs and the lower trunk drain upward into the inferior vena cava. Because the leg veins are especially susceptible to dysfunction, they warrant special attention.

The *deep veins* of the legs carry about 90% of the venous return from the lower extremities. They are well supported by surrounding tissues.

In contrast, the *superficial veins* are located subcutaneously, and are supported relatively poorly. The superficial veins include (1) the *great saphenous vein,* which originates on the dorsum of the foot, passes just in front of the medial malleolus, and then continues up the medial aspect of the leg to join the deep venous system (the femoral vein) below the inguinal ligament; and (2) the *small saphenous vein,* which begins at the side of the foot and passes upward along the back of the leg to join the deep system in the popliteal space. Anastomotic veins connect the two saphenous veins superficially and, when dilated, are readily visible. In addition, *communicating (or perforating) veins* connect the saphenous system with the deep venous system.

Deep, superficial, and communicating veins all have one-way valves within them. These allow venous blood to flow from the superficial to the deep system and toward the heart, but not in the opposite directions. Muscular activity contributes importantly to venous blood flow. As calf muscles contract in walking, for example, blood is squeezed upward against gravity, and competent valves keep it from falling back again.

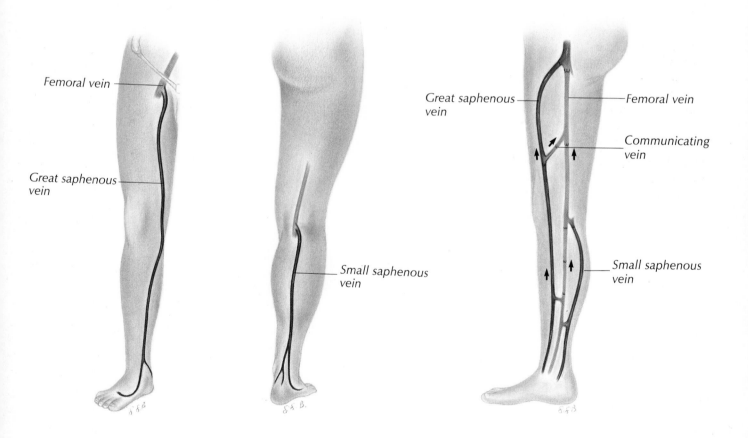

THE LYMPHATIC SYSTEM AND LYMPH NODES

The lymphatic system comprises an extensive vascular network that drains fluid, called lymph, from bodily tissues and returns it to the venous circulation. The system starts peripherally as blind lymphatic capillaries and continues centrally as thin vascular vessels and then collecting ducts that finally empty into major veins at the root of the neck. The lymph transported in these channels is filtered through lymph nodes that are interposed along the way.

Lymph nodes are round, oval, or bean-shaped structures that vary in size according to their location. Some lymph nodes, such as the preauriculars, if palpable at all, are typically very small. The inguinal nodes, in contrast, are relatively large—often 1 cm in diameter or occasionally even 2 cm in an adult.

In addition to its vascular functions, the lymphatic system plays an important role in the body's immune system. Cells within the lymph nodes engulf foreign substances and produce antibodies.

Only the superficial lymph nodes are accessible to physical examination. These include the cervical nodes (p. 168), the axillary nodes (p. 326), and nodes in the arms and legs.

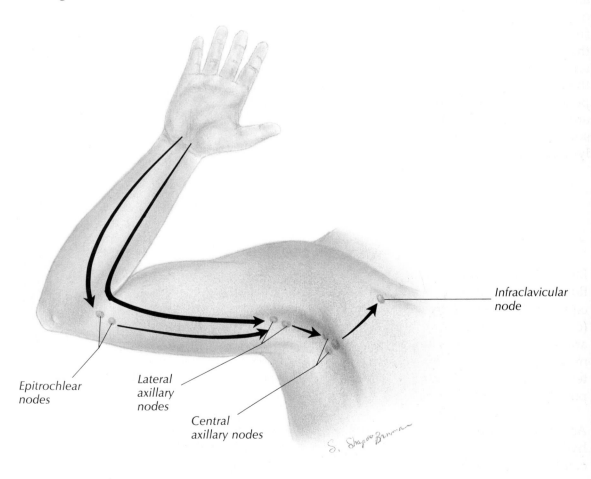

Epitrochlear nodes

Lateral axillary nodes

Central axillary nodes

Infraclavicular node

Recall that the axillary lymph nodes drain most of the arm. Lymphatics from the ulnar surface of the forearm and hand, the little and ring fingers, and the adjacent surface of the middle finger, however, drain first into the *epitrochlear nodes.* These are located on the medial surface of the arm about 3 cm above the elbow. Lymphatics from the rest of the arm drain mostly into the axillary nodes. A few may go directly to the infra-claviculars.

The lymphatics of the lower limb, following the venous supply, consist of both deep and superficial systems. Only the superficial nodes are palpable. The *superficial inguinal nodes* include two groups. The *horizontal group* lies in a chain high in the anterior thigh below the inguinal ligament. It drains the superficial portions of the lower abdomen and buttock, the external genitalia (but not the testes), the anal canal and perianal area, and the lower vagina.

The *vertical group* clusters near the upper part of the saphenous vein and drains a corresponding region of the leg. In contrast, lymphatics from the portion of leg drained by the small saphenous vein (the heel and outer aspect of the foot) join the deep system at the level of the popliteal space. Lesions in this area, therefore, are not usually associated with palpable inguinal lymph nodes.

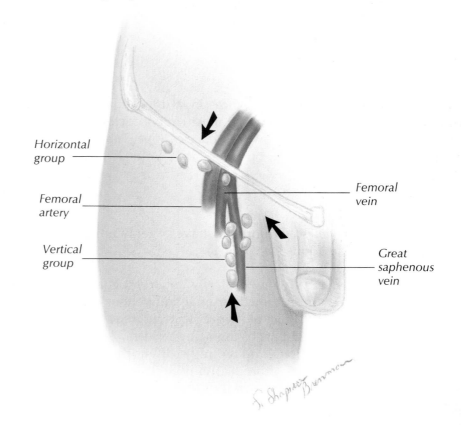

Horizontal group

Femoral artery

Vertical group

Femoral vein

Great saphenous vein

FLUID EXCHANGE AND THE CAPILLARY BED

Blood circulates from arteries to veins through the capillary bed. Here fluids diffuse across the capillary membrane, maintaining a dynamic equilibrium between the vascular and interstitial spaces. Blood pressure (or hydrostatic pressure) within the capillary bed, especially near the arteriolar end, forces fluid out into the tissue spaces. In effecting this movement, it is aided by the relatively weak osmotic attraction of proteins within the tissues (interstitial colloid osmotic pressure) and is opposed by the hydrostatic pressure of the tissues.

As blood continues through the capillary bed toward the venous end its hydrostatic pressure falls, and another force gains dominance. This is the colloid osmotic pressure of plasma proteins, which pulls fluid back into the vascular tree. Net flow of fluid, which was directed outward on the arteriolar side of the capillary bed, reverses itself and turns inward on the venous side. Lymphatic capillaries, which also play an important role in this equilibrium, remove excessive fluid, including protein, from the interstitial space.

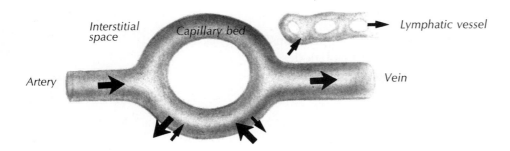

Lymphatic dysfunction or disturbances in hydrostatic or osmotic forces can all disrupt this equilibrium. The most common clinical result is the increased interstitial fluid known as edema. (See Table 16-1, Mechanisms and Patterns of Edema, pp. 455–456.)

CHANGES WITH AGE

Children and young adolescents normally have larger lymph nodes relative to body size than do adults (see p. 561).

Aging itself brings relatively few clinically important changes to the peripheral vascular system. Although arterial and venous disorders, especially atherosclerosis, do afflict older people more frequently, they probably cannot be considered part of the aging process. Age lengthens the arteries, makes them tortuous, and typically stiffens their walls, but these changes develop with or without atherosclerosis and therefore lack diagnostic specificity. Loss of arterial pulsations is not a part of normal aging, however, and demands careful evaluation. Skin may get thin and dry with age, nails may grow more slowly, and hair on the legs often becomes scant. Because these changes are common, they are not specific for arterial insufficiency, although they are classically associated with it.

Techniques of Examination

Assessment of the peripheral vascular system relies primarily on inspection of the arms and legs, palpation of the pulses, and a search for edema. See Chapter 4 for a method of integrating these techniques into your examination of the limbs. Additional maneuvers may be useful when you suspect an abnormality.

ARMS

Inspect both arms from the fingertips to the shoulders. Note:

- Their size, symmetry, and any swelling
- The venous pattern
- The color of the skin and nail beds and the texture of the skin

Palpate the *radial pulse* with the pads of your fingers on the flexor surface of the wrist laterally. Compare the pulses in both arms.

Edema of an arm with prominent veins suggests venous obstruction.

Lymphedema of arm and hand may follow radical mastectomy with axillary node dissection.

In Raynaud's disease, wrist pulses are typically normal, but spasm of more distal arteries causes episodes of sharply demarcated pallor of the fingers.

Pulses here or elsewhere in the body may be described as increased, normal, diminished, or absent. If an artery is widely dilated, it is aneurysmal.

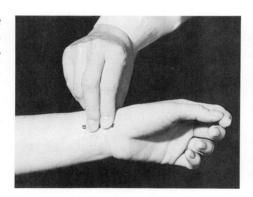

If you suspect arterial insufficiency, feel for the *brachial pulse*. Flex the patient's elbow slightly, and with the thumb of your opposite hand palpate the artery just medial to the biceps tendon at the antecubital crease. The brachial artery can also be felt higher in the arm in the groove between the biceps and triceps muscles.

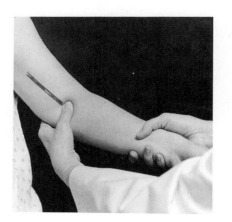

Feel for one or more *epitrochlear nodes*. With the patient's elbow flexed to about 90° and the forearm supported by your hand, reach around behind the arm and feel in the groove between the biceps and triceps muscles, about 3 cm above the medial epicondyle. If a node is present, note its size, consistency, and tenderness.

Epitrochlear nodes are difficult or impossible to identify in most normal people.

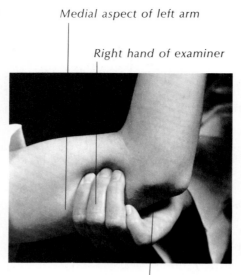

Medial aspect of left arm

Right hand of examiner

Medial epicondyle of humerus

An enlarged epitrochlear node may be secondary to a lesion in its drainage area or may be associated with generalized lymphadenopathy.

LEGS

The patient should be lying down and draped so that the external genitalia are covered and the legs fully exposed. A good examination is impossible through stockings or socks!

Inspect both legs from the groin and buttocks to the feet. Note:

- Their size, symmetry, and any swelling
- The venous pattern and any venous enlargement
- Any pigmentation, rashes, scars, or ulcers
- The color and texture of the skin, the color of the nail beds, and the distribution of hair on the lower legs, feet, and toes

Palpate the *superficial inguinal nodes*, including both the horizontal and the vertical groups. Note their size, consistency, and discreteness, and note any tenderness. Nontender, discrete inguinal nodes up to 1 cm or even 2 cm in diameter are frequently palpable in normal people.

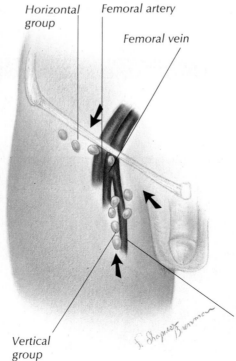

Horizontal group　*Femoral artery*

Femoral vein

Vertical group

Great saphenous vein

See Color Plate 16-1, Chronic Insufficiency of Arteries and Veins (p. 453).

See Color Plate 16-2, Common Ulcers of the Feet and Ankles (p. 454).

Lymphadenopathy refers to enlargement of the nodes, with or without tenderness. Try to distinguish between local and generalized lymphadenopathy, respectively, by finding either (1) a causative lesion in the drainage area, or (2) enlarged nodes in at least two other noncontiguous lymph node regions.

Palpate the pulses in order to assess the arterial circulation.

● *The femoral pulse.* Press deeply, below the inguinal ligament and about midway between the anterior superior iliac spine and the symphysis pubis. As in deep abdominal palpation, the use of two hands, one on top of the other, may facilitate this examination, especially in obese patients.

Significant decrease in or absence of arterial pulses in the legs is most commonly due to arteriosclerosis obliterans. When a pulse is diminished or absent, it indicates partial or complete arterial occlusion proximally. A decreased or absent femoral pulse, for example, suggests disease at the aortic or iliac level. All pulses distal to the occlusion are typically affected. Chronic arterial occlusion causes intermittent claudication (pp. 88–89), postural color changes (pp. 450–451), and trophic changes in the skin (p. 453).

An exaggerated, widened femoral pulse suggests a femoral aneurysm, a pathologic dilatation of the artery.

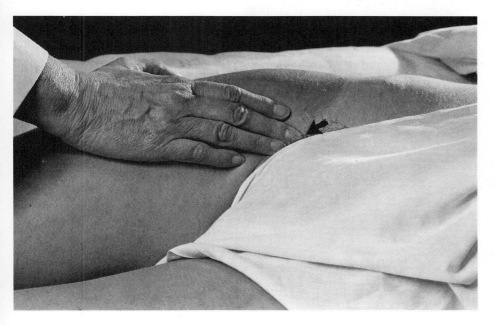

● *The popliteal pulse.* The patient's knee should be somewhat flexed, the leg relaxed. Place the fingertips of both hands so that they just meet in the midline behind the knee and press them deeply into the popliteal fossa. The popliteal pulse is frequently more difficult to find than other pulses. It is deeper and feels more diffuse.

An exaggerated, widened popliteal pulse suggests an aneurysm of the popliteal artery. Neither popliteal nor femoral aneurysms are common. They are usually due to arteriosclerosis, and occur primarily in men over 50.

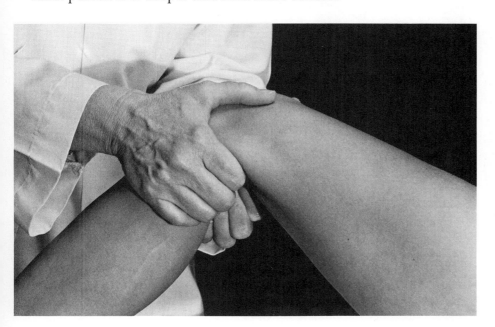

If you cannot feel the popliteal pulse with this approach, try feeling for it with the patient prone. Flex the patient's knee to about 90°, let the lower leg relax against your shoulder or upper arm, and press your two thumbs deeply into the popliteal fossa.

Arteriosclerosis obliterans most commonly obstructs arterial circulation in the thigh. The femoral pulse is then normal, the popliteal decreased or absent.

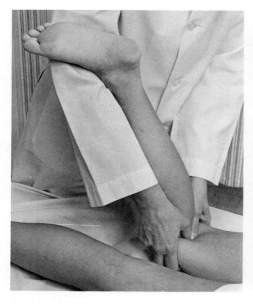 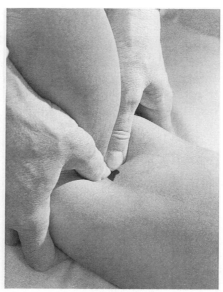

- *The dorsalis pedis pulse.* Feel the dorsum of the foot (not the ankle) just lateral to the extensor tendon of the great toe. If you cannot feel a pulse, explore the dorsum of the foot more laterally.

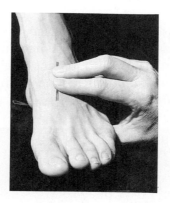

The dorsalis pedis artery may be congenitally absent or may branch higher in the ankle. Search for a pulse more laterally.

Decreased or absent foot pulses (assuming a warm environment) with normal femoral and popliteal pulses suggest occlusive disease in the lower popliteal artery or its branches—a pattern often associated with diabetes mellitus.

- *The posterior tibial pulse.* Curve your fingers behind and slightly below the medial malleolus of the ankle. (This pulse may be hard to feel in a fat or edematous ankle.)

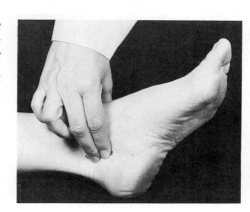

Sudden arterial occlusion, as by embolism or thrombosis, causes pain and numbness or tingling. The limb distal to the occlusion becomes cold, pale, and pulseless. Emergency treatment is required. If collateral circulation is good, only numbness and coolness may result.

Tips on feeling difficult pulses: (1) Position your own body and examining hand comfortably; awkward positions decrease your tactile sensitivity. (2) Place your hand properly and linger there, varying the pressure of your fingers to pick up a weak pulsation. If unsuccessful, then explore the area deliberately. Avoid flitting about. (3) Do not confuse the patient's pulse with your own pulsating fingertips. If you are unsure, count your own heart rate and compare it with the patient's. The rates are usually different. Your carotid pulse is convenient for this comparison.

Note the temperature of the feet and legs with the backs of your fingers. Compare one side with the other. Bilateral coldness is most often due to a cold environment or anxiety.

Coldness, especially when unilateral or associated with other signs, suggests arterial insufficiency, an inadequate arterial circulation.

Look for edema. Compare one foot and leg with the other, noting their relative size and the prominence of veins, tendons, and bones.

Edema causes swelling that may obscure the veins, tendons, and bony prominences.

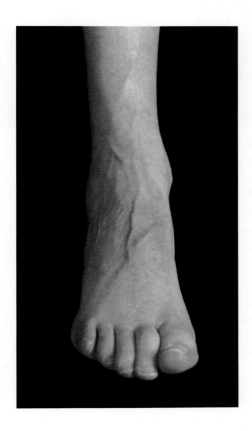

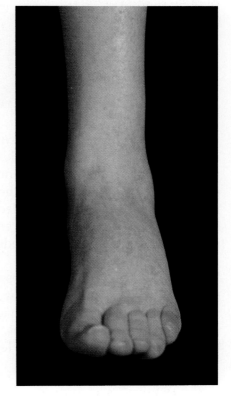

Check for pitting edema. Press firmly but gently with your thumb for at least 5 seconds (1) over the dorsum of each foot (see p. 446), (2) behind each medial malleolus, and (3) over the shins. Look for pitting—a depression caused by your pressure. Normally there is none. The severity of edema is graded on a four-point scale, from slight to very marked.

See Table 16-1, Mechanisms and Patterns of Edema (pp. 455–456).

See Table 16-2, Some Peripheral Causes of Edema (p. 457).

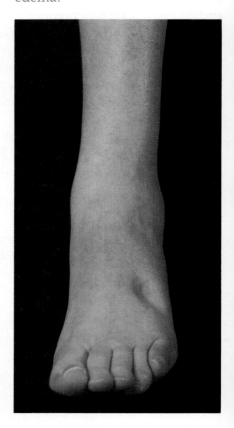

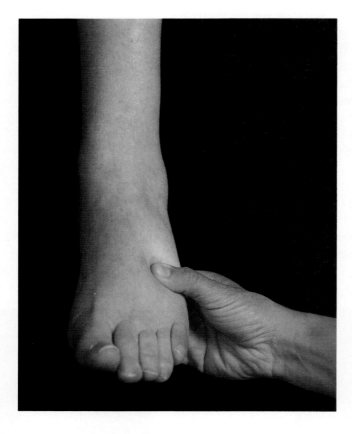

If you suspect edema, *measurement of the legs* may help you to identify it and to follow its course. With a flexible tape, measure (1) the forefoot, (2) the smallest possible circumference above the ankle, (3) the largest circumference at the calf, and (4) the midthigh a measured distance above the patella with the knee extended. Compare one side with the other. A difference of over 1 cm just above the ankle or 2 cm at the calf is unusual in normal people and suggests edema.

Conditions such as muscular atrophy can also cause different circumferences in the legs.

If edema is present, look for possible causes in the peripheral vascular system. These include (1) recent deep venous thrombosis, (2) chronic venous insufficiency due to previous deep venous thrombosis or to incompetence of the venous valves, and (3) lymphedema. Note the extent of the swelling. How far up the leg does it go?

In deep venous thrombosis, the extent of edema suggests the location of the occlusion: the calf when the lower leg or the ankle is swollen, the iliofemoral veins when the entire leg is swollen.

Is the swelling unilateral or bilateral? Are the veins unusually prominent?

Venous distention suggests a venous cause of edema.

Try to identify any venous tenderness that may accompany deep venous thrombosis. Palpate the groin just medial to the femoral pulse for tenderness of the femoral vein. Next, with the patient's leg flexed at the knee and relaxed, palpate the calf. With your fingerpads, gently compress the

A painful, pale, swollen leg, together with tenderness of the femoral vein, suggests deep iliofemoral thrombosis. Tender-

calf muscles against the tibia, and search for any tenderness or cords. Deep venous thrombosis, however, may have no demonstrable signs, and diagnosis often depends on other kinds of tests.

Note the color of the skin.

Is there a local area of redness? If so, note its temperature, and gently try to feel the firm cord of a thrombosed vein in the area. The calf is most often involved.

Are there brownish areas near the ankles?

Note any ulcers in the skin. Where are they?

Feel the thickness of the skin.

Ask the patient to stand, and *inspect the saphenous system for varicosities.* The standing posture allows any varicosities to fill with blood and makes them visible. You can easily miss them when the patient is in a supine position. Feel for any varicosities, noting any signs of thrombophlebitis.

ness and cords deep in the calf suggest deep thrombosis there. Calf tenderness, however, may be present without thrombosis.

Local swelling, redness, warmth, and a subcutaneous cord suggest superficial thrombophlebitis.

A brownish color or ulcers just above the ankle suggest chronic venous insufficiency.

Thickened (brawny) skin occurs in lymphedema and advanced venous insufficiency.

Varicose veins are dilated and tortuous. Their walls may feel somewhat thickened.

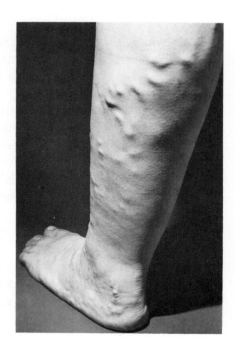

SPECIAL MANEUVERS

EVALUATING THE COMPETENCY OF VENOUS VALVES. When varicose veins are present, two tests are useful in assessing the competency of the venous valves, *i.e.,* their ability to prevent the retrograde flow of blood.

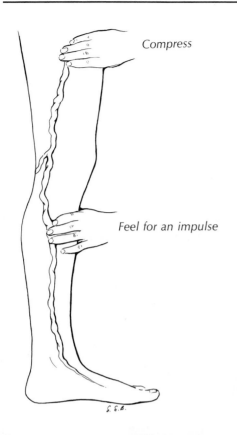

Compress

Feel for an impulse

The manual compression test gives information about the valves in the saphenous system. With the fingertips of one hand, feel the dilated vein. With your other hand at least 20 cm higher in the leg, compress the vein firmly. Feel for an impulse transmitted to your lower hand. Competent saphenous valves should block the transmission of any impulse.

The small saphenous vein can be tested in the same way. Because valves are closer together in the lower leg, your hands need not be so far apart.

A palpable impulse transmitted to the lower hand indicates incompetency of the valve(s) in that portion of the vein between your two hands.

Incompetent valves allow blood to flow backward in the veins, thus increasing hydrostatic pressure in the legs and causing edema—a condition called venous insufficiency. When the valvular incompetency is limited to the saphenous veins (superficial venous insufficiency), severe symptoms seldom ensue.

The retrograde filling (Trendelenburg) test helps to assess valvular competency in the communicating veins as well as in the saphenous system. Elevate the patient's leg to 90° to empty it of venous blood.

Next, occlude the great saphenous vein in the upper thigh by either (1) manual compression, or (2) a tourniquet wrapped tightly enough to occlude this vein but not the deeper vessels. Ask the patient to stand. While you keep the vein occluded, watch for venous filling in the leg. Normally the saphenous vein fills from below, taking about 35 seconds as blood flows through the capillary bed into the venous system.

Rapid filling of the superficial veins while the saphenous vein is occluded indicates incompetent valves in the communicating veins. Blood flows quickly in a retrograde direction from the deep to the saphenous system.

After the patient has stood for 20 seconds, release the compression and look for any sudden additional venous filling. Normally there is none: competent valves in the saphenous vein block retrograde flow. Slow venous filling continues.

Sudden additional filling of superficial veins after release of compression indicates incompetent valves in the saphenous vein.

When both steps of this test are normal, the response is termed negative–negative. Negative–positive and positive–negative responses may also occur.

When both steps are abnormal, the test is positive–positive.

EVALUATING THE BEDFAST PATIENT. People who are confined to bed, especially when they are emaciated, elderly, or have neurologic impairment, are particularly susceptible to skin damage and ulceration.

Pressure sores result when sustained compression obliterates arteriolar and capillary blood flow to the skin. Sores may also result from the shearing forces created by bodily movements. When a person slides down in bed from a partially sitting position, for example, or is dragged rather than lifted up from a supine position, the movements may distort the soft tissues of the buttocks and close off the arteries and arterioles within. Friction and moisture further increase the risk.

The assessment of every susceptible patient should include careful inspection of the skin overlying the sacrum, buttocks, greater trochanters, knees, and heels. Roll the patient onto one side to get a good view of the sacrum and buttocks.

Local redness of the skin warns of impending necrosis, although some deep pressure sores develop without antecedent redness. Ulcers may be seen.

Use this position also to evaluate a patient for *sacral edema*. Press firmly for at least 5 seconds in the sacral area and look for any pitting. If you find it, check other areas higher on the back.

Dependent edema may accumulate in the back of a bed patient and not appear in the legs.

EVALUATING THE ARTERIAL SUPPLY TO THE HAND. If you suspect arterial insufficiency in the arm or hand, try to feel the *ulnar pulse* as well as the radial and brachial pulses. Feel for it deeply on the flexor surface of the wrist medially. The pulse of a normal ulnar artery, however, may not be palpable.

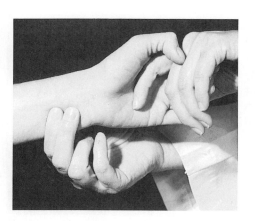

Arterial insufficiency is much less common in the arms than in the legs. Thromboangiitis obliterans (Buerger's disease) or acute arterial occlusion (as from an embolus) may cause it, producing diminished or absent pulses at the wrist.

The *Allen test* gives further information. This test is also useful to assure the patency of the ulnar artery before puncturing the radial artery for blood samples. The patient should rest with hands in lap, palms up.

Ask the patient to make a tight fist with one hand, and compress both radial and ulnar arteries firmly between your thumbs and fingers. Then ask the patient to open the hand into a relaxed, slightly flexed position. The palm is pale.

Extending the hand fully may cause pallor and a falsely positive test.

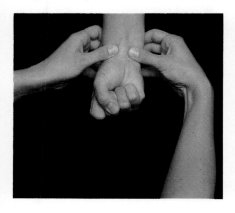 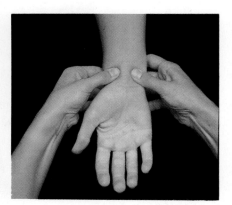

Release your pressure over the ulnar artery. If the ulnar artery is patent, the palm flushes within about 3 to 5 seconds.

Persisting pallor indicates occlusion of the ulnar artery or its distal branches.

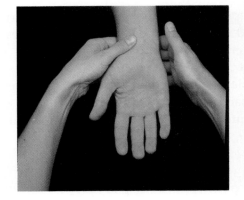
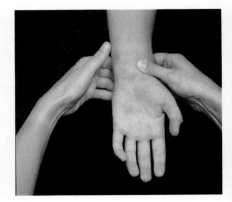

Patency of the radial artery may be tested by the same method, but this time release the radial artery while still compressing the ulnar.

POSTURAL COLOR CHANGES OF CHRONIC ARTERIAL INSUFFICIENCY. If pain or diminished pulses suggest arterial insufficiency (an inadequate arterial circulation), look for postural color changes. Raise both legs, as shown at the right, to about 60° until maximal pallor of the feet develops—usually within a minute. In light-skinned persons, either maintenance of normal color, as seen in this right foot, or slight pallor is normal.

Marked pallor on elevation suggests arterial insufficiency.

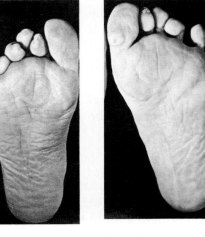
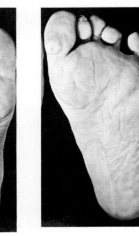

Then ask the patient to sit up with legs dangling down. Compare both feet, noting the time required for:

This foot is still pale and the veins are just beginning to fill —signs of arterial insufficiency.

- Return of pinkness to the skin, normally about 10 seconds or less
- Filling of the veins of the feet and ankles, normally about 15 seconds

This right foot has normal color and the veins on the feet have filled. These are normal responses, suggesting an adequate circulation.

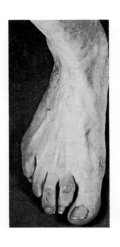
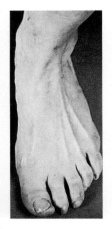

Normal responses accompanied by diminished arterial pulses suggest that a good collateral circulation has developed around an arterial occlusion.

Look for any unusual rubor (dusky redness) to replace the pallor of the dependent foot. Rubor may take a minute or more to appear.

These changes may be difficult to see in black persons. Inspect the soles of the feet for color changes, and use tangential lighting to visualize the veins.

(Source of foot photos: Kappert A, Winsor T: Diagnosis of Peripheral Vascular Diseases, p 33. Philadelphia, FA Davis, 1972)

Persisting rubor on dependency suggests arterial insufficiency. When veins are incompetent, dependent rubor and the timing of color return and venous filling are not reliable tests of arterial insufficiency.

Color Plate 16-1   Chronic Insufficiency of Arteries and Veins

CHRONIC ARTERIAL INSUFFICIENCY *(Advanced)*

CHRONIC VENOUS INSUFFICIENCY *(Advanced)*

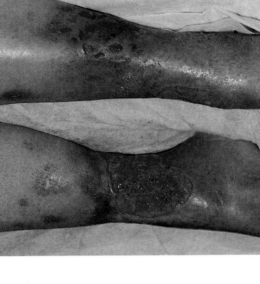

Rubor

Ulcer

	CHRONIC ARTERIAL INSUFFICIENCY *(Advanced)*	CHRONIC VENOUS INSUFFICIENCY *(Advanced)*
PAIN	Intermittent claudication, progressing to rest pain	None to an aching pain on dependency
PULSES	Decreased or absent	Normal, though may be difficult to feel through edema
COLOR	Pale, especially on elevation; dusky red on dependency	Normal, or cyanotic on dependency. Petechiae, then brown pigmentation appear with chronicity.
TEMPERATURE	Cool	Normal
EDEMA	Absent or mild; may develop as the patient tries to relieve rest pain by lowering the leg	Present, often marked
SKIN CHANGES	Thin, shiny, atrophic skin; loss of hair over foot and toes; nails thickened and ridged (trophic changes)	Often brown pigmentation around the ankle, stasis dermatitis, and possible thickening of the skin and narrowing of the leg as scarring develops
ULCERATION	If present, involves toes or points of trauma on feet	If present, develops at sides of ankle, especially medially
GANGRENE	May develop	Does not develop

(Sources of photos: *Arterial Insufficiency*—Kappert A, Winsor T: Diagnosis of Peripheral Vascular Diseases, p 15. Philadelphia, FA Davis, 1972; *Venous Insufficiency*—Marks R: Skin Disease in Old Age, p 224. Philadelphia, JB Lippincott, 1987)

Color Plate 16-2   Common Ulcers of the Feet and Ankles

	ARTERIAL INSUFFICIENCY	CHRONIC VENOUS INSUFFICIENCY	TROPHIC ULCER
LOCATION	Toes, feet, or possibly in areas of trauma (e.g., the shin)	Inner, sometimes outer ankle	Pressure points in areas with diminished sensation, as in diabetic polyneuropathy
SKIN AROUND THE ULCER	No callus or excess of pigment, may be atrophic	Pigmented, sometimes fibrotic	Calloused
PAIN	Often severe, unless neuropathy masks it	Not severe	Absent (and therefore the ulcer may go unnoticed)
ASSOCIATED GANGRENE	May be present	Absent	In uncomplicated trophic ulcer, absent
ASSOCIATED SIGNS	Decreased pulses, trophic changes, pallor of the foot on elevation, dusky rubor on dependency	Edema, pigmentation, stasis dermatitis, and possibly cyanosis of the foot on dependency	Decreased sensation, absent ankle jerks

(Source of photos: Marks R: Skin Disease in Old Age, pp 224, 233, 235. Philadelphia, JB Lippincott, 1987)

Table 16-1 Mechanisms and Patterns of Edema

Causes of edema may be divided roughly into two groups: (1) *general or systemic causes*, including congestive heart failure, hypoalbuminemia, and excessive renal retention of salt and water; and (2) *local causes*, such as venous stasis, lymphatic stasis, and prolonged dependency. Increased capillary permeability may be either local or general in distribution.

	MECHANISM OF EDEMA	DISTRIBUTION OF EDEMA	OTHER SIGNS MAY INCLUDE—
RIGHT-SIDED CONGESTIVE HEART FAILURE	Decreased ability of the heart to accept venous blood increases the hydrostatic pressure in the veins and capillaries, producing congestion and loss of fluid into the tissues.	Edema first appears in the dependent areas of the body where hydrostatic pressure is highest (*i.e.*, the feet and the legs). When the patient is bedridden, the low back is dependent and becomes edematous.	Increased jugular venous pressure, an enlarged and often tender liver, an enlarged heart, S_3
HYPOALBUMINEMIA	Decreased colloid osmotic pressure in the plasma allows excessive fluid to escape into the interstitial space. Causes include cirrhosis, the nephrotic syndrome, and severe malnutrition.	Edema may appear first in the loose subcutaneous tissues of the eyelids, especially after the patient lies down at night, but may also show first in the feet and legs. In cirrhosis, ascites often appears first. When cirrhosis is more advanced, edema may become generalized.	Signs of chronic liver disease such as ascites, spider angiomas, and jaundice. Signs of the nephrotic syndrome vary with its causes. Serum albumin is low.
EXCESSIVE RENAL RETENTION OF SALT AND WATER	The kidneys may initiate edema by retaining excessive amounts of salt and water, some of which pass into the interstitial space. Drugs such as corticosteroids, estrogens, and some antihypertensives may be responsible.	Edema usually starts in the dependent areas and may become generalized.	Usually none

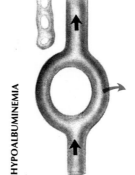

▶ *Continued*

Table 16-1   *Mechanisms and Patterns of Edema*

Table 16-1 (Cont'd.)

	Mechanism	Location	Characteristics
VENOUS STASIS SECONDARY TO OBSTRUCTION OR INSUFFICIENCY 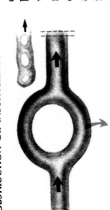	Thrombophlebitis may block venous drainage. Venous valves may be damaged by thrombophlebitis or become incompetent because of varicose veins. Less commonly, veins may be compressed from the outside, as by a tumor or fibrosis. In any case, hydrostatic pressure rises in the veins and capillaries, producing excessive loss of fluid into the tissues.	Edema is limited to the area of blockage, often one leg or, less commonly, both legs or an arm. A blocked superior vena cava may cause edema in the entire upper part of the body.	Local swelling and increased tissue turgor. When large veins such as the superior vena cava or the iliofemoral veins are involved, an increased venous pattern of dilated veins may be visible. Tenderness sometimes accompanies phlebitis. Signs of venous insufficiency
LYMPHATIC STASIS (LYMPHEDEMA)	Lymph channels may be congenitally abnormal or they may be obstructed by tumor, fibrosis, or inflammation.	Local, often involving one or both legs. Lymphedema of an arm may follow radical mastectomy.	Indurated skin in the involved area. Except in the early phases, lymphedema is characteristically nonpitting.
ORTHOSTATIC EDEMA	Prolonged sitting or standing, without sufficient muscular activity to promote venous flow, increases the pressure in the veins and capillaries and thus increases the flow of fluid into the interstitial spaces.	The dependent areas (*e.g.,* the legs)	None. Get a good history, including long bus or train trips. People who get up after prolonged bed rest are at first especially susceptible to orthostatic edema.
INCREASED CAPILLARY PERMEABILITY 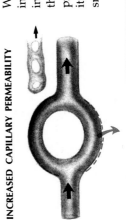	When capillary permeability increases, protein leaks into the interstitial spaces and, by increasing the interstitial colloid osmotic pressure, draws excessive fluid with it. Causes vary, including burns, snake bite, and allergy.	Usually local, depending on the cause; may be generalized	Variable

Table 16-2   Some Peripheral Causes of Edema

Table 16-2   Some Peripheral Causes of Edema

ORTHOSTATIC EDEMA — *Foot swollen*, *Pitting*

LYMPHEDEMA — *Skin thick*, *No pitting*, *Foot swollen*

LIPEDEMA — *No pitting*, *Foot spared*

CHRONIC VENOUS INSUFFICIENCY* — *Pigment*, *Ulcer*, *Pitting*, *Advanced*

	ORTHOSTATIC EDEMA	LYMPHEDEMA	LIPEDEMA	CHRONIC VENOUS INSUFFICIENCY*
PROCESS	Edema from prolonged sitting or standing	Lymphatic obstruction	Fatty deposition in legs (not true edema)	Chronic obstruction or valvular incompetence of the deep veins
NATURE OF EDEMA	Soft, pits on pressure	Soft early, becomes hard and nonpitting	Minimal, if any	Soft, pits on pressure; later may become brawny (hard)
SKIN THICKENING	Absent	Marked	Absent	Occasional
ULCERATION	Absent	Rare	Absent	Common
PIGMENTATION	Absent	Absent	Absent	Common
FOOT INVOLVEMENT	Present	Present	Absent	Present
BILATERALITY	Always	Often	Always	Occasionally

* The advanced state described here is seen in *deep venous insufficiency*, also called postphlebitic syndrome or post-thrombotic syndrome. *Superficial venous insufficiency* seldom progresses to this state; mild bilateral edema is its chief manifestation.

Chapter 17
The Musculoskeletal System

Anatomy and Physiology

This section reviews briefly the structure and function of joints and describes the anatomical landmarks of several clinically important joints. Identify these landmarks first on yourself or on a fellow student. Range of motion at each joint varies greatly with age and health. The figures given here are intended to be general guides, not absolute standards.

STRUCTURE AND FUNCTION OF JOINTS

A typical *freely movable joint* is diagrammed at the right.

Note that the bones themselves do not touch each other within the joint but are covered by articular cartilage that forms a cushion between the bony surfaces. At the margins of the articular cartilage is attached the synovial membrane. This membrane is pouched or folded to allow for joint movement. It encloses the synovial cavity and secretes into it a small amount of viscous lubricating fluid—the synovial fluid.

The synovial membrane is surrounded by a fibrous joint capsule, which in turn is strengthened by ligaments extending from bone to bone.

Some joints, such as those between the vertebral bodies illustrated here, are *slightly movable joints*. Here the bones are separated not by a synovial cavity but by a fibrocartilaginous disc. At the center of each disc is the nucleus pulposus, fibrogelatinous material that forms a cushion or shock absorber between the vertebral bodies.

Bursae are disc-shaped, fluid-filled synovial sacs that occur at points of friction around joints and facilitate movement. They lie between the skin and the convex surface of a bone or joint (*e.g.,* the prepatellar bursa, p. 468) or in areas where tendons or muscles rub against bone, ligaments, or other tendons or muscles (*e.g.,* the subacromial bursa, p. 464).

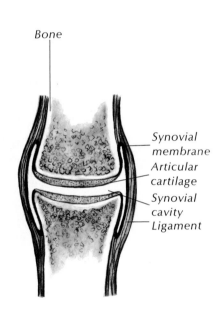

Bone
Synovial membrane
Articular cartilage
Synovial cavity
Ligament

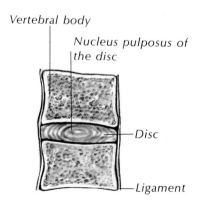

Vertebral body
Nucleus pulposus of the disc
Disc
Ligament

SPECIFIC JOINTS

TEMPOROMANDIBULAR JOINT. The temporomandibular joint forms the articulation between mandible and skull. Feel for it just in front of the tragus of each ear as the jaw is opened and closed.

WRISTS AND HANDS. At the wrist, identify the bony tips of the radius (laterally) and the ulna (medially). On the dorsum of the wrist, palpate the groove of the radiocarpal or wrist joint.

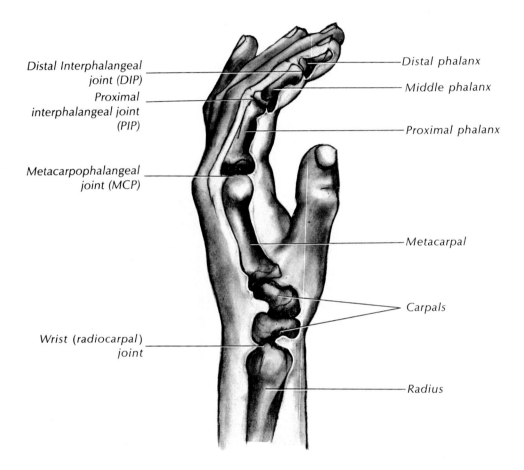

Distal Interphalangeal joint (DIP)
Proximal interphalangeal joint (PIP)
Metacarpophalangeal joint (MCP)
Wrist (radiocarpal) joint

Distal phalanx
Middle phalanx
Proximal phalanx
Metacarpal
Carpals
Radius

The carpal bones within the hand cannot be readily identified clinically. However, palpate each of the five metacarpals and the proximal, middle, and distal phalanges. (The thumb lacks a middle phalanx.) Flex the hand somewhat and find the groove marking the metacarpophalangeal joint of each finger. It is distal to the knuckle and can be felt best on either side of the extensor tendon.

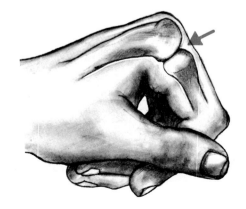

Many tendons pass across the wrist and hand to insert on the fingers. Through much of their course these tendons travel in synovial sheaths or tunnels. Although not normally palpable, these sheaths may become swollen or inflamed.

Illustrated below and at the right is the *range of motion at the wrists*—

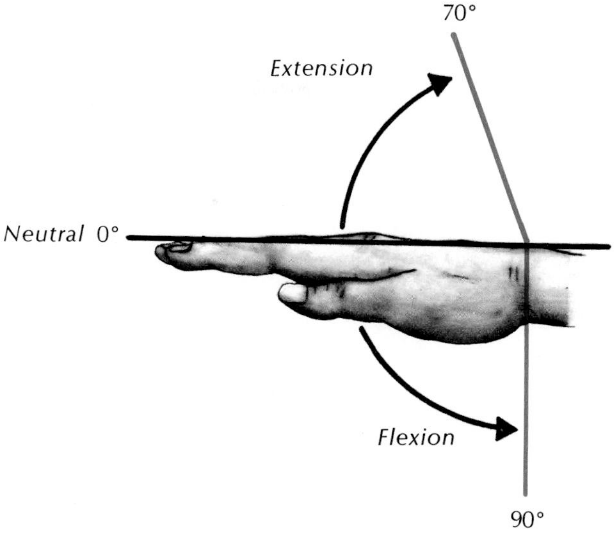

70°

Extension

Neutral 0°

Flexion

90°

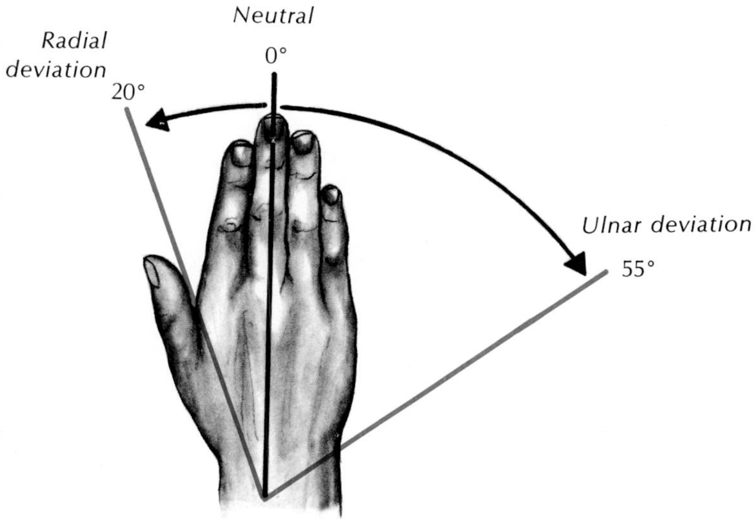

Neutral
0°

Radial deviation
20°

Ulnar deviation
55°

And *at the joints of the fingers*—

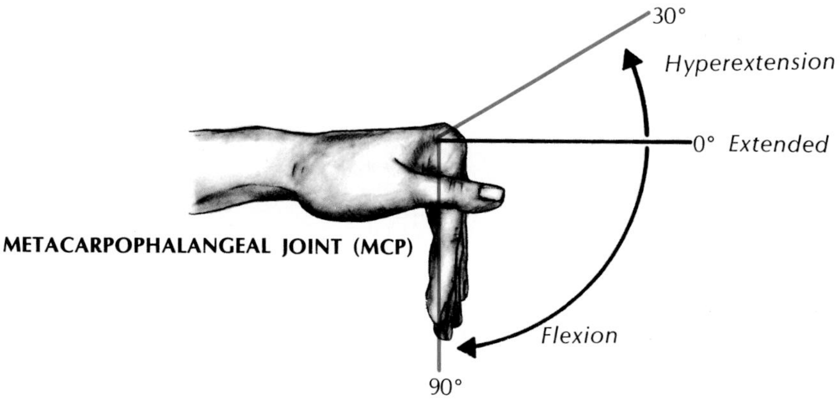

30°

Hyperextension

0° *Extended*

METACARPOPHALANGEAL JOINT (MCP)

Flexion

90°

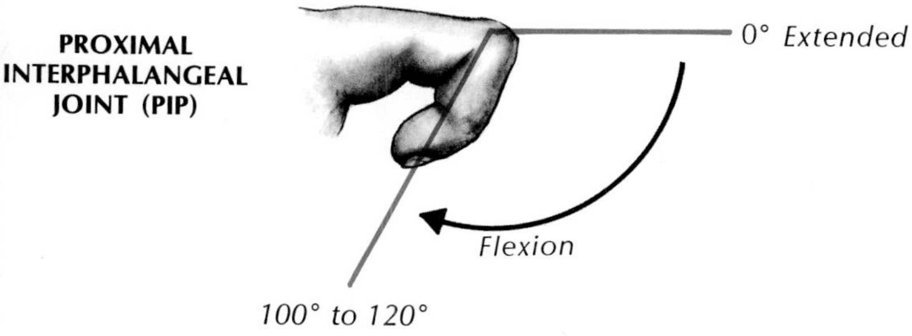

PROXIMAL INTERPHALANGEAL JOINT (PIP)

0° *Extended*

Flexion

100° to 120°

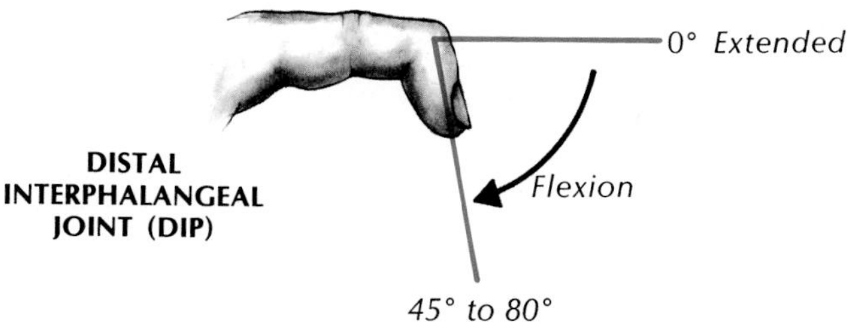

0° *Extended*

DISTAL INTERPHALANGEAL JOINT (DIP)

Flexion

45° to 80°

ELBOWS. Identify the medial and lateral epicondyles of the humerus and the olecranon process of the ulna. A bursa (not illustrated) lies between the olecranon process and the skin. The synovial membrane is most accessible to examination between the olecranon and the epicondyles. Neither bursa nor synovium is normally palpable.

The sensitive ulnar nerve can be felt posteriorly between olecranon and medial epicondyle.

Movements at the elbow are illustrated below.

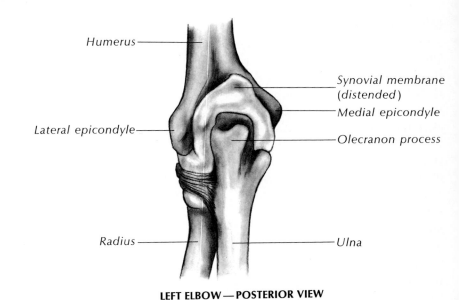

LEFT ELBOW—POSTERIOR VIEW

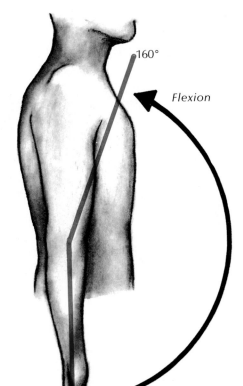

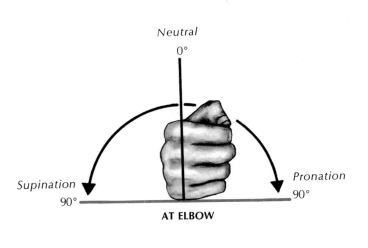

SHOULDERS AND ENVIRONS. Identify the following landmarks: (1) the manubrium of the sternum, (2) the sternoclavicular joint, and (3) the clavicle. With your fingers, trace the clavicle laterally—over its medial two thirds, which is convex, and its lateral third, which is concave. Now, from behind, follow the bony spine of the scapula laterally and upward until it becomes the *acromion*, the summit of the shoulder. Its upper surface is rough and slightly convex. Identify the anterior surface, or tip, of the acromion and mark it with ink. With your index finger on top of the acromion, just behind its tip, press medially to find the slightly elevated ridge that marks the distal end of the clavicle. This junction marks the acromioclavicular joint (shown by the arrow). Now, from the top of the acromion again, move your finger laterally and down a short step to the next bony prominence, the *greater tubercle of the humerus.* Mark this with ink. Now sweep your finger medially a few centimeters until you feel a large bony prominence, the *coracoid process* of the scapula. Mark this also. These three points—(1) the tip of the acromion, (2) the greater tubercle of the humerus, and (3) the coracoid process—orient you to the anatomy of the shoulder.

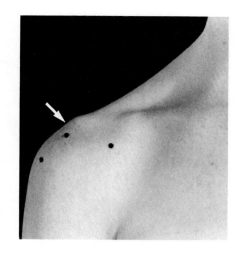

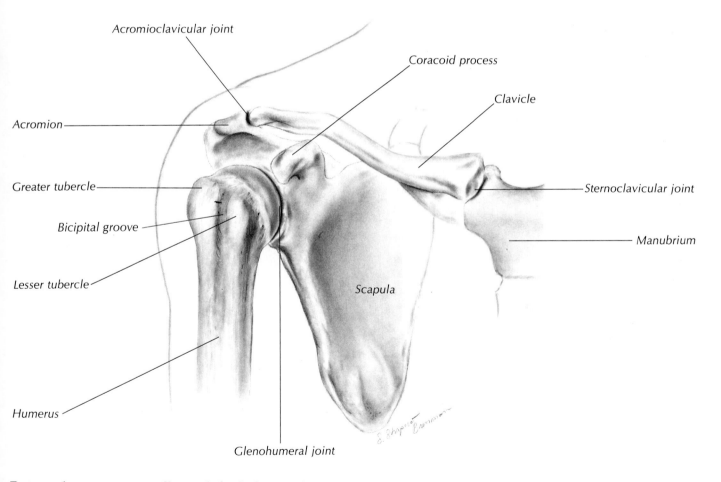

Rotate the arm externally and find the tendinous cord that runs just medial to the greater tubercle. Roll it under your fingers. This is the tendon of the long head of the biceps. It runs in the bicipital groove between the greater and lesser tubercles.

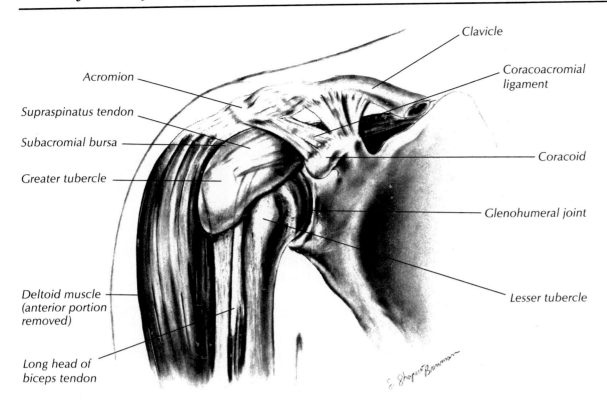

Clavicle

Acromion

Coracoacromial
ligament

Supraspinatus tendon

Subacromial bursa

Greater tubercle

Coracoid

Glenohumeral joint

Deltoid muscle
(anterior portion
removed)

Lesser tubercle

Long head of
biceps tendon

The glenohumeral joint, between the scapula and the humerus, is deeply situated and not normally palpable. Its fibrous capsule is reinforced by the tendons of four muscles, which together are called the *rotator cuff*. The supraspinatus, which runs above the joint, and the infraspinatus and teres minor, which cross it posteriorly, all insert on the greater tubercle of the humerus.

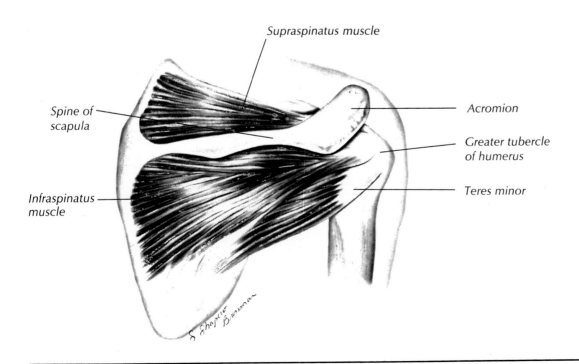

Supraspinatus muscle

Spine of
scapula

Acromion

Greater tubercle
of humerus

Infraspinatus
muscle

Teres minor

The subscapularis (the fourth rotator cuff muscle, not illustrated), originates on the anterior surface of the scapula, crosses the joint anteriorly, and inserts on the lesser tubercle.

The arch formed by the acromion, the coracoid, and the coracoacromial ligament protects the glenohumeral joint, as illustrated on page 464. Deep to this arch and extending anterolaterally under the deltoid muscle lies the subacromial bursa. It overlies the supraspinatus tendon. Although you normally cannot feel either the bursa or the supraspinatus tendon, tenderness originating there can be found just below the tip of the acromion.

The normal *range of motion at the shoulder* is illustrated below.

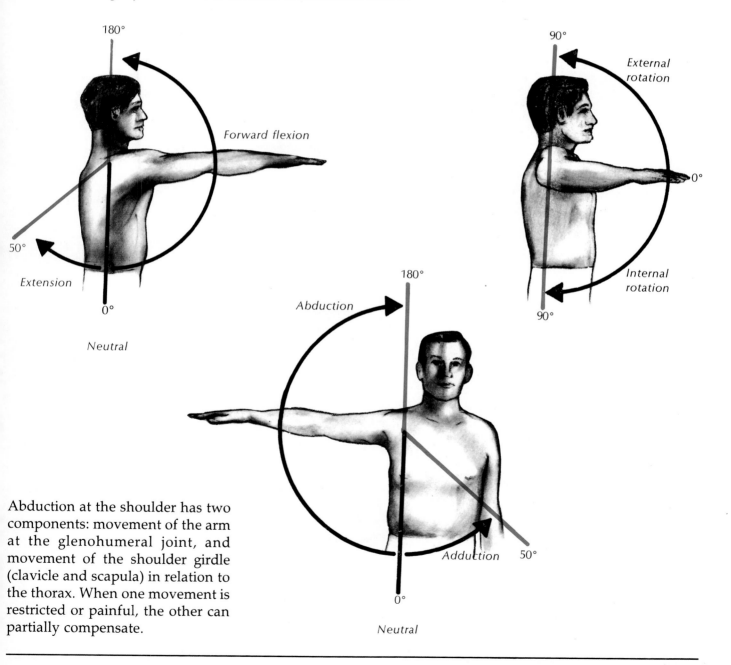

Abduction at the shoulder has two components: movement of the arm at the glenohumeral joint, and movement of the shoulder girdle (clavicle and scapula) in relation to the thorax. When one movement is restricted or painful, the other can partially compensate.

ANKLES AND FEET. The principal landmarks of the ankle are (1) the medial malleolus, the bony prominence at the distal end of the tibia, and (2) the lateral malleolus, the distal end of the fibula. Ligaments extend from each malleolus onto the foot. The strong Achilles tendon inserts on the heel posteriorly.

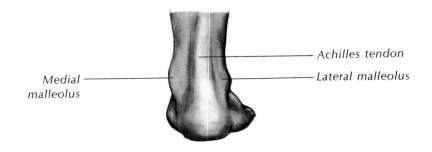

Motions at the ankle joint itself (the tibiotalar joint) are limited to dorsiflexion and plantar flexion.

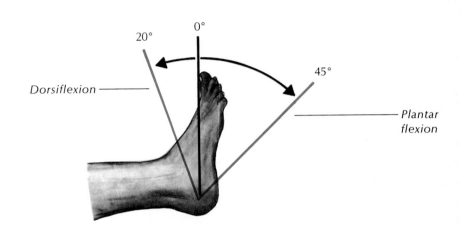

Inversion and eversion of the foot are functions of the subtalar (talocalcaneal) and transverse tarsal joints.

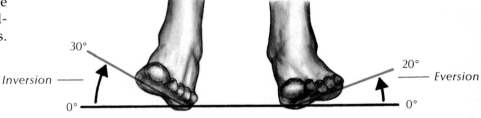

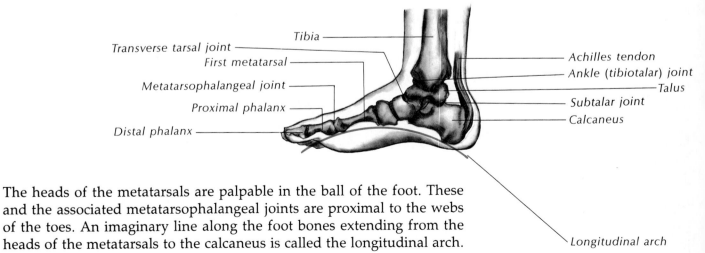

The heads of the metatarsals are palpable in the ball of the foot. These and the associated metatarsophalangeal joints are proximal to the webs of the toes. An imaginary line along the foot bones extending from the heads of the metatarsals to the calcaneus is called the longitudinal arch.

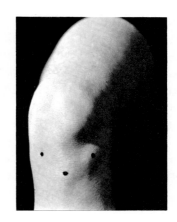

THE KNEE. The knee joint involves three bones: the femur, the tibia, and the patella (or kneecap). It also has three articular surfaces: two between femur and tibia (the medial and lateral compartments of the tibiofemoral joint) and one between patella and femur (the patellofemoral compartment).

Landmarks in and around the knee will orient you to this complicated joint. Identify the flat medial surface of the tibia—the shin. Follow its anterior border upward to the tibial tuberosity. Mark this point with a dot of ink. Now follow the medial border of the tibia upward until it merges into a bony prominence—the medial condyle of the tibia. This is somewhat higher than the tibial tuberosity. In a comparable location on the other side of the knee, find a similar prominence—the lateral condyle. Mark both condyles with ink. These three points form an isosceles triangle. On the lateral surface of the knee, somewhat below the level of the lateral tibial condyle, find the head of the fibula.

Now identify three parts of the femur. Bring your fingertips firmly down the medial surface of the thigh along a line analogous to the inner seam of a pant leg. Your fingers will run up against an abrupt bony prominence, the adductor tubercle. Just below this is the medial epicondyle. The lateral epicondyle can be found comparably situated on the other side.

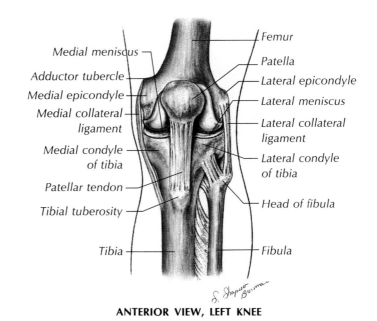

ANTERIOR VIEW, LEFT KNEE

The patella rests on the anterior articulating surface of the femur, roughly midway between the epicondyles. It lies within the tendon of the quadriceps muscle. This tendon continues below the knee joint as the patellar tendon and inserts on the tibial tuberosity.

Two collateral ligaments, one on each side of the knee, give medial and lateral stability to the joint. To feel the lateral collateral ligament, cross one leg so that the ankle rests on the opposite knee and find the firm cord that runs from the lateral epicondyle of the femur to the head of the fibula. The medial collateral ligament is not palpable. Two cruciate ligaments (not illustrated) cross obliquely within the knee and give it anteroposterior stability.

With the knee flexed about 90°, you can press your thumbs—one on each side of the patellar tendon—into the groove of the tibiofemoral joint. Note that the patella lies just above this joint line. As you press your thumbs downward you can feel the edge of the tibial plateau, the upper surface of the tibia. Follow it medially, then laterally until you are stopped by the converging femur and tibia. The medial and lateral menisci, crescent-shaped fibrocartilaginous pads that lie on the tibial plateaus, form cushions between tibia and femur. By moving your thumbs upward and toward the midline to the top of the patella, you can follow the articulating surface of the femur and identify the margins of the joint.

The soft tissue in front of the joint space, on either side of the patellar tendon, is the infrapatellar fat pad.

Several bursae lie near the knee. The prepatellar bursa lies between the patella and the overlying skin, while the superficial infrapatellar bursa lies anterior to the patellar tendon.

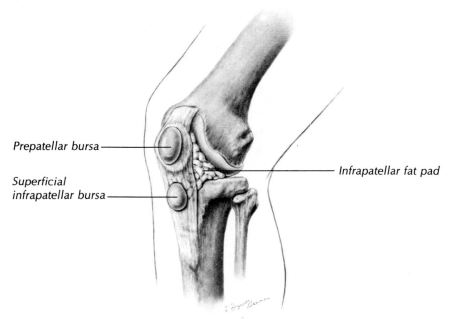

Prepatellar bursa

Superficial infrapatellar bursa

Infrapatellar fat pad

Observe the concavities that are usually evident at each side of the patella and also above it. Occupying these areas is the synovial cavity of the knee joint. This cavity includes an extension upward and deep to the quadriceps muscle—the suprapatellar pouch. Although the synovium is not normally detectable, these areas may become swollen and tender when the joint is inflamed.

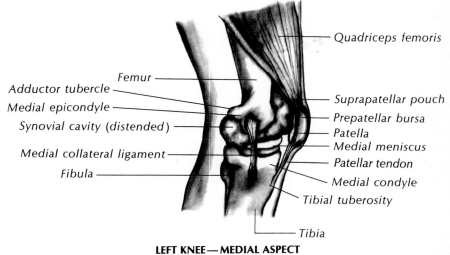

Femur
Adductor tubercle
Medial epicondyle
Synovial cavity (distended)
Medial collateral ligament
Fibula

Quadriceps femoris
Suprapatellar pouch
Prepatellar bursa
Patella
Medial meniscus
Patellar tendon
Medial condyle
Tibial tuberosity
Tibia

LEFT KNEE—MEDIAL ASPECT

The principal *movements of the knee* are extension, flexion, and sometimes hyperextension.

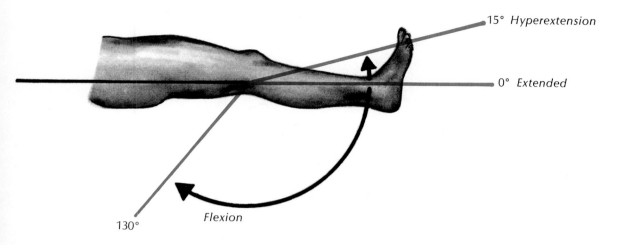

PELVIS AND HIPS. The hip joint lies deep and is not directly palpable. The greater trochanter of the femur can be felt about a palm's breadth below the iliac crest. The superficial trochanteric bursa lies on the posterolateral surface of the greater trochanter.

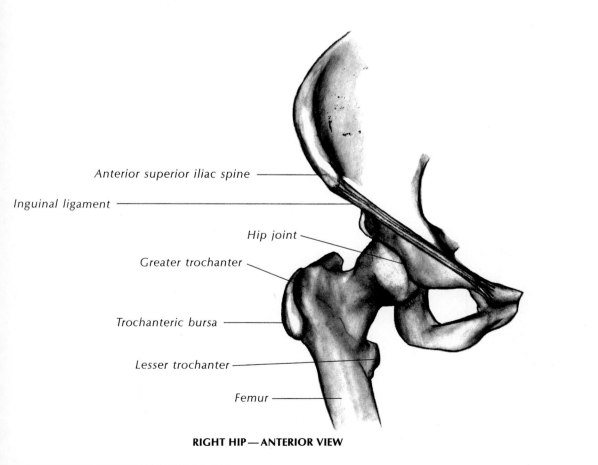

RIGHT HIP—ANTERIOR VIEW

Movements of the hip are illustrated below.

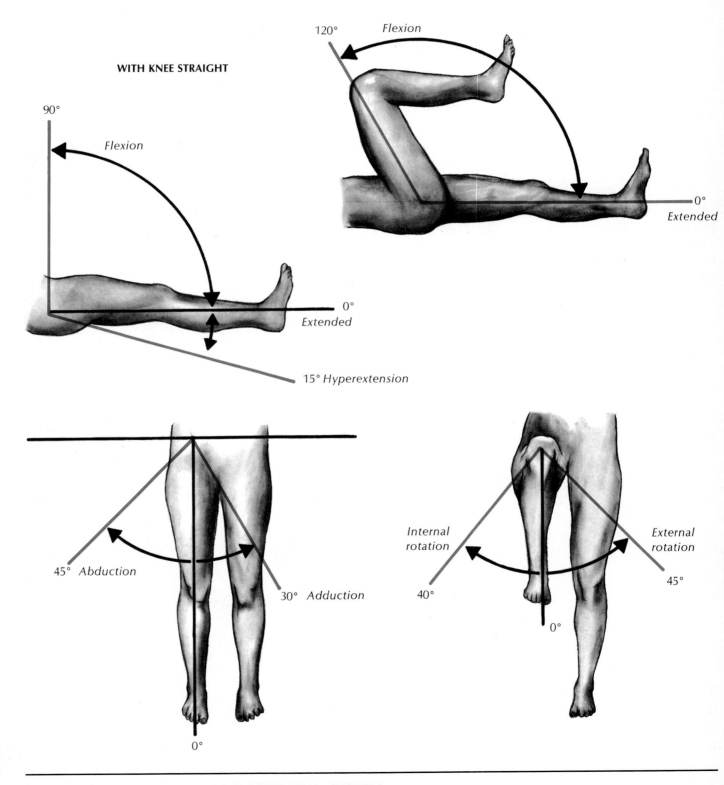

WITH KNEE FLEXED

120°

Flexion

0°
Extended

WITH KNEE STRAIGHT

90°

Flexion

0°
Extended

15° *Hyperextension*

45° *Abduction*

30° *Adduction*

0°

Internal rotation

40°

External rotation

45°

0°

SPINE. Viewing the patient from behind, identify the following landmarks: (1) the spinous processes, which become more evident on forward flexion, (2) the paravertebral muscles on either side of the midline, (3) the scapulae, (4) the iliac crests, and (5) the posterior superior iliac spines, usually marked by skin dimples. The spinous processes of C7 and often T1 are unusually prominent. A line drawn between the iliac crests crosses the spinous process of L4.

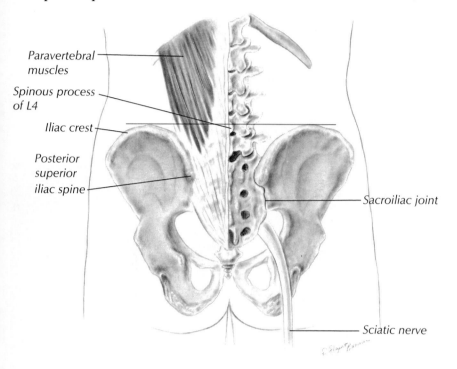

Paravertebral muscles

Spinous process of L4

Iliac crest

Posterior superior iliac spine

Sacroiliac joint

Sciatic nerve

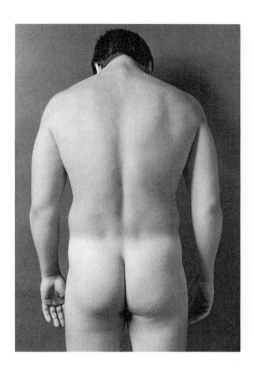

Viewed laterally, the spine has cervical and lumbar concavities and a thoracic convexity. The sacral curve forms a second convexity.

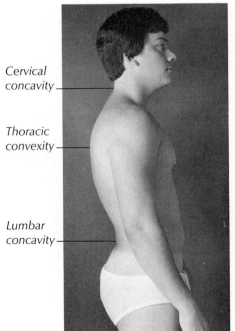

Cervical concavity

Thoracic convexity

Lumbar concavity

The most mobile portion of the spine is the neck. Flexion and extension occur chiefly between the head and the 1st cervical vertebra, rotation occurs primarily between the 1st and 2nd vertebrae, and lateral bending involves the cervical spine from the 2nd to the 7th vertebra.

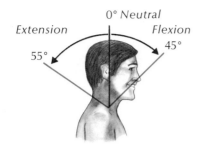

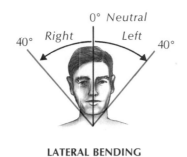

LATERAL BENDING

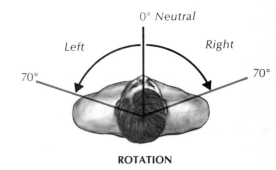

ROTATION

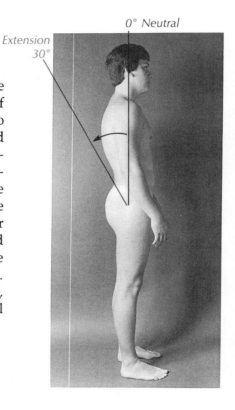

Movements of the rest of the spine (*i.e.,* from the sacrum to the base of the neck) are more difficult to measure than those in the neck and are subject to considerable individual variation. What looks like spinal flexion takes place partly at the hips. For this reason, and because people differ in the length of their limbs, flexion cannot be estimated accurately by noting the distance of their fingertips from the floor. As the patient flexes forward, watch the lumbar area. Its normal concavity should flatten out.

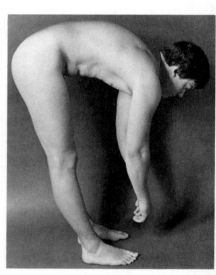

FLEXION

LATERAL BENDING

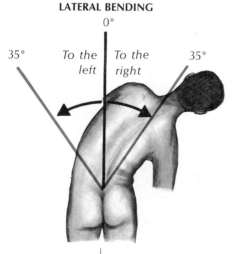

ROTATION

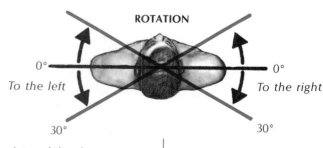

Excluding the neck, with pelvis stabilized

CHANGES WITH AGE

Adolescence. The musculoskeletal system changes importantly during adolescence—in size, proportion, and strength. Between the approximate ages of 12.5 and 15 years, boys undergo an adolescent growth spurt, gaining an average of 8 inches in height and more than 40 pounds in weight. On the average, the growth spurt in girls occurs about 2 years earlier and is smaller in magnitude. Bodily proportions change in fairly regular sequence: the legs elongate, the hips and the chest widen, the shoulders broaden, and finally the trunk lengthens and the chest deepens. Shoulders broaden more in boys, while in girls an increase in the bony pelvis produces relatively greater widening of the hips. Muscles increase in size and strength, especially in boys. For illustrations of these changes, see page 130.

As in sexual maturation, adolescents vary widely in their musculoskeletal development. Those who mature relatively late in relation to their peers face competitive disadvantages even though they are entirely normal. Adolescent changes in height, musculoskeletal development, and sex maturity correlate well with each other and provide a better basis for counseling teenagers than does a normative concept based on chronological age alone.

Aging. Musculoskeletal changes continue through the adult years. Soon after maturity adults begin to lose height subtly, and significant shortening becomes obvious in old age. Most loss of height occurs in the trunk as intervertebral discs become thinner and the vertebral bodies shorten or even collapse because of osteoporosis. Flexion at the knees and the hips may contribute to the shortened stature. The limbs of an elderly person thus tend to look long in proportion to the trunk.

The alterations in discs and vertebrae contribute too to the kyphosis of aging and increase the antero-posterior diameter of the chest, especially in women.

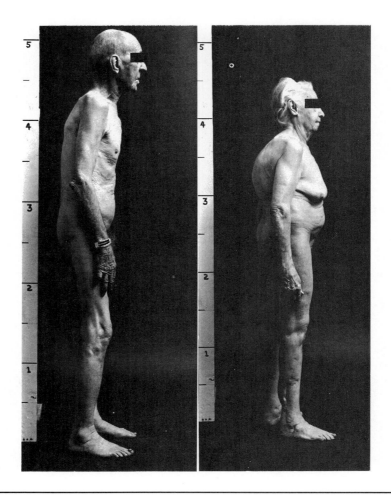

With aging, skeletal muscles decrease in bulk and power, as described in the next chapter (p. 512), and ligaments lose some of their tensile strength. Range of motion diminishes, partly because of osteoarthritis, a condition that usually accompanies the repetitive and accumulated stresses of the passing years.

Techniques of Examination

GENERAL APPROACH

While examining the musculoskeletal system, direct your attention to function as well as to structure. During the interview, you should have evaluated the patient's abilities to carry out normal activities of daily living. Also keep these abilities in mind during your physical examination.

In your initial survey of the patient you have assessed general appearance, bodily proportions, and ease of movement. Now, using inspection and palpation, you will examine individual joints or groups of joints, their range of motion, and the tissues surrounding them.

Note particularly:

- Any *limitation* in the normal *range of motion* or any unusual *increase* in the *mobility* of a joint (instability). Range of motion varies among individuals and decreases with aging.

  Decreased range of motion in arthritis, inflammation of tissues around the joint, fibrosis in or around a joint, or bony fixation (ankylosis)

- Any *signs of inflammation* such as:

  Swelling in or around the joint. Swelling may involve the synovial membrane, which then feels boggy, or doughy, to your fingers, or may be produced by excessive synovial fluid within the joint space. Swelling sometimes originates not in the joint itself but in tissues around it, such as bones, tendons, tendon sheaths, bursae, and fat. Trauma to any of these structures may also cause swelling.

  Palpable bogginess, or doughiness, of the synovial membrane indicates synovitis. Palpable joint fluid indicates an effusion in the joint. Synovitis and joint fluid often coexist.

  Tenderness in or around the joint. Try to define the specific anatomic structure that is tender. Trauma may also cause tenderness.

  Arthritis, tendonitis, bursitis, osteomyelitis

  Increased *heat.* Use the backs of your fingers to compare the joint with the symmetrical joint on the opposite side or, if both joints are involved, with the tissues near them.

  Tenderness and warmth over a thickened synovium suggest rheumatoid arthritis.

  Redness of the overlying skin. This is the least common sign of inflammation near the joints.

  Redness of the skin over a tender joint suggests septic or gouty arthritis, or possibly rheumatic fever.

- *Crepitus (crepitation),* a palpable or even audible crunching or grating produced by movement of a joint or tendon. Crepitus is more significant when it is associated with other symptoms or signs than when it exists by itself. Cracking or snapping sounds, which result from movement of tendons or ligaments over bone, may occur in normal joints such as the knees.

  Fine, soft crepitus may be felt over inflamed joints. Coarser crepitus suggests roughened articular cartilages, as in an inflamed joint or osteoarthritis. A creaking, leathery crepitus may arise in inflamed tendon sheaths.

- *Deformities*, including:

  Those produced by a restriction in the range of motion at a joint

  Malalignment of articulating bones

  An abnormality in the relationship between two articulating surfaces

- The *condition of the surrounding tissues*, including muscle atrophy, subcutaneous nodules, and skin changes

- *Muscular strength.* Testing of muscular strength is described in Chapter 18.

- *Symmetry* of involvement. Note whether arthritic changes involve several joints symmetrically on both sides of the body or affect only one or perhaps two joints.

Flexion deformity of the hip (see p. 485)

Ulnar deviation of the fingers in rheumatoid arthritis (see p. 491); bowlegs

Dislocation, a complete loss of contact between the two surfaces, and subluxation, a partial loss of contact

Subcutaneous nodules in rheumatoid arthritis or rheumatic fever

Muscular weakness and atrophy in rheumatoid arthritis

Involvement of only one joint increases the likelihood of bacterial arthritis. Rheumatoid arthritis typically involves several joints, symmetrically distributed.

When handling a person with painful joints, be gentle and move slowly. Often patients can move more comfortably by themselves. Let them show you how they manage.

The detail with which you examine the musculoskeletal system will vary widely. You will be able to do the examination described in this chapter in only 3 to 4 minutes. Its thoroughness is appropriate to a patient with joint complaints. An even briefer survey for those without musculoskeletal symptoms is outlined in Chapter 4. Patients with extensive or severe musculoskeletal problems will require more time.

WITH THE PATIENT SITTING UP

HEAD AND NECK

THE TEMPOROMANDIBULAR JOINT. Place the tip of your index finger just in front of the tragus of each ear and ask the patient to open his or her mouth. The tips of your fingers should drop into the joint spaces as the mouth opens. Observe the range of motion, feel for swelling, and note any tenderness. Snapping or clicking may be felt and heard in normal people.

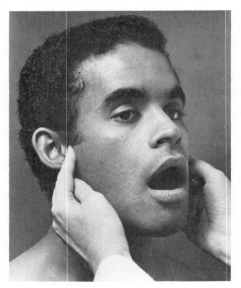

Swelling, tenderness, and decreased range of motion suggest arthritis.

THE CERVICAL SPINE

Inspection. Observe the neck for deformities and abnormal posture.

Palpation. Feel the spinous processes of the cervical spine and the related soft tissues, including the trapezius muscles, the muscles between the scapulae, and the sternomastoids. Identify any areas of tenderness.

Range of Motion. Ask the patient to:

- Touch chin to chest (flexion)
- Touch chin to each shoulder (rotation)
- Touch each ear to the corresponding shoulder without raising the shoulder (lateral bending)
- Put the head back (extension)

See Table 2-16, Pains in the Neck (p. 93). Late ankylosing spondylitis may cause an immobile neck with a characteristic deformity. The head and neck are thrust forward, contrasting with a kyphotic thorax.

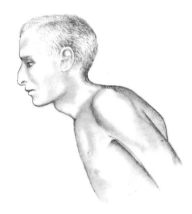

HANDS AND WRISTS

RANGE OF MOTION. Ask the patient to:

- *Make a fist* with each hand, thumb across the knuckles, and then extend and spread the fingers. A person should be able to make tight fists and extend and spread the fingers smoothly and easily.

Conditions that impair range of motion include arthritis, inflammation of the tendon sheaths (tenosynovitis), and fibrosis in the palmar fascia (Dupuytren's contracture). See Table 17-1, Swellings and Deformities of the Hands (pp. 491–493).

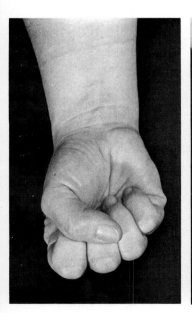
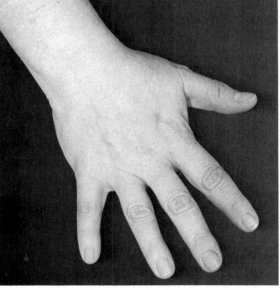

- *Flex and extend the wrists.* Because grip is strongest when the wrist is partly extended, impaired extension is especially important.
- With palms down, *move the hands laterally and medially* (ulnar and radial deviation).

INSPECTION. Look for any swelling, redness, nodules, deformity, or muscular atrophy.

Osteoarthritis of the distal interphalangeal joints appears as hard dorsolateral nodules called Heberden's nodes.

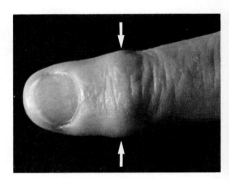

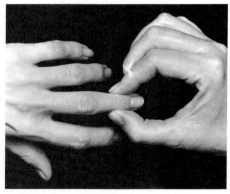

PALPATION. Feel the medial and lateral aspects of each *distal interphalangeal joint* (DIP) between your thumb and index finger, noting any swelling, bogginess, bony enlargement, or tenderness.

In a like manner, palpate each *proximal interphalangeal joint* (PIP).

The proximal interphalangeal joints are affected less often. Rheumatoid arthritis commonly involves the proximal joints.

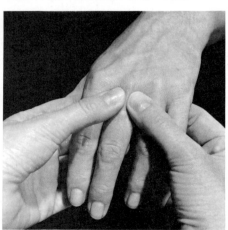

With your thumbs, palpate the *metacarpophalangeal joints* (the MCPs), just distal to and on each side of the knuckle. Note any swelling, bogginess, or tenderness.

Rheumatoid arthritis often involves the metacarpophalangeal joints; osteoarthritis rarely does.

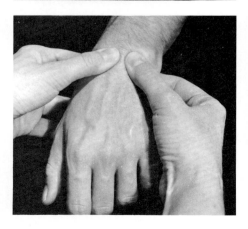

Palpate each *wrist joint*, with your thumbs on the dorsum of the wrist, your fingers beneath it. Note any swelling, bogginess, or tenderness.

Swelling suggests rheumatoid arthritis if it is bilateral and lasts for several weeks.

Gonococcal infection may involve the wrist joint (arthritis) or the tendon sheaths at the wrist (gonococcal tenosynovitis).

ELBOWS

RANGE OF MOTION. Ask the patient to bend and straighten the elbows. With arms at sides and elbows flexed (so that shoulder movements cannot simulate those of the forearm), the patient should then turn palms up (supination) and down (pronation).

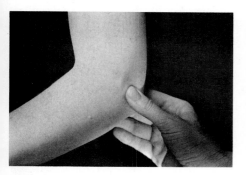

INSPECTION AND PALPATION. Support the patient's forearm with your opposite hand so that the elbow is flexed to about 70°. Examine the elbow, including the extensor surface of the ulna and the olecranon process, noting any nodules or swelling. Palpate the groove on either side of the olecranon as illustrated, noting any thickening, swelling, or tenderness.

Press on the lateral and medial epicondyles, noting any tenderness.

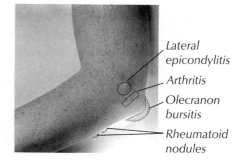

Lateral epicondylitis
Arthritis
Olecranon bursitis
Rheumatoid nodules

See Table 17-2, Swollen or Tender Elbows (p. 494).

SHOULDERS AND RELATED STRUCTURES

RANGE OF MOTION. Ask the patient to (1) raise both arms to a vertical position at the sides of the head, (2) place both hands behind the neck, with elbows out to the side (external rotation and abduction), and (3) place both hands behind the small of the back (internal rotation). By cupping your hand over the shoulder during these movements, note any crepitus.

INSPECTION. Observe the shoulders and shoulder girdle anteriorly, and inspect the scapulae and related muscles posteriorly. Note any swelling, deformity, or muscular atrophy.

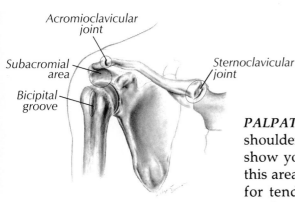

Acromioclavicular joint
Subacromial area
Bicipital groove
Sternoclavicular joint

PALPATION. If there is a history of shoulder pain, ask the patient to show you just where it is. Palpate this area and the following regions for tenderness: (1) the sternoclavicular joint, (2) the acromioclavicular joint, (3) the subacromial area, and (4) the bicipital groove.

The most common cause of shoulder pain is rotator cuff tendinitis (the impingement syndrome). See Table 17-3, Painful Shoulders (pp. 495–496).

WITH THE PATIENT LYING DOWN
ANKLES AND FEET

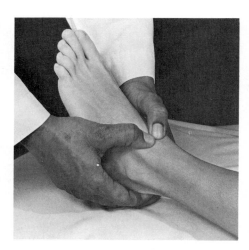

INSPECTION AND PALPATION. Observe all surfaces of the ankles and feet, noting any deformities, nodules, or swellings, and any calluses or corns.

See Table 17-4, Abnormalities of the Feet and Toes (pp. 497–498).

Ankle Joint. With your thumbs, palpate the anterior aspect of each ankle joint, as shown on the left, noting any bogginess, swelling, or tenderness.

Localized tenderness in arthritis of the ankle

Feel along the Achilles tendon for nodules and tenderness.

Rheumatoid nodules; tenderness of Achilles tendinitis or bursitis

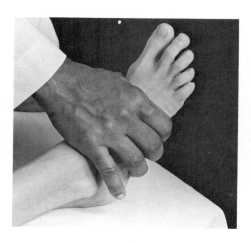

Metatarsophalangeal Joints. Screen for tenderness of these joints by compressing the forefoot between your thumb and fingers. Exert your pressure just proximal to the heads of the 1st and 5th metatarsals.

Tenderness on compression of the metatarsophalangeal joints is an early sign of rheumatoid arthritis. Acute inflammation of the first metatarsophalangeal joint suggests gout.

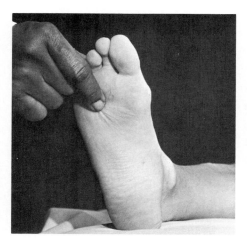

To evaluate the metatarsophalangeal joints individually, firmly palpate the heads of the five metatarsals and the grooves between them with your thumb and index finger. Place your thumb on the dorsum of the foot and your index finger on the plantar surface. Note any tenderness.

Pain and tenderness, called metatarsalgia, have many causes.

RANGE OF MOTION

The Ankle (Tibiotalar) Joint. Dorsiflex and plantar flex the foot at the ankle.

The Subtalar Joint. Stabilize the ankle with one hand, grasp the heel with the other, and invert and evert the foot.

These four maneuvers help to identify which joints of an arthritic foot are involved.

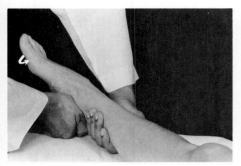

INVERSION

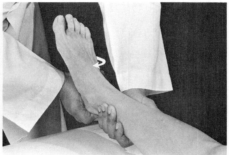

EVERSION

The Transverse Tarsal Joint. Stabilize the heel and invert and evert the forefoot.

An arthritic joint is frequently painful when moved in any direction, while a ligamentous sprain produces maximal pain when the ligament is stretched. For example, in a common form of sprained ankle, inversion and plantar flexion of the foot cause pain, while eversion and dorsiflexion are relatively pain-free.

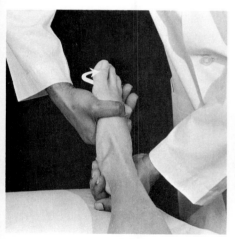

INVERSION

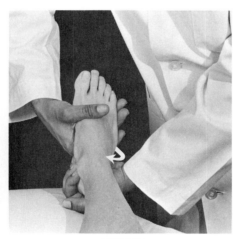

EVERSION

The Metatarsophalangeal Joints. Flex the toes in relation to the feet.

KNEES AND HIPS

INSPECTION OF THE KNEES. Note their alignment and any deformity. Observe any atrophy of the quadriceps muscles. Look for loss of the normal hollows around the patella (an early sign of swelling in the knee joint and suprapatellar pouch), and note any other swelling in or around the knee.

Bowlegs (genu varum), knock-knees (genu valgum), or flexion contracture (inability to extend fully)

PALPATION OF THE KNEES. Try to feel any thickening or swelling in the suprapatellar pouch and along the sides of the patella. Starting about 10 cm above the superior border of the patella (well above the pouch), feel the soft tissues between your thumb and fingers. Move your hand distally in progressive steps, trying to identify the pouch. Continue your palpation along the sides of the patella. Note any tenderness or any warmth greater than that of surrounding tissues. The synovial membrane of the suprapatellar pouch and knee joint is not normally palpable.

Swelling above and adjacent to the patella suggests synovial thickening or fluid in the knee joint.

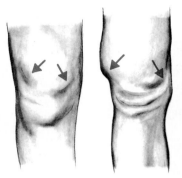

Moderate   Marked
swelling   swelling

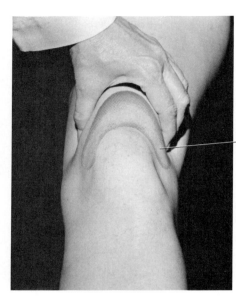

Suprapatellar pouch

Thickening, bogginess, tenderness, and warmth in these areas indicates synovial inflammation. Nontender effusions are common in osteoarthritis.

Bursitis causes a more localized swelling, as in prepatellar bursitis (housemaid's knee).

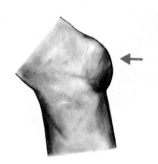

FURTHER STEPS TO DETECT FLUID IN THE KNEE JOINT IF YOU SUSPECT IT

The Bulge Sign. With the ball of your hand, milk the medial aspect of the knee firmly upward two or three times to displace any fluid.

Then press or tap the knee just behind the lateral margin of the patella.

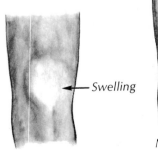

Swelling

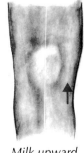

Milk upward

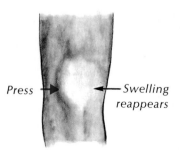

Press   Swelling reappears

A bulge of returning fluid indicates an effusion within the knee joint.

Watch for a bulge of returning fluid in the hollow medial to the patella. Normally none is seen.

A bulge sign is especially useful in detecting small effusions. It may be absent in large effusions.

Ballottement of a "Floating Patella." Firmly grasp the thigh just above the patella with one hand, thus forcing fluid out of the suprapatellar pouch into the space between the patella and the femur. Place the fingers of your other hand on the patella and push it sharply back against the femur. Feel for a palpable click. In the absence of fluid, none is felt because the patella is already snug against the femur.

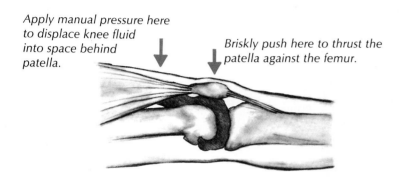

Apply manual pressure here to displace knee fluid into space behind patella.

Briskly push here to thrust the patella against the femur.

When the patella is separated from the femur by excessive joint fluid, the sharp backward thrust makes it collide against the femur with a palpable click.

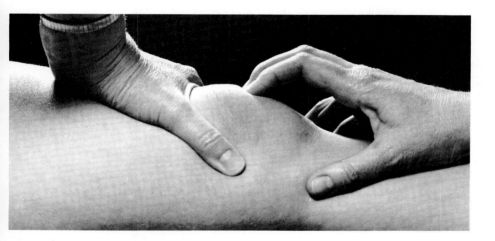

Ballottement is especially useful in identifying large effusions; it is insensitive to small ones.

THE PATELLOFEMORAL COMPARTMENT. Compress the patella and move it against the underlying femur. Then push the patella distally and ask the patient to tighten the knee against the table, thus contracting the quadriceps. Note any pain or crepitus with these maneuvers. Crepitus alone has little significance.

Pain and crepitus occur in osteoarthritis and in chondromalacia patellae, a similar condition that affects younger people.

THE TIBIOFEMORAL JOINT. Now flex the patient's knee to about 90° so that you can better palpate this joint. The patient's foot should rest on the examining table. With your thumbs, press into the joint and palpate along the tibial margins from the patellar tendon toward each side of the knee. Then palpate along the course of each collateral ligament. Identify any points of tenderness. Note any irregular bony ridges along the joint margins.

Tenderness from damaged menisci or collateral ligaments. The fat pad, when injured, may also be tender.

Bony ridges along the joint margins may be felt in osteoarthritis.

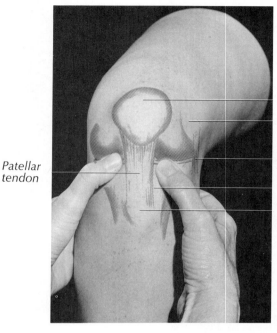

Patellar tendon

Patella
Lateral epicondyle
Lateral collateral ligament
Tibia
Tibial tuberosity

THE TIBIAL TUBEROSITY. In an adolescent with knee pain, press on the tibial tuberosity and note any swelling or tenderness.

A tender, swollen tibial tuberosity in an adolescent suggests Osgood–Schlatter disease.

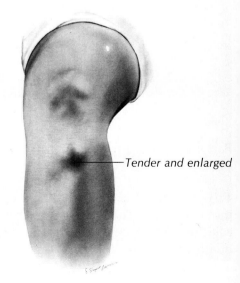

Tender and enlarged

Palpation of the posterior aspects of the knees is done best when the patient stands (see p. 487).

RANGE OF MOTION AT THE HIPS AND THE KNEES

Flexion of Knees and Hips. Ask the patient to bend each knee in turn up to the chest and pull it firmly against the abdomen.

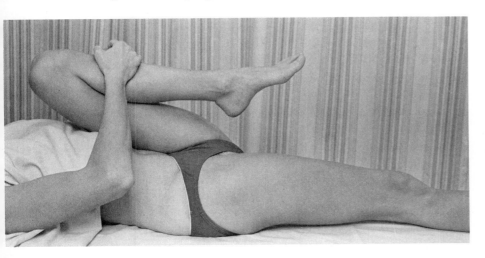

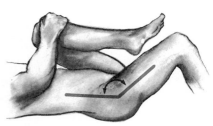

Flexion of the opposite thigh indicates a flexion deformity of that hip.

Observe the degree of flexion at hip and knee. In addition, note whether the opposite thigh remains on the table, fully extended at the hip.

Rotation of the Hips. Flex the leg to 90° at hip and knee, stabilize the thigh with one hand, grasp the ankle with the other, and swing the lower leg—medially for external rotation at the hip, and laterally for internal rotation.

Restriction of internal rotation is an especially sensitive indicator of hip disease such as arthritis. External rotation is often restricted also.

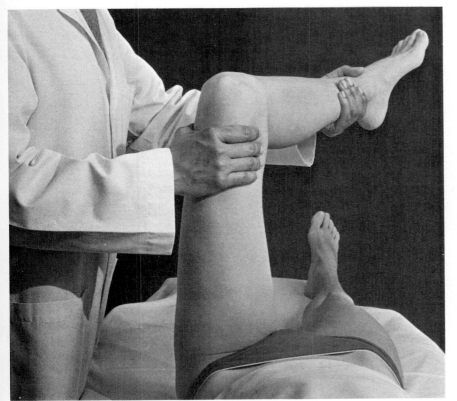

EXTERNAL ROTATION

Rotation may also be tested with the patient's legs extended. From the foot of the table, grasp the ankle and rotate the leg internally and externally. Judge the range of movement by watching the patella. Rotation in this position is normally somewhat less than with the hip flexed to 90°.

Abduction of the Hips. Stabilize the pelvis by pressing down on the opposite anterior superior iliac spine with one hand. With the other hand, grasp the ankle and abduct the extended leg until you feel the iliac spine move. This movement marks the limit of hip abduction.

Restricted abduction is common in hip disease.

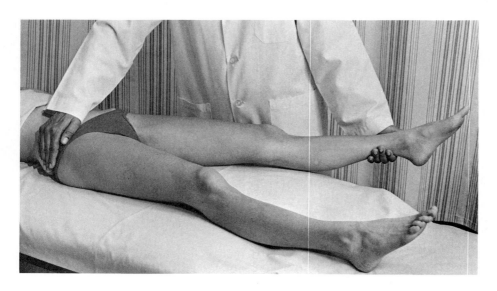

Alternatively, stand at the foot of the table, grasp both ankles, and abduct both extended legs at the hips.

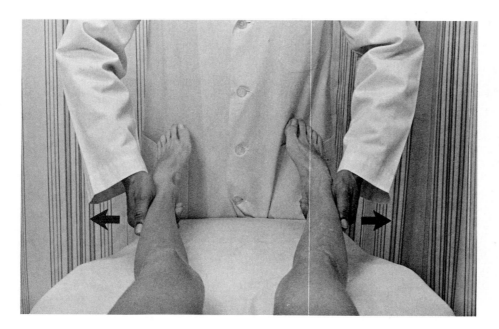

This method allows easy comparison of the two sides when movements are restricted.

WITH THE PATIENT STANDING

INSPECTION OF THE LEGS AND THE FEET. Note any deformities of the knees, any swellings in the popliteal spaces, and other deformities such as flat feet.

Bowlegs, knock-knees, popliteal swelling of a Baker's cyst (usually a swollen bursa)

THE SPINE

INSPECTION. The gown should allow adequate visualization of the patient's spine. Observe the spine—

- From the side, noting the cervical, thoracic, and lumbar curves

See Table 17-5, Abnormal Spinal Curvatures (pp. 499–500).

- From behind, noting any lateral curves. Look for any differences in the heights of the shoulders, the iliac crests, and the skin creases below the buttocks. Note whether an imaginary line dropped from the spinous process of T1 falls, as it should, through the gluteal cleft.

Unequal heights of the iliac crests (a pelvic tilt) suggest unequal lengths of the legs. Such a tilt is abolished by placing supports under one foot. Scoliosis and adduction or abduction deformities of the hip may also cause a pelvic tilt.

Scoliosis often becomes evident during adolescence, before symptoms appear.

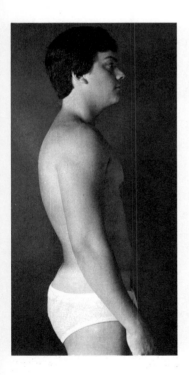
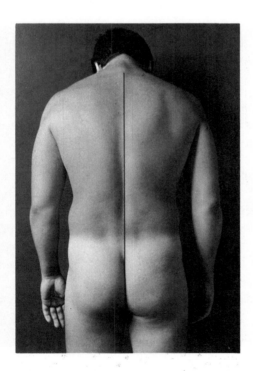

RANGE OF MOTION. Ask the patient to bend forward to touch the toes (flexion). Note the smoothness and symmetry of movement, the range of motion, and the curve in the lumbar area. As flexion proceeds, the lumbar concavity should flatten out.

Paravertebral muscle spasm and ankylosing spondylitis may prevent flattening; the lumbar concavity persists.

Sit down, stabilize the patient's pelvis with your hands, and ask the patient to (1) bend sideways (lateral bending), (2) bend backwards to-

Decreased spinal mobility in osteoarthritis and ankylosing

ward you (extension), and (3) twist the shoulders one way and then the other (rotation).

PALPATION. From a sitting or standing position, palpate the spinous processes with your thumb. In the lower lumbar area, determine whether one spinous process seems unusually prominent in relation to the one above it. Identify any tenderness.

You may also wish to percuss the spine for tenderness by thumping it (not too roughly) with the ulnar surface of your fist.

Inspect and palpate the paravertebral muscles for tenderness and spasm. Palpate for tenderness in any other areas that are suggested by the patient's symptoms. Try to identify the underlying structures involved. A skin dimple usually overlies the posterior superior iliac spine and guides you toward the sacroiliac area.

spondylitis, among other conditions

A spinous process of L5 or possibly L4 that feels unusually prominent in relation to the one above it suggests spondylolisthesis of the prominent vertebra.

Percussion may produce pain when osteoporosis, malignancy, or infection involves the spine.

A paravertebral muscle in spasm looks prominent, feels tight, and is usually tender.

Remember that tenderness in the costovertebral angles may signify kidney infection rather than a musculoskeletal problem.

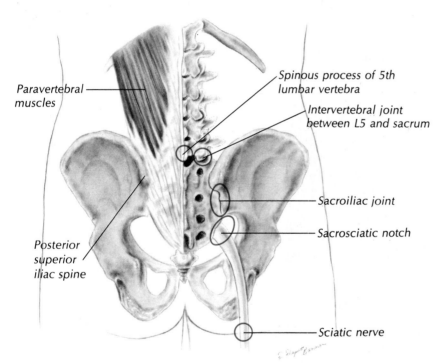

Paravertebral muscles

Spinous process of 5th lumbar vertebra

Intervertebral joint between L5 and sacrum

Sacroiliac joint

Sacrosciatic notch

Posterior superior iliac spine

Sciatic nerve

Herniated intervertebral discs, most common between L5 and S1 or between L4 and L5, may produce tenderness of the spinous processes, the intervertebral joints, the paravertebral muscles, the sacrosciatic notch, and the sciatic nerve.

Rheumatoid arthritis may also cause tenderness of the intervertebral joints. Ankylosing spondylitis may produce sacroiliac tenderness.

See Table 2-15, Low Back Pain (p. 92).

See pages 489–490 for further testing of low back pain with leg radiation.

SPECIAL MANEUVERS

FOR THE CARPAL TUNNEL SYNDROME. Pain and numbness in the hand, especially at night, suggest compression of the median nerve in the carpal tunnel. This tunnel is a narrow channel in the palm of the hand, between the carpal bones dorsally and a band of more superficial fascia ventrally.

Through the tunnel run the flexor tendons and the median nerve. Two clinical tests are used:

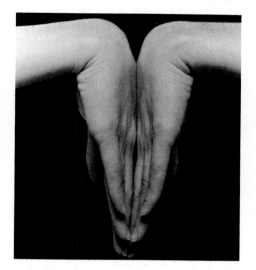

Phalen's Test. Hold the patient's wrists in acute flexion for 60 seconds. Alternatively, ask the patient to press the backs of both hands together to form right angles.

If numbness and tingling develop over the distribution of the median nerve (*e.g.*, the palmar surface of the thumb, and the index, middle, and part of the ring fingers), the sign is positive, suggesting the carpal tunnel syndrome.

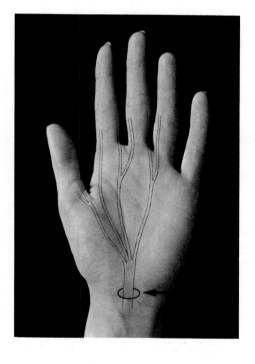

Tinel's Sign. With your finger, percuss lightly over the course of the median nerve in the carpal tunnel at the spot indicated by the arrow.

Tingling or electric sensations in the distribution of the median nerve constitute a positive test, suggesting the carpal tunnel syndrome.

FOR LOW BACK PAIN WITH RADIATION INTO THE LEG. If the patient has noted low back pain that radiates down the leg, check straight leg raising on each side in turn. Raise the patient's relaxed and straightened leg until pain occurs. Then dorsiflex the foot.

Record the degree of elevation at which pain occurs, the quality and distribution of the pain, and the effects of dorsiflexion. Tightness and mild discomfort in the hamstrings with these maneuvers are common and do not indicate radicular pain.

Sharp pain radiating from the back down the leg in an L5 or S1 distribution (radicular pain) suggests tension on or compres-

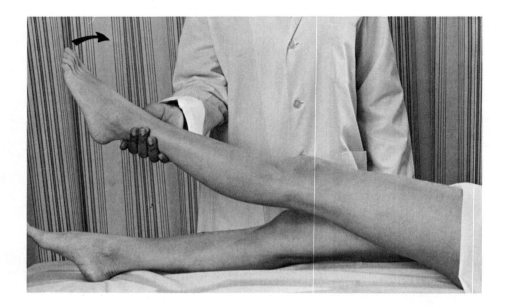

sion of the nerve root(s), often caused by a herniated lumbar disc. Dorsiflexion of the foot increases the pain. Increased pain in the affected leg when the opposite leg is raised strongly confirms radicular pain and constitutes a positive *crossed straight leg-raising sign.*

MEASURING THE LENGTH OF LEGS. If you suspect that the patient's legs are unequal in length, measure them. Get the patient relaxed in the supine position and symmetrically aligned with legs extended. With a tape, measure the distance between the anterior superior iliac spine and the medial malleolus. The tape should cross the knee on its medial side.

Unequal leg length may explain a scoliosis.

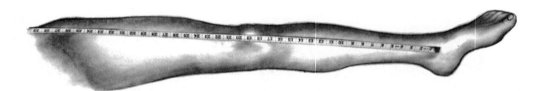

DESCRIBING LIMITED MOTION OF A JOINT. Although precise measurement of motion is not routinely necessary, limitations can be described in degrees. Pocket goniometers are available for this purpose. In the two examples shown below, the red lines indicate the range of the patient's movement and the black lines show the normal range.

Your observations may be described in several ways. The numbers in parentheses are suitably abbreviated recordings.

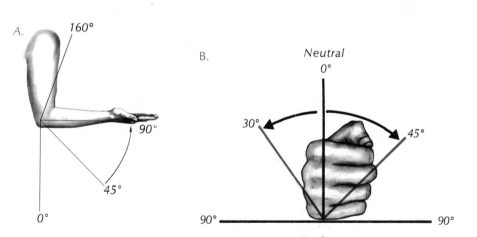

A. The elbow flexes from 45° to 90° (45° → 90°),

-or-

The elbow has a flexion deformity of 45° and can be flexed farther to 90° (45° → 90°).

B. Supination at elbow = 30° (0° → 30°)
Pronation at elbow = 45° (0° → 45°)

Table 17-1   Swellings and Deformitites of the Hands

Table 17-1   Swellings and Deformities of the Hands

OSTEOARTHRITIS (Degenerative Joint Disease)

Nodules on the dorsolateral aspects of the distal interphalangeal joints, called Heberden's nodes, are due to the bony overgrowth of osteoarthritis. Usually hard and painless, they affect the middle-aged or elderly and often, although not always, are associated with arthritic changes in other joints. Flexion and deviation deformities may develop. Similar nodules on the proximal interphalangeal joints, called Bouchard's nodes, are less common. The metacarpophalangeal joints are spared.

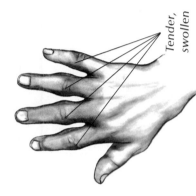

Radial deviation of distal phalanx

Heberden's node

Bouchard's node

Metacarpophalangeal joints uninvolved

ACUTE RHEUMATOID ARTHRITIS

Tender, painful, stiff joints characterize rheumatoid arthritis. Symmetrical involvement on both sides of the body is typical. The proximal interphalangeal, metacarpophalangeal, and wrist joints are frequently affected; the distal interphalangeal joints are rarely so. Patients with acute disease often have fusiform or spindle-shaped swelling of the proximal interphalangeal joints.

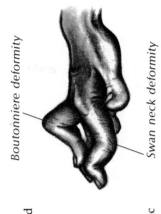

Tender, swollen

CHRONIC RHEUMATOID ARTHRITIS

As the arthritic process continues and worsens, chronic swelling and thickening of the metacarpophalangeal and proximal interphalangeal joints appear. Range of motion becomes limited and the fingers may deviate toward the ulnar side. The interosseous muscles atrophy. The fingers may show "swan neck" deformities (*i.e.,* hyperextension of the proximal interphalangeal joints with fixed flexion of the distal interphalangeal joints). Less common is a boutonniere deformity (*i.e.,* persistent flexion of the proximal interphalangeal joint with hyperextension of the distal interphalangeal joint).

Rheumatoid nodules may accompany either the acute or the chronic stage.

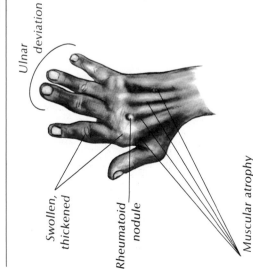

Boutonniere deformity

Swan neck deformity

Ulnar deviation

Swollen, thickened

Rheumatoid nodule

Muscular atrophy

◆ *Continued*

Table 17-1   Swellings and Deformitites of the Hands

Table 17-1   (Cont'd.)

CHRONIC TOPHACEOUS GOUT

The deformities that develop in long-standing chronic tophaceous gout can sometimes mimic those of rheumatoid and osteoarthritis. Joint involvement is usually not so symmetrical as in rheumatoid arthritis. Acute inflammation may be present. Knobby swellings around the joints sometimes ulcerate and discharge white chalklike urates.

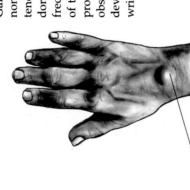

Swollen

Knobby swelling

Draining tophus

GANGLION

Ganglia are cystic, round, usually nontender swellings located along tendon sheaths or joint capsules. The dorsum of the hand and wrist is a frequent site of involvement. Flexion of the wrist makes ganglia more prominent; extension tends to obscure them. Ganglia may also develop elsewhere on the hands, wrists, ankles, and feet.

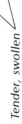

Cystic swelling

TENDON SHEATH AND PALMAR SPACE INFECTIONS

ACUTE TENOSYNOVITIS

Infection of the flexor tendon sheaths (acute tenosynovitis) may follow local injury, even of apparently trivial nature. Unlike arthritis, tenderness and swelling develop not in the joint but along the course of the tendon sheath, from the distal phalanx to the level of the metacarpophalangeal joint. The finger is held in slight flexion; attempts to extend it are very painful.

Pain on extension

Swelling and tenderness along tendon sheath

Finger held in slight flexion

ACUTE TENOSYNOVITIS AND THENAR SPACE INVOLVEMENT

If the infection progresses, it may escape the bounds of the tendon sheath to involve one of the adjacent fascial spaces within the palm. Infections of the index finger and thenar space are illustrated.

Early diagnosis and treatment are important.

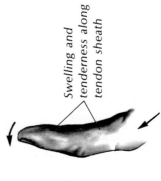

Puncture wound

Tender, swollen

Table 17-1 Swellings and Deformitites of the Hands

FELON

Injury to the fingertip may result in infection in the enclosed fascial spaces of the finger pad. Severe pain, localized tenderness, swelling, and dusky redness are characteristic. Early diagnosis and treatment are important.

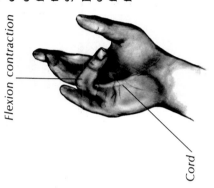

Puncture wound

Swollen, tender, dusky red

DUPUYTREN'S CONTRACTURE

The first sign of a Dupuytren's contracture is a thickened plaque overlying the tendon of the ring finger and possibly the little finger at the level of the distal palmar crease. Subsequently the skin in this area puckers, and a thickened fibrotic cord develops between palm and finger. Flexion contracture of the fingers may gradually ensue.

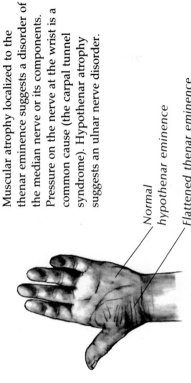

Flexion contraction

Cord

TRIGGER FINGER

A trigger finger is caused by a painless nodule in a flexor tendon in the palm, near the head of the metacarpal. The nodule is too big to enter easily into the tendon sheath when the person tries to extend the fingers from a flexed position. With extra effort or assistance, the finger extends with a palpable and audible snap as the nodule pops through the narrow area. This snap may also be evident during flexion. Watch and listen as the patient flexes and extends the fingers, and feel for both the nodule and the snap.

THENAR ATROPHY

Muscular atrophy localized to the thenar eminence suggests a disorder of the median nerve or its components. Pressure on the nerve at the wrist is a common cause (the carpal tunnel syndrome). Hypothenar atrophy suggests an ulnar nerve disorder.

Normal hypothenar eminence

Flattened thenar eminence

Table 17-2 Swollen or Tender Elbows

OLECRANON BURSITIS

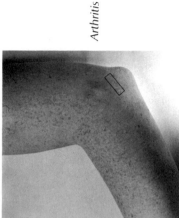

Olecranon bursitis

Swelling and inflammation of the olecranon bursa may result from trauma or may be associated with rheumatoid or gouty arthritis. The swelling is superficial to the olecranon process.

RHEUMATOID NODULES

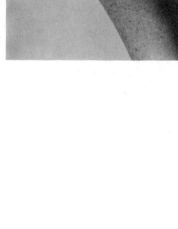

Rheumatoid nodules

Subcutaneous nodules may develop at pressure points along the extensor surface of the ulna in patients with rheumatoid arthritis. They are firm and nontender, and are not attached to the overlying skin. They may or may not be attached to the underlying periosteum. Although they may develop in the area of the olecranon bursa, they often occur more distally.

ARTHRITIS OF THE ELBOW

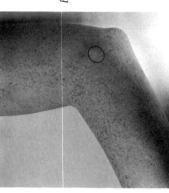

Arthritis

Synovial inflammation or fluid is felt best in the grooves between the olecranon process and the epicondyles on either side. Palpate for a boggy, soft, or fluctuant swelling and for tenderness.

EPICONDYLITIS

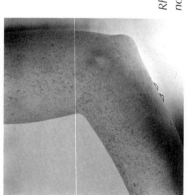

Epicondylitis

Lateral epicondylitis (tennis elbow) follows repetitive extension of the wrist or pronation–supination of the forearm. Pain and tenderness develop at the lateral epicondyle and possibly in the extensor muscles close to it. When the patient tries to extend the wrist against resistance, pain increases.

Medial epicondylitis (pitcher's or Little League elbow) follows repetitive wrist flexion, as in throwing. Tenderness is maximal at the medial epicondyle. Wrist flexion against resistance increases the pain.

Table 17-3   Painful Shoulders

Table 17-3   Painful Shoulders

ROTATOR CUFF TENDINITIS
(Impingement Syndrome)

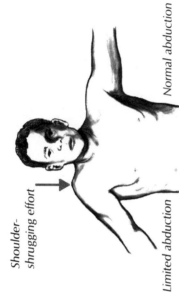

When the arm is raised, the rotator cuff may impinge against the under surface of the acromion and the coracoacromial ligament. Repeated impingement of this kind, as in throwing or swimming, can cause edema and hemorrhage followed by inflammation and fibrosis, most often involving the supraspinatus tendon. Acute, recurrent, or chronic pain may result, often aggravated by activity. Sharp catches of pain may occur as the arm is elevated into an overhead position. When the supraspinatus tendon is involved, tenderness is maximal just below the tip of the acromion. The patients tend to be young (teens to 40 years) and are often, though not necessarily, athletically active.

ROTATOR CUFF TEARS

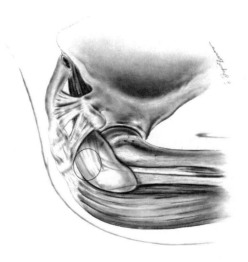

Shoulder-shrugging effort

Limited abduction

Normal abduction

Repeated impingement (or other conditions) may weaken the rotator cuff and eventually cause partial or complete tears in it, usually after the age of 40 years. Injury, such as falling, may precipitate a tear. Manifestations include weakness, atrophy of the supraspinatus and infraspinatus muscles, pain, and tenderness. In a complete tear of the supraspinatus tendon (illustrated), active abduction at the glenohumeral joint is severely impaired. Efforts to abduct the arm produce a characteristic shoulder shrugging instead.

CALCIFIC TENDINITIS

Calcific tendinitis refers to a degenerative process in the tendon that is associated with the deposition of calcium salts. Like rotator cuff tendinitis, it usually involves the supraspinatus tendon. Acute, disabling attacks of shoulder pain may occur, usually in patients over 30 years of age and more often in women. The arm is held close to the side, and all motions are severely limited by pain. Tenderness is maximal below the tip of the acromion. The subacromial bursa, which overlies the supraspinatus tendon, may become involved in the inflammation. Chronic, less severe pain may also occur.

► Continued

Table 17-3   Painful Shoulders

Table 17-3 (Cont'd.)

BICIPITAL TENDINITIS	ACROMIOCLAVICULAR ARTHRITIS	ADHESIVE CAPSULITIS *(Frozen Shoulder)*
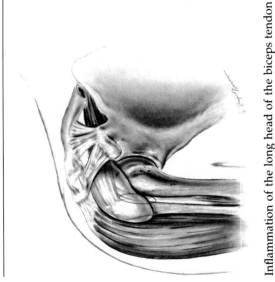	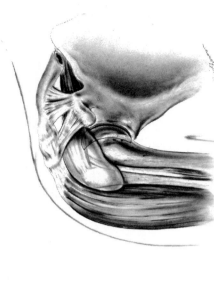	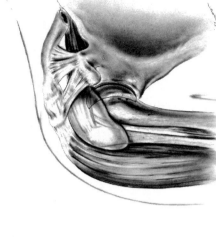

BICIPITAL TENDINITIS

Inflammation of the long head of the biceps tendon and its sheath causes anterior shoulder pain that may resemble rotator cuff tendinitis and may coexist with it. This tendon, like the cuff, may suffer impingement injury. Tenderness is maximal in the bicipital groove. By externally rotating and abducting the arm, you can more easily separate this area from the subacromial tenderness of supraspinatus tendinitis. With the patient's arm at the side, elbow flexed to 90°, ask the patient to supinate the forearm against your resistance. Increased pain in the bicipital groove confirms this condition.

ACROMIOCLAVICULAR ARTHRITIS

Acromioclavicular arthritis is not a common cause of shoulder pain. When present, it usually is the result of direct injury to the shoulder girdle with resulting degenerative changes. Tenderness is localized over the acromioclavicular joint. Although motion in the glenohumeral joint is not painful in acromioclavicular arthritis, as it is in many other painful conditions of the shoulder, movements of the scapula, such as shoulder shrugging, are.

ADHESIVE CAPSULITIS *(Frozen Shoulder)*

Adhesive capsulitis refers to a mysterious fibrosis of the glenohumeral joint capsule, manifested by diffuse, dull, aching pain in the shoulder and progressive restriction of motion, but usually no localized tenderness. The condition is usually unilateral and occurs in persons aged 50 to 70. There is often an antecedent painful disorder of the shoulder or possibly another condition (such as myocardial infarction) that has decreased shoulder movements. The course is chronic, lasting months to years, but the disorder often resolves spontaneously, at least partially.

Table 17-4   Abnormalities of the Feet and Toes

Table 17-4   Abnormalities of the Feet and Toes

ACUTE GOUTY ARTHRITIS	HALLUX VALGUS	FLAT FEET
		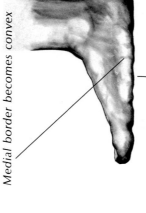 *Medial border becomes convex* *Sole touches floor*
Hot, red, tender, swollen		
The metatarsophalangeal joint of the great toe may be the first joint involved in acute gouty arthritis. It is characterized by a very painful and tender, hot, dusky red swelling that extends beyond the margin of the joint. It is easily mistaken for a cellulitis. Acute gout may also involve the dorsum of the foot.	In hallux valgus, the great toe is abnormally abducted in relationship to the first metatarsal, which itself is deviated medially. The head of the first metatarsal may enlarge on its medial side and a bursa may form at the pressure point. This bursa may become inflamed.	Signs of flat feet may be apparent only when the patient stands, or they may become permanent. The longitudinal arch flattens so that the sole approaches or touches the floor. The normal concavity on the medial side of the foot becomes convex. Tenderness may be present from the medial malleolus down along the medial-plantar surface of the foot. Swelling may develop anterior to the malleoli. Inspect the shoes for excess wear on the inner side of the soles and heels.

➡ *Continued*

Table 17-4   Abnormalities of the Feet and Toes

Table 17-4   (Cont'd.)

INGROWN TOENAIL

Red, tender

Granulation tissue

The sharp edge of the great toenail may dig into and injure the skin fold, resulting in inflammation and infection. A tender, reddened, overhanging nail fold, sometimes with granulation tissue and purulent discharge, results.

HAMMER TOE

Hyperextended

Flexed

Most commonly involving the second toe, a hammer toe is characterized by hyperextension at the metatarsophalangeal joint with flexion at the proximal interphalangeal joint. A corn frequently develops at the pressure point over the proximal interphalangeal joint.

CORN

Red, thickened

A corn is a painful conical thickening of skin that results from recurrent pressure on normally thin skin. The apex of the cone points inward and causes pain. Corns characteristically occur over bony prominences (*e.g.,* the 5th toe). When located in moist areas (*e.g.,* at pressure points between the 4th and 5th toes), they are called soft corns.

CALLUS

Like a corn, a callus is an area of greatly thickened skin that develops in a region of recurrent pressure. Unlike a corn, however, a callus involves skin that is normally thick, such as the sole, and is usually painless. If a callus is painful, suspect an underlying plantar wart.

PLANTAR WART

A plantar wart is a common wart (verruca vulgaris) located in the thickened skin of the sole. It may look somewhat like a callus or even be covered by one. Look for the characteristic small dark spots that give a stippled appearance to a wart. Normal skin lines stop at the wart's edge.

NEUROTROPHIC ULCER

When pain sensation is diminished or absent (as in diabetic neuropathy, for example), neurotrophic ulcers may develop at pressure points on the feet. Although often deep, infected, and indolent, they are painless. Callus formation about the ulcer is diagnostically helpful. Like the ulcer itself, it results from chronic pressure.

Table 17-5   Abnormal Spinal Curvatures

Table 17-5   *Abnormal Spinal Curvatures*

NORMAL SPINAL CURVATURES	FLATTENING OF THE LUMBAR CURVE	LUMBAR LORDOSIS	KYPHOSIS
Note the gentle curves of the normal spine—concavities in the cervical and lumbar regions and a convexity in the thorax.	When you see flattening of the lumbar curve, look for muscle spasm in the lumbar area and for decreased spinal mobility. This combination of signs suggests the possibility of a herniated lumbar disc or, especially in men, ankylosing spondylitis.	Lordosis—an accentuation of the normal lumbar curve—develops to compensate for the protuberant abdomen of pregnancy or marked obesity (as illustrated here). It may also compensate for kyphosis and flexion deformities of the hips. A deep midline furrow may be seen between the lumbar paravertebral muscles.	Kyphosis—a rounded thoracic convexity—is common in aging, especially in women. In adolescent patients, consider Scheuermann's disease.

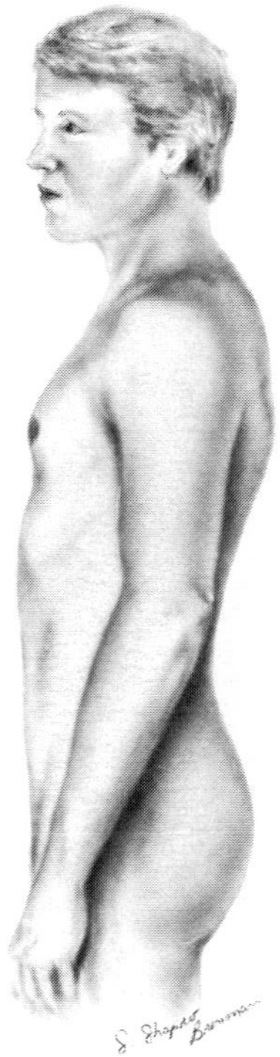

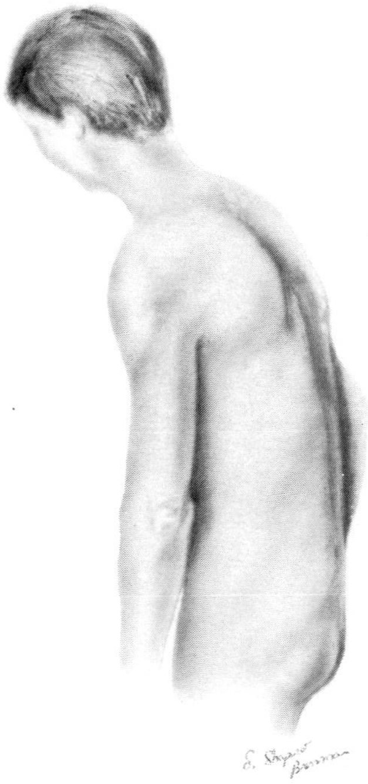

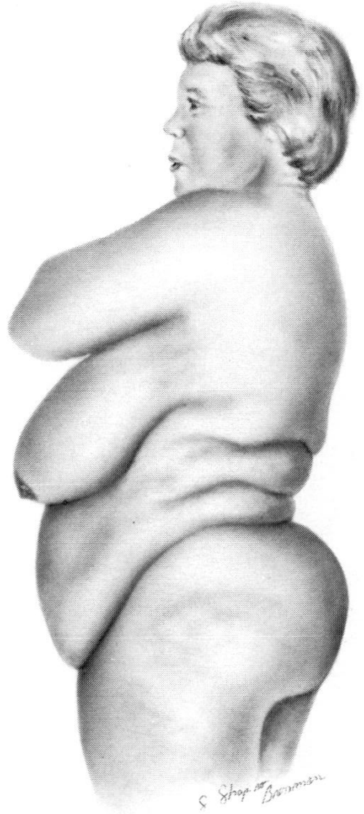

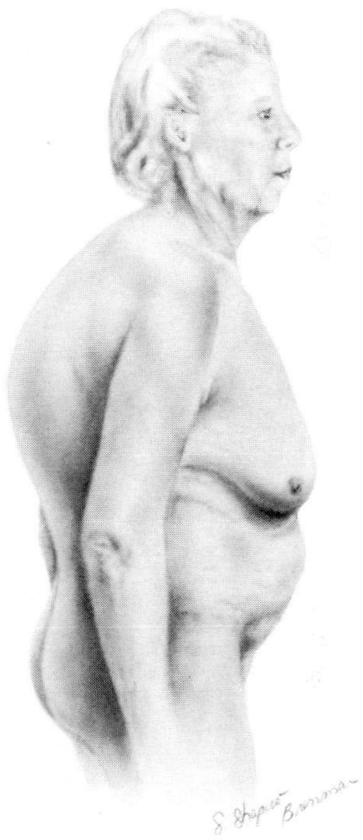

► *Continued*

Table 17-5   Abnormal Spinal Curvatures

Table 17-5   (Cont'd.)

GIBBUS	LIST	SCOLIOSIS

Gibbus is an angular deformity of a collapsed vertebra. Causes include metastatic cancer and tuberculosis of the spine.

List is a lateral tilt of the spine. When a plumb line dropped from the spinous process of T1 falls to one side of the gluteal cleft, a list is present. Causes include a herniated disc and painful spasms of the paravertebral muscles. Scoliosis (a lateral curve of spine) is inherent in a list but has not been fully compensated for by a spinal deviation in the opposite direction.

Scoliosis—a lateral curvature of the spine—is shown here with a thoracic convexity to the right. The body has compensated for the curve and a plumb line from T1 drops through the gluteal cleft. Scoliosis may be structural, as illustrated, or functional.

Structural scoliosis is typically associated with rotation of the vertebrae upon each other, and the rib cage is accordingly deformed. This deformity is seen best when the patient flexes forward. On the side of the thoracic convexity, the ribs bulge posteriorly and are widely separated. On the opposite side, they are displaced anteriorly and are close together.

Functional scoliosis compensates for other abnormalities such as unequal leg lengths. It involves neither vertebral rotation nor thoracic deformity. The scoliosis disappears with forward flexion.

Chapter 18
The Nervous System

Anatomy and Physiology

This section deals briefly with some of the anatomy and physiology that relate directly to the neurologic examination. After a short description of the brain, it discusses the spinal cord and the simplest level of nervous response—the reflex arc. It then summarizes the motor pathways that initiate voluntary action, coordinate movements, and maintain posture and balance. Sensory pathways are considered next, and then the cranial nerves with both their motor and their sensory functions. The section concludes with variations in neurologic findings that are associated with age.

THE BRAIN

The brain has four regions: the cerebrum, the diencephalon, the brainstem, and the cerebellum.

The cerebral hemispheres constitute the greatest mass of brain tissue. Their outer layers are formed by the cellular gray matter known as the cerebral cortex.

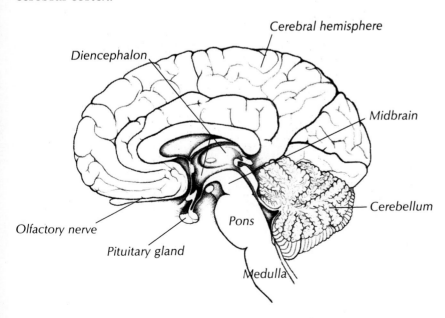

Consciousness depends on interaction between intact cerebral hemispheres and an activating (or arousal) system that lies in the diencephalon and upper brainstem. Either extensive disease of the cerebral cortex or damage to the activating system may impair consciousness to the point of coma.

The cerebellum is primarily concerned with coordination.

The brainstem, which continues down to the spinal cord, has three sections: the midbrain, the pons, and the medulla.

The paired cranial nerves 2 through 12 emerge from the diencephalon and the brainstem, as illustrated on the right. The olfactory nerves (really nerve tracts) emerge from the cerebral hemispheres. Observable abnormalities in the functions of specific cranial nerves help to identify the location of lesions in the nervous system. The functions of the cranial nerves are summarized on pages 511 and 512.

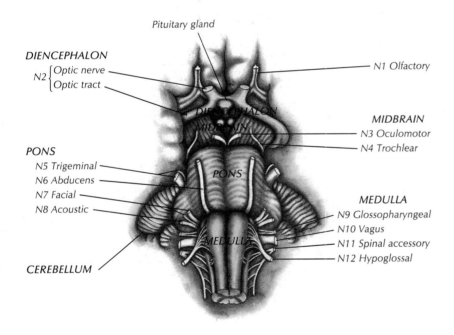

Pituitary gland

DIENCEPHALON

N2 { Optic nerve
    { Optic tract

N1 Olfactory

MIDBRAIN
N3 Oculomotor
N4 Trochlear

PONS
N5 Trigeminal
N6 Abducens
N7 Facial
N8 Acoustic

MEDULLA
N9 Glossopharyngeal
N10 Vagus
N11 Spinal accessory
N12 Hypoglossal

CEREBELLUM

THE SPINAL CORD AND REFLEX ARC

The spinal cord is a cylindrical mass of nervous tissue that is encased within the bony vertebral column. It contains long tracts that connect the brain with the peripheral nervous system, and it also mediates reflex activity.

A reflex is an involuntary bodily response involving three basic components: a receiving apparatus, a nerve center, and a responding apparatus.

Deep tendon (muscle stretch) reflexes in the arms and legs illustrate this fundamental organization.

To elicit a deep tendon reflex, one briskly taps the tendon of a partially stretched muscle. By stretching the muscle farther, such a tap stimulates special sensory endings in the muscle and generates an impulse that travels up each of many *sensory* nerve fibers* to the spinal cord. Each sensory fiber travels with other sensory and motor nerve fibers in a *peripheral nerve.*

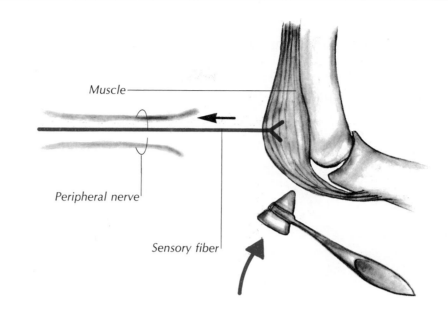

A peripheral nerve may carry nerve fibers supplying a fairly large area of the body. As the nerve fibers approach the cord, they are reorganized on a segmental basis into 31 pairs of *spinal nerves* (8 cervical, 12 thoracic, 5 lumbar, 5 sacral, and 1 coccygeal). Within the vertebral canal, each spinal nerve separates into posterior (dorsal) and anterior (ventral) roots. The *posterior root* contains the sensory fibers. The sensory nerve impulse for the deep tendon reflex is carried on through the sensory fiber into the spinal cord, where it synapses with a *motor neuron*, or *anterior horn cell.*

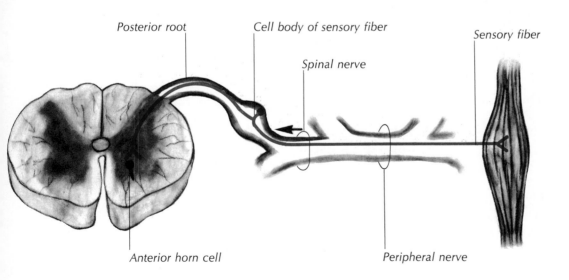

* The word "sensory," as used here, does not necessarily imply conscious sensation, although many authors prefer to use the term in this restricted sense. It would be more precise to use the term "afferent," indicating the direction in which the nerve impulse travels (*i.e.*, toward the spinal cord or brain). The term "efferent" (away from the cord or brain) would then be used instead of "motor."

After stimulation across the synapse, an impulse is then transmitted down the motor neuron, traversing in turn the motor *anterior nerve root*, the spinal nerve, and the peripheral nerve. By transmitting an impulse across the neuromuscular junction, it then stimulates the muscle to a brisk contraction, completing the reflex arc.

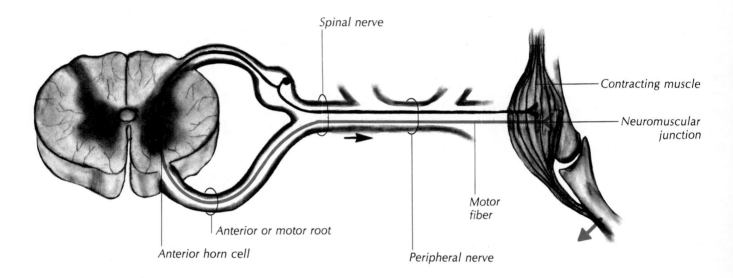

A deep tendon reflex is thus dependent on (1) intact sensory (afferent) nerve fibers, (2) functional synapses in the spinal cord, (3) intact motor (efferent) nerve fibers, (4) functional neuromuscular junctions, and (5) competent muscle fibers.

A single deep tendon reflex characteristically involves only a few spinal segments together with their sensory and motor fibers. An abnormality in such a reflex, therefore, helps to locate a pathologic lesion. You should know the segmental levels of the following deep tendon reflexes:

Biceps reflex	Cervical 5,6
Supinator (brachioradialis) reflex	Cervical 5,6
Triceps reflex	Cervical, 6,7
Knee reflex	Lumbar 2,3,4
Ankle reflex	Sacral 1 primarily

Reflexes may be initiated by stimulating skin as well as muscle. Stroking the skin of the abdomen, for example, produces a localized muscular twitch. These superficial (cutaneous) reflexes (and the spinal segments from which they come) include:

Abdominal reflexes—upper	Thoracic 8,9,10
—lower	Thoracic 10,11,12
Plantar responses	Lumbar 5, sacral 1

MOTOR PATHWAYS

Higher motor pathways of three kinds impinge on the anterior horn cells: the corticospinal (pyramidal) tract, the extrapyramidal system, and the cerebellar system.

● *The corticospinal (pyramidal) tract.** Voluntary movements originate in the motor cortex of the brain. Fibers from nerve cells there travel down through the corticospinal tract to the brainstem. Here most of them cross over to the opposite side and then continue down the spinal cord, where they synapse with anterior horn cells or with intermediate neurons. The corticospinal tracts not only mediate voluntary movement but also integrate skilled, complicated, or delicate movements by grading the motor responses and by stimulating selected muscular actions while inhibiting others. They also carry impulses that inhibit muscle tone, the slight tension maintained by a normal muscle even when it is relaxed. Fibers similar to corticospinal fibers connect with motor nerve cells in the cranial nerves and are then termed corticobulbar. Both corticospinal and corticobulbar neurons are often called upper motor neurons.

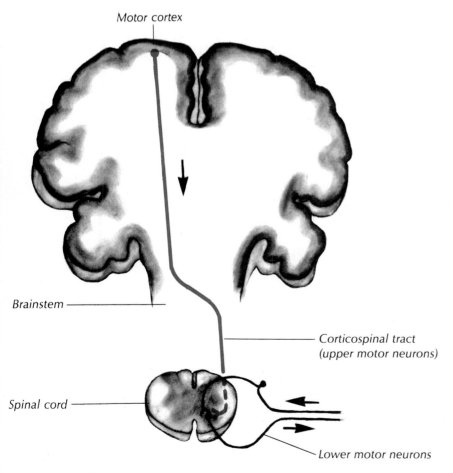

Motor cortex

Brainstem

Corticospinal tract
(upper motor neurons)

Spinal cord

Lower motor neurons

* Strictly speaking the corticospinal tract, the pyramidal tract, and upper motor neurons are not synonymous, but clinically the terms are often used interchangeably.

- *The extrapyramidal system.* This exceedingly complex system includes motor pathways between the cerebral cortex, basal ganglia, brainstem, and spinal cord but is outside the corticospinal (pyramidal) tract system. It helps to maintain muscle tone and to control body movements, especially gross automatic movements such as walking.
- *The cerebellar system.* The cerebellum receives both sensory and motor input and coordinates muscular activity, maintains equilibrium, and helps to control posture.

All three of these higher motor pathways affect motor activity only through the lower motor neurons—sometimes called the "final common pathway." Any movement, whether initiated voluntarily in the cortex, "automatically" in the basal ganglia, or reflexly in the sensory receptors, must ultimately be translated into action via the anterior horn cells, the lower motor neurons. A lesion in any of these areas will produce effects on movement or reflex activity.

When the corticospinal tract is damaged or destroyed, its functions are reduced or lost below the level of injury. An affected limb becomes weak or paralyzed, and skilled, complicated, or delicate movements are performed especially poorly when compared to gross movements. Muscle tone is increased and deep tendon reflexes are exaggerated. If the tract is damaged below its crossover in the brainstem, unilateral motor impairment occurs on the same (ipsilateral) side of the body. If the damage occurs above the tract's crossover, motor impairment develops on the opposite (contralateral) side.

Damage to the lower motor neurons causes ipsilateral weakness and paralysis, but in this case muscle tone and reflexes are decreased or absent.

Neither extrapyramidal nor cerebellar disease causes paralysis, but each can be disabling. Damage to the extrapyramidal system (specifically the basal ganglia) produces changes in muscle tone (most often an increase), disturbances in posture and gait, a slowness or lack of spontaneous and automatic movements (bradykinesia), and a variety of involuntary movements. Cerebellar damage impairs coordination, gait, and equilibrium, and decreases muscle tone.

SENSORY PATHWAYS

Sensory impulses not only participate in reflex activity, as previously described, but also give rise to conscious sensation.

Sensation is initiated by stimulation of sensory receptors located in skin, mucous membranes, muscles, tendons, and viscera. An impulse generated by one of these receptors travels along a sensory nerve fiber toward the spinal cord. In its course it usually travels with other sensory and motor nerve fibers in a peripheral nerve. The peripheral nerve is reorganized centrally on a segmental basis, divides into posterior and anterior roots, and enters the spinal cord. The sensory nerve fiber follows the posterior (or dorsal) root. After entry into the spinal cord, the sensory impulse proceeds along one of two courses: (1) the spinothalamic tracts, or (2) the posterior columns.

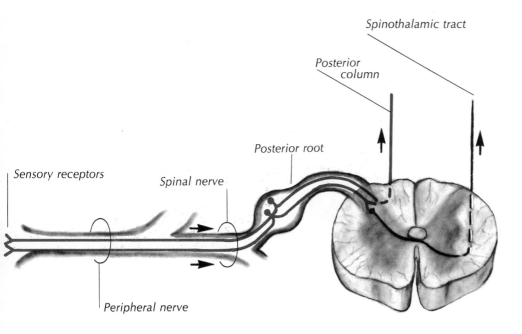

Within one or two spinal segments from their entry into the cord, fibers conducting the sensations of *pain* and *temperature* pass into the posterior horn of the spinal cord and synapse with secondary sensory neurons. These secondary neurons then cross to the opposite side just anterior to the central canal and pass upward in the lateral spinothalamic tract of the cord.

Fibers conducting the sensations of *position* and *vibration* pass directly into the *posterior columns* of the cord and travel upward to the medulla, where they then synapse with secondary sensory neurons. These secondary neurons cross over to the other side at the medullary level and continue on to the thalamus.

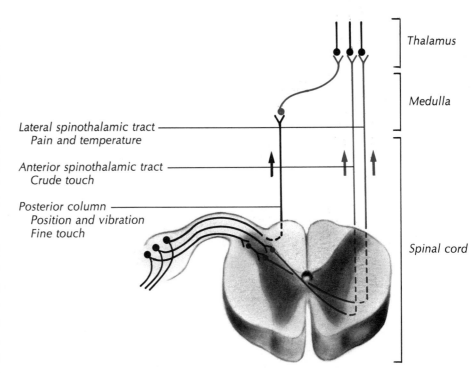

Nerve fibers carrying the sensation of *light touch* take one of two pathways. Some fibers conduct *fine touch*—touch that is accurately localized and finely discriminating. These fibers travel in the posterior column together with fibers that carry position and vibration sense. A second group transmits *crude touch*—a sensation perceived as light touch but without accurate localization. These fibers synapse in the posterior horn with secondary neurons that cross to the opposite side and ascend in the anterior spinothalamic tract to the thalamus. Because touch impulses originating on one side of the body travel up both sides of the cord, touch sensation is often preserved despite partial damage to the cord.

At the thalamic level, the general quality of sensation is perceived (*e.g.,* pain, cold, pleasant and unpleasant), but fine distinctions are not made. For full perception, a third group of sensory neurons carries impulses from synapses in the thalamus to the sensory cortex of the brain. Here stimuli are localized and discriminations made among them.

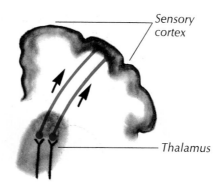

Lesions at different points in the sensory pathways produce different kinds of sensory loss. Patterns of sensory loss, together with their associated motor findings, are therefore helpful in figuring out where the causative lesions might be. A lesion in the sensory cortex may not impair the perception of pain, touch, and position, for example, but does impair finer discriminations. A person so affected cannot appreciate the size, shape, or texture of an object by feeling it and therefore cannot identify it. Loss of position and vibration sense with preservation of other sensations points to disease of the posterior columns, while loss of all sensations from the waist down, together with paralysis and hyperactive reflexes in the legs, indicates transection of the spinal cord (see Table 18-6, pp. 558–559).

A knowledge of dermatomes also aids in localizing neurologic lesions. A dermatome is the band of skin innervated by the sensory nerve root of a single spinal segment. Dermatome patterns are mapped in the next two figures. Their levels are considerably more variable than the diagrams suggest, and dermatomes overlap each other. The sensory nerves from each side of the body overlap slightly across the midline.

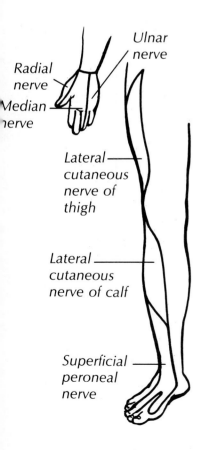

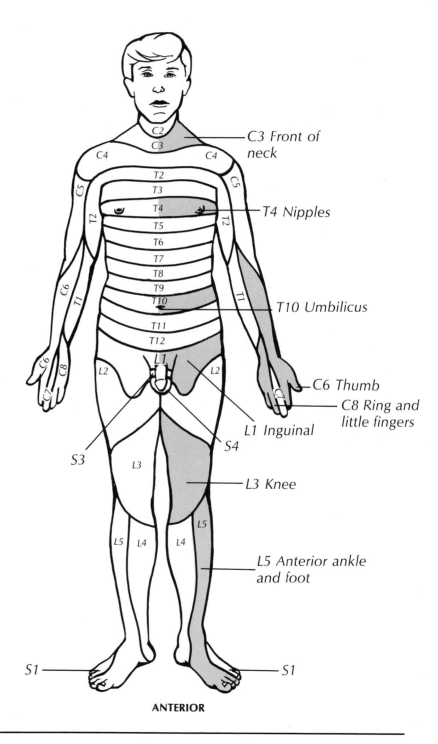

ANTERIOR

Do not try to memorize all the dermatomes. It is useful, however, to remember the locations of some, such as those shaded in red on the right side of the diagrams. The distribution of a few key peripheral nerves is shown in the inserts on the left.

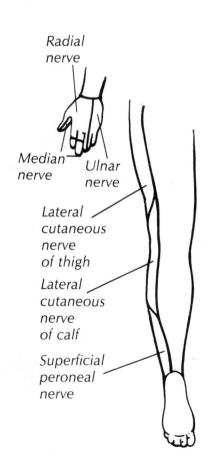

Radial nerve

Median nerve

Ulnar nerve

Lateral cutaneous nerve of thigh

Lateral cutaneous nerve of calf

Superficial peroneal nerve

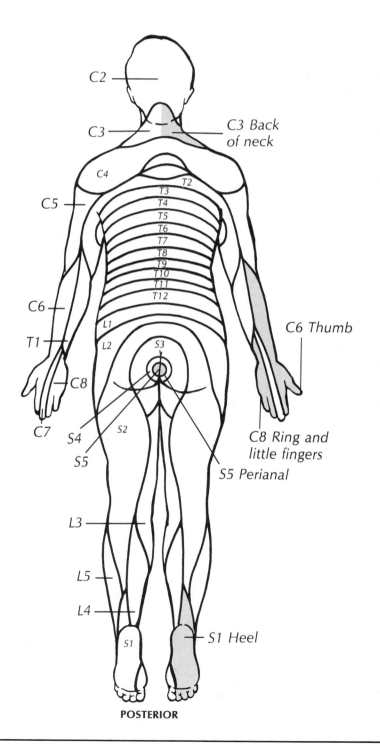

C2

C3

C3 Back of neck

C4

C5

T2
T3
T4
T5
T6
T7
T8
T9
T10
T11
T12

C6

T1

L1

L2

S3

C6 Thumb

C8

C7

S4

S5

S2

S5 Perianal

C8 Ring and little fingers

L3

L5

L4

S1

S1 Heel

POSTERIOR

THE CRANIAL NERVES

Nerves that emerge from the central nervous system within the head rather than from the vertebral column are called cranial nerves. There are 12 pairs. Functions of the cranial nerves most relevant to physical examination are summarized below.

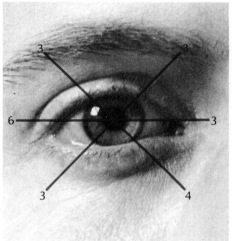

RIGHT EYE (N3, N4, N6)

NO.	NERVE	FUNCTION
N1	Olfactory	Sense of smell
N2	Optic	Vision
N3	Oculomotor	Pupillary constriction, opening the eye, and most extraocular movements
N4	Trochlear	Downward, inward movement of the eye
N6	Abducens	Lateral deviation of the eye
N5	Trigeminal	*Motor*—temporal and masseter muscles (jaw clenching), also lateral movement of the jaw

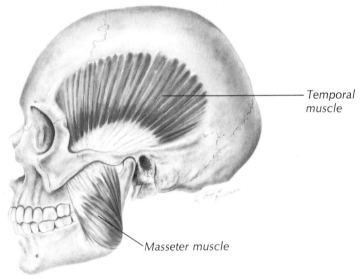

— Temporal muscle

—Masseter muscle

N5 MOTOR

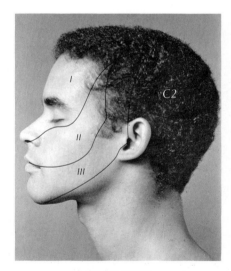

N5 SENSORY

		Sensory—facial. The nerve has three divisions: I. ophthalmic, II. maxillary, and III. mandibular.
N7	Facial	*Motor*—facial movements, including those of facial expression, closing the eye, and closing the mouth
		Sensory—taste for salty, sweet, sour, and bitter substances on the anterior two thirds of the tongue
N8	Acoustic	Hearing (cochlear division) and balance (vestibular division)
N9	Glossopharyngeal	*Sensory*—posterior portions of the eardrum and ear canal, the pharynx, and the posterior tongue, including taste (salty, sweet, sour, bitter)
		Motor—pharynx

(continued)

NO.	NERVE	FUNCTION
N10	Vagus	*Sensory*—pharynx and larynx
		Motor—palate, pharynx, and larynx
N11	Spinal accessory	*Motor*—the sternomastoid and upper portion of the trapezius

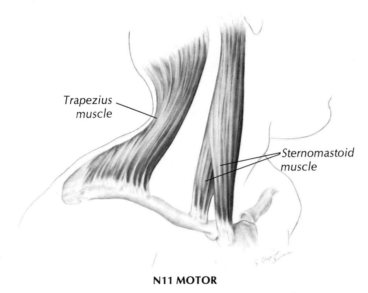

Trapezius muscle

Sternomastoid muscle

N11 MOTOR

N12	Hypoglossal	*Motor*—tongue

CHANGES WITH AGE

Aging. In assessing the nervous system of an elderly person, it is sometimes difficult to distinguish the changes of normal aging from those of age-related or other diseases. Some findings that you would consider abnormal in younger people, however, occur often enough in the elderly that you may attribute them to aging alone. Alterations in hearing, vision, extraocular movements, and pupillary size, shape, and reactivity have been described in Chapter 7 (see pp. 170–171).

Changes in the motor system are common. Elderly persons move and react with less speed and agility than younger ones, and skeletal muscles decrease in bulk. The hands of an aged person often look thin and bony because their small muscles have atrophied. Look for such muscular wasting in the backs of the hands, where atrophy of the dorsal interosseous muscles may leave concavities or grooves. As illustrated on page 524, this change is often most evident between the thumb and the hand (1st and 2nd metacarpals) but may also be seen between the other metacarpals. Atrophy of small muscles may also flatten the thenar and hypothenar eminences of the palms. Muscle strength, though diminished, is relatively well maintained. Arm and leg muscles may also show atrophy. This sometimes exaggerates the apparent size of adjacent joints.

Occasionally, an aged person develops a benign essential tremor (p. 554). Head, jaw, lips, or hands may tremble at a rate and amplitude suggesting parkinsonism (p. 554). The tremor is usually slightly faster, however, and there is no muscular rigidity.

Old age may also alter some of the reflexes. The gag reflex may be diminished or absent. Ankle reflexes may be symmetrically decreased or absent, even when reinforced. Less commonly, knee reflexes are similarly affected. Abdominal reflexes may diminish or disappear and, partly because of musculoskeletal changes in the feet, the plantar responses become less obvious and more difficult to interpret.

Vibration sense is frequently decreased or lost in the feet and ankles (but not in the fingers or over the shins). Less commonly, position sense may diminish or disappear.

If changes such as those described are accompanied by other neurologic abnormalities, or if atrophy and reflex changes are asymmetrical, you should search for an explanation other than age alone.

Techniques of Examination

GENERAL APPROACH

The detail of an appropriate neurologic examination varies widely. In apparently healthy persons screening is adequate, and some methods are recommended both in this chapter and in Chapter 4. If a person has symptoms possibly due to neurologic disease, however, you will need to use further techniques, tailored to the patient's problem. This section includes a practicable and reasonably inclusive examination that will give you additional techniques to use as needed. Be aware that many other techniques may be useful in specific situations. Consult textbooks of neurology as the need arises.

For efficiency, you should integrate certain portions of the neurologic assessment with other parts of your examination. Survey the patient's mental status and speech during the interview, for example, even though you may wish to do further testing after your neurologic evaluation. Assess some of the cranial nerves as you examine the head and neck, and inspect the arms and legs for neurologic abnormalities while you also observe the peripheral vascular and musculoskeletal systems. Chapter 4 provides an outline for this kind of integrated approach. Think about and describe your findings, however, in terms of the nervous system as a unit.

Organize your thinking into five categories: (1) mental status and speech, (2) cranial nerves, (3) the motor system, (4) the sensory system, and (5) reflexes.

For abnormalities of mental status and speech, see Chapter 3, Mental Status.

THE CRANIAL NERVES

SCREENING. From the more comprehensive tests of cranial nerves described below, the following constitutes a thorough survey:

- Visual acuity, visual fields, and ocular fundi (N2)
- Pupillary reactions (N2,3)
- Extraocular movements (N3,4,6)
- Corneal reflexes* and jaw movements (N5)
- Facial movements (N7)
- Hearing (N8)
- Swallowing and rise of the palate (N9,10)
- Voice (N10) and speech (N5,7,10,12)
- Inspection of the tongue (N12)

---

* Substitute light touch sensation on the face if the patient uses contact lenses.

FIRST CRANIAL NERVE (OLFACTORY). Test the *sense of smell* by presenting the patient with familiar and nonirritating odors. First be sure that each nasal passage is open by compressing one side of the nose and asking the patient to sniff through the other. The patient should then close both eyes. Occlude one nostril and under the other hold one of several substances such as cloves, coffee, soap, or vanilla. Ask if the patient smells anything and, if so, what. Test the other side. A person should normally perceive odor on each side, and can often identify it.

SECOND CRANIAL NERVE (OPTIC). Test *visual acuity.* (See pp. 172–173.)

Inspect the *optic fundi* ophthalmoscopically, with special attention to the optic discs. (See pp. 180–184.)

Determine the *visual fields by confrontation.* (See pp. 173–174.)

Now test for *extinction of vision* on one side. With both the patient's eyes open, wiggle your fingers simultaneously in both upper temporal quadrants. Your fingers should be outside the binocular field of vision. The stimulus on the patient's left side is thus seen only by the left eye and that on the right only by the right eye, as diagrammed below. Ask the patient to point to your movements. Both stimuli should be seen. Repeat in the lower temporal quadrants. This test is designed to detect extinction, a subtle suppression of vision when the vision itself, as evaluated directly by confrontation, is normal. Patterns of abnormality resemble homonymous hemianopsias and quadrantic defects.

Bilateral decrease in or loss of smell has many causes, including nasal disease, excessive smoking, and the use of cocaine. It may be congenital. Unilateral loss of smell without nasal disease suggests a lesion in the frontal lobe of the brain.

Optic atrophy, papilledema

See Table 7-2, Visual Field Defects (p. 198).

Perception of movement on only one side suggests extinction, signifying a lesion of the parietal cortex. Below, for example, the only stimuli perceived are those on the patient's right. Those on the left are extinguished.

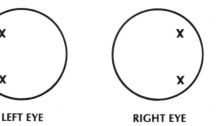

LEFT EYE   **RIGHT EYE**

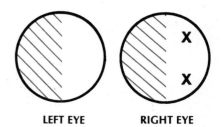

LEFT EYE   **RIGHT EYE**

THIRD, FOURTH, AND SIXTH CRANIAL NERVES (OCULOMOTOR, TROCHLEAR, AND ABDUCENS). (See pp. 179–180.) Inspect the size and shape of the pupils, and compare one side with the other. Test the *pupillary reactions to light;* if these are abnormal, examine the *near response* also.

Test the *extraocular movements* in the six cardinal fields of gaze, and look for loss of conjugate movements in any of the six directions. Check convergence of the eyes. Identify any nystagmus, noting the field of gaze in which it appears, the plane in which movements occur (horizontal, vertical, rotary, or mixed), and the direction of the quick and slow components.

See Table 7-7, Pupillary Abnormalities (pp. 203–204).

See Table 7-8, Deviations of the Eyes (p. 205).

See Table 18-1, Nystagmus (pp. 548–549).

Look for ptosis of the upper eyelids. A slight difference in the width of the palpebral fissures may be noted in about one third of all normal people.

Ptosis in 3rd nerve palsy, Horner's syndrome, myasthenia gravis

FIFTH CRANIAL NERVE (TRIGEMINAL)

Motor. While palpating the temporal and masseter muscles in turn, ask the patient to clench his or her teeth. Note the strength of muscle contraction.

Weak or absent contraction of the temporal and masseter muscles on one side suggests a lesion of the 5th cranial nerve. Bilateral weakness may result from upper or lower motor neuron involvement. When the patient has no teeth, this test may be difficult to interpret.

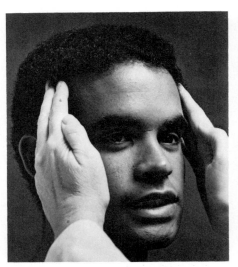

PALPATING TEMPORAL MUSCLES

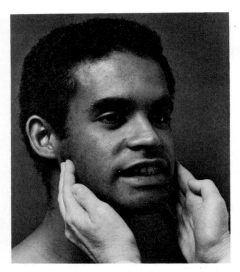

PALPATING MASSETER MUSCLES

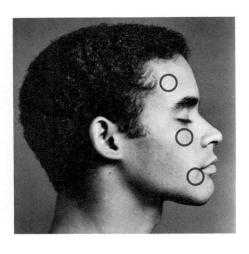

Sensory. After explaining what you plan to do, test the forehead, cheeks, and jaw on each side for *pain* sensation. Suggested areas are indicated by the circles. The patient's eyes should be closed. Use a safety pin or other suitable sharp object,* occasionally substituting the blunt end for the point as a stimulus. Ask the patient to report whether it is "sharp" or "dull" and to compare sides. (*Note:* You have actually tested for pain only in areas touched with the point of the pin.)

Unilateral decrease in or loss of facial sensation suggests a lesion of the 5th cranial nerve or of interconnecting higher sensory pathways. Such a sensory loss may also be associated with a conversion reaction.

---

* A safety pin is easy to handle and can be closed safely. Common pins are also used. Needles are too sharp. Sharp wood splinters can be made from breaking an applicator stick or twisting and breaking a tongue blade into two long sections, but the wood often dulls quickly. Any tool must be removed from the examining area after use and discarded safely.

If you find an abnormality, confirm it by testing *temperature* sensation. Two test tubes, filled with hot and ice-cold water are the traditional stimuli. A tuning fork may also be used. It usually feels cool. If you are near running water, the fork is easily made colder or warm. Dry it before use. Touch the skin and ask the patient to identify "hot" or "cold."

Then test for *light touch*, using a fine wisp of cotton. Ask the patient to respond whenever you touch the skin.

Test *the corneal reflex*. Ask the patient to look up and away from you. Approaching from the other side, out of the patient's line of vision, and avoiding the eyelashes, touch the cornea (not just the conjunctiva) lightly with a fine wisp of cotton. If the patient is apprehensive, however, first touching the conjunctiva may allay fear.

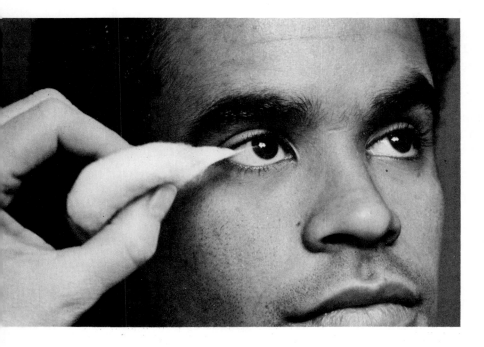

Look for blinking of the eyes, the normal reaction to this stimulus. (The sensory limb of this reflex is carried in the 5th cranial nerve, the motor response in the 7th.)

Absence of blinking suggests a lesion of the 5th cranial nerve. A lesion of the 7th cranial nerve (the nerve to the muscles that close the eyes) may also impair this reflex. Use of contact lenses frequently diminishes or abolishes this reflex.

SEVENTH CRANIAL NERVE (FACIAL). Inspect the face, both at rest and during conversation with the patient. Note any asymmetry (*e.g.*, of the nasolabial folds), and observe any tics or other abnormal movements.

Flattening of the nasolabial fold and drooping of the lower eyelid suggest facial weakness.

Ask the patient to:

1. Raise both eyebrows.
2. Frown.   *frowned*
3. Close both eyes tightly so that you cannot open them. Test muscular strength by trying to open them, as illustrated.
4. Show both upper and lower teeth.
5. Smile.
6. Puff out both cheeks.

Note any weakness or asymmetry.

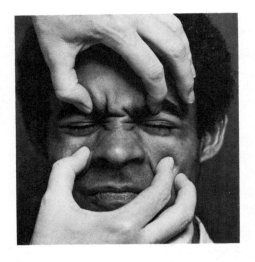

A lower motor neuron lesion, such as Bell's palsy, affects both the upper and the lower face; an upper motor neuron (or central) lesion affects mainly the lower face. See Table 18-2, Types of Facial Paralysis (pp. 550–551).

In unilateral facial paralysis, the mouth is pulled away from the paralyzed side when the patient smiles or shows some teeth.

EIGHTH CRANIAL NERVE (ACOUSTIC). Assess *hearing*. If hearing loss is present, (1) test for *lateralization*, and (2) compare *air and bone conduction*. (See pp. 187–188.)

See Table 7-15, Patterns of Hearing Loss (pp. 220–221).

Specific tests of *vestibular function* are seldom included in the usual neurologic examination, although nystagmus may indicate vestibular dysfunction. Consult textbooks of neurology or otolaryngology as the need arises.

NINTH AND TENTH CRANIAL NERVES (GLOSSOPHARYNGEAL AND VAGUS). Listen to the patient's *voice*. Is it hoarse or does it have a nasal quality?

Hoarseness in vocal cord paralysis; a nasal voice in paralysis of the palate

Is there difficulty in swallowing?

Pharyngeal or palatal weakness

Ask the patient to say "ah" or to yawn as you watch the *movements of the soft palate and the pharynx*. The soft palate normally rises symmetrically, the uvula remains in the midline, and each side of the posterior pharynx moves medially, like a curtain. The slightly curved uvula seen occasionally in a normal person should not be mistaken for a uvula deviated by a 10th nerve lesion.

The palate fails to rise with a bilateral lesion of the vagus nerve. In unilateral paralysis, one side of the palate fails to rise and, together with the uvula, is pulled toward the normal side (see p. 228).

Warn the patient that you are going to test the *gag reflex*. Stimulate the back of the throat lightly on each side in turn and note the gag reflex. It may be symmetrically diminished or absent in some normal people.

Unilateral absence of this reflex suggests a lesion of the 9th or perhaps the 10th cranial nerve.

ELEVENTH CRANIAL NERVE (SPINAL ACCESSORY). From behind, look for atrophy or fasciculations in the trapezius muscles, and compare one side with the other. Ask the patient to shrug both shoulders upward against your hands. Note the strength and contraction of the trapezii.

Weakness with atrophy and fasciculations indicates lower motor neuron disease. When the trapezius is paralyzed, the

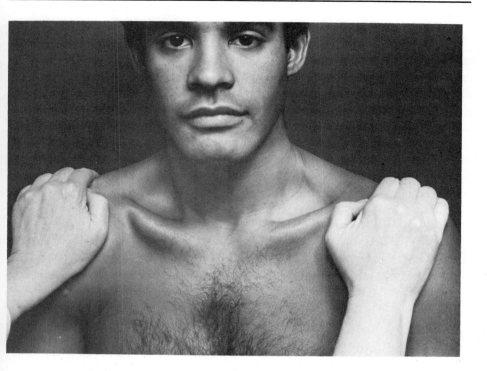

shoulder droops and the scapula is displaced downward and laterally.

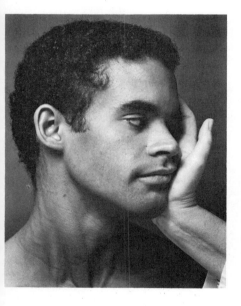

Ask the patient to turn the head to each side against your hand. Observe the contraction of the opposite sternomastoid and note the force of the movement against your hand.

A supine patient with bilateral weakness of the sternomastoids has difficulty raising the head off the pillow.

TWELFTH CRANIAL NERVE (HYPOGLOSSAL). Listen to the articulation of the patient's words. This depends on cranial nerves 5, 7, and 10 as well as N12.

Inspect the patient's tongue as it lies on the floor of the mouth. Look for any atrophy or fasciculations. Some coarser restless movements are often seen in a normal tongue. Then, with the patient's tongue protruded, look for asymmetry, atrophy, or deviation from the midline. Ask the patient to move the tongue from side to side, and note the symmetry of the movement. In ambiguous cases, ask the patient to push the tongue against the inside of each cheek in turn as you palpate externally for strength.

For poor articulation (dysarthria), see page 114. Atrophy and fasciculations suggest lower motor neuron disease. If unilateral, the protruded tongue deviates toward the involved side. It feels strong when pressing toward the involved side but weak on the normal side.

NEUROLOGIC SCREENING

By observing the patient during the interview and early parts of the examination, you should already have gathered tentative information about the nervous system. Additional screening procedures may either affirm good functions or suggest impairments that guide your further assessment.

GAIT AND LEGS. Ask the patient to:

● *Walk across the room* or down the hall, then turn, and come back. Observe posture, balance, swinging of the arms, and movements of the legs. Normally balance is easy, the arms swing at the sides, and turns are smoothly accomplished.

A gait that lacks coordination, with reeling and instability, is called ataxic. Ataxia may be due to cerebellar disease, loss of position sense, or intoxication. See Table 18-3, Abnormalities of Gait and Posture (pp. 552–553).

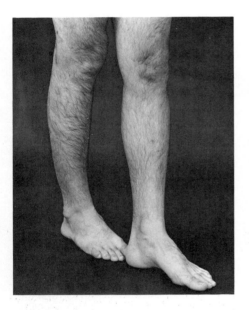

● *Walk heel-to-toe* in a straight line —a pattern called *tandem walking*.

Tandem walking may reveal an ataxia not previously obvious.

● *Walk on the toes*, then *on the heels*—sensitive tests respectively for plantar flexion and dorsiflexion of the ankles, as well as for balance.

Walking on toes and heels may reveal distal muscular weakness in the legs. Further, weak dorsiflexion is a sensitive test for upper motor neuron weakness.

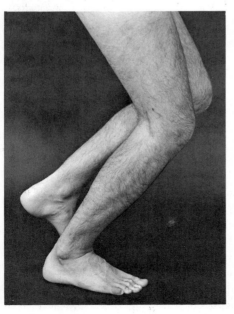

● *Hop in place* on each foot in turn (if the patient is not too old or ill). Hopping involves the proximal muscles of the legs as well as the distal ones and requires both good position sense and normal cerebellar function.

Difficulty with hopping may be due to weakness, lack of position sense, or cerebellar dysfunction.

● *Do a shallow knee bend*, first on one leg, then on the other. Supporting the patient's elbow lightly may be helpful.

Difficulty here suggests proximal weakness (extensors of the hip), weakness of the quadriceps (the extensor of the knee), or both.

Rising from a sitting position without arm support and *stepping up* on a sturdy stool are more suitable tests than hopping or knee bends when patients are old or less robust.

People with proximal muscle weakness involving the pelvic girdle and legs have difficulty rising from a chair and stepping up onto a stool.

ROMBERG TEST. This is a functional test of position sense. The patient should first stand with feet together and eyes open, then close both eyes for 20 to 30 seconds without support. Note the patient's ability to maintain an upright posture, and be sure not to allow a fall. Normally only minimal swaying occurs.

In ataxia due to loss of position sense, vision compensates for the sensory loss. The patient can stand fairly well with eyes open but loses balance when they are closed, thus demonstrating a *positive Romberg sign.* In cerebellar ataxia, the patient has difficulty standing with feet together whether the eyes are open or closed.

ARMS, SHOULDERS, AND HANDS. *Check for a pronator drift.* Usually this test can be combined with a Romberg test. Ask the patient to hold both arms straight forward, palms up, and then to close both eyes and maintain this position for 20 to 30 seconds. A normal person can hold this position well. Stand close enough to protect the patient from falling. Alternatively, the patient may sit during this test.

The tendency of one forearm to pronate suggests a mild hemiparesis; downward drift of the arm with flexion of fingers and elbow may also occur. These movements are called a *pronator drift,* shown below.

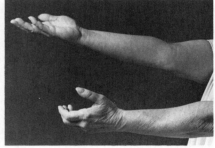

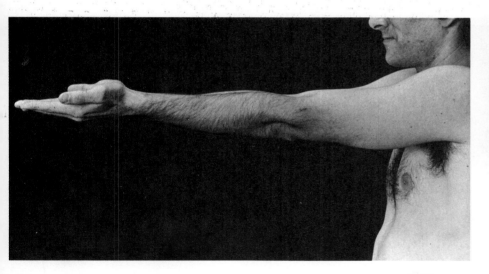

A sideward or upward drift, sometimes with searching, writhing movements of the hands, suggests loss of position sense.

Now, instructing the patient to keep the arms up and eyes shut, as shown above, *tap the arms briskly downward.* The arms normally return smoothly to the horizontal position. This response requires muscular strength, coordination, and a good sense of position.

A weak arm is easily displaced and often remains so. When position sense is lacking, the patient may not recognize the displacement and, if told to correct it, does so poorly. In cerebellar incoordination, the arm returns to its original position but with overshooting and bounces.

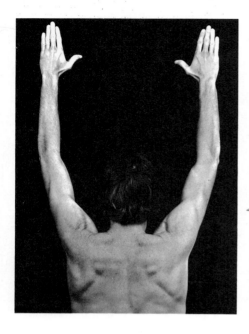

Then ask the patient to *raise both arms overhead* with palms forward for 20 to 30 seconds. Again, observe the maintenance of this position.

Try to force the arms down to the sides against the patient's resistance. Note any weakness.

Drifting or weakness on one side suggests hemiparesis. Shoulder girdle disease may also cause drifting or weakness.

Watch for winging as the patient slowly lowers both arms forward and down to the sides. Winging is a backward displacement of the scapula away from the chest wall. Alternatively, look for winging as the patient pushes with arms extended forward against a wall or against your hand. The normal appearance is shown at right.

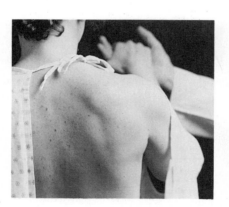

In winging, shown below, the medial border of the scapula juts backward. It suggests weakness of the serratus anterior muscle.

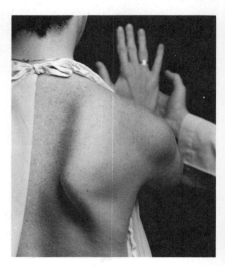

In very thin but normal people, the scapulae may look somewhat winged in the absence of weakness.

Test the grip. Ask the patient to squeeze two of your fingers as hard as possible and not let them go. (To avoid getting hurt by hard squeezes,

A weak grip may be due to either upper or lower motor

place your own middle finger on top of your index finger.) You should normally have difficulty removing your fingers from the patient's grip.

neuron disease. It may also result from painful disorders of the hands.

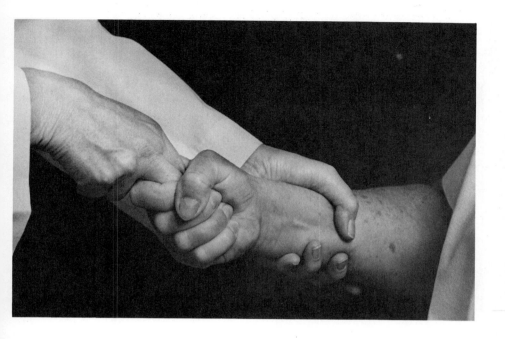

Testing both grips simultaneously facilitates comparison.

THE MOTOR SYSTEM

Assessment of the motor system focuses on five components: involuntary movements, muscle bulk, muscle tone, muscle strength, and coordination. These components are described below in sequence. You may either use this sequence or check each component in the arms, trunk, and legs in turn. Throughout this assessment, note the patient's bodily positions at rest and during movement. If you see any abnormalities, note their nature and the parts of the body involved.

SCREENING. In addition to the procedures described in the previous section,

- Look for involuntary movements or abnormal positions.
- Observe muscle bulk.
- Assess muscle tone.
- Test rapid alternating movements in the hands.

INVOLUNTARY MOVEMENTS. Watch for any involuntary movements, noting their location, quality, rate, rhythm, amplitude, and relation to posture, activity, fatigue, emotion, or other factors.

MUSCLE BULK. Note the size and contours of the muscles. Have normal muscular convexities become flattened or concave, suggesting atrophy?

Abnormal positions alert you to neurologic deficits. For example, unilateral flexion of the elbow, wrist, and fingers, with plantar flexion of the foot, suggests hemiparesis or hemiplegia (see pp. 552, 560).

See Table 18-4, Involuntary Movements (pp. 554–556).

When looking for atrophy, pay particular attention to the shoulder and pelvic girdles and the hands. The thenar and hypothenar eminences should be full and convex, and the spaces between the metacarpals, where the dorsal interosseous muscles lie, should be full or only slightly depressed. Atrophy of hand muscles may occur with normal aging, however, as shown on the right below.

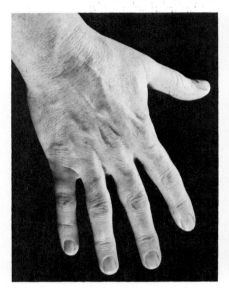
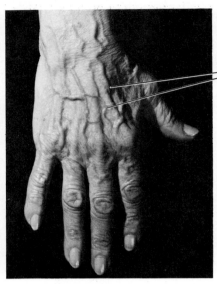

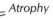 — Atrophy

Hand of a 44-year-old woman

Hand of an 84-year-old woman

Muscular *atrophy* refers to a loss of muscle bulk (wasting). It results from lower motor neuron disease and disease of the muscle itself. *Hypertrophy* refers to an increase in bulk with proportionate strength, while increased bulk with diminished strength is called *pseudohypertrophy* (seen in the Duchenne form of muscular dystrophy).

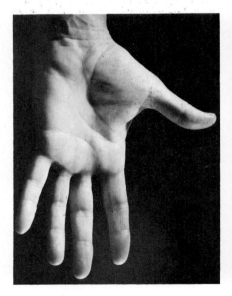
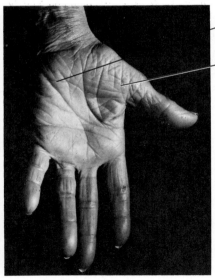

— Hypothenar eminence

— Flattening of the thenar eminence due to mild atrophy

Hand of a 44-year-old woman

Hand of an 84-year old woman

Flattening of the thenar and hypothenar eminences and concavities or furrowing between the metacarpals suggest atrophy. Localized atrophy of the thenar and hypothenar eminences suggests damage to the median and ulnar nerves, respectively.

Other causes of muscular atrophy include motor neuron diseases, disuse of the muscles, rheumatoid arthritis, and protein-calorie malnutrition.

Be alert for fasciculations (fine, flickering, irregular movements) in atrophic muscles. If you see none, a tap on the muscle with a reflex hammer may stimulate them.

MUSCLE TONE. When a normal muscle with an intact nerve supply is relaxed voluntarily, it maintains a slight residual tension known as muscle tone. This can be assessed best by feeling the muscle's resistance to passive stretch. Persuade the patient to relax. Take one hand with yours and, while supporting the elbow, flex and extend the patient's fingers, wrist, and elbow, and put the shoulder through a moderate range of motion. With practice, these actions can be combined into a single smooth movement. On each side, note muscle tone—the resistance offered to your movements. Tense patients may show increased resistance. You will learn the feel of normal resistance only with repeated practice.

If you suspect decreased resistance, hold the forearm and shake the hand loosely back and forth. Normally the hand moves back and forth freely but is not completely floppy.

If resistance is increased, determine whether it varies as you move the limb or whether it persists throughout the range of movement and in both directions, *e.g.*, during both flexion and extension. Feel for any jerkiness in the resistance.

To assess muscle tone in the legs, support the patient's thigh with one hand, grasp the foot with the other, and flex and extend the patient's knee and ankle on each side. Note the resistance to your movements.

MUSCLE STRENGTH. Normal individuals vary widely in their strength, and your standard of normal, while admittedly rough, should allow for such variables as age, sex, and muscular training. A person's dominant side is usually slightly stronger than the other side. Keep this difference in mind when you compare sides. Remember too that a muscle is strongest when shortest, weakest when longest. Use this difference either to gain advantage over strong muscles or to give advantage to weak ones.

You usually test muscle strength by asking the patient to move actively against your resistance or to resist your movement. Watch for muscular contraction and feel for the strength exerted. Some muscles may be too weak to overcome resistance. You can then test them against gravity alone or with gravity eliminated. When the forearm rests in a pronated position, for example, dorsiflexion at the wrist can be tested against

The presence of fasciculations supports lower motor neuron damage as the cause of atrophy.

Resistance to passive stretch is decreased when the reflex arc is interrupted by a lesion affecting the sensory or the lower motor neuron. It may also be decreased in muscular and cerebellar disease and in the acute stages of a spinal cord injury or cerebrovascular accident.

Marked floppiness indicates hypotonic (flaccid) muscles.

Increased resistance that varies, commonly worse at the extremes of the range, is called *spasticity*. High resistance, followed by sudden relaxation as the limb is moved, is called *clasp-knife spasticity*. Spasticity indicates upper motor neuron disease. Resistance that persists throughout the range and in both directions is called *lead-pipe rigidity*. A superimposed ratchetlike jerkiness is *cogwheel ridigity*. Both kinds of rigidity may be felt in parkinsonism.

Impaired strength is called weakness or paresis. Absence of strength is called paralysis or plegia. *Hemiparesis* refers to weakness of one half of the body; *hemiplegia* to paralysis of

gravity alone. When the forearm is midway between pronation and supination, dorsiflexion at the wrist can be tested with gravity eliminated. Finally, you may be able to see or feel a weak muscular contraction even if it fails to move the body part.

Muscle strength is graded on a 0 to 5 scale:

    0—No muscular contraction detected
    1—A barely detectable flicker or trace of contraction
    2—Active movement of the body part with gravity eliminated
    3—Active movement against gravity
    4—Active movement against gravity and some resistance
    5—Active movement against full resistance without evident fatigue.
       This is normal muscle strength.

Many clinicians make further distinctions by using plus or minus signs toward the stronger end of this scale. Thus +4 indicates good but not full strength, while −5 means a trace of weakness.

Described below are methods of testing some major muscle groups, the spinal levels for which are shown in parentheses. To localize lesions in the spinal cord or the peripheral nervous system more precisely, however, very discrete testing may be necessary. For these specialized methods, refer to detailed texts of neurology.

Test flexion (C5,6) *and extension* (C6,7,8) *at the elbow* by having the patient pull and push against your hand.

one half of the body. *Paraplegia* means paralysis of the legs; *quadriplegia,* paralysis of all four limbs.

See Table 18-5, Differentiation of Motor Disorders (p. 557).

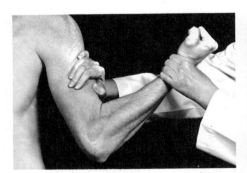

FLEXION

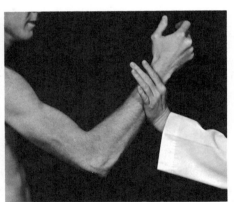

EXTENSION

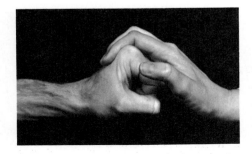

Test extension at the wrist (C6,7,8, radial nerve) by asking the patient to make a fist and resist your pulling it down.

Weakness of extension is seen in lower motor neuron disease (*e.g.,* radial nerve damage) and upper motor neuron disease (*e.g.,* hemiplegia).

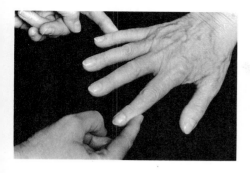

Test finger abduction (C8, T1, ulnar nerve). Position the patient's hand with palm down and fingers spread. Instructing the patient not to let you move the fingers, try to force them together.

Weak finger abduction in ulnar nerve disorders

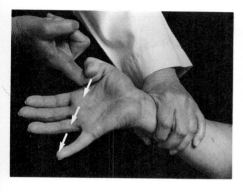

Test opposition of the thumb (C8, T1, median nerve). The patient should try to touch the tip of the little finger with the thumb, against your resistance.

Weak opposition of the thumb in median nerve disorders such as the carpal tunnel syndrome

Assessment of *muscle strength of the trunk* may already have been made in other segments of the examination. It includes:

● Flexion, extension, and lateral bending of the spine, and
● Thoracic expansion and diaphragmatic excursion during respiration

Test flexion at the hip (L2,3,4) by placing your hand on the patient's thigh and asking the patient to raise the leg against it.

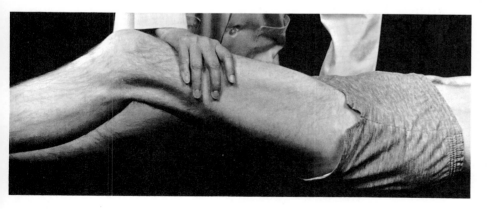

Test abduction at the hips (L4,5, S1). Place your hands firmly on the bed outside the patient's knees. Ask the patient to spread both legs against your hands.

Test adduction at the hips (L2,3,4). Place your hands firmly on the bed between the patient's knees. Ask the patient to bring both legs together.

Symmetrical weakness of the proximal muscles suggests a myopathy (a disorder of muscles); symmetrical weakness of distal muscles suggests a polyneuropathy (a disorder of peripheral nerves).

Test extension at the knee (L2,3,4) by supporting the knee in flexion and asking the patient to straighten the leg against your hand.

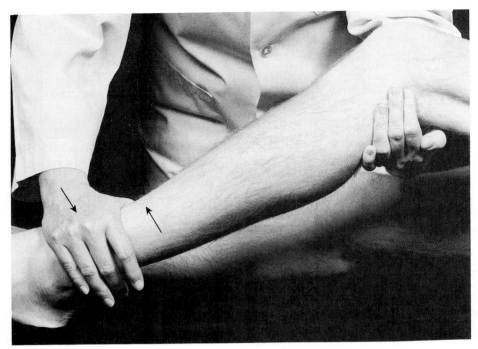

EXTENSION AT THE KNEE

Test flexion at the knee (L4,5, S1,2) as shown below. Place the patient's leg so that the knee is flexed with the foot resting on the bed. Tell the patient to keep the foot down as you try to straighten the leg.

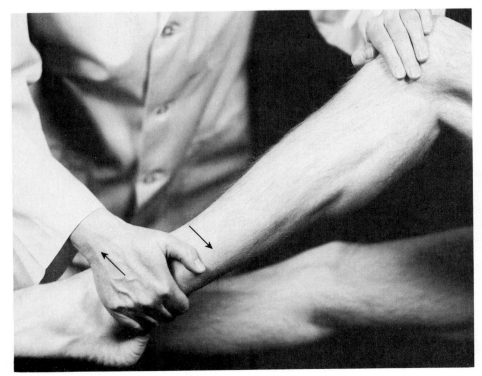

FLEXION AT THE KNEE

Test dorsiflexion (mainly L4,5) *and plantar flexion* (mainly S1) *at the ankle* by asking the patient to pull up and push down against your hand.

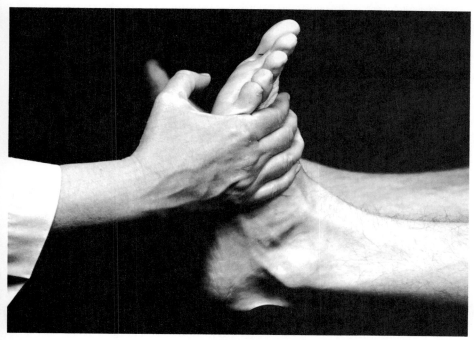

DORSIFLEXION

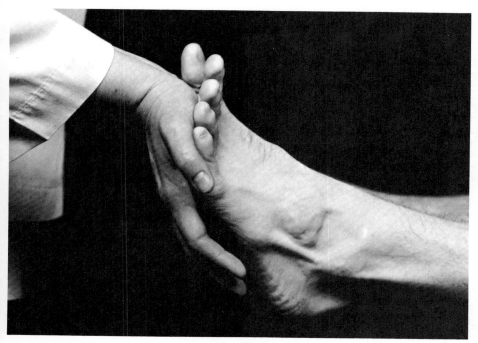

PLANTAR FLEXION

COORDINATION. During the motor screening examination, you have already done a preliminary assessment of coordination. Now test it further by two methods. The sitting position is preferable for testing the arms.

1. *Rapid Alternating Movements.* Show the patient how to strike one hand on the thigh, raise the hand, turn it over, and then strike the back of the hand down on the same place. Urge the patient to repeat these alternating movements as rapidly as possible.

Observe the speed, rhythm, and smoothness of the movements. Repeat with the other hand. The nondominant hand often performs somewhat less well.

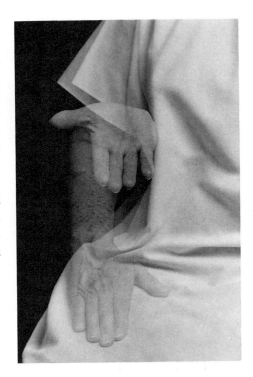

In cerebellar disease, one movement cannot be followed quickly by its opposite and movements are slow, irregular, and clumsy. This abnormality is called *dysdiadochokinesis.* Upper motor neuron weakness and extrapyramidal disease may also impair rapid alternating movements, but not in the same manner.

Show the patient how to tap the distal joint of the thumb with the tip of the index finger, again as rapidly as possible. Again, observe the speed, rhythm, and smoothness of the movements. The nondominant side often performs less well.

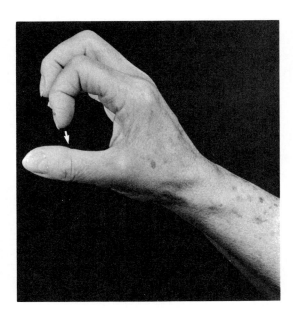

2. *Point-to-Point Testing.* Ask the patient to touch your index finger and then his or her nose alternately several times. Move your finger about so that the patient has to alter directions and extend the arm fully to reach it. Observe the accuracy and smoothness of movements and watch for any tremor.

In cerebellar disease, movements are clumsy, unsteady, and inappropriately varying in their speed, force, and direction. The finger may initially overshoot its mark, but finally reaches it fairly well. Such movements are termed *dysmetria*. An intention tremor may appear toward the end of the movement (see p. 554).

Now hold your finger in one place so that the patient can touch it with one arm and finger outstretched. Ask the patient to raise the arm overhead and lower it again to touch your finger. After several repeats, ask the patient to close both eyes and try several more times. Repeat on the other side. Normally a person can touch the examiner's finger successfully with eyes open or closed. These maneuvers test position sense and the functions of both the labyrinth and the cerebellum.

Cerebellar disease causes incoordination that may get worse with eyes closed. Inaccuracy that appears with eyes closed suggests loss of position sense. Repetitive and consistent deviation to one side (referred to as *past pointing*), worse with the eyes closed, suggests cerebellar or vestibular disease.

To assess the legs, the patient should be lying down.

1. *Rapid Alternating Movements.* Ask the patient to tap your hand as quickly as possible with the ball of each foot in turn. Note any slowness or awkwardness. The feet normally perform less well than the hands.

Dysdiadochokinesis in cerebellar disease

2. *Point-to-Point Testing.* Ask the patient to place one heel on the opposite knee, and then run it down the shin to the big toe. Note the smoothness and accuracy of the movements. Repetition with the patient's eyes closed tests for position sense. Repeat on the other side.

In cerebellar disease, the heel may overshoot the knee and then oscillate from side to side down the shin. When position sense is lost, the heel is lifted too high and the patient tries to look. With eyes closed, performance is poor.

REFLEXES

To *elicit a deep tendon reflex,* persuade the patient to relax, position the limbs properly and symmetrically, and strike the tendon briskly, using a wrist movement. Your strike should be quick and direct, not glancing. You may use either the pointed or the flat end of the hammer. The pointed end is useful in striking small areas, such as your finger, as it overlies the biceps tendon, while the flat end gives the patient less discomfort over the brachioradialis. Hold the reflex hammer between your thumb and

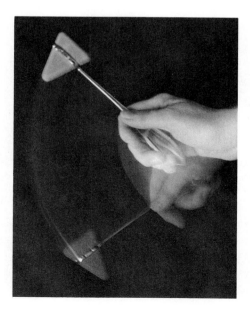

index finger so that it swings freely within the limits set by your palm and other fingers. Note the speed, force, and amplitude of the reflex response. Always compare one side with the other.

Reflexes are usually graded on a 0 to 4+ scale:

4+ Very brisk, hyperactive; often indicative of disease; often associated with clonus (rhythmic oscillations between flexion and extension)

3+ Brisker than average; possibly but not necessarily indicative of disease

2+ Average; normal

1+ Somewhat diminished; low normal

0 No response

Hyperactive reflexes suggest upper motor neuron disease. Sustained clonus confirms it. Reflexes may be diminished or absent when sensation is lost, when the relevant spinal segments are damaged, or when the lower motor neurons are damaged. Diseases of muscles and neuromuscular junctions may also decrease reflexes.

Reflex response depends partly on the force of your stimulus. Use no more force than you need to provoke a definite response. Differences between sides are usually easier to assess than symmetrical changes. Symmetrically diminished or even absent reflexes may be found in normal people.

If the patient's reflexes are symmetrically diminished or absent, use *reinforcement*, a technique involving isometric contraction of other muscles that may increase reflex activity. In testing arm reflexes, for example, ask the patient to clench his or her teeth or to squeeze one thigh with the opposite hand. If leg reflexes are diminished or absent, reinforce them by asking the patient to lock fingers and pull one hand against the other. Tell the patient to pull just before your strike the tendon.

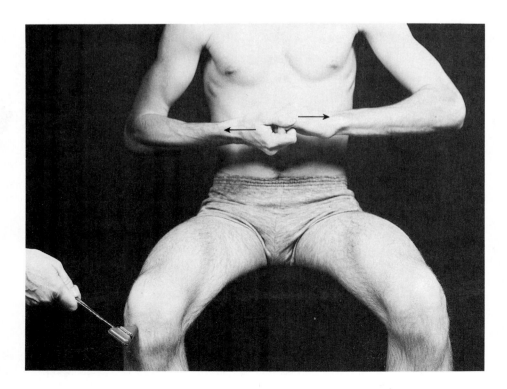

THE BICEPS REFLEX (C5, C6). The patient's arm should be partially flexed at the elbow with palm down. Place your thumb or finger firmly on the biceps tendon. Strike with the reflex hammer so that the blow is aimed directly through your digit toward the biceps tendon.

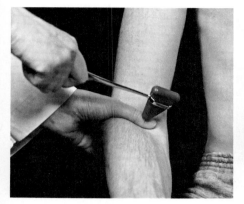
PATIENT SITTING

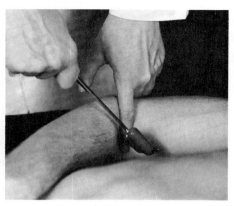
PATIENT LYING DOWN

Observe flexion at the elbow, and watch for and feel the contraction of the biceps muscle.

THE TRICEPS REFLEX (C6, C7). Flex the patient's arm at the elbow, with palm toward the body, and pull it slightly across the chest. Strike the triceps tendon above the elbow. Use a direct blow from directly behind it. Watch for contraction of the triceps muscle and extension at the elbow.

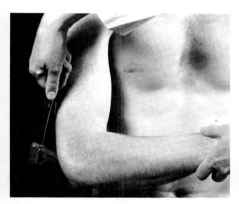
PATIENT SITTING

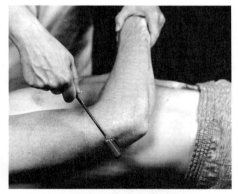
PATIENT LYING DOWN

When it is difficult to get a sitting patient relaxed enough to test for a triceps reflex, an alternate method may help. Support the upper arm as illustrated, and ask the patient to let it go limp as if it were "hung up to dry." Then strike the triceps tendon.

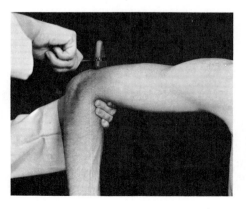

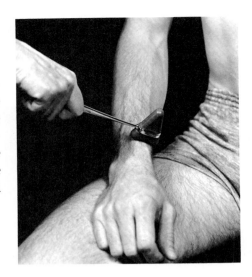

THE SUPINATOR OR BRACHIO-RADIALIS REFLEX (C5, C6). The patient's hand should rest on the abdomen or the lap, with the forearm partly pronated. Strike the radius about 1 to 2 inches above the wrist. Watch for flexion and supination of the forearm.

THE ABDOMINAL REFLEXES. Test the abdominal reflexes by lightly but briskly stroking each side of the abdomen, above (T8, T9, T10) and below (T10, T11, T12) the umbilicus, in the directions illustrated. Use a key, the wooden end of a cotton-tipped applicator, or a tongue blade twisted so that it is split longitudinally. Note the contraction of the abdominal muscles and deviation of the umbilicus toward the stimulus. Obesity may mask an abdominal reflex. In this situation, use your finger to retract the patient's umbilicus away from the side to be stimulated. Feel with your retracting finger for the muscular contraction.

Abdominal reflexes may be absent in both upper and lower motor neuron disorders.

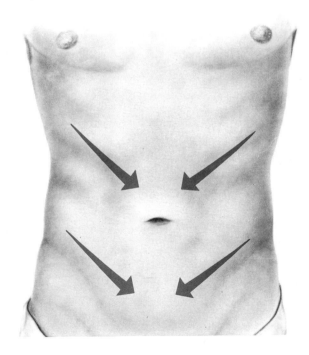

THE KNEE REFLEX (L2, L3, L4). The patient may be either sitting or lying down as long as the knee is flexed. Briskly tap the patellar tendon just below the patella. Note contraction of the quadriceps with extension at the knee. A hand on the patient's anterior thigh lets you feel this reflex.

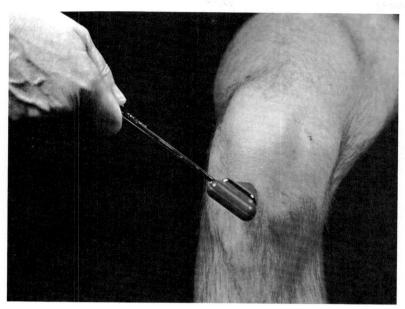

PATIENT SITTING

Two methods are useful in examining the supine patient. Supporting both knees at once, as shown below on the left, allows you to assess small differences between knee reflexes by repeatedly testing one reflex, then the other. Sometimes, however, supporting both legs is uncomfortable for both the examiner and the patient. A comfortable alternative method by which your supporting arm is in turn supported by the patient's opposite leg is shown below on the right. Some patients are better able to relax with this method.

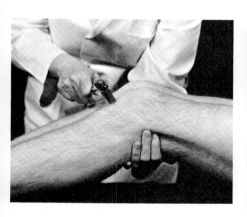 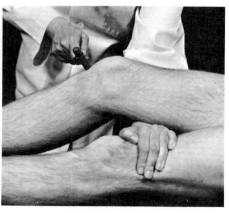

THE ANKLE REFLEX (PRIMARILY S1). With the leg somewhat flexed at the knee, dorsiflex the foot at the ankle. Persuade the patient to relax. Strike the Achilles tendon. Watch and feel for plantar flexion at the ankle. Note also the speed of relaxation after muscular contraction.

The slowed relaxation phase of reflexes in hypothyroidism is

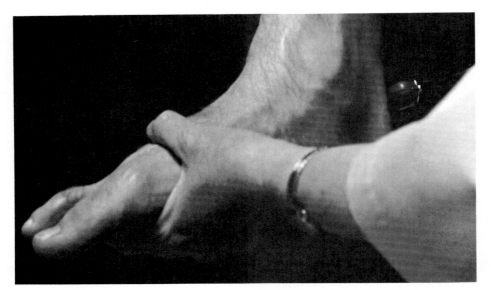

PATIENT SITTING

often easily seen and felt in the ankle reflex.

When the patient is lying down, flex one leg at both hip and knee and rotate it externally so that the lower leg rests across the opposite shin. Then dorsiflex the foot at the ankle and strike the Achilles tendon.

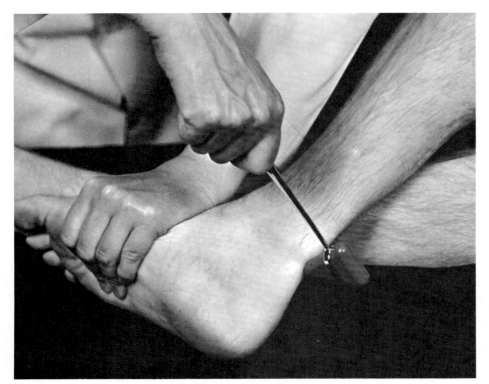

PATIENT LYING DOWN

THE PLANTAR RESPONSE (L5, S1). With an object such as a key or the wooden end of an applicator stick, stroke the lateral aspect of the sole from the heel to the ball of the foot, curving medially across the ball. Use

Dorsiflexion of the big toe, often accompanied by fanning of the other toes, constitutes a

the lightest stimulus that will provoke a response, but be increasingly firm if necessary. Note movement of the toes, normally flexion.

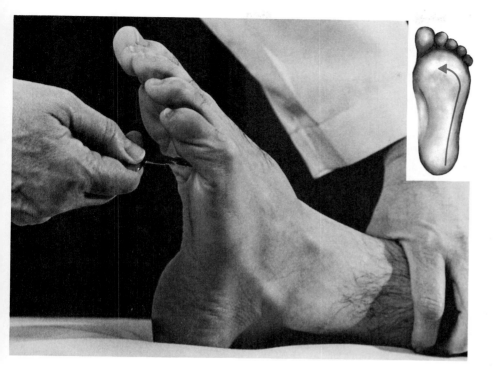

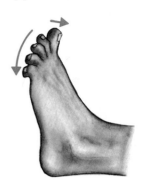

Babinski response. It often indicates upper motor neuron dis-

ease. Unconscious states, due to drug and alcohol intoxication or subsequent to an epileptic seizure, may also cause it.

Some patients withdraw from this stimulus by flexing the hip and the knee. Hold the ankle, if necessary, to complete your observation. It is sometimes difficult to distinguish withdrawal from a Babinski response.

A marked Babinski response is occasionally accompanied by reflex flexion at hip and knee.

CLONUS. If the reflexes are hyperreactive, test for *ankle clonus.* Support the knee in a partly flexed position. With your other hand, dorsiflex and plantar flex the foot a few times while encouraging the patient to relax,

Sustained clonus indicates upper motor neuron disease. The ankle plantar flexes and dorsiflexes repetitively and rhythmically.

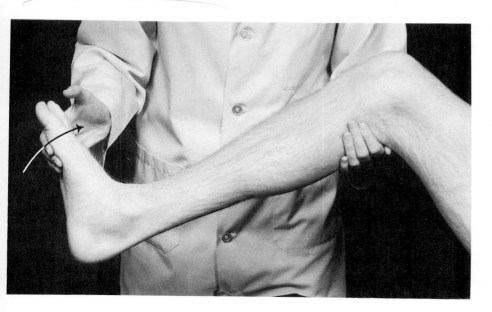

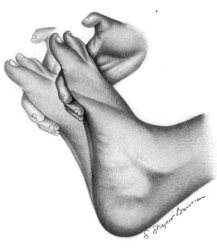

and then sharply dorsiflex the foot and maintain it in dorsiflexion. Look and feel for rhythmic oscillations between dorsiflexion and plantar flexion. In most normal people, the ankle does not react to this stimulus. A few clonic beats may be seen and felt, especially when the patient is tense or has exercised.

Clonus may also be elicited at other joints. A sharp downward displacement of the patella, for example, may elicit patellar clonus in the extended knee.

THE SENSORY SYSTEM

To evaluate the sensory system, you will test several kinds of sensation:

- Pain and temperature, impulses for which are carried in the spinothalamic tracts of the cord
- Position and vibration, impulses for which are carried in the posterior columns
- Light touch, impulses for which are carried along both of these pathways, and
- Discriminative sensations, which depend on some of the above sensations but also require cortical judgments

Familiarize yourself with each kind of test so that you can use it as indicated.

Two patterns of testing are described—one for screening, the other for a more detailed evaluation.

SCREENING

- Check pain sensation in the hands and the feet.
- Check vibration sense in the hands and the feet.
- Briefly compare light touch on both arms and on both legs.
- Assess stereognosis in the hands.

PATTERNS OF TESTING. Because sensory testing quickly fatigues many patients and then produces unreliable results, conduct the examination as efficiently as possible. Pay special attention to those areas (1) where there are symptoms such as numbness or pain, (2) where there are motor or reflex abnormalities that suggest a lesion of the spinal cord or periph-

Meticulous sensory mapping helps to establish the level of a spinal cord lesion and to determine the location of a more peripheral lesion, such as in a

eral nervous system, and (3) where there are trophic changes (*e.g.*, absent or excessive sweating, atrophic skin, or cutaneous ulceration). Repeated testing at another time is often required to confirm abnormalities.

The following patterns of testing help you to identify sensory deficits accurately and efficiently.

1. Compare symmetrical areas on the two sides of the body, including the arms, legs, and trunk.

2. When testing pain, temperature, and touch, also compare the distal with the proximal areas of the extremities. Further, scatter the stimuli so as to sample most of the dermatomes and major peripheral nerves (see pp. 509–510). One suggested pattern includes both shoulders (C4), the inner and outer aspects of the forearms (C6 and T1), the thumbs and little fingers (C6 and C8), the fronts of both thighs (L2), the medial and lateral aspects of both calves (L4 and L5), the little toes (S1), and the medial aspect of each buttock (S3).

3. When testing vibration and position, first test the fingers and toes. If these are normal, you may safely assume that more proximal areas will also be normal.

4. Vary the pace of your testing so that the patient does not merely respond to your repetitive rhythm.

5. When you detect an area of sensory loss or hypersensitivity, map out its boundaries in detail. Stimulate first at a point of reduced sensation and move by progressive steps until the patient detects the change. An example is shown at right.

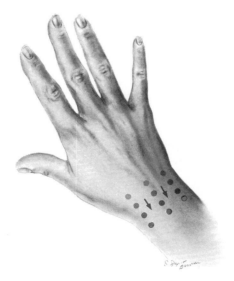

By identifying the distribution of sensory abnormalities and the kinds of sensations affected, you can infer where the causative lesion might be. Any motor deficit or reflex abnormality also helps in this localizing process.

Before each kind of test, show the patient what you plan to do and what responses you want. Unless otherwise specified, the patient's eyes should be closed during actual testing.

Examples of Abnormalities column:

nerve root or in a major peripheral nerve or one of its branches.

Hemisensory loss due to a lesion in the spinal cord or higher pathways

Symmetrical distal sensory loss suggests a polyneuropathy, as described in the example below. You may miss this finding unless you compare distal and proximal areas.

Here all sensation in the hand is lost. Repetitive testing in a proximal direction reveals a gradual change to normal sensation at the wrist. This pattern fits neither a peripheral nerve nor a dermatome (see p. 509). If bilateral, it suggests the "glove and stocking" sensory loss of a polyneuropathy.

See Table 18-6, Patterns of Sensory Loss (pp. 558–559).

PAIN. Use a sharp safety pin or other suitable tool, as described on page 516. Occasionally, substitute the blunt end for the point. Ask the patient, ''Is this sharp or dull?'' or, when making comparisons, ''Does this feel the same as this?'' Use as light a stimulus as the patient can perceive as sharp, and try not to draw blood.

To prevent any chance of transmitting a blood-borne infection, remember to discard the pin or other device safely, and do not reuse it on another person.

TEMPERATURE. (This is often omitted if pain sensation is normal, but include it if there is any question.) Use two test tubes, filled with hot and cold water, or a tuning fork heated or cooled by water. Touch the skin and ask the patient to identify ''hot'' or ''cold.''

LIGHT TOUCH. With a fine wisp of cotton, touch the skin lightly, avoiding pressure. Ask the patient to respond whenever a touch is felt, and to compare one area with another. Calloused skin is normally relatively insensitive and should be avoided.

VIBRATION. Use a relatively low-pitched tuning fork of 128 Hz or 256 Hz. Tap it on the heel of your hand and place it firmly over a distal interphalangeal joint of the patient's finger, then over the interphalangeal joint of the big toe. Ask what the patient feels. If you are uncertain whether it is pressure or vibration, ask the patient to tell you when the vibration stops, and then touch the fork to stop it. If vibration sense is impaired, proceed to more proximal bony prominences (*e.g.,* wrist and elbow or medial malleolus, patella, anterior superior iliac spine, spinous processes, and clavicles).

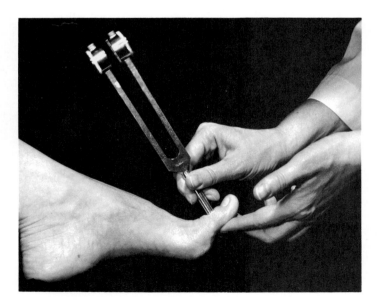

POSITION. Grasp the patient's big toe, holding it by its sides between your thumb and index finger, and then pull it away from the other

Analgesia refers to absence of pain sensation, *hypalgesia* to decreased sensitivity to pain, and *hyperalgesia* to increased sensitivity.

Anesthesia is absence of touch sensation, *hypesthesia* is decreased sensitivity, and *hyperesthesia* is increased sensitivity.

Vibration sense is often the first sensation to be lost in a peripheral neuropathy. Common causes include diabetes and alcoholism. Vibration sense is also lost in posterior column disease. It is here where testing vibration sense in the trunk may be useful in estimating the level of a cord lesion. Remember that aging may also be associated with decreased vibration sense.

Loss of position sense, like loss of vibration sense, suggests

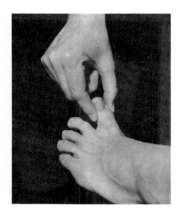

toes so as to avoid friction. (These precautions prevent extraneous tactile stimuli from indicating to the patient a change of position that might not otherwise be detected.) Show what you mean by "up" and "down" as you move the patient's toe clearly upward and downward. Then, with the patient's eyes closed, ask for an "up" or "down" response as you move the toe in a small arc.

either posterior column disease or a lesion of the peripheral nerve or root.

Repeat several times on each side, avoiding simple alternation of the stimuli. If position sense is impaired, move proximally to test it at the ankle joint. In a similar fashion, test position in the fingers, moving proximally if indicated to the metacarpophalangeal joints, wrist, and elbow.

DISCRIMINATIVE SENSATIONS. Several additional maneuvers test the ability of the sensory cortex to correlate, analyze, and interpret sensations. Because discriminative sensations are dependent on touch and position sense, they are useful only when these sensations are either intact or only slightly impaired.

Screen a patient with stereognosis, and proceed to the other methods if indicated. The patient's eyes should be closed during all these maneuvers.

When touch and position sense are normal or only slightly impaired, a disproportionate decrease in or loss of discriminative sensations suggests disease of the sensory cortex. Stereognosis, number identification, and two-point discrimination are also impaired by posterior column disease.

1. *Stereognosis.* Stereognosis refers to the ability to identify an object by feeling of it. Place in the patient's hand a familiar object such as a

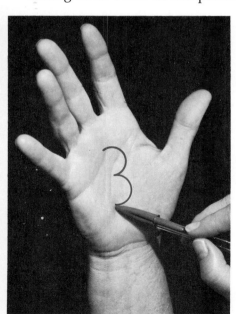

coin, paper clip, key, pencil, or cotton ball, and ask the patient to tell you what it is. Normally a patient will manipulate it skillfully and identify it correctly. Asking the patient to distinguish "heads" from "tails" on a coin is a sensitive test of stereognosis.

2. *Number identification (graphesthesia).* When motor impairment, arthritis, or other conditions prevent the patient from manipulating an object well enough to identify it, test the ability to identify numbers. With the blunt end of a pen or pencil, draw a large number in

Astereognosis refers to the inability to recognize objects placed in the hand.

The inability to recognize numbers, like astereognosis, suggests a lesion in the sensory cortex.

the patient's palm. A normal person can identify most such numbers.

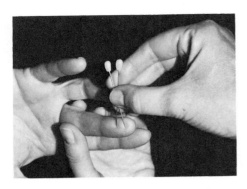

3. *Two-point discrimination.* Using the sides of two pins or the two ends of an opened paper clip, touch a finger pad in two places simultaneously. Alternate the double stimulus irregularly with a one-point touch. Be careful not to cause pain.

Find the minimal distance at which the patient can discriminate one from two points (normally less than 5 mm on the finger pads). This test may be used on other parts of the body, but normal distances vary widely from one body region to another.

Lesions of the sensory cortex increase the distance between two recognizable points.

4. *Point localization.* Briefly touch a point on the patient's skin. Then ask the patient to open both eyes and point to the place touched. Normally a person can do so accurately. This test, together with that for extinction, is especially useful on the trunk and the legs.

Lesions of the sensory cortex impair the ability to localize points accurately.

5. *Extinction.* Simultaneously stimulate corresponding areas on both sides of the body. Ask where the patient feels your touch. Normally both stimuli are felt.

With lesions of the sensory cortex, only one stimulus may be recognized. The stimulus on the side opposite the damaged cortex is extinguished.

SPECIAL MANEUVERS

MENINGEAL SIGNS. Testing for meningeal signs is not part of a routine examination, but should be done when you suspect inflammation of the meninges—the result of infection (meningitis) or bleeding (subarachnoid hemorrhage). (See also pp. 593–594 and 626–627.)

With the patient recumbent, place your hands behind the patient's head and flex the neck forward, until the chin touches the chest if possible. Note resistance or pain. Watch also for flexion of the patient's hips and knees in reaction to your maneuver—a response that constitutes a *Brudzinski's sign*.

Pain in the neck and resistance to flexion suggest meningeal inflammation but may be due to arthritis or neck injury. Flexion of hips and knees suggests meningeal inflammation.

Flex one of the patient's legs at both hip and knee, then straighten the knee. Note any unusual resistance or pain. Resistance to full extension, with discomfort behind the knee, occurs in many normal people.

Pain and increased resistance to extending the knee constitutes a *Kernig's sign.* When bilateral, it suggests meningeal irritation.

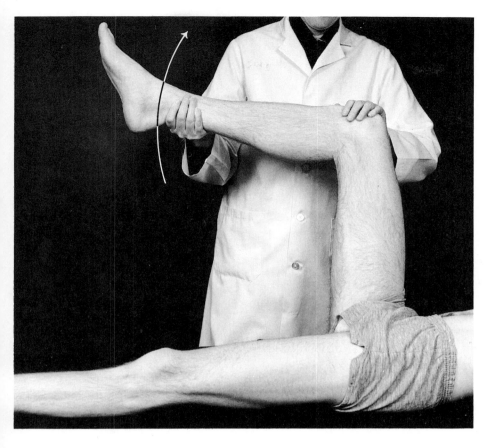

Compression of a lumbosacral
nerve root may also cause resistance, together with pain in the
low back and the posterior
thigh. Only one leg is usually
involved.

ASTERIXIS. Asterixis is useful in identifying a metabolic encephalopathy
in patients whose mental functions are impaired. Ask the patient to hold
both arms forward, with hands cocked up and fingers spread. Watch for
1 to 2 minutes, coaxing the patient as necessary to maintain this position.

Sudden, brief, nonrhythmic
flexion of the hands and fingers
indicates asterixis (p. 556).

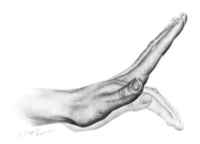

THE STUPOROUS OR COMATOSE PATIENT. Survey the patient
quickly. Make sure that the airway is clear, and look for evidence of
bleeding and shock. Assess the vital signs, including pulse, blood pressure, and rectal temperature. (Laboratory studies and emergency management are beyond the scope of this text.)

Without neglecting further observations of the patient, make every effort
possible to get a history from relatives or friends or from witnesses of the
developing illness. Try to determine the speed with which unconsciousness developed; any premonitory symptoms, precipitating factors, or

previous episodes; the duration of the unconsciousness; and the appearance and behavior of the patient during it. A history of past medical or psychiatric illnesses is also useful.

Despite the atmosphere of emergency, take several minutes and carefully observe:

● The rate and rhythm of respirations

See Table 8-1, Abnormalities in Rate and Rhythm of Breathing (p. 256).

● Posture and motor activity, noting especially position in bed

See Table 18-7, Abnormal Postures in the Comatose Patient (p. 560).

● The position of head and eyes, and any spontaneous movements

● Any odors

Alcohol, liver failure, uremia

● Any abnormalities of the skin, including color, moisture, evidence of bleeding disorders, and needlemarks or other lesions

Jaundice, cyanosis, cherry red color of carbon monoxide poisoning

As you go on with your examination, take two *important precautions:*

● If there is any question of trauma to the head or neck, do not bend the neck until x-ray examination has ruled out a fracture of the cervical spine.

● In examining the ocular fundi, do not dilate the pupils with a mydriatic solution. It could mask important eye signs.

Proceed to a *general and neurologic examination,* with special attention to the following:

● Examine the head carefully for signs of trauma.

Bruises, lacerations, swelling

● Test for meningeal signs.

Meningitis, subarachnoid hemorrhage

● Examine the eyes, especially:
  The fundi

Papilledema, hypertensive retinopathy

  The pupils and their reaction to light

See Table 7-7, Pupillary Abnormalities (pp. 203–204). In deep coma, the presence of pupillary reflexes favors a metabolic cause; their absence favors a structural cause.

The extraocular movements, if possible

The corneal reflexes. Bilateral loss of these reflexes may be due to the coma itself or to prior use of contact lenses.

Reflex loss in lesions affecting the 5th or 7th cranial nerves.

- Inspect the ears and nose.

Blood or cerebrospinal fluid in the nose or the ears suggests a skull fracture; otitis media suggests a possible brain abscess.

- Watch for facial asymmetry.
- Inspect the mouth and the throat.

Tongue injury suggests a seizure.

- Examine the heart, lungs, and abdomen.

- Complete a neurologic examination, insofar as you are able.

Four additional maneuvers may be especially helpful:

1. *Assess the response to stimuli,* increasing the strength of the stimulus as follows:

   a. Give a simple command.
   b. Call the patient's name.
   c. Produce pain—for example, by pressing the bony ridges above the eyes, or by pinching the sides of the neck or the inner portions of upper arms and thighs. Start gently.

Avoidance movements persist in stupor and light coma but are lost in deeper coma.

Observe how strong a stimulus is required to produce a response. Note whether:

   a. Motor responses are confined to one side of the body.

Motor responses confined to one side suggest paralysis of the other side.

   b. Stimuli from both sides or only one side of the body produce a response.

When a stimulus on one side of the body produces a response but a similar stimulus on the opposite side does not, suspect a sensory deficit on the latter side.

2. *Look for flaccid paralysis,* as in acute hemiplegia, by grasping each forearm near the wrist and raising it to a vertical position. Note the position of the hand, usually only slightly flexed at the wrist.

The hemiplegia of sudden cerebral accidents is usually flaccid at first. A flaccid hand droops

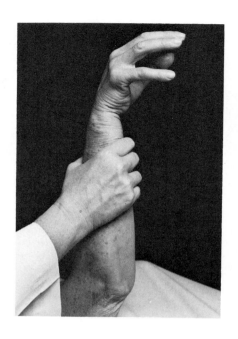

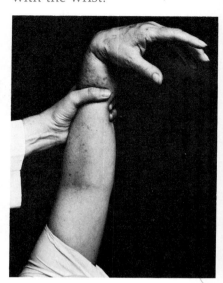

limply to form a right angle with the wrist.

Then lower the arms to about 12 or 18 inches off the bed and drop them. Watch how they fall. A normal arm drops somewhat slowly.

A flaccid arm drops rapidly, like a flail.

Flex the patient's knees and support them on your arm. Then extend one leg at a time at the knee and drop it to the bed. Compare the speed with which each leg falls.

In hemiplegia, the flaccid leg falls more rapidly.

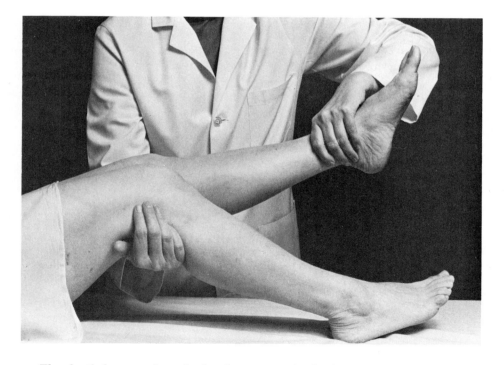

Flex both legs so that the heels rest on the bed and release them. The normal leg returns slowly to its original extended position.

In hemiplegia, the flaccid leg falls rapidly into extension with external rotation at the hip.

3. *Test for the oculocephalic reflex (doll's eye movements).* Holding open the upper eyelids so that you can see the eyes, turn the head quickly, first to one side and then to the other. Flex the neck forward, and then extend it. Observe the eye movements.

In a comatose patient with an intact brainstem, the patient's eyes move in the opposite direction as if still gazing ahead in their initial position (doll's eye movements), shown below.

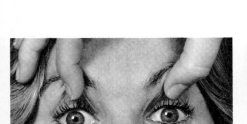 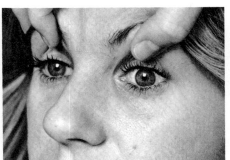 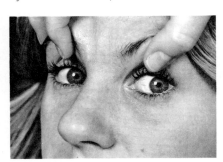

Unless consciously fixing their gaze, fully conscious patients move their eyes unpredictably or only slightly in a direction opposite to your movement. As illustrated above, for example, you have turned the patient's head to her right, and her eyes have moved slightly to her left.

Loss of doll's eye movements in a comatose patient suggests a lesion of midbrain or pons, or very deep coma, shown below.

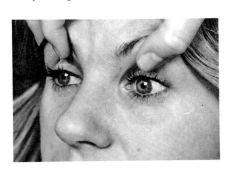

4. *Test the oculovestibular reflex with caloric stimulation.* Make sure that the eardrums are intact and the canals clear. Elevate the patient's head to 30°, and place a kidney basin under the ear to catch any overflowing water. With a large syringe, inject icewater through a small catheter that is lying in (but not plugging) the ear canal. Watch for eye movements. The normal awake patient responds with nystagmus, with the quick jerking component moving away from the irrigated ear. Although a few milliliters of ice water often produce a response in a normal person, you may need to use up to 200 ml in a comatose patient. Repeat on the opposite side, waiting 3 to 5 minutes if necessary for the first response to disappear.

A comatose patient with an intact brainstem responds by conjugate deviation of the eyes toward the irrigated ear. Loss of this reflex (no response to stimulation) suggests a brainstem lesion.

Table 18-1 Nystagmus

Table 18-1 Nystagmus

Nystagmus is a rhythmic oscillation of the eyes. Analogous to a tremor in other parts of the body, it is essentially a disorder of ocular posture. Its causes are multiple, including impairment of vision in early life, disorders of the labyrinth and the cerebellar system, and drug toxicity. Nystagmus occurs normally when a person watches a rapidly moving object (*e.g.*, a passing train). Observe the three characteristics of nystagmus listed below and on the following page. Then refer to textbooks of neurology for differential diagnosis.

Nystagmus is usually quicker in one direction than in the other, and is then defined by its quicker phase. For example, if the eyes jerk quickly to the patient's left and drift back slowly to the right, the patient is said to have nystagmus to the left.

Occasionally, nystagmus consists only of coarse oscillations without quick and slow components. It is then said to be *pendular.*

The movements of nystagmus may occur in one or more planes (*i.e.*, horizontal, vertical, or rotary). It is the plane of the movements, not the direction of the gaze, that defines this variable.

DIRECTION OF THE QUICK AND SLOW COMPONENTS

EXAMPLE: NYSTAGMUS TO THE LEFT—A SLOW DRIFT TO THE RIGHT, THEN A QUICK JERK TO THE LEFT IN EACH EYE

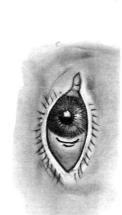
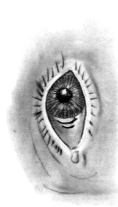

PLANE OF THE MOVEMENTS

HORIZONTAL NYSTAGMUS

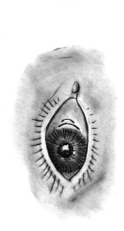

VERTICAL NYSTAGMUS

ROTARY NYSTAGMUS

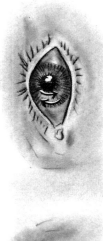
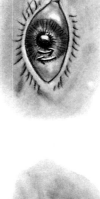
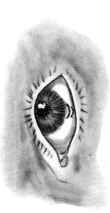
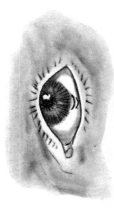
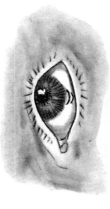
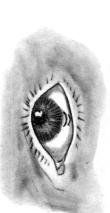
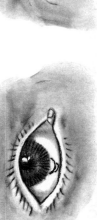

Table 18-1   *Nystagmus*

FIELD OF GAZE IN WHICH NYSTAGMUS APPEARS

EXAMPLE: NYSTAGMUS ON RIGHT LATERAL GAZE

NYSTAGMUS PRESENT

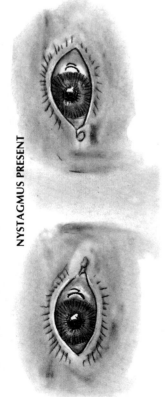

NYSTAGMUS NOT PRESENT

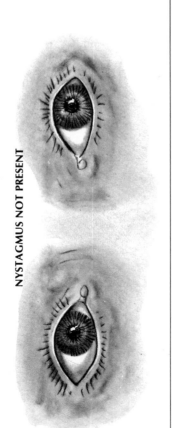

Although nystagmus may be present in all fields of gaze, it may instead appear or become accentuated only on deviation of the eyes (*e.g.,* to the side or upward). On extreme lateral gaze, the normal person may show a few beats resembling nystagmus. Avoid making assessments in such extreme positions, and observe for nystagmus only within the field of full binocular vision.

Table 18-2   Types of Facial Paralysis

Facial weakness or paralysis may result either (1) from a lesion of the facial nerve itself, anywhere from its origin in the pons to its periphery in the face, or (2) from a lesion involving the upper motor neurons anywhere between the cortex and the pons. A lesion of the facial nerve (the lower motor neuron), exemplified here by a Bell's palsy, is compared with an upper motor neuron lesion, exemplified by a hemiplegia. Note their different effects on the upper part of the face, by which they can be distinguished.

LOWER MOTOR NEURON PARALYSIS

Damage to the right facial nerve paralyzes the entire right side of the face, including the forehead.

CLOSING EYES

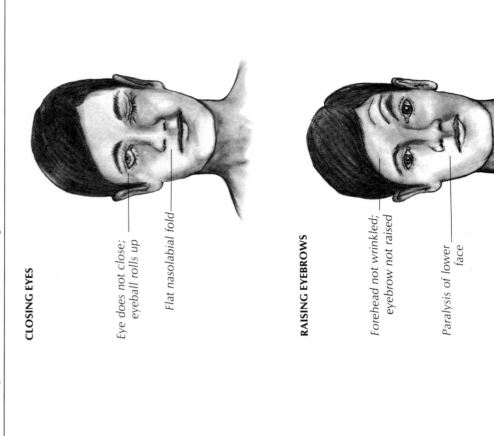

Eye does not close; eyeball rolls up

Flat nasolabial fold

RAISING EYEBROWS

Forehead not wrinkled; eyebrow not raised

Paralysis of lower face

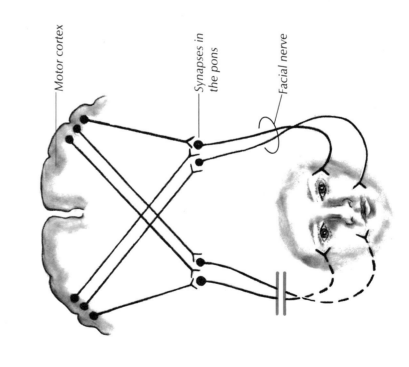

Motor cortex

Synapses in the pons

Facial nerve

Table 18-2   Types of Facial Paralysis

UPPER MOTOR NEURON PARALYSIS

The lower part of the face normally is controlled by upper motor neurons located on only one side of the cortex—the opposite side. Left-sided damage to these upper motor neurons, as in a stroke, paralyzes the right lower face. The upper face, however, is controlled by upper motor neurons from both sides of the cortex. Even though the upper motor neurons on the left are destroyed, others on the right remain and the right upper face continues to function fairly well.

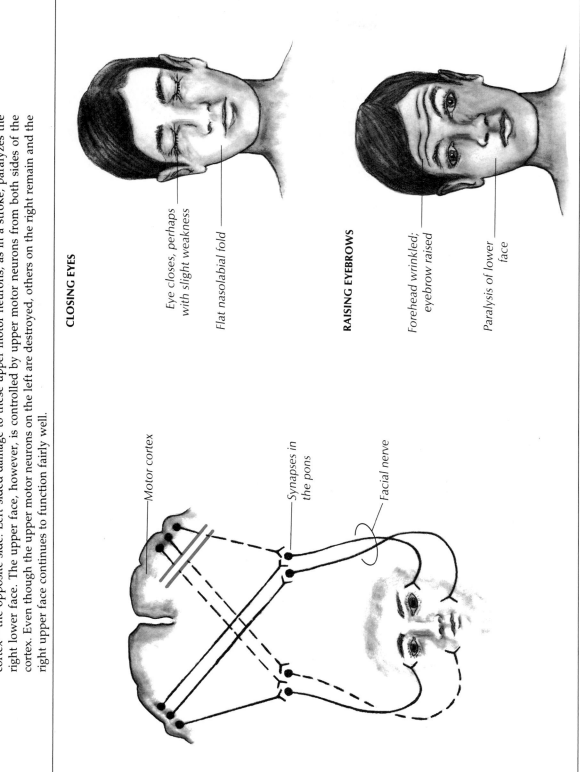

CLOSING EYES

Eye closes, perhaps with slight weakness

Flat nasolabial fold

RAISING EYEBROWS

Forehead wrinkled; eyebrow raised

Paralysis of lower face

Motor cortex

Synapses in the pons

Facial nerve

Table 18-3   Abnormalities of Gait and Posture

	SPASTIC HEMIPARESIS	SCISSORS GAIT	STEPPAGE GAIT
UNDERLYING DEFECT	Associated with unilateral upper motor neuron disease, as with a stroke	Associated with bilateral spastic paresis of the legs	Associated with foot drop, usually secondary to lower motor neuron disease
DESCRIPTION	One arm is held immobile and close to the side, with elbow, wrist, and interphalangeal joints flexed. The leg is extended, with plantar flexion of the foot. On walking, the patient either drags the foot, often scraping the toe, or circles it stiffly outward and forward (circumduction).	The gait is stiff. Each leg is advanced slowly and the thighs tend to cross forward on each other at each step. The steps are short. The patient appears to be walking through water.	These patients either drag their feet or lift them high, with knees flexed, and bring them down with a slap onto the floor, thus appearing to be walking up stairs. They are unable to walk on their heels. The steppage gait may involve one or both sides.

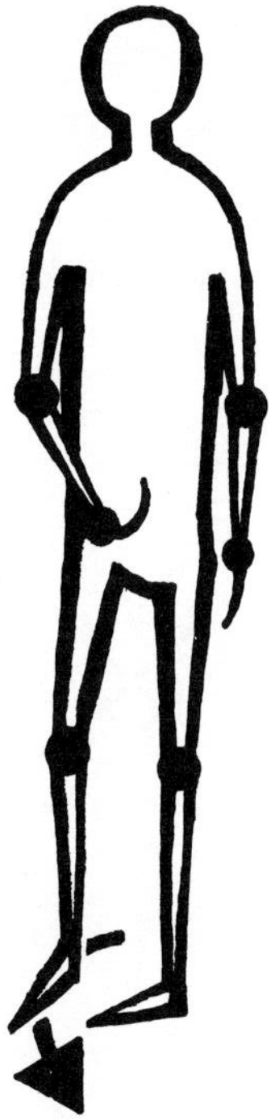

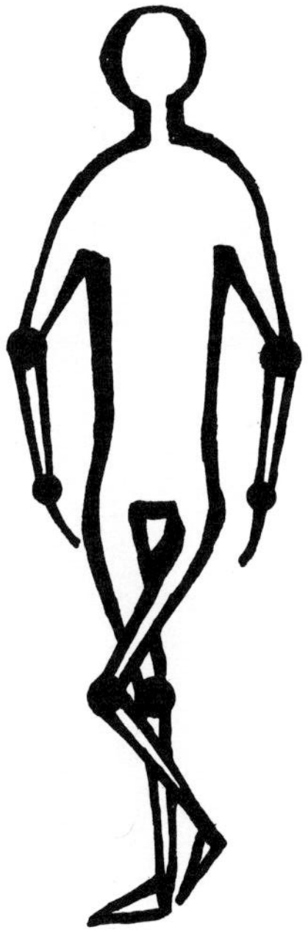

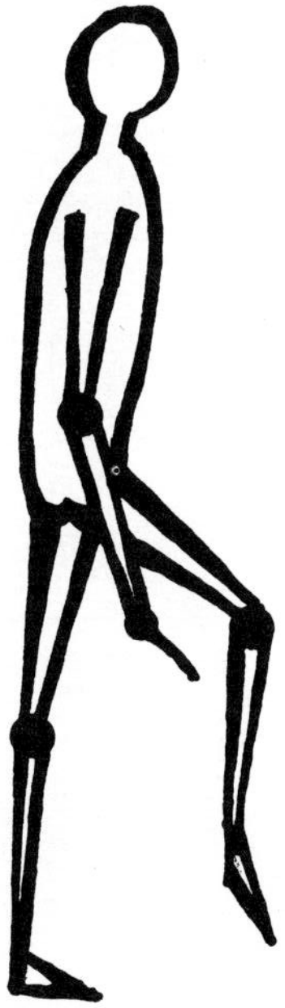

Table 18-3   Abnormalities of Gait and Posture

	SENSORY ATAXIA	CEREBELLAR ATAXIA	PARKINSONIAN GAIT	GAIT OF OLD AGE
UNDERLYING DEFECT	Associated with loss of position sense in the legs, as from polyneuropathy or posterior column damage	Associated with disease of the cerebellum or associated tracts	Associated with the basal ganglia defects of Parkinson's disease	The aging process
DESCRIPTION	The gait is unsteady and wide-based (with feet wide apart). These patients throw their feet forward and bring them outward and bring them down, first on the heels and then on the toes, with a double tapping sound. They watch the ground for guidance while walking. With eyes closed, they cannot stand steadily with feet together (a positive Romberg sign) and the staggering gait worsens.	The gait is staggering, unsteady, and wide-based, with exaggerated difficulty on the turns. These patients cannot stand steadily with feet together, whether their eyes are open or closed.	The posture is stooped, with head and neck forward and hips and knees slightly flexed. Arms are flexed at elbows and wrists. The patient is slow in getting started. Steps are short and often shuffling. Arm swings are decreased and the patient turns around stiffly—"all in one piece."	Speed, balance, and grace decrease with aging. Steps become short, uncertain, and even shuffling. The legs may be flexed at hips and knees. A cane may bolster lost confidence.

Table 18-4 Involuntary Movements

TREMORS

Tremors are relatively rhythmic oscillatory movements which may be roughly subdivided into three groups: resting (or static) tremors, intention tremors, and postural tremors.

RESTING (OR STATIC) TREMORS	INTENTION TREMORS	POSTURAL TREMORS
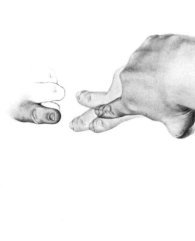		

These tremors are most prominent at rest, and may decrease or disappear with voluntary movement. Illustrated is the common, relatively slow, fine, pill-rolling tremor of parkinsonism, about 5 per second.

Intention tremors, absent at rest, appear with activity and often get worse as the target is neared. Causes include disorders of cerebellar pathways, as in multiple sclerosis.

These tremors appear when the affected part is actively maintaining a posture. Examples include the fine, rapid tremor of hyperthyroidism and the tremors of anxiety and fatigue. The most common form is benign essential (and sometimes familial) tremor. It may worsen somewhat with intention.

FASCICULATIONS

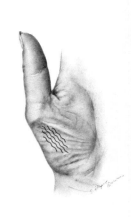

Fasciculations are fine, rapid, flickering or twitching movements originating in relatively small groups of muscle fibers (fascicles, or muscle bundles). They vary irregularly in frequency and extent, but, unlike tremors, rarely move a joint. When seen in muscles that are undergoing atrophy, they indicate lower motor neuron disease.

Table 18-4 Involuntary Movements

TICS

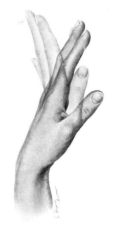

Tics are brief, repetitive, stereotyped, coordinated movements occurring at irregular intervals. Examples include repetitive winking, grimacing, and shoulder shrugging.

CHOREA

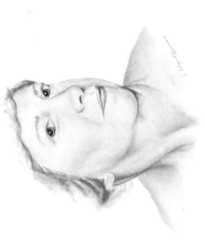

Choreiform movements are brief, rapid, jerky, irregular, and unpredictable. They occur at rest or interrupt normal coordinated movements. Unlike tics, they seldom repeat themselves. The face, head, lower arms, and hands are often involved. Causes include Sydenham's chorea (with rheumatic fever) and Huntington's disease.

ATHETOSIS

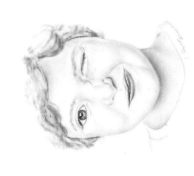

Athetoid movements are slower and more twisting and writhing than choreiform movements, and have a larger amplitude. They most commonly involve the face and the distal extremities. Athetosis is often associated with spasticity. Causes include cerebral palsy.

DYSTONIA

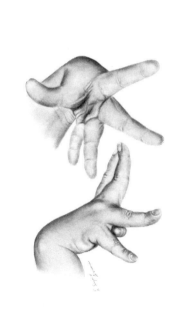

Dystonic movements are somewhat similar to athetoid movements, but often involve larger portions of the body, including the trunk. Grotesque, twisted postures may result. Causes include drugs such as phenothiazines, dystonia musculorum deformans, and, as illustrated, spasmodic torticollis.

➡ *Continued*

Table 18-4 Involuntary Movements

Table 18-4 (Cont'd.)

ASTERIXIS

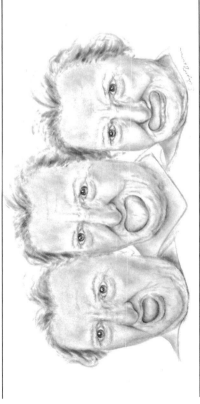

Asterixis is classified as a negative myoclonus (with sudden muscular inhibitions rather than contractions). The extended wrist or fingers flex suddenly, briefly, and nonrhythmically, then return to their original position. Movements occur every 2 to 30 seconds. In a mentally impaired patient, asterixis favors metabolic encephalopathy over psychiatric or structural brain disease.

MYOCLONUS

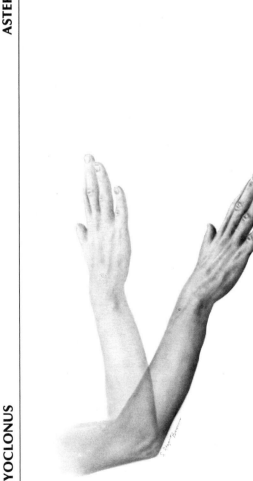

Myoclonic movements are sudden, brief, rapid, unpredictable muscular contractions that usually involve the limbs or the trunk. They may be single or repetitive. Myoclonus may occur in a normal person who is falling asleep, but is also associated with a variety of neurologic disorders, including metabolic encephalopathies.

ORAL–FACIAL DYSKINESIAS

Oral–facial dyskinesias are rhythmic, repetitive, bizarre movements that chiefly involve the face, mouth, jaw, and tongue: grimacing, pursing of the lips, protrusions of the tongue, opening and closing of the mouth, and deviations of the jaw. The limbs and trunk are involved less often. These movements may be a late complication of psychotropic drugs such as phenothiazines, and have then been termed *tardive* (late) dyskinesias. They also occur in long-standing psychoses, in some elderly individuals, and in some edentulous persons.

Table 18-5   Differentiation of Motor Disorders

Table 18-5   Differentiation of Motor Disorders

	LOWER MOTOR NEURON DISORDERS	UPPER MOTOR NEURON DISORDERS	PARKINSONISM (an Extrapyramidal Disorder)	CEREBELLAR DISORDERS
DESCRIPTION	Muscle strength, tone, and reflexes are decreased or lost. Deficits are limited to areas supplied by the spinal segment(s), root(s), or nerve(s) involved. In peripheral polyneuropathy, weakness is more prominent distally.	Weakness involves whole groups of muscles such as the abductors and extensors of the arms and the flexors of the legs. Deep tendon reflexes and muscle tone, in contrast to strength, are increased.	Movements are diminished and slowed, with little or no real weakness. Muscle tone is increased, causing rigidity which, when marked, may impair the deep tendon reflexes. A resting tremor is typical.	Balance and coordination are impaired, as manifested by dysarthria, an ataxic gait, intention tremors, and poor performance of rapid alternating movements and point-to-point tests. Muscle tone is decreased.
INVOLUNTARY MOVEMENTS	Often fasciculations	No fasciculations	Resting tremors	Intention tremors
MUSCLE BULK	Atrophy	Normal, or mild atrophy due to disuse	Normal	Normal
MUSCLE TONE	Decreased to absent	Increased, spastic	Increased, rigid	Decreased
MUSCLE STRENGTH	Decreased or lost	Decreased or lost	Normal or slightly decreased	Normal or slightly decreased
COORDINATION	Unimpaired, although limited by weakness. Finger tapping on the thumb is accurate within the limits of residual strength.	Slowed and limited by weakness. Fine movements such as finger tapping are particularly impaired, but without cerebellar deficits.	Relatively unimpaired, although movements are slowed and often tremulous. Fine movements often remain surprisingly accurate.	Inappropriate speed and force of movements, overshooting, and clumsy turns. Intention tremors may further impair fine movements.
REFLEXES IN AFFECTED AREAS				
DEEP TENDON	Decreased or absent	Hyperactive	Normal, though may be impaired by rigidity	Normal. Knee jerks may be swinging (pendular).
PLANTAR	Flexor or absent	Extensor (Babinski response)	Flexor	Flexor
ABDOMINAL	Absent	Absent	Normal	Normal

Table 18-6   Patterns of Sensory Loss

Table 18-6 Patterns of Sensory Loss

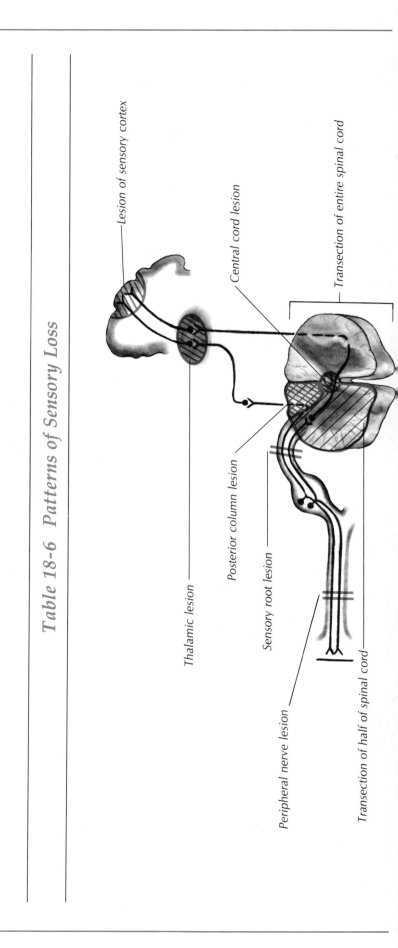

Lesion of sensory cortex

Central cord lesion

Transection of entire spinal cord

Thalamic lesion

Posterior column lesion

Sensory root lesion

Peripheral nerve lesion

Transection of half of spinal cord

Table 18-6   Patterns of Sensory Loss

LOCATION OF THE LESION	SENSORY DEFICIT	ASSOCIATED MOTOR CHANGES
PERIPHERAL NERVE	Usually a loss of all sensations in the distribution of a peripheral nerve on the involved side, but different sensations may be affected differently	Often signs of a lower motor neuron lesion in the muscles supplied by the involved nerve
MULTIPLE PERIPHERAL NERVES (*Peripheral Polyneuropathy*)	Usually a loss of all sensations in a distal and symmetrical distribution, with gradual shading from normal to diminished sensation	Often lower motor neuron signs similarly distributed, but a peripheral neuropathy may be purely sensory
SENSORY ROOT(S)	Loss of all sensations in the spinal segments involved and on the same side. More than one root must usually be affected.	None from a sensory root lesion alone
CENTRAL CORD (*as in Early Syringomyelia*)	Loss of pain and temperature sensations in one or several dermatomes. Other sensations are preserved unless sensory tracts in the cord become involved.	Lower motor neuron signs involving the same spinal segments may be present. Later, upper motor neuron signs below the level of the lesion may appear.
POSTERIOR COLUMN	Loss of position and vibration, stereognosis, number-writing, and two-point discrimination, on the involved side. Loss is often bilateral.	None unless upper motor pathways in the cord are also affected
TRANSECTION OF HALF OF THE SPINAL CORD (*Brown–Séquard Syndrome*)	Loss of position and vibration sensations below the level of the lesion on the involved side. Loss of pain and temperature sensations on the opposite side from one or two dermatomes below the level of the lesion downward. Touch is relatively unaffected.	Upper motor neuron signs below the level of the lesion on the involved side
TRANSECTION OF THE ENTIRE SPINAL CORD	Bilateral loss of sensation below the level of the lesion	Bilateral upper motor neuron signs below the level of the lesion
THALAMUS	Decrease in all sensations over the entire half of the body on the side opposite the lesion. Diffuse pain may be present in the area of sensory loss.	Upper motor neuron signs (hemiparesis) on the side opposite the lesion may occur if the adjacent corticospinal tract is involved.
SENSORY CORTEX	Loss of discriminative sensations on the opposite side of the whole body. There may be some decrease in other sensations, but less prominently.	If motor pathways are involved by the lesion, upper motor neuron signs on the side opposite the lesion

Table 18-7　Abnormal Postures in the Comatose Patient

HEMIPLEGIA (Early)

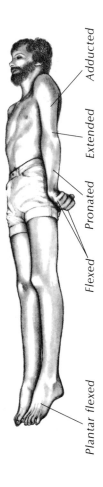

Externally rotated

Flaccid

Sudden unilateral brain damage involving the corticospinal tract may produce a hemiplegia, or one-sided paralysis, which early in its course is flaccid. Spasticity will develop later. The paralyzed arm and leg are slack. They fall loosely and without tone when raised and dropped to the bed. Spontaneous movements or responses to noxious stimuli are limited to the opposite side. The leg may lie externally rotated. One side of the lower face may be paralyzed, and that cheek puffs out on expiration. Both eyes may be turned away from the paralyzed side.

DECORTICATE RIGIDITY

Flexed

Adducted

Flexed

Internally rotated

Plantar flexed

In decorticate rigidity, the upper arms are held tight to the sides with elbows, wrists, and fingers flexed. The legs are extended and internally rotated. The feet are plantar flexed. This posture implies a destructive lesion of the corticospinal tracts within or very near the cerebral hemispheres. When unilateral, this is the posture of chronic spastic hemiplegia.

DECEREBRATE RIGIDITY

Flexed　Pronated　Extended　Adducted

Plantar flexed

In decerebrate rigidity, the jaws are clenched and the neck is extended. The arms are adducted and stiffly extended at the elbows, with forearms pronated, wrists and fingers flexed. The legs are stiffly extended at the knees, with the feet plantar flexed. This posture may occur spontaneously or only in response to external stimuli such as light, noise, or pain. It is caused by a lesion in the diencephalon, midbrain, or pons, although severe metabolic disorders such as hypoxia or hypoglycemia may also produce it.

Chapter 19
The Physical Examination of Infants and Children

Robert A. Hoekelman

The anatomy and physiology, the techniques of examination, and the normal and abnormal findings presented in the foregoing sections of this book focus primarily on the adult patient. Most of this material is also applicable to infants and children. Developmentally, however, children are anatomically and physiologically unique. Consequently, many of the techniques, the physical findings, and the significance of the findings differ in younger patients.

The purpose of this section is to describe how to conduct those parts of the physical examination of infants and children that require different approaches and techniques than those used for examining adults. Emphasis is placed on the normal, variations of normal, and those accompanying common pathologic conditions of infancy and childhood. Uncommon pathologic conditions are not presented, except for the few that require specific examination techniques for detection. The texts listed in the bibliography should be consulted for complete differential diagnoses of abnormal physical findings.

When assessing an infant or a child, always consider where the patient is on the continuum of growth and development, as well as the age range in which that point is normally reached. You must also reflect upon the different rates of growth of the various systems of the body. For example, growth and development of the central nervous system, the lymphatic system, and the reproductive system parallel neither general somatic growth nor each other. The figure at the right illustrates these differences.

You must be well acquainted, therefore, with the normal and abnormal patterns of growth and development. You should be aware, for example, that a physical finding such as a Babinski response is abnormal beyond the age of 2 years, but may be found in as many as 10% of normal subjects before that age.

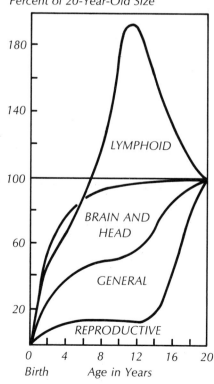

GROWTH PATTERNS OF VARIOUS SYSTEMS

Percent of 20-Year-Old Size

The developmental milestones measured by the Denver Developmental Screening Test are discussed on page 570 and illustrated on pages 571 and 572. Texts dealing with more comprehensive developmental information are listed in the bibliography.

Measurement of length, weight, and head circumference at various ages is very useful in comparing a patient's physical growth with norms for infants, children, and adolescents. The grids for length and weight on page 563 are used for females and those on page 564 for males. Similar grids are available for head circumference measurements. Entries on these grids should be made at each well-child visit, scheduled more frequently during the first 2 years of life than thereafter (see page 565 for Guidelines for Health Supervision recommended by the American Academy of Pediatrics). Measurements should be recorded more often when a patient is not keeping pace with or begins to exceed these expected patterns of growth.

The examination described in this chapter is divided into regions or systems similar to those in the rest of the book. Each section discusses three somewhat different approaches tailored to different *developmental levels:* infancy (the first year), early childhood (1 year through 4 years), and late childhood (5 years through 12 years). The physical examination of adolescents (13 years through 20 years) is conducted essentially like that of the adult.

Because treatment of individual systems here is brief, sections on *techniques of examination* **are set off in boldface rather than presented separately, as in the earlier chapters.**

The reader should first return to Chapter 4, *Physical Examination: Approach and Overview,* to recall the methods and sequence of examining an adult patient. By and large, the methods used to examine adults are applied to the examination of infants and children. The exceptions are noted in the sections that follow. The examination sequence for infants and children differs in that potentially painful or distressing maneuvers are performed near the end of the examination and relatively non-disturbing maneuvers early on. For example, palpating the head and neck, determining the range of motion of the extremities at each joint, and auscultating the heart and lungs are best done early because they are less threatening than looking into the ears and mouth or palpating the abdomen, which are done near the end of the examination. Areas of the body in which the patient, by history, is having pain are usually examined last.

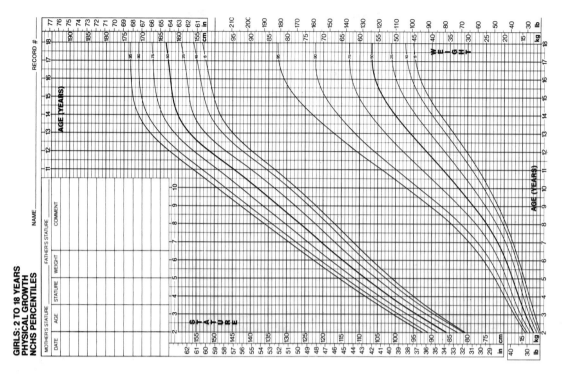

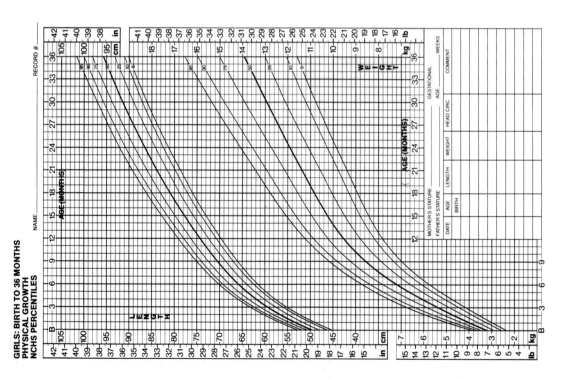

(Adapted from Hamill PVV, Drizd TA, Johnson CL, Reed RB, Roche AF, Moore AM: Physical growth: National Center for Health Statistics percentiles, Am J Clin Nutr 32:607–629, 1979. Data from the National Center for Health Statistics [NCHS], Hyattsville, MD. Figures provided through the courtesy of Ross Laboratories, Columbus, OH.)

BOYS: 2 TO 18 YEARS
PHYSICAL GROWTH
NCHS PERCENTILES

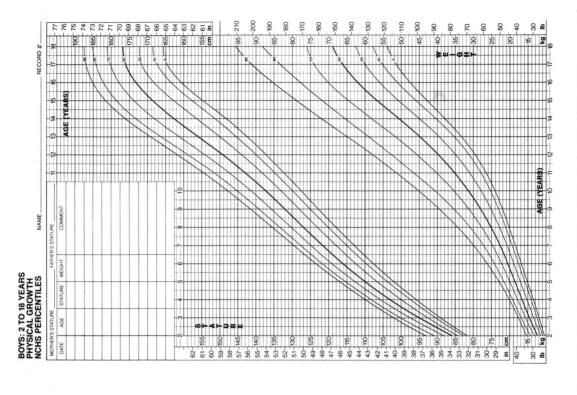

BOYS: BIRTH TO 36 MONTHS
PHYSICAL GROWTH
NCHS PERCENTILES

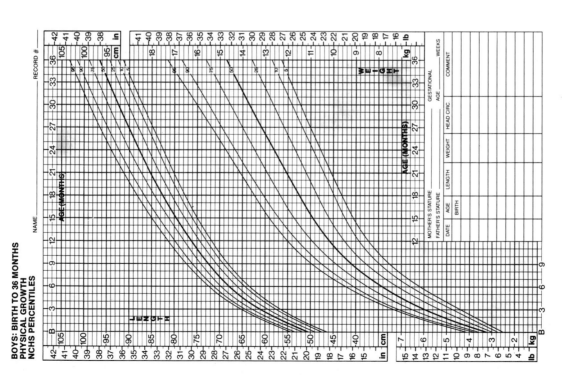

(Adapted from Hamill PVV, Drizd TA, Johnson CL, Reed RB, Roche AF, Moore AM: Physical growth: National Center for Health Statistics percentiles, Am J Clin Nutr 32:607–629, 1979. Data from the National Center for Health Statistics [NCHS], Hyattsville, MD. Figures provided through the courtesy of Ross Laboratories, Columbus, OH.)

Guidelines for Health Supervision

ITEM	INFANCY						EARLY CHILDHOOD					LATE CHILDHOOD					ADOLESCENCE			
AGE	By 1 mo.	2 mos.	4 mos.	6 mos.	9 mos.	12 mos.	15 mos.	18 mos.	24 mos.	3 yrs.	4 yrs.	5 yrs.	6 yrs.	8 yrs.	10 yrs.	12 yrs.	14 yrs.	16 yrs.	18 yrs.	20+ yrs.
HISTORY Initial/Interval	●	●	●	●	●	●	●	●	●	●	●	●	●	●	●	●	●	●	●	●
MEASUREMENTS Height and Weight	●	●	●	●	●	●	●	●	●	●	●	●	●	●	●	●	●	●	●	●
Head Circumference	●	●	●	●	●	●														
Blood Pressure										●	●	●	●	●	●	●	●	●	●	●
SENSORY SCREENING Vision	S	S	S	S	S	S	S	S	S	S	O	O	O	O	S	O	O	S	O	O
Hearing	S	S	S	S	S	S	S	S	S	S	O	O	S	S	S	O	S	S	O	S
DEVELOPMENT/BEHAVIOR ASSESSMENT	●	●	●	●	●	●	●	●	●	●	●	●	●	●	●	●	●	●	●	●
PHYSICAL EXAMINATION	●	●	●	●	●	●	●	●	●	●	●	●	●	●	●	●	●	●	●	●
PROCEDURES Hereditary/Metabolic Screening	●																			
Immunization		●	●	●			●	●				●					●			
Tuberculin Test	←———————————●→						←———●———→					←———●———→					←———●———→			
Hematocrit or Hemoglobin	←————————●——→						←——●————→					←———●———→					←————●——→			
Urinalysis	←——————●————→						←————●——→					←———●———→					←————●——→			
ANTICIPATORY GUIDANCE	●	●	●	●	●	●	●	●	●	●	●	●	●	●	●	●	●	●	●	●
INITIAL DENTAL REFERRAL									●											

Key: = ● to be performed: S = subjective, by history: O = objective, by a standard testing method; arrows indicate that the test should be performed once within that period.

These guidelines, promulgated in 1987 by the American Academy of Pediatrics' Committee on Practice and Ambulatory Care, recommended the frequency with which visits for health supervision of infants, children, and adolescents should occur and the various activities and procedures that should be included during each visit.

In general, neophyte (and some veteran) examiners are intimidated by the thought of approaching a tiny baby or a screaming child, especially if the physical examination is performed under the critical eyes of anxious parents. Although it takes a bit of courage to overcome this feeling, one soon comes to accept this challenge easily and to enjoy almost all such encounters.

APPROACH TO THE PATIENT

Infancy

The first year of life, infancy, is divided into the neonatal period (the first 28 days) and the postneonatal period (29 days to 1 year). This distinction is important only for reporting mortality rates for those age groups.

EXAMINATION OF THE NEWBORN INFANT

The next few pages deal with (1) the classification of newborn infants according to birth weight and gestational age, (2) their immediate adaptation to extrauterine life, using basic clinical signs to predict immediate survival and long-term morbidity, and (3) special techniques used in the general assessment. Methods used in examining the organ systems of newborns are for the most part identical to those used during the rest of infancy.

The newborn should be examined briefly immediately after birth to determine the general condition of cardiorespiratory, neurologic, and gastrointestinal systems and to detect any gross congenital abnormalities.

Newborn infants may be classified according to their birth weight, their gestational age (maturity), or a combination of these two dimensions.

- *Classification by Birth Weight*

    Premature = birth weight < 2500 grams
    Full-term = birth weight ≥ 2500 grams

- *Classification by Gestational Age*

    Pre-term = gestation ≤ 37 weeks
    Term = gestation 38 to 42 weeks
    Post-term = gestation ≥ 42 weeks

- *Classification by Birth Weight and Gestational Age*

    Weight Small for Gestational Age (SGA) = birth weight < 10th percentile on the intrauterine growth curve
    Weight Appropriate for Gestational Age (AGA) = birth weight within the 10th and 90th percentiles on the intrauterine growth curve

Weight Large for Gestational Age (LGA) = birth weight > 90th percentile on the intrauterine growth curve

The figure below depicts nine possible categories of maturity for newborn infants, based on birth weight and gestational age: pre-term SGA, AGA, and LGA; term SGA, AGA, and LGA; and post-term SGA, AGA, and LGA.

Each of these categories has a different mortality rate, highest for pre-term SGA and AGA infants and lowest for term AGA infants. Furthermore, pre-term AGA infants are more prone to hyaline membrane disease, apnea, patent ductus arteriosus with left-to-right shunt, and infection, while pre-term SGA infants are more likely to experience asphyxia, hypoglycemia, and hypocalcemia.

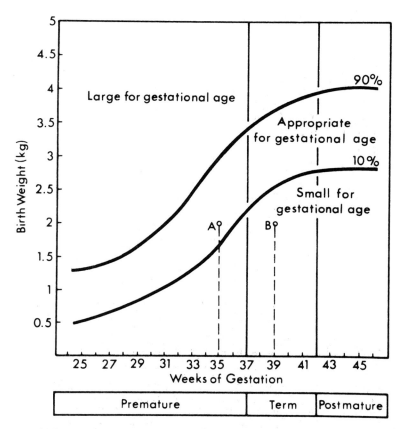

Level of intrauterine growth based on birth weight and gestational age of liveborn, single, white infants. Point A represents a premature infant, while point B indicates an infant of similar birth weight who is mature but small for gestational age; the growth curves are representative of the 10th and 90th percentiles for all of the newborns in the sampling. (Adapted for publication in the Merck Manual 15th edition, 1987, from Sweet YA: Classification of the low-birth-weight infant. In Klaus MH, Fanaroff AA: Care of the High-Risk Neonate, 3rd ed. Philadelphia, WB Saunders, 1986. Reproduced with permission.)

Several physical and neurologic characteristics of newborns, defined by Dubowitz, Dubowitz, and Goldberger, can also be used to estimate an infant's gestational age fairly accurately. (See the bibliography.)

The Apgar Scoring System: the infant's immediate adaptation to extrauterine life can be assessed with a set of five clinical signs, each scored on a 3-point scale (0, 1, or 2). The Apgar scores may range from 0 to 10, if the method of scoring shown in Table 19-1 is used. Each infant should be

One-minute Apgar scores of 7 or less usually indicate nervous system depression. Scores of 4 or less indicate severe depres-

scored at 1 minute and 5 minutes following birth. If at 5 minutes the Apgar score is 8 or more, a more complete examination should then be conducted.

sion requiring immediate resuscitation. Five-minute Apgar scores of less than 7 place the infant at high risk for subsequent central nervous system dysfunction.

Table 19-1   The Apgar Scoring System

	ASSIGNED SCORE		
CLINICAL SIGN	0	1	2
HEART RATE	Absent	<100	>100
RESPIRATORY EFFORT	Absent	Slow and irregular	Good; crying
MUSCLE TONE	Flaccid	Some flexion of the arms and legs	Active movement
REFLEX IRRITABILITY*	No responses	Crying	Crying vigorously
COLOR	Blue, pale	Pink body, blue extremities	Pink all over

* Reaction to insertion of a soft rubber catheter into the external nares

Listen to the anterior thorax with your stethoscope, palpate the abdomen, and inspect the head, face, oral cavity, extremities, genitalia, and perineum. Pass a small tube through the nose, nasopharynx, and esophagus into the stomach to establish their patency. To be sure that the tube is in the stomach, palpate the epigastrium for the tip itself; if the tip cannot be felt, feel or listen there for the emergence of an air bubble blown by mouth through the tube into the stomach. Aspirate the gastric contents in premature babies and babies born by cesarean section in order to prevent regurgitation and aspiration.

Failure to pass the tube through the nasopharynx suggests *posterior nasal (choanal) atresia.*

Failure to pass the tube into the stomach suggests *esophageal atresia,* usually with an associated *tracheoesophageal fistula.*

A more extensive examination of the newborn should be conducted within 12 hours of birth and again at approximately 72 hours of age when the effects of anesthesia and shock of birth have subsided.

Observe the baby first as it is lying undisturbed in the bassinet and then completely undressed on an examining table.

Best results, in terms of responsiveness, are obtained 2 or 3 hours after a feeding when the baby neither is too satiated (and therefore less responsive) nor too hungry (and therefore more agitated).

Observe the baby's color, size, body proportions, nutritional status, and posture as well as respirations and movements of the head and extremities.

Normal newborns lie in a symmetrical position with the limbs semiflexed and the legs partially abducted at the hip. The head is slightly flexed and positioned in the midline or turned to one side. Normal newborns have spontaneous motor activity of flexion and extension, alternating between the arms and the legs. The forearms supinate with flexion at the elbow

In *breech babies* the legs and head are extended, and the legs of a *frank breech baby* are abducted and externally rotated.

and pronate with extension. The fingers are usually flexed in a tight fist, but may extend in slow athetoid posturing movements. Low amplitude and high-frequency tremors of the arms, legs, and body are seen with vigorous crying and even at rest during the first 48 hours of life.

Most newborn infants are cooperative during the examination unless it is close to feeding time.

Make sure that the baby is quiet when you auscultate the heart and lungs and palpate the abdomen, since these maneuvers are more difficult to perform if the baby is crying. Place a sugar nipple, a bottle of formula, or the tip of one of your fingers in a crying baby's mouth to silence the baby long enough to complete these portions of the examination.

Hereafter, the order of examination is relatively unimportant, except that hip abduction (pp. 623–624) should be performed at the end because it usually causes the baby to cry.

By 4 days after birth, however, tremors occurring at rest signal central nervous system disease. Asymmetrical movements of the arms or legs at any time should alert the clinician to the possibility of central or peripheral neurologic deficits, birth injuries, or congenital anomalies.

EXAMINATION OF OLDER INFANTS

After the newborn period and throughout the rest of infancy, little difficulty should be encountered in performing the complete physical examination. The key to success is distraction. Since infants usually attend to only one thing at a time, it is relatively easy to bring the baby's attention to something other than the examination being performed.

Use a moving object, a flashing light, a game of peek-a-boo, tickling, or any sort of noise to distract the baby.

Infants usually do not object to removal of their clothing. Indeed, most seem to prefer being nude, perhaps because it allows for greater tactile stimulation. It is wise, however, in the interest of keeping yourself and your surroundings dry, to leave the diaper in place throughout the examination, removing it only to examine the genitalia, rectum, lower spine, and hips.

You can perform much of the examination with the infant lying or sitting in the parent's lap or held in an upright position against the parent's chest, although this usually is not necessary except with tired, hungry, or acutely ill babies. Occasionally, most of the physical examination can be completed without waking a sleeping infant.

Observing the parent–infant interaction is important. The parent's affect in talking about the infant, manner of holding, moving, and dressing the baby, and response to situations that may produce discomfort for the infant should be noted. A breast or a bottle feeding should be observed.

Such observations may identify maladaptive nurturing patterns on the parent's part and are important in assessing "failure to

Before performing the general physical examination of older infants, you should test for attainment of developmental milestones, such as the ability to reach for a toy, transfer a cube from one hand to the other, and use the thumb and forefinger pincer grasp in picking up a small object.

The standard for measuring the attainment of developmental milestones throughout infancy and childhood is the Denver Developmental Screening Test (DDST). The DDST is designed to detect developmental delays in personal-social, fine motor-adaptive, language, and gross motor dimensions from birth through 6 years of age. It can be administered easily and rapidly.

The form used for recording the specific observations made is shown on page 571 and directions for its use are on page 572. Each test item is represented on the DDST form under the appropriate age by a bar, which indicates when 25, 50, 75, and 90 percent of children attain the developmental milestone depicted. It must be emphasized that the DDST is only a measure of developmental attainment in the dimensions indicated and not a measure of intelligence.

Early Childhood

One of the most difficult challenges facing the professional who cares for children in this age group is completing the examination without producing a physical struggle, a crying child, or a distraught parent. When this is accomplished successfully, it provides a great measure of satisfaction to all involved and comes close to "art" in the practice of pediatrics.

Gaining the confidence and dispersing the fears of the child begin at the moment of encounter and continue throughout the entire visit. The approach may vary with the place and circumstances of the visit; however, a health supervision visit for a well child will probably allow greater development of rapport than will a visit at the office, in the home, or in the hospital emergency room when the child is acutely ill.

During the interview children should usually remain dressed. This may prolong the visit, but avoids apprehension on their part and affords the opportunity later to observe their response to being undressed or their ability to undress themselves. Children are also more apt to play quietly and interact with the parent and examiner more appropriately if fully clothed.

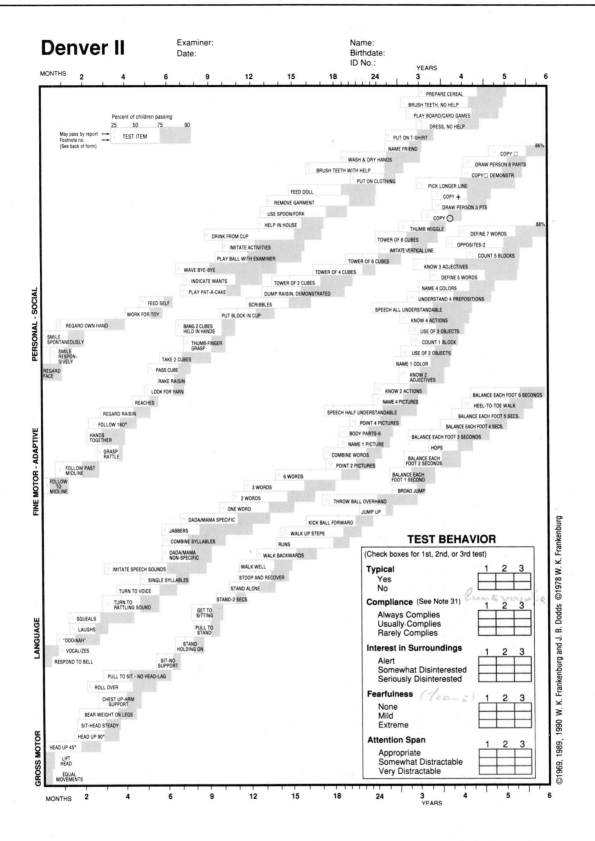

Denver II

Examiner:
Date:

Name:
Birthdate:
ID No.:

DIRECTIONS FOR ADMINISTRATION

1. Try to get child to smile by smiling, talking or waving. Do not touch him/her.
2. Child must stare at hand several seconds.
3. Parent may help guide toothbrush and put toothpaste on brush.
4. Child does not have to be able to tie shoes or button/zip in the back.
5. Move yarn slowly in an arc from one side to the other, about 8" above child's face.
6. Pass if child grasps rattle when it is touched to the backs or tips of fingers.
7. Pass if child tries to see where yarn went. Yarn should be dropped quickly from sight from tester's hand without arm movement.
8. Child must transfer cube from hand to hand without help of body, mouth, or table.
9. Pass if child picks up raisin with any part of thumb and finger.
10. Line can vary only 30 degrees or less from tester's line.
11. Make a fist with thumb pointing upward and wiggle only the thumb. Pass if child imitates and does not move any fingers other than the thumb.

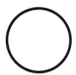   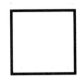

12. Pass any enclosed form. Fail continuous round motions.
13. Which line is longer? (Not bigger.) Turn paper upside down and repeat. (pass 3 of 3 or 5 of 6)
14. Pass any lines crossing near midpoint.
15. Have child copy first. If failed, demonstrate.

When giving items 12, 14, and 15, do not name the forms. Do not demonstrate 12 and 14.

16. When scoring, each pair (2 arms, 2 legs, etc.) counts as one part.
17. Place one cube in cup and shake gently near child's ear, but out of sight. Repeat for other ear.
18. Point to picture and have child name it. (No credit is given for sounds only.)
    If less than 4 pictures are named correctly, have child point to picture as each is named by tester.

 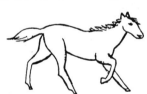 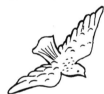 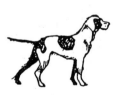 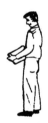

19. Using doll, tell child: Show me the nose, eyes, ears, mouth, hands, feet, tummy, hair. Pass 6 of 8.
20. Using pictures, ask child: Which one flies?... says meow?... talks?... barks?... gallops? Pass 2 of 5, 4 of 5.
21. Ask child: What do you do when you are cold?... tired?... hungry? Pass 2 of 3, 3 of 3.
22. Ask child: What do you do with a cup? What is a chair used for? What is a pencil used for?
    Action words must be included in answers.
23. Pass if child correctly places <u>and</u> says how many blocks are on paper. (1, 5).
24. Tell child: Put block **on** table; **under** table; **in front of** me, **behind** me. Pass 4 of 4.
    (Do not help child by pointing, moving head or eyes.)
25. Ask child: What is a ball?... lake?... desk?... house?... banana?... curtain?... fence?... ceiling? Pass if defined in terms of use, shape, what it is made of, or general category (such as banana is fruit, not just yellow). Pass 5 of 8, 7 of 8.
26. Ask child: If a horse is big, a mouse is __? If fire is hot, ice is __? If the sun shines during the day, the moon shines during the __? Pass 2 of 3.
27. Child may use wall or rail only, not person. May not crawl.
28. Child must throw ball overhand 3 feet to within arm's reach of tester.
29. Child must perform standing broad jump over width of test sheet (8 1/2 inches).
30. Tell child to walk forward, ⚬⚬⚬⚬⚬➔ heel within 1 inch of toe. Tester may demonstrate.
    Child must walk 4 consecutive steps.
31. In the second year, half of normal children are non-compliant.

OBSERVATIONS:

Instructions printed on the back of the DDST form (p. 571) for administering some of the items contained in the Denver Developmental Screening Test. (Reprinted with permission from William K. Frankenburg, M.D.)

Engage children in conversation appropriate to their ages and ask simple questions about their health or illness. Compliment them about their appearance, dress, or performance, tell a story, or play a simple trick to help "break the ice."

If children respond to conversation and questions directed to them by silence, shielding of the eyes, or apprehension, it is wise to ignore them temporarily.

Include in your observations during the interview a general assessment of the degree of sickness or wellness, mood, state of nutrition, speech, cry, respiratory pattern, facial expression, apparent chronologic and emotional age, posture (particularly as it may reflect discomfort), and developmental skills. In addition, closely observe the parent–child interaction, including the amount of separation tolerated, displays of affection, and response to discipline.

Specific developmental testing (such as building towers with blocks, playing ball with the examiner, and performing hop, skip, and jump maneuvers) is best accomplished at the end of the interview, just before the formal physical examination. This "fun and games" interlude is likely to improve the child's view of the examiner and enhance cooperation during the examination.

The actual performance of the physical examination, with certain exceptions, need not take place on the examining table. In fact, some parts of the examination can best be accomplished with the child standing, sitting on the parent's lap, or even sitting on the examiner's lap. Also, it is not essential that the child be completely undressed throughout the examination; often, exposing only the part of the body being examined will suffice and most likely avert objection by the child. Occasionally, a child is reluctant to undress because the examining room is cool and the examining table and instruments (including the examiner's hands) are cold, rather than because of apprehension or modesty. When two or more siblings are to be examined, it is wise to begin with the oldest, who is most likely to cooperate and set a good example for the younger children.

Actually, only a few children resist undressing. Most will allow themselves to be stripped to their underpants and placed, sitting, on the examining table without objection.

During the examination, ask the parent to stand at the head of the examining table, to the right of the child and to your left as you face the examining table. As with infants, distraction is the key to gaining

This dialogue will indicate the child's level of receptive and expressive function and will direct the approach by the examiner.

Abusing parents often pay little or no attention to their abused child, treating him or her more like a piece of property than a person. By the same token, an abused child usually demonstrates no separation anxiety when physically and environmentally removed from the parents. On the other hand, both child and parents may appear overaffectionate to one another in an attempt to hide the abuse.

the patient's cooperation. The child in this age group, however, is not as easily distracted as the infant; therefore, approach the patient pleasantly and, whenever possible, explain each step of the examination before performing it. Demonstrate the procedure on yourself or on a doll or toy animal. This also helps the child understand what is to be done. For example, you can place the otoscope in your ear, flash the light into your open mouth, or place the stethoscope on your chest. Allow the child to play with the examining instruments to create an atmosphere of trust. Play at blowing out the examining light or use the stethoscope bell as a telephone to create attractive diversions.

The initial ''laying on of the hands'' is the most crucial point of the examination; if resistance is encountered, it will most likely be at this point. Therefore, the first contact should be in nonvulnerable areas.

Hold the patient's hand, count the fingers, and palpate the wrist and elbow while talking gently to place the patient at ease.

Having both of the examiner's hands in contact with the patient's body whenever possible has a comforting effect on the patient and is less apt to produce involuntary withdrawal than is the use of one hand or a few probing fingers.

For example, when examining the heart, place your left hand on the patient's right shoulder while your right hand, holding the stethoscope, makes contact with the chest wall.

In a sense, the left hand acts as both a distracting and a comforting force. The examiner who moves unhesitatingly, firmly, and gracefully, and who talks pleasantly and reassuringly throughout the examination is not apt to provoke apprehension.

Use a firm voice and unequivocal instructions when asking a child to perform an act pertaining to the examination. Tell the child what to do rather than asking the child to do it. For example, say "Roll over on your belly" rather than "Will you roll over on your belly for me?"

Some children stop resisting when spoken to sharply, but most increase their resistance. Often they will sit or lie passively on the examining table covering both eyes with their hands, because they think the examiner cannot see them if they cannot see the examiner. This posture can be tolerated, because it does not interfere with the examination. The eyes can easily be examined after the child has dressed.

Base the order of your examination on performing the least distressing procedures first and the most distressing last. Thus, perform those parts of the examination that can be accomplished while the child is sitting—for example, palpation, percussion, and auscultation of the

heart and lungs—before the child lies down. Since lying down may make the child feel more vulnerable and resist further examination, accomplish this with great care. Often you can avert apprehension by supporting the head and back with your arm while the child lies down. Once the child is supine, examine the abdomen first, the throat and ears next to last, and the genitalia and rectum last. Examination of the genitalia and perineum, when a rectal examination is not performed, is usually less disturbing to the child than is the examination of the throat. However, in light of the fastidious and perhaps modest nature of some parents, leave these portions of the examination to last.

The child's comfort should be paramount in conducting the examination. Immediately before an examination maneuver the child should be told kindly, but matter-of-factly, of the likelihood of pain or other unpleasant sensations that might result. In instances when the child is extremely apprehensive about one portion of the examination (*e.g.*, the examination of the throat), it is helpful to do this first. Indeed, to ensure a reasonable interview, it may be necessary to complete the entire physical examination before obtaining the history. Distasteful portions of the examination should be accomplished quickly to minimize the child's discomfort. The examiner should remember, however, that the physical examination is designed to gather essential information and that the child's comfort may need to be sacrificed somewhat to achieve this end. A completed examination is a comfort and reassurance to the parent and examiner; an incomplete examination is a frustration and a source of dissatisfaction to both.

Obviously there will be resistance to the examination at times. Some children will scream throughout the examination but offer no physical resistance. Most, however, will fight the examination and strive to gain an upright position and the comfort and security of a parent's arms. Parents can be helpful here in orally reassuring children and in actually restraining their movements for certain parts of the examination. It is sometimes necessary to ask a parent who is overly sympathetic and ineffective in calming the child to leave the room. Surprisingly, the parent may be happy to leave; if the request to leave is refused, however, the examiner should obtain the assistance of a neutral person to help restrain the child, and make the best of it.

Rarely, for the child's sake or the parent's, it is necessary to discontinue the examination before it is completed and return to it another time.

Using another person, in addition to the parent, to restrain the child is often helpful under ordinary circumstances; however, using other kinds of restraints or mummying methods has no place in the physical examination procedure.

The examiner should not convey feelings of frustration or anger, but should reassure the parent that the child's resistance is usual. Embarrassment may cause the parent to compound the problem by scolding the child. Some parents feel that the examiner is at fault when their child is uncooperative while being examined. Others feel that such resistance is a reflection of the child's level of independence.

Neophyte examiners are apt to be less successful in examining very young children than in examining older ones. However, with practice, perseverance, and patience they should succeed. It is difficult to teach "how to approach a reluctant child." Examiners must learn which techniques work best for them as individuals and which approach they find most comfortable.

Late Childhood

There is usually little difficulty in examining most children after they reach school age. Some, however, may have unpleasant memories of previous encounters with examiners and offer resistance.

Question children to determine their orientation to time and place, their knowledge, and their language and number skills. Use intelligence screening tests, such as the Goodenough draw-a-man, the Durrell, and the Bender, when there is some element of doubt concerning the child's intellectual capacity. Keep these tests to a minimum, however, to avoid errors due to familiarity with their content, should formal psychological testing be necessary. Observe motor skills involved in writing, tying shoelaces, buttoning shirt fronts, and using scissors, and determine right–left discrimination for self (attained at age 6 or 7 years) and for others (attained at age 8 or 9 years).

A child's modesty may be the greatest deterrent to a successful examination. Therefore girls, as early as age 6 or 7, should be gowned. For both boys and girls, leave underpants on until their removal is required, even if the lower half of the body is draped. It is usually wise for examiners who are of the opposite sex from their preadolescent and adolescent patients to leave the room while the patient disrobes. Younger children often request that siblings of the opposite sex depart, and older boys frequently prefer that their mothers leave during the examination.

The order of examination in late childhood can follow that used with adults. At any age it is important, however, to withhold examination of painful areas until last.

THE GENERAL SURVEY

Observing infants and children carefully over time is extremely rewarding, as is noting general physical and behavioral signs. This section covers the measurement of vital signs and body size, which is particularly important in infants and children because deviations from the normal are apt to be the first and only indicators of disease.

TEMPERATURE

For infants and children younger than 7 years, rectal temperatures should be used almost exclusively because accurate oral temperature readings are difficult to obtain. For premature infants, axillary temperatures are satisfactory for close monitoring of temperature regulation, although electronic thermometers for continuous temperature recordings are used in neonatal intensive care units. Otherwise, electronic thermometers are rarely used with infants and children because of the expense and fragility of the instruments. Temperature recordings should be obtained in any situation in which an infectious, collagen vascular, or malignant disease is suspected. For patients in whom no disease is suspected (*e.g.*, for well-child visits) it is not necessary to determine the body temperature.

The technique of obtaining the rectal temperature is relatively simple. Place the infant or child prone on the examining table, on the parent's lap, or on your own lap. While you separate the buttocks with the thumb and forefinger of one hand, with the other hand gently insert a well lubricated rectal thermometer (inclined approximately 20° from the table or lap) through the anal sphincter approximately 1 inch into the rectum. One method for holding a child while obtaining the rectal temperature is demonstrated in the illustration on the right.

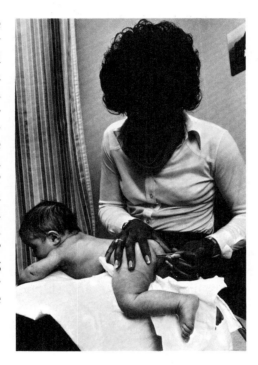

Body temperature in infants and children is less constant than that in adults. The average rectal temperature is higher in infancy and early childhood, usually not falling below 99.0°F (37.2°C) until after the third year. At 18 months 50% of children have mean rectal temperatures of 100°F (37.8°C) or higher. Ranges in body temperature of children may be as much as 3 or more degrees Fahrenheit during the course of a single day. Rectal temperature recordings may approach 101°F (38.3°C) in normal children, particularly in late afternoon after a full day of activity.

Anxiety may elevate the body temperature, as demonstrated by the frequency with which elevated temperatures are found in children on elective hospital admission.

In overwhelming infection, an infant's temperature may be normal or subnormal. On the other hand, during early childhood extremely high temperature recordings (103° to 105°F, 39.5° to 40.5°C) are common, even with minor infections.

PULSE

The heart rate in infants and children is quite labile and more sensitive to the effects of illness, exercise, and emotion than that in adults. The average heart rates for pediatric patients, according to age, are shown in Table 19-2.

Obtain the heart rate in infants by observing the pulsations of the anterior fontanelle, by palpating the carotid or the femoral arteries, or by directly auscultating the heart if the rate is very rapid. Palpate the radial artery at the wrist in older children and in young children who are cooperative.

Beyond the neonatal period a pulse greater than 180 usually indicates *paroxysmal auricular tachycardia.*

Table 19-2   Average Heart Rate of Infants and Children at Rest

AGE	AVERAGE RATE	TWO STANDARD DEVIATIONS
Birth	140	50
1st 6 months	130	50
6–12 months	115	40
1–2 years	110	40
2–6 years	103	35
6–10 years	95	30
10–14 years	85	30

RESPIRATORY RATE

As with the heart rate, the respiratory rate in infants and children has a greater range and is more responsive to illness, exercise, and emotion than that in adults. The rate of respirations per minute ranges between 30 and 80 in the newborn, 20 and 40 during early childhood, and 15 and 25 during late childhood, reaching adult levels at age 15 years.

Respiratory rates that exceed 100 per minute are seen in diseases associated with lower respiratory tract obstruction (for example, *bronchiolitis* and *bronchial asthma*).

The respiratory rate may vary appreciably from moment to moment in premature and full-term newborn infants, with periods of rapid breathing alternating with spells of apnea. The respiratory pattern in these circumstances should therefore be observed for more than the usual 30 to 60 seconds to determine the true rate.

Apnea of greater than 20 seconds in duration can occur in both premature infants and seemingly healthy newborns. These infants may be at risk for *Sudden Infant Death Syndrome (SIDS).*

In infancy and early childhood, diaphragmatic breathing is predominant and thoracic excursion is minimal; therefore, you can more easily ascertain the respiratory rate by observing abdominal rather than chest excursions. Auscultation of the chest and placement of the stethoscope in front of the mouth and external nares are also useful for counting respirations in this age group. In older children, observe the thoracic movement directly or palpate the thorax to determine the respiratory rate.

BLOOD PRESSURE

Measuring the blood pressure in infants and children is often omitted because it has erroneously been judged to be too difficult to obtain from an active child. When the procedure is explained and demonstrated beforehand, however, most children 3 years of age and older are fascinated by the sphygmomanometer and are very cooperative. Obtaining the blood pressure measurement should be part of the physical examination of every child of this age and of any infant or toddler whose history or physical examination suggests that the blood pressure may be high or low (rare).

Elevations of blood pressure levels in normal individuals occur due to exercise, crying, and emotional upset. Because children may be anxious about the entire physical examination as well as the blood pressure procedure *per se*, some clinicians prefer to obtain the blood pressure near the end of the examination. Others repeat the determination at the end of the formal examination if the initial pressure was high.

Anxiety may produce elevated systolic blood pressure readings.

Use the sphygmomanometer to determine blood pressures in children as you would in adults. The inflatable rubber bag cuff should be long enough to encircle the upper arm or the leg completely, with or without overlap. It should be wide enough to cover approximately 75% of the upper arm or the leg. A narrower cuff elevates the pressure reading, while a wider cuff lowers it and interferes with proper placement of the stethoscope's bell over the artery as it traverses the antecubital space or the popliteal space.

With children, unlike adults, the point at which the sounds first become muffled (not the disappearance point) is recorded as the diastolic pressure. At times, especially in early childhood, the Korotkoff sounds are not audible due to a narrow or deeply placed brachial artery; in such instances, palpate the radial artery at the wrist to determine the blood pressure. The point at which the pulse is first felt is recorded as the systolic pressure. This is approximately 10 mm Hg lower than the systolic pressure determined by auscultation. The diastolic pressure cannot be determined by using the radial pulse method.

In infants and very young children, small extremities and lack of cooperation preclude the use of auscultatory and palpation techniques to determine the blood pressure. However, a value lying somewhere between the systolic and diastolic pressures can be obtained by using the *flush technique*.

With the cuff in place, wrap an elastic bandage snugly around the elevated arm, proceeding from the fingers to the antecubital space. This essentially empties the capillary and venous network. Inflate the cuff to a pressure above the expected systolic reading, remove the bandage, and place the pallid arm at the patient's side. Allow the cuff

pressure to fall slowly until the sudden flush of normal color returns to the forearm, hand, and fingers. The endpoint is strikingly clear. This method may also be used in the leg.

A more accurate measure of the systolic blood pressure of infants and very young children is obtained with an electronic sphygmomanometer (Doppler), which senses arterial blood flow vibrations, converts them to systolic blood pressure levels, and transmits them to a digital read-out device. Purchase and maintenance costs limit their use to neonatal and pediatric intensive care units and cardiac diagnostic centers.

The level of systolic blood pressure increases gradually throughout infancy and childhood. Measured in mm Hg, normal systolic pressure in males is in the vicinity of 70 mm Hg at birth, 85 at 1 month, 90 at 6 months, 95 at 5 years, 100 at 8 years, 110 at 13 years, and 120 at 18 years. The diastolic pressure reaches about 55 mm Hg at 1 year of age and gradually increases throughout childhood and adolescence to approximately 70 mm Hg at age 18. Normal systolic and diastolic pressures in females are approximately 5 mm Hg lower than those in males at all these age levels.

The 1987 Task Force on Blood Pressure Control in Children defined *Normal Blood Pressure* as systolic and diastolic BPs < 90th percentile for age and sex; *High Normal Blood Pressure* as average systolic and/or average diastolic BPs between the 90th and 95th percentiles for age and sex;

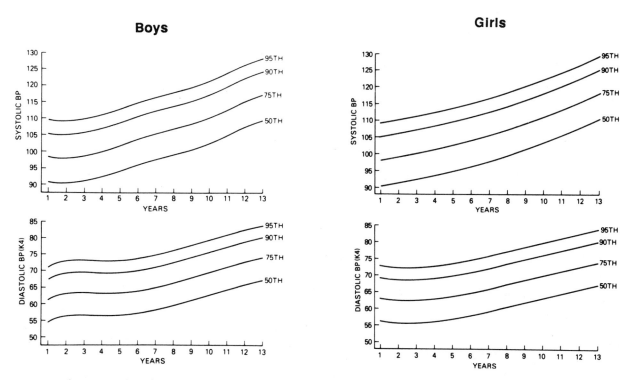

Age-specific percentiles of BP measurements in boys and girls 1 to 13 years of age. K4 = Korotkoff phase IV sound (low-pitched and muffled). (From the Second Task Force on Blood Pressure Control in Children of the National Heart, Lung, and Blood Institute. Pediatrics [Suppl] 79:1–25, 1987. Reproduced with permission.)

and *High Blood Pressure* (hypertension) as average systolic and/or diastolic BPs ≥ 95th percentile for age and sex with measurements obtained on at least three occasions. The figures on p. 580 provide the age-specific percentiles needed to make these assessments.

Children who have hypertension should be evaluated extensively to determine its cause. For infants and young children, a specific cause can usually be found. In older children and adolescents, however, the etiology may be obscure, and in many instances observed elevated blood pressure may be a developmental phenomenon that disappears over time.

Renal disease (78%), renal arterial disease (12%), coarctation of the aorta (2%), and pheochromocytoma are the most common causes of hypertension during infancy and early childhood. Primary hypertension becomes increasingly prevalent beyond age 6 years.

SOMATIC GROWTH

Growth, reflected in increases in body weight and length along expected pathways and within certain limits, is probably the best indicator of health (see pp. 563–564). The significance of any measure is determined by relating it to prior measurements of the same dimension, to mean values and standard deviations for that dimension as they occur in other individuals, and to measures of other dimensions in the same patient. Measures of somatic growth in infants and children, therefore, should be plotted on standard growth charts so that those comparisons can be made.

Measurements of height and weight above the 97th percentile or below the 3rd percentile on standard growth charts may indicate a growth disturbance and require investigation.

HEIGHT. **Measure the body length of infants by placing them supine on a measuring board or in a measuring tray, as illustrated below. If these are not available, measure the distance between marks made on**

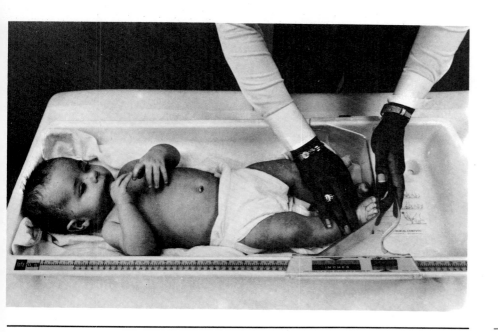

the examining table paper indicating the crown and the heel of the infant. Direct measurement of the infant in this way or with a tape is inaccurate, unless an assistant holds the baby still with its legs extended. Measure the height in older children by standing the child with heels, back, and head against a wall marked with a centimeter or inch rule. Hold a small board flat against the top of the child's head and at right angles to the rule to complete the measure.

Weighing scales equipped with a height measure are not as satisfactory because children are less likely to stand erect when not against a wall; many younger children also fear standing on a scale's slightly raised, unsteady base.

WEIGHT. **Weigh infants directly with an infant scale, rather than indirectly by holding them while you stand on the scale and subtracting your weight from the total weight registered. Remove all clothing, except for underpants in children beyond infancy and dressing gowns provided for girls in late childhood. Use balance rather than spring scales, and whenever possible weigh the child on the same scale at each visit.**

HEAD CIRCUMFERENCE. The head circumference should be determined at every physical examination during the first 2 years of life, at least biennially thereafter, and at any *initial* examination at whatever age, to determine the rate of growth and the absolute growth of the head.

A cloth or soft plastic centimeter tape is preferred for this procedure, but disposable paper tapes are satisfactory.

Place the tape over the occipital, parietal, and frontal prominences to obtain the greatest circumference. During infancy and early childhood this is done best with the patient supine.

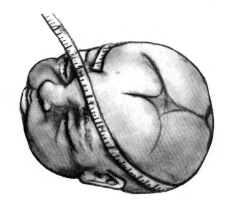

The head circumference reflects the rate of growth of the cranium and its contents.

If growth is delayed, *premature closure of the sutures* or *microcephaly* should be considered.

Measurements of chest circumference and the abdominal circumference are, in general, inaccurate and have no clinical use.

THE SKIN

Infancy

The newborn infant's skin has many unique characteristics. The texture is soft and smooth. In white infants an erythematous flush, giving the entire surface of the skin the appearance of a "boiled lobster," is present during the first 8 to 24 hours, after which the normal pale pink coloring predominates. Vasomotor changes in the dermis and subcutaneous tissue—a response to cooling or chronic exposure to radiant heat—produce a mottled appearance (*cutis marmorata*), particularly on the trunk, arms, and legs. In normal newborns a striking color change is often seen: one side of the body is red, the other pale, and an abrupt border separates the two sides at the midline. This phenomenon (*harlequin dyschromia*) is transient and its etiology unknown. The hands and feet are "blue" (*acrocyanosis*) at birth and may remain so for several days. This may recur throughout early infancy under chilling conditions. After 4 or 5 hours the cyanosis in the hands becomes less marked than in the feet.

Melanotic pigmentation of the skin is not intense in most black newborns, except in the nailbeds and the skin of the scrotum. Ill-defined blackish blue areas located over the buttocks and lower lumbar regions are often seen, especially in black, Native American, and Oriental babies. These areas, called *Mongolian spots,* are due to the presence of pigmented cells in the deeper layers of the skin. The spots become less noticeable as the pigment in the overlying cells becomes more prominent, and they eventually disappear in early childhood.

There is a fine, downy growth of hair called *lanugo* over the entire body, but mostly on the shoulders and back. The amount and length vary from baby to baby, and are unusually prominent in prematures. Most of this hair is shed within 2 weeks. The amount of hair on the head of a newborn varies considerably, being absent entirely in some and abundant in others. All the original hair is shed within a few months and replaced with a new crop, sometimes of a different color.

Desquamation of the skin is often present at birth, varying in degree from a scattered flakiness to complete shedding of entire areas in large sheets of cornified epidermis. Also, a cheesy white material, composed of sebum and desquamated epithelial cells and called *vernix caseosa,* covers the body in varying degrees at birth. It is always present in the vaginal

Generalized pallor indicates either anoxia, in which the pulse will be slowed, or severe anemia, in which the pulse will be very rapid.

This marbled, or dappled, reticular pattern is especially prominent in premature infants and *cretins* (congenital hypothyroidism) and in infants with *Down's syndrome.*

If acrocyanosis does not disappear within 8 hours, cyanotic congenital heart disease should be considered.

labial folds and under the fingernails. A certain amount of puffiness and edema, even to the point of pitting over the hands, feet, lower legs, pubis, and sacrum, may be present but usually disappears by the second or third day.

Normal "physiologic" jaundice, which occurs in approximately 50% of all babies, appears on the second or third day and usually disappears within a week, but may persist for as long as a month.

Use natural daylight rather than artificial light when evaluating for the presence of jaundice at any age. In borderline cases, press a glass slide against the infant's cheek to help you detect the presence of jaundice by producing a blanched background for contrast.

Older infants who are fed yellow vegetables (carrots, sweet potatoes, and squash) may develop a pale, yellow orange color that is sometimes mistaken for jaundice. However, the pigmentation in this condition, called *carotenemia*, is limited to the palms, soles, nose, and nasolabial folds. The conjunctivas are not involved.

Three dermatologic conditions are seen in newborns often enough to deserve description. None is of clinical significance. *Milia*, pinhead-sized, smooth, white, raised areas without surrounding erythema, on the nose, chin, and forehead, are caused by retention of sebum in the openings of the sebaceous glands. Milia may be present at birth but more often appear within the first few weeks of life and disappear spontaneously over several weeks. *Miliaria rubra* consists of scattered vesicles on an erythematous base, usually on the face and the trunk, caused by sweat gland duct obstruction. This rash also disappears spontaneously within 1 to 2 weeks. *Erythema toxicum*, which usually appears on the second or third day of life, consists of erythematous macules with central urticarial wheals or vesicles scattered diffusely over the entire body, appearing much like flea bites. The cause is unknown and the lesions disappear spontaneously within a week.

Irregular reddened areas frequently are found over the nape of the neck ("stork's beak" mark) and on the upper eyelids, the forehead, and the upper lip ("angel kisses"). This redness is due to proliferation of the skin's capillary bed, and is variously called *capillary hemangioma, nevus flammeus, nevus vasculosus,* and *telangiectatic nevus.* The lesions invariably disappear at about a year of age, although they may occasionally reappear, even in adulthood, when the skin is flushed from anger or embarrassment. Such lesions appearing on other areas of the skin are larger, darker (purplish), more sharply demarcated, and may involve the mucosa of the mouth or the vagina. These "port-wine stains" are not likely to fade.

In general, jaundice that appears within 24 hours of birth should alert one to the possible presence of hemolytic disease; jaundice that persists beyond 2 weeks of age should raise suspicions of biliary obstruction. Jaundice may indicate severe infection at any time in infancy, particularly in the newborn.

When a port wine stain affects the skin innervated by the ophthalmic portion of the trigeminal nerve, the vascular network of the meninges and ocular orbit may also be affected. This can result in seizures, hemiparesis, mental retardation, and glaucoma—the *Sturge–Weber syndrome.*

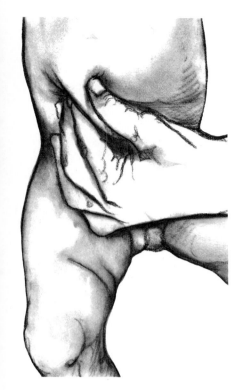

The examination of the skin should go beyond observation and include palpation.

Roll a fold of loosely adherent skin on the abdominal wall between your thumb and forefinger to determine its consistency, the amount of subcutaneous tissue, and the degree of hydration.

The skin in well-hydrated infants and children returns to its normal position immediately upon release.

Delay in return, a phenomenon called *tenting*, usually occurs in dehydrated patients.

Early and Late Childhood

The normal child's skin beyond the first year does not vary significantly. The techniques of examination and the general classification of pathologic lesions for this age are as with the adult.

THE HEAD AND NECK

Infancy

The *head* accounts for one fourth of the body length and one third of the body weight at birth, whereas at full maturity it only accounts for one eighth of the body length and, for most, one tenth of the body weight. The bones of the skull are separated from one another by membranous tissue spaces called *sutures*. The areas where the major sutures intersect in the anterior and posterior portions of the skull are known as *fontanelles*. The sutures and fontanelles, shown in this figure, form the basis for much of the physical assessment of the infant's head.

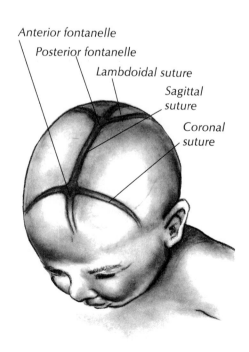

Anterior fontanelle
Posterior fontanelle
Lambdoidal suture
Sagittal suture
Coronal suture

The sutures feel like slightly depressed ridges and the fontanelles like soft concavities. The anterior fontanelle at birth measures 4 cm to 6 cm in its largest diameter and normally closes between 4 and 26 months of age; 90% close between 7 and 19 months. The posterior fontanelle measures 1 cm to 2 cm at birth and usually closes by 2 months of age. The intracranial pressure is reflected in the amount of tenseness and fullness seen and felt in the anterior fontanelle. Increased intracranial pressure produces a bulging, full anterior fontanelle. This is normally seen when a baby cries, coughs, or vomits. Pulsations of the fontanelle reflect the peripheral pulse.

Increased intracranial pressure is found in infectious and neoplastic diseases of the central nervous system and with obstruction to the circulation of cerebrospinal fluid within the ventricles of the brain. Decreased intracranial pressure, reflected in a depressed fontanelle, is a sign of dehydration in infants.

For best results examine the anterior fontanelle for tenseness and fullness while the baby is sitting quietly or being held upright.

The anterior fontanelle is such an important indicator of high or low intracranial pressure and of serious disease of the central nervous system that seasoned clinicians palpate it before doing any other part of the physical examination on an acutely ill baby.

Dilated scalp veins are indicative of long-standing increased intracranial pressure.

The newborn infant's cranial bones may overlap at the sutures to a certain degree. This phenomenon, called *molding*, results from passage of the head through the birth canal and disappears within 2 days. It is not seen in babies born by cesarean section.

A newborn baby's scalp often is swollen from edema and bruising over the occipitoparietal region. This is the *caput succedaneum*, caused by the drawing of that portion of the scalp into the cervical os when the amniotic sac ruptures. The negative pressure or vacuum effect caused by the loss of amniotic fluid produces distended capillaries with local extravasation of blood and fluid. These findings subside within the first 24 hours of life.

A second type of localized swelling involving the scalp, the *cephalohematoma*, often is seen in newborns. (see Table 19-3, p. 589).

When examining the infant's head, ascertain the shape and symmetry of the skull and the face.

Asymmetry of the cranial vault (*plagiocephaly*) occurs when an infant lies constantly on one side. Such positioning results in a flattening of the occiput on the dependent side and a prominence of the frontal region on the opposite side. It disappears as the baby becomes more active and spends less time in one position. In almost all instances, symmetry is restored when the position of the head becomes less constant. *In utero* positioning may result in transient facial asymmetries. If the head is flexed on the sternum, a shortened chin (*micrognathia*) may result; pressure of the shoulder on the jaw may create a temporary lateral displacement of the mandible.

Plagiocephaly is apt to be more prominent in infants with *torticollis* secondary to injury to the sternomastoid muscle at birth, in the mentally and physically handicapped, and in understimulated infants.

The premature infant's head at birth is relatively long in the occipitofrontal diameter and narrow in the bitemporal diameter. This relation-

The shape of the head may be altered by premature closure of

ship continues for most of the first year. An abnormally large head (*hydrocephaly*, see Table 19-3, p. 589, or *megacephaly*) and an abnormally small head (*microcephaly*) should be recognized easily, but either condition initially requires frequent observation, including measurements, for early diagnosis and treatment.

If, in palpating the newborn's skull, you press your thumb or forefinger too firmly over the temporoparietal or parieto-occipital areas, you may feel the underlying bone give momentarily, much as a ping-pong ball responds to similar pressure.

This condition, known as *craniotabes,* is due to osteoporosis of the outer table of the involved membranous bone. It may be found in some normal infants. Purposeful elicitation of this finding is not recommended.

Percuss the parietal bone on each side by tapping your index or middle finger directly against its surface.

This will produce a "cracked-pot" sound (*Macewen's sign*) in normal infants prior to closure of their cranial sutures.

Percuss at the top of the cheek just below the zygomatic bone in front of the ear, using the tip of your index or middle finger.

One or two contractions of the facial muscles in response to percussion are present in many newborn infants and can persist normally throughout infancy and early childhood (*Chvostek's sign*).

Transillumination of the skull is useful and should be part of every initial examination of an infant.

In a completely darkened room place a standard three-battery flashlight, with a soft rubber collar attached to the lighted end, flush against the skull at various points (see Table 19-3, p. 589). In normal infants a 2-cm halo of light is present around the circumference of the flashlight when it is placed over the frontoparietal area, and a 1-cm halo is present when the flashlight is placed over the occipital area.

one or more of the cranial sutures (*craniosynostosis*). The nature of the resultant skull deformity depends on the sutures involved. Although palpation of affected sutures may reveal a raised bony ridge in the final stages, early diagnosis is made by a roentgenogram.

Craniotabes may result from increased intracranial pressure, as in *hydrocephaly*, from metabolic disturbances such as *rickets*, and from infection such as *congenital syphilis.*

Macewen's sign can be elicited in older infants and children who have increased intracranial pressure that causes closed cranial sutures to separate, *e.g.*, in *lead encephalopathy* and *brain tumor.*

Chvostek's sign is quite striking, and its elicitation may produce repeated contractions of the facial muscle in *hypocalcemic tetany* and *tetanus* (newborns and older children) and *tetany due to hyperventilation* (children and adolescents).

Uniform transillumination of the entire head occurs when the cerebral cortex is partially absent or thinned. Localized bright spots may be seen with *subdural effusion* and *porencephalic cysts.*

Routine auscultation of the skull to detect the presence of a *bruit* is of little use until late childhood because a systolic or continuous bruit may be heard over the temporal areas in normal children until the age of 5. Similar findings may be found in older children who are significantly anemic.

The *neck* of the newborn is relatively short.

While the infant is supine, palpate the neck with your thumb and forefinger, feeling for masses, lymph nodes, cysts, and the position of the thyroid cartilage and the trachea. Move the head through its full range of motion at the neck (extension, flexion, lateral bending, and rotation 90° to the left and right). Palpate the clavicles for evidence of a fracture (shortening, break in contour, and crepitus at the fracture site).

The neck is supple and easily mobile in all directions throughout infancy. Its musculature is not sufficiently developed to enable the infant to turn its head from side to side until 2 weeks of age, to lift its head 90° when lying prone until 2 months of age, or to hold its head upright when sitting until 3 months of age.

Bruits heard in nonanemic older children suggest increased intracranial pressure or an intracranial arteriovenous shunt or aneurysm.

A *thyroglossal duct fistula* or *cyst* may be seen or felt in the midline immediately superior to the thyroid cartilage. Thyroglossal duct cysts are rarely found at birth but may appear in early infancy. They are usually small, rounded, and firm, and can be differentiated from midline subcutaneous lesions in that they move with swallowing.

Cervical lymphadenopathy is not seen often during infancy. When it is, the cause is usually due to viral or bacterial infection.

Remnants of the three lower branchial clefts may be seen as skin tags, cysts, or fistulas along the anterior border of the sternomastoid muscle.

Injury to the sternomastoid muscle with bleeding into the muscle as it is stretched during the birth process results in wry neck (*torticollis*). The head is tilted and twisted toward the injured side, and in 2 or 3 weeks a firm fibrous mass is felt within the muscle. This ordinarily disappears in 3 to 4 months and rarely requires excision.

Table 19-3 Abnormal Enlargement of the Head in Infancy

Table 19-3   Abnormal Enlargement of the Head in Infancy

CEPHALOHEMATOMA

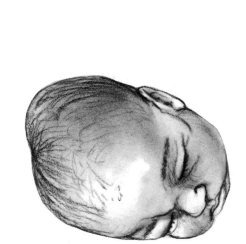

Although not present at birth, cephalohematomas appear within the first 24 hours and are due to subperiosteal hemorrhage involving the outer table of one of the cranial bones. The swelling (see illustration above, which shows a cephalohematoma overlying the left parietal bone), unlike the caput succedaneum and hematomas associated with skull fractures, does not extend across a suture. It may be small and well localized or may involve the entire bone. Occasionally, bilateral symmetrical swellings occur after difficult deliveries. Although initially soft, the swellings develop a raised bony margin within 2 to 3 days, due to the rapid deposition of calcium at the edges of the elevated periosteum. The entire process usually disappears within a few weeks, but may remain as a residual osteoma that is not resorbed for a year or two.

HYDROCEPHALY

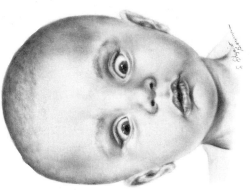

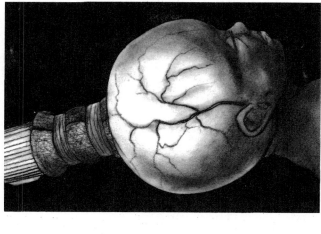

In hydrocephaly, the eyes are deviated downward, revealing the upper scleras and creating the *"setting sun"* sign as shown in the figure above. The setting sun sign is also seen briefly in some normal newborns. (Redrawn from Paine RS: Neurological examination of infants and children. Pediatr Clin North Am 7:476, 1960)

Transillumination of the skull in advanced cases of hydrocephaly produces a glow of light over the entire cranium, as illustrated above.

Table 19-4   Diagnostic Facies in Childhood

Table 19-4   *Diagnostic Facies in Childhood*

FETAL ALCOHOL SYNDROME	CONGENITAL SYPHILIS	CRETINISM	FACIAL NERVE PALSY
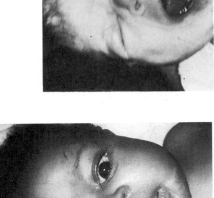	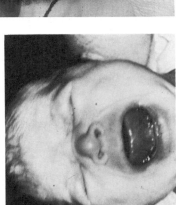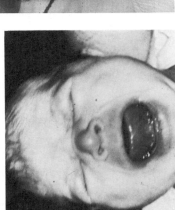	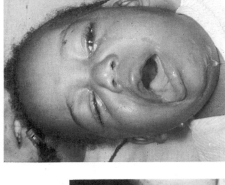	

FETAL ALCOHOL SYNDROME

Babies born to women who are chronic alcoholics are at increased risk for growth deficiency, microcephaly, and mental retardation. Facial characteristics shown here include short palpebral fissures, a wide and flattened philtrum (the space between the external nares and the upper lip's vermilion border), and thin lips. (Illustration reproduced with permission from Clark DA, Thompson JE: Pathology of the Neonate. Philadelphia, Wyeth Laboratories, 1986)

CONGENITAL SYPHILIS

In utero infection by *Treponema pallidum* usually occurs after the 16th week of gestation and affects virtually all fetal organs. If it is not treated, 25% of infected babies will die before birth and another 30% shortly thereafter. Signs of illness appear in survivors within the first month of life. Facial stigmata shown here include bulging of the frontal bones and nasal bridge depression (saddle nose), both due to periostitis; rhinitis from weeping nasal mucosal lesions; and a circumoral rash. Mucocutaneous inflammation and fissuring of the mouth and lips (rhagades), not shown here, may also occur as stigmata of congenital syphilis, as may tibial periostitis (saber shins) and dental dysplasia (Hutchinson's teeth—see Table 7-19, p. 226).

CRETINISM

The child with cretinism (congenital hypothyroidism) has coarse facial features, a low-set hair line, sparse eyebrows, and an enlarged tongue. Associated features include a hoarse cry, umbilical hernia, dry and cold extremities, myxedema, mottled skin, and mental retardation. (A black-and-white print of a color photograph, reproduced with permission from Gellis S, Feingold M: Syndromes in Pediatrics, Part I. In Famous Teachings in Modern Medicine. Medcom, Inc, 1969)

FACIAL NERVE PALSY

Peripheral (lower motor neuron) paralysis of the facial nerve may occur due to (1) an injury to the nerve from pressure over the stylomastoid foramen during labor and delivery, (2) inflammation during episodes of acute or chronic otitis media of the portion of the nerve that traverses the middle ear, or (3) unknown causes (Bell's palsy). See page 518 and Table 18-2, Types of Facial Paralysis (pp. 550–551). The nasolabial fold on the affected side is flattened and the eye does not close. This is accentuated during crying, as shown here. Full recovery occurs in ≥90% of those affected, usually within a few weeks.

Table 19-4   *Diagnostic Facies in Childhood*

HYPERTHYROIDISM

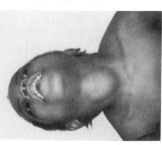
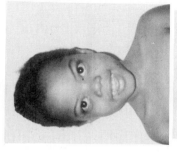

Thyrotoxicosis (Graves' disease) occurs in approximately 2 per 1,000 children under the age of 10 years. Affected children exhibit hypermetabolism and accelerated linear growth. Facial characteristics shown in this 6-year-old girl are "staring" eyes (not true exophthalmos, which is rare in children) and an enlarged thyroid gland (goiter). See Table 7-22 (p. 229).

PERENNIAL ALLERGIC RHINITIS

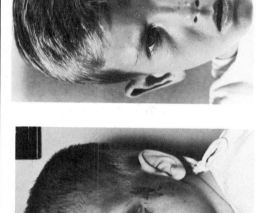

The child suffering from perennial allergic rhinitis has an open mouth (cannot breath through the nose) and edema and discoloration of the lower orbitopalpebral grooves ("allergic shiners"). Such a child is often seen to push the nose upward and backward with a hand ("allergic salute") and to grimace (wrinkle the nose and mouth) to relieve nasal itching and obstruction. (Illustration reproduced with permission from Marks MB: Allergic shiners: Dark circles under the eyes in children. Clin Pediatr 5:656, 1966).

BATTERED-CHILD SYNDROME

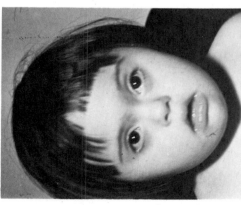

The child who has been physically abused (battered) usually has old *and* fresh bruises about the head and face and may either look sad and forlorn or be actively seeking to please, sometimes even particularly involved with and attentive to the abusing parent. Other stigmata include: bruises in areas not usually subject to injury (axilla and groin); x-ray evidence of fractures of the skull, ribs, and long bones in various stages of healing; and skin lesions that are morphologically similar to implements used to inflict trauma (hand, belt buckle, strap, rope, coat hanger, or lighted cigarette).

DOWN'S SYNDROME

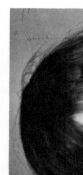

The child who has Down's syndrome (Trisomy 21) usually has a small, rounded head, a flattened nasal bridge, oblique palpebral fissures, prominent epicanthal folds, small, low-set, shell-like ears, and a relatively large tongue. Associated features include generalized hypotonia, transverse palmar creases (simian lines), shortening and incurving of the 5th fingers (clinodactyly), Brushfield's spots (see p. 596), and mental retardation. (A black-and-white print of a color photograph, reproduced with permission from Dynski–Klein M: Color Atlas of Pediatrics, p 309. London, Year Book Medical Publishers/Wolfe Medical Publications, 1975)

Early and Late Childhood

Beyond infancy the head and neck, except as previously mentioned, should be examined with the procedures used in examining the adult. There are diagnostic facies in childhood that reflect chromosomal abnormalities, endocrine defects, social disease, chronic illness, and other categories of disease (see Table 19-4, pp. 590–591 for examples).

A swollen parotid gland may be difficult to detect during the early stages of mumps.

With your index finger palpate along a line extending from the outer canthus of the eye to the lower tip of the pinna.

Inspect the orifice of the parotid (Stenson's) duct, which emerges from the midportion of the buccal mucosa.

Parotid swelling and tenderness strongly suggest *mumps*.

Tenderness is elicited when mumps is present.

Redness and swelling are usually present with mumps.

Parotid gland swelling, from any cause, extends above and below the mandible at the angle of the jaw; the swelling due to *cervical adenitis* occurs only below these landmarks.

The adult lymphatic system, including the lymph nodes, is described on pages 168–169 (head and neck), 326–327 (axillae and breasts), 370 (male genitalia), 387 (female genitalia), and 438–439 (arms and legs).

Cervical lymphadenopathy may occur in a variety of circumstances, including:

As shown in the figure on page 561, the child's lymphatic system reaches its zenith of growth at 12 years of age; the size of its various components (lymph nodes and the tonsils and adenoids, in particular) is greater between the ages of 6 and 20 years than at other ages. Parents and clinicians who are unaware of this may become unduly concerned that large and even not so large visible nodes, especially in the neck, may be malignant. However, most lymph nodes, cervical or otherwise, that are enlarged in children are either just "normally so" or are due to local infections (mostly viral) and not to malignant disease. This is particularly the case if the node is less than 2 cm in diameter, if it is not hard or fixed to the skin or underlying tissues, and, in the case of cervical lymph nodes, if the chest x-ray findings are normal. Concern regarding malignancy is raised when a supraclavicular lymph node is enlarged, when fever lasting more than a week without apparent cause accompanies the lymphadenopathy, and when there has been a weight loss of 5 pounds or more within the previous 6 months.

1. *Acute anterior cervical lymphadenitis* of bacterial origin, with or without preceding or concomitant acute tonsillitis or pharyngitis. The tonsillar lymph node on the affected side is most often involved and is very swollen and tender.

2. *Acute posterior cervical lymphadenitis* secondary to acute otitis externa, acute or chronic mastoiditis (rare), and scalp lesions (*pediculosis capitis, tinea capitis*)

3. *Infectious mononucleosis* caused by Epstein–Barr virus.

Generalized lymphadenopathy may occur, but the cervical lymph nodes are most prominently involved and may be quite large and tender.

4. *Kawasaki's disease* (mucocutaneous lymph node syndrome) of unknown cause. Again, generalized lymphadenopathy is usual when lymphadenopathy is present and the cervical lymph nodes are then likely to be involved to a marked or minimal degree.

5. Malignant disease, including *leukemia, Hodgkin's disease, non-Hodgkin's lymphoma*, and *metastatic cancer*, may appear with enlarged cervical lymph nodes or enlarged lymph nodes in other regions of the body.

Occipital lymphadenopathy may also occur with scalp lesions and is usually present with rubella.

Neck mobility is important when central nervous system diseases, especially meningitis, are considered, because the neck may be less supple than normal when such diseases are present.

With the child supine, cradle the head in your hands so that you provide complete support (p. 594). Move the head gently in all directions to determine any resistance to motion, especially to flexion. Normally, the head moves freely.

In infancy and early childhood, this is a more reliable test for nuchal rigidity and meningeal irritation than *Brudzinski's sign* or *Kernig's sign* (see pp. 542–543). The infant's neck may retain its mobility, even when meningeal irritation, as with meningitis, is present.

Nuchal rigidity, or marked resistance to movement of the head in any direction, suggests meningeal irritation, which may exist with central nervous system infections, bleeding, and tumors.

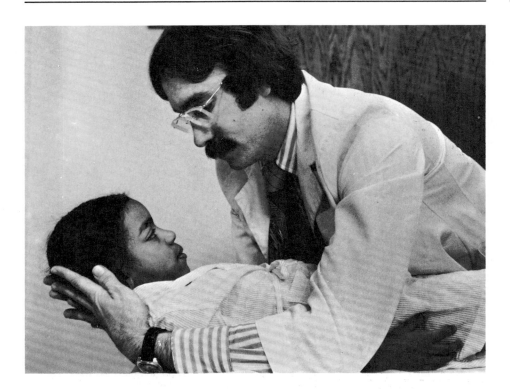

To detect nuchal rigidity in early and late childhood, ask the child to sit with legs extended on the examining table. Normally children should be able to sit upright and touch their chins to their chests. Younger children may be persuaded to flex their necks forward by getting them to look at a small toy or a light beam placed on their upper sternum.

When meningeal irritation is present, the child assumes the *tripod position* and is unable to assume a full upright position to perform the chin-to-chest maneuver.

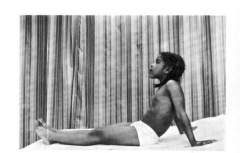

THE EYE

Infancy

It is somewhat difficult to examine the newborn's eyes because the lids are ordinarily held tightly closed. Attempts at separating the lids usually increase the contraction of the orbicularis oculi muscles. Because bright light causes infants to blink their eyes, the newborn's eyes should be examined in subdued lighting.

Hold the baby upright in your extended arms, fixing the head in the midline with your thumbs as illustrated on p. 595. Rotate yourself with the baby slowly in one direction. This usually causes the baby's eyes to open, providing a clear view of the scleras, pupils, irises, and

extraocular movements. The eyes look in the direction you are turning. When the rotation stops, the eyes look in the opposite direction, following a few unsustained nystagmoid movements.

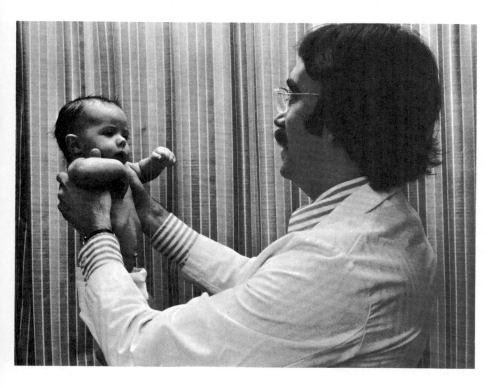

Conjugate eye movements develop rapidly after birth, but definitive following movements are not seen for a few weeks. Nystagmus in one or many directions is common immediately after birth. During the first 10 days of life the eyes remain fixed, staring in one direction as the head is moved slowly through the full range of motion (*doll's eye test*). Intermittent alternating convergent strabismus is frequently seen or reported by parents during the first 6 months of life.

Small subconjunctival, scleral, and retinal hemorrhages are common in newborns. Because pupillary reactivity to light is poor during the first 4 to 5 months, reactions are best observed by first shading one eye and then uncovering it. The *optical blink reflex*, wherein the infant blinks the eyes and extends the head in response to a bright light, is normally present in all newborns and may be used to test light perception. Inequality of pupil size in both bright and subdued light is common, but should be considered significant if constant over time and associated with other ocular or central nervous system findings. The corneal reflex is always present at birth.

Each iris should be inspected for the presence of a cleft (*coloboma*) and for *Brushfield's spots*. The latter appear as white specks, usually scattered around the entire circumference of the iris; although present in some normal infants, they strongly suggest *Down's syndrome*. The presence of prominent inner epicanthal folds along with an upward outer slant to the eyelids also suggests this malady (see Table 19-4, p. 591). Chemical conjunctivitis, caused by placement of silver nitrate in the eyes at birth as a prophylaxis against gonorrheal conjunctivitis (*ophthalmia neonatorum*), occurs frequently in normal infants and is characterized by edema of the lids and inflammation of the conjunctivas with a purulent discharge.

Dacryocystitis and *nasolacrimal duct obstruction* with ocular discharge and tearing may follow chemical conjunctivitis due to silver nitrate instillation.

Demonstrate the red retinal (or fundus) reflex by setting the ophthalmoscope at 0 diopters and viewing the pupil at a distance of approximately 10 inches. Normally a red or an orange color is reflected from the fundus through the pupil.

A *funduscopic examination* should be performed on all infants. Normally the examination can be postponed until between 2 and 6 months of age, when the infant is most cooperative, unless the ocular or neurologic examination indicates that it should be done immediately. Such examinations are not difficult to perform if one exercises patience and persistence. However, a mydriatic solution may be required.

Both retinal anomalies and opacities of the cornea, anterior chamber, or lens interrupt the light pathway and give a partial red or a completely dark reflex. In infants, *cataracts*, a *persistent posterior lenticular fibrovascular sheath*, and *retinopathy of prematurity* (retrolental fibroplasia) may cause a dark light reflex. Beyond infancy, *retinal detachment*, *chorioretinitis*, and *retinoblastoma* should be suspected when a white retinal reflex is encountered (leukokoria).

Instill a sterile mydriatic (2.5% phenylephrine with 0.5% cyclopentolate—one drop in each eye) for proper visualization. This can be repeated after 45 minutes if pupillary dilatation has not occurred. Place the baby supine on the examining table or on the parent's lap, or have the parent hold the baby upright over his or her shoulder. If the baby needs calming, use a sugar nipple. Retract the lids, if necessary, with your thumb and first finger. Funduscopic examination is otherwise the same as in adults. The cornea can ordinarily be seen at +20 diopters, the lens at +15 diopters, and the fundus at 0 diopters. Babies with acute central nervous system disease should not have their pupils dilated, except as directed by a child neurologist or ophthalmologist.

The optic disc is pale in infants, the peripheral vessels are not well developed, and the foveal light reflection is absent. *Papilledema* is rarely seen, even with markedly increased intracranial pressure, because the fontanelles and open sutures absorb the increased pressure, sparing the optic discs. Until age 3 years the sutures will separate sufficiently to prevent papilledema. If vascular or optic disc anomalies are found, the parents' fundi should be examined to determine a possible genetic origin and a prognosis.

Retinal hemorrhages associated with intracranial bleeding are accompanied by dilated, congested, tortuous retinal veins. Pigmentary changes occur in the retina in newborns with congenital *toxoplasmosis*, *cytomegalic inclusion disease*, and *rubella* infections.

The development of central vision progresses from birth, when only light perception is thought to be present, to adult visual levels attained at approximately 6 years of age.

Vision assessment in the newborn is based on the presence of visual reflexes—direct and consensual pupillary constriction in response to light, and blinking in response to bright light and to quick movement of an object toward the eyes.

Those visual reflexes imply that both light perception and some degree of visual acuity are present shortly after birth. Opticokinetic nystagmus (produced by the rapid movement of vertical black lines across the visual fields), used as a test of vision on one group of newborns 1½ to 5 days after birth, demonstrated a visual acuity of at least 20/670 in 93%. That this acuity improves is evident even without refractive measurement references. At 2 to 4 weeks of age, fixation on objects occurs; at 5 to 6 weeks, coordinated eye movements in following an object are seen; at 3 months, the eyes converge and the baby begins to reach for various-sized objects at various distances as eye–hand coordination and the ability to focus are accomplished. At the age of 1 year, normal visual acuity is in the range of 20/200.

Failure to progress along these lines may indicate mental deficiency as well as diminished or absent vision.

Early Childhood

When examining a child in this age group, the most important condition the examiner must detect is *amblyopia ex anopsia.* This is not the most serious ophthalmologic disease, but in comparison with others of significance it is the most prevalent and offers, with early intervention, the best prognosis. Improvement in this condition is unlikely if treatment is instituted after the sixth year of life. Amblyopia means reduced vision in an otherwise normal eye, and the reduced vision in this situation is caused by disuse. In essence, because of disconjugate fixation, one of the two images received by the optic cortex is suppressed to avoid diplopia or images of unequal clarity. One eye then becomes "lazy" and stops functioning to its full capacity; visual acuity in that eye is reduced markedly by suppression of central (foveal) vision. Since the two most common causes of amblyopia ex anopsia are *strabismus* and *anisometropia* (an eye with a refractive error 1.5 diopters or more greater than its pair), it is important to be able to test accurately for muscle weakness and visual acuity.

Obstructive amblyopia is secondary to a *cataract, corneal opacity,* or severe *ptosis.*

Muscle weakness causing one eye to deviate inwardly (*esotropia*) or outwardly (*exotropia*) may be detected by the *Hirschberg test* or the *cover test.*

The *Hirschberg test* ascertains the location of a light reflection on the cornea of each eye. Attract the patient's attention to a light held at your midforehead. While the patient's eyes are fixed on the light, note the light's reflection on each cornea. First hold the patient's head fixed in the midline and then turn it to the left and the right while the child's eyes remain fixed on the light.

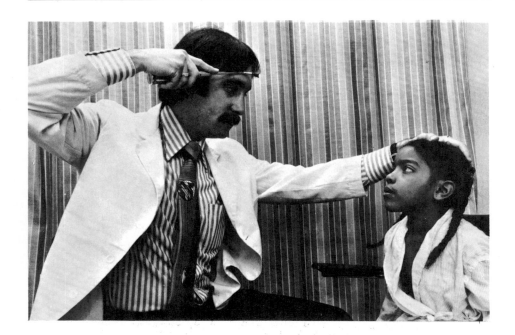

NORMAL PATTERN

RIGHT ESOTROPIA

RIGHT EXOTROPIA

To detect esotropia and exotropia, look for a change in the corneal reflection pattern on lateral gaze. The reflections on each cornea should be symmetrical; the type and degree of tropia can be determined by the pattern of asymmetrical placement of the reflections. The normal pattern and those with esotropia and exotropia are shown at the right. The light patterns should also be noted with upward, downward, and upper-outer and downward-outer movements of the eyes, although these are much less likely to reveal muscle imbalances.

The *cover test* is more sophisticated because it detects frank strabismus, differentiates the type of deviation, and determines the characteristics of any latent deviation. Attract the patient's attention once more to the mid-forehead light. Place your other hand on top of the child's head and your thumb in front of one eye while observing the other for movement. Then remove your thumb and observe both eyes for movement. If either or both eyes move, a strabismus is present. Repeat the test, covering and uncovering the other eye with your thumb.

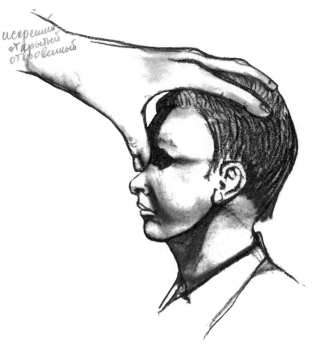

The combination of movements observed allows for a differential diagnosis of the strabismus in question. The results of using the cover test, more properly called the cover–uncover test, in monocular right esotropia are shown at the right.

Testing visual acuity in early childhood is not simple. The variables of the child, the examiner, the test environment, and the test itself all contribute significantly to the outcome and should be carefully considered if valid results are to be obtained. Unfortunately, there is no test that accurately measures visual acuity in children under the age of 3 years. Since each eye must be tested separately to detect amblyopia, one eye must be covered by an elastoplast bandage to ensure complete occlusion. Resistance to placement of the patch may be overcome by calling it a "pirate's patch." A child with amblyopia might accept the patch on the amblyopic eye, but *not* on the good eye.

Opticokinetic testing is the most accurate method for testing visual acuity in this age group; however, this method requires too much technical equipment to use in most settings. Two other simpler *tests of visual acuity* are of some worth.

The *miniature toy test* uses identical sets of small toys representing familiar objects (a cube, a marble, a coin, etc.). Give the child one set and keep the other. Ask the child to match each toy shown at a distance of 10 feet. *Worth's test* uses five balls ranging from ½ to 1½ inches in diameter. Beginning with the largest, throw each on the floor and ask the child to retrieve it. These tests, at best, detect only *grossly* impaired vision rather than the degree of such impairment.

In children over the age of 3 years, the *Snellen E chart* (a form of direct visual testing) is very adequate. Most youngsters cooperate in indicating the direction of the E, either orally or by pointing. For those who initially have difficulty with this test, an E card can be sent home with the child for practice. Charts with pictures instead of Es are often used but have no special advantage, nor have any other testing methods generally available. The normal visual acuity at age 3 years is ±20/40, at age 4 to 5 years, ±20/30, and at 6 to 7 years, 20/20.

The *visual fields* can be examined in infants and young children with the child sitting on the parent's lap.

Hold the head in the midline while bringing an object, such as a measuring tape case or a small toy, into the child's field of vision from several points behind, above, and below. Eyes deviating in its direction indicate that the child has seen the object.

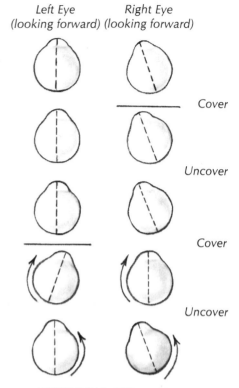

Left Eye
(looking forward)

Right Eye
(looking forward)

Cover

Uncover

Cover

Uncover

MONOCULAR RIGHT ESOTROPIA

Late Childhood

The eye problems and methods of examining the eye for this age group have been covered in the adult section. In general, vision testing machines used for mass screening in schools tend to underrate visual acuity and produce over-referrals.

You can distinguish a simple refractive error from organic causes of diminished vision by asking the child to look through a pinhole punched in a card. Visual acuity improves by using the pinhole card when refractive errors are present, but not when organic ocular disease exists.

THE EAR

Infancy

Note the position of the ears in relation to the eyes. Normally the upper portion of the auricle (pinna) joins the scalp on or above the extension of a line drawn across the inner and outer canthus of the eye.

Small, deformed, or low-set auricles may indicate associated congenital defects, especially renal agenesis or anomalies.

Examination of the ear in the immediate neonatal period establishes only the patency of the ear canal, because the tympanic membranes are obscured by accumulated vernix caseosa for the first 2 or 3 days of life. In infancy the ear canal is directed downward from the outside; therefore, **the auricle should be pulled gently downward** for the best visualization of the ear drum. The light reflex on the tympanic membrane is diffuse and does not become cone-shaped for several months.

Inspect the ear and surrounding skin. Test the infant's hearing by eliciting the *acoustic blink reflex*. This is positive (and indicates that the infant can hear) when one observes blinking eyes in response to a sudden sharp sound produced at a distance of about 12 inches from the ear by snapping the fingers, clapping the hands, or using a bell or other kinds of mechanical noisemaking devices. Be sure that in generating the sound you do not produce an airstream that could cause the baby to blink.

A small skin tab, cleft, or pit is frequently found just forward of the tragus and represents a remnant of the first branchial cleft.

The acoustic blink reflex is difficult to elicit during the first 2 or 3 days of life, and may disappear temporarily after it is elicited a few times. This test is crude at best, and the absence of blinking in response to sound is not diagnostic of deafness nor does its presence assure normal hearing. At 2 weeks of age the infant may jump in response to a sudden noise; at 10 weeks the infant may cease body movements momentarily. Between 3 and 4 months of age the eyes and head will turn toward the sound. Even before this, the respiratory rate may increase when familiar sounds, generating anticipation of forthcoming pleasures, are heard.

The parents' impression of the baby's auditory acuity is usually correct. When they believe that their baby cannot hear, it should be assumed that they are correct until proven otherwise.

Screening of infants for hearing loss is very costly and produces unacceptable levels of false-positive and false-negative results. Selective screening of newborn infants who are at high risk for hearing deficits by virtue of family history, physical findings, or perinatal difficulties should be performed using brainstem evoked response audiometry.

Early Childhood

The examination of the ear becomes more difficult as children grow. They resist because their ear canals are sensitive and they cannot observe the procedure.

Often it is helpful if you initially place the otoscopic speculum gently into the external auditory canal of one ear, remove it instantly, and repeat the procedure on the other. Then you can begin again, taking the necessary time in the actual examination, because the child's apprehensions have probably been allayed.

The ears can be examined successfully even in struggling children if you restrain them carefully and manipulate both ear and otoscope gently.

Place the patient supine and ask the parent or an assistant to hold the child's arms extended and close to the sides of the head, thus limiting movement from side to side. Approach from the child's right side and lean across the lower chest and upper abdomen to restrict movements of the trunk. A third person may be needed to hold the feet and legs if the child struggles unduly; however, this is rarely necessary.

This same restraining procedure may be used in examining the eyes, nose, and throat, as illustrated below.

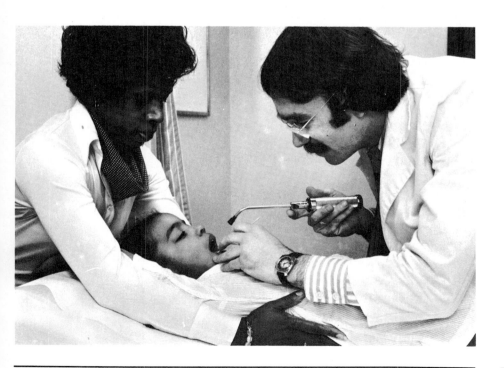

When examining the right ear, turn the child's head to the left and hold it firmly with the lateral aspect of your right hand and wrist. Hold the otoscope inverted in your right hand and manipulate the auricle with your left hand, the lateral aspect of which can be used to help keep the child's head still. In this age group, the external auditory canal is directed upward and backward from the outside and the auricle must be pulled upward, outward, and backward to afford the best visualization. The thumb and forefinger of your right hand, which holds the otoscope, should be buffered from sudden movements of the child's head by your restraining right hand and your forearm, which rests firmly on the examining table. See the illustration below.

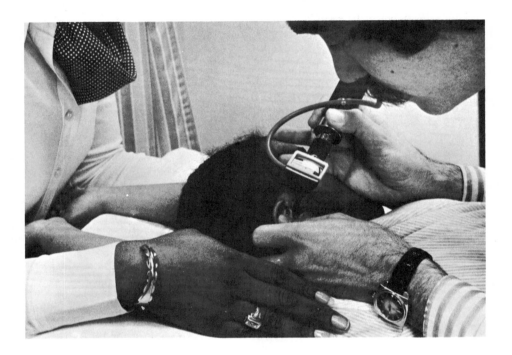

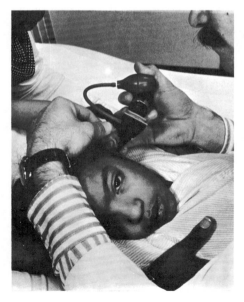

When examining the left ear, turn the patient's head to the right and hold it firmly with the lateral aspect of your left hand and wrist. The thumb and forefinger of your left hand should manipulate the auricle and your right hand should hold the otoscope inverted. The lateral aspect of the fifth finger of your right hand is held against the patient's head to provide a buffer against sudden movement by the patient. This procedure is illustrated at the left.

The speculum of the otoscope should be as large in diameter as will allow for comfortable ¼- to ½-inch penetration into the external auditory canal. This provides maximum visualization of the canal and drum and a reasonable seal for observing the effects of pneumatic otoscopy. Some examiners attach a rubber tip to the end of the speculum to gain a tighter, more comfortable seal.

Pneumatic otoscopy should be part of every otoscopic examination; it is accomplished by observing the tympanic membrane as the pressure in the external auditory canal is increased or decreased. You can do this by introducing and removing air from the canal—by applying positive and negative pressures with a rubber squeeze bulb (as shown in the figure here and the second figure on p. 602) or by blowing and sucking on a rubber tube attached to the otoscope (shown in the first figure on p. 602).

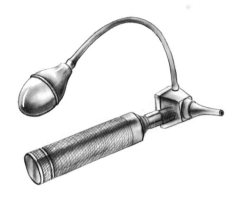

When air is introduced into the normal ear canal, the tympanic membrane and its light reflex move inward. When air is removed, the tympanic membrane moves outward, toward the examiner. This to-and-fro movement of the tympanic membrane has been likened to the luffing of a sail.

This movement is absent in chronic middle ear infection (serous otitis media), and diminished in some cases of acute otitis media.

Accumulation of cerumen in the ear canal commonly obscures the view of a child's tympanic membrane. Very often this accumulation is unilateral. There are several instruments and ear-washing techniques that may be used to remove ear wax comfortably. (These are described in DeWeese DD et al (eds): Otolaryngology—Head and Neck Surgery. St Louis, CV Mosby, 1988.)

Purulent material and debris in the ear canal are found both in otitis externa and in otitis media with a ruptured tympanic membrane. Washing out the ear canal is contraindicated, in the first instance because of the pain created by the procedure and in the second instance because the cleansing fluid and canal debris are forced into the middle ear through the perforated tympanic membrane.

Simple auditory screening in this age group can be accomplished by whispering at a distance of 8 feet.

Otitis media and *otitis externa* may be differentiated clinically by gently moving the pinna, which will cause exquisite pain in otitis externa but no discomfort in purulent otitis media. Acute *mastoiditis* in children is accompanied by a forward protrusion of the auricle of the affected ear, in addition to redness, swelling, and tenderness overlying the mastoid bone.

Ask the child questions or give commands, taking care that lip reading is not possible. In addition, you can use a tuning fork to screen for hearing, using your own auditory acuity as the control.

If these screening methods reveal any diminution of hearing, full audiometric testing should be performed. Furthermore, all children should be given a full-scale acoustic screening test with an audiometer before beginning school, as should any child at whatever age with delayed speech development. Because of their complexity, audiometric screening devices used for older children are often unsatisfactory for use in early childhood; when speech is delayed or defective, direct referral to a hearing and speech center may be more appropriate.

Significant, temporary hearing loss for as long as 4 months may follow an episode of otitis media.

Late Childhood

As the child grows, the ease and techniques of examining the ears and testing the hearing approach the levels and methods used for adults. There are no ear abnormalities or variations of normal unique to this age group. A possible exception is the "selective deafness" some children and adolescents demonstrate in hearing only what they choose when spoken to in either soft or loud voices by their parents and teachers.

THE NOSE AND THROAT

Infancy

Test the patency of the nasal passages by occluding each nostril alternately while holding the infant's mouth closed. This will not cause stress in a normal baby, since most newborns are nasal breathers. On the other hand, occluding both nares simultaneously and allowing the mouth to open will cause considerable distress. Indeed, some infants are unable to breathe through their mouths (*obligate nasal breathers*). Obstructed posterior nasal passage(s) can be confirmed by attempting to pass a number-14 French catheter through each nostril into the posterior nasopharynx.

The nasal passages in newborns may be obstructed in *choanal atresia* and by displacement of the nasal cartilage during delivery.

The newborn's *mouth* is edentulous. The gums are smooth with a raised, 1-mm, serrated fringe of tissue on the buccal margins. Occasionally, pearl-like retention cysts are seen along the ridges and are easily mistaken for teeth—they disappear spontaneously within a month or two.

Petechiae are commonly found on the soft palate after birth.

Rarely, *supernumerary teeth* are found. These are soft, have no enamel, and shed within a few days. They should be removed, however, to prevent their aspiration into the lower respiratory tract.

The frenulum of the upper lip may be quite thick and extend from the superior aspect of the inner lip to the posterior portion of the upper gum, creating a deep notch in the gum's midline. The frenulum of the tongue varies in consistency from a thin, filamentous membrane to a thick,

Epstein's pearls, pinhead-sized, white or yellow, rounded elevations that are located along the midline of the hard palate near

fibrous cord. Its length varies, such that it may attach midway on the undersurface of the tongue or at its very tip. A heavy fibrous frenulum that extends to the tip of the tongue may interfere with its protrusion (*tongue tie*). No difficulties will be encountered with nursing or speech, however, if the tongue can be extended as far as the alveolar ridge, which is usually possible.

its posterior border, are caused by retained secretions and disappear within a few weeks or months.

The *pharynx* can best be visualized while the baby is crying. This is true throughout infancy and early childhood. A tongue blade produces strong reflex elevation of the base of the tongue and obstructs the view of the infant's pharynx. Tonsillar tissue is not seen in the newborn.

Oral moniliasis (*thrush*) is a common malady in infants, usually contracted from mothers with vaginal moniliasis. In thrush, a lacy white material with an erythematous base is seen on the surface of the oral mucous membranes. Difficulty in removing it distinguishes it from milk curds, which wipe away.

Little saliva is produced during the first 3 months of life. As infants begin to produce saliva, drooling occurs because there are no lower teeth to provide a dam for retention.

The presence of large amounts of saliva in the newborn suggests a *tracheoesophageal fistula.*

Listen to the infant's *breathing* and the *quality of the cry*.

A shrill or high-pitched cry in infancy may indicate increased intracranial pressure. Such cries also occur in newborn infants born to narcotic-addicted mothers. A hoarse cry should make one suspect hypocalcemic *tetany* or *cretinism;* absence of any cry suggests severe illness or profound mental retardation. A continuous inspiratory and expiratory stridor may be caused by a relatively small larynx (*infantile laryngeal stridor*) or by delay in the development of the cartilage in the tracheal rings (*tracheomalacia*).

Early and Late Childhood

Visualize the anterior portion of the *nose* by pushing up its tip. Use a large-bore speculum attached to the otoscope to look deeper into the nostrils.

Examination of the *mouth* may present difficulties in early childhood, and restraints are usually needed (see figure on p. 601). The

The presence of *Koplik's spots* on the buccal mucosa opposite

young child may be more comfortable sitting in the parent's lap, as shown below.

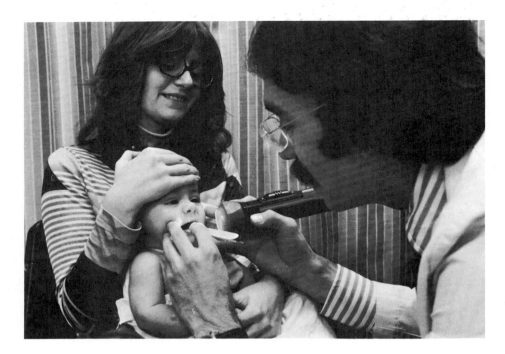

the first and second molars in a child with fever, coryza, and cough is proof positive of prodromal measles (*rubeola*), and the appearance of a generalized maculopapular rash within 24 hours is certain. Koplik's spots appear as grains of salt on individual erythematous bases. Their number varies according to when in the course of the illness they are observed. When three or more appear in a particular spot, they are easily recognized.

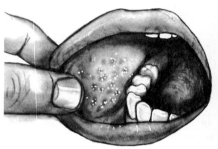

When children clamp their teeth and purse their lips, gently push the tongue blade through the lips along the buccal mucosa and between the alveolar ridges behind the molars. This produces a gag reflex and, with it, complete visualization of the *pharynx*.

A direct assault on the front teeth will only meet with failure and a splintered tongue blade. Most children, however, are not that resistant and can be enticed easily to open their mouths, especially if they do not see a throat stick in the examiner's hand. Children who can stick out their tongues and say "ahhh!" do not require further manipulation for complete visualization of the pharynx. A good examiner can determine all that needs to be known with one quick look. Older children will permit placement of the tongue blade on one side of the base of the tongue and then the other. A transilluminator attachment to the oto-ophthalmoscopic handle is more useful than the standard penlight or flashlight in that its giraffe-like configuration allows for delivery of concentrated light in the recesses of the oral cavity and the pharynx.

The transilluminator may also be used, of course, to transilluminate the sinuses when sinusitis is suspected. This requires a completely dark room and a cooperative child.

Transilluminate the frontal sinuses **by firmly placing the tip of the light above each eye against the inner aspect of the supraorbital ridge of the frontal bone.**

Normally, one sees a faint glow of light transmitted through the bone outlining the frontal sinus on the same side.

Transilluminate the maxillary sinuses by placing the neck and head of the light in the patient's mouth and pressing the tip against first one side and then the other of the hard palate. Instruct the patient to seal both lips around the shaft of the transilluminator attachment while you look for the maxillary sinus glow on the corresponding side of the face. Cleanse the transilluminator before and after using it.

The *teeth* should be examined for timing and sequence of eruption, number, character, condition, and position. Abnormalities of the enamel may reflect past or present, general or localized disease. Malocclusion should be looked for in late childhood. Most malocclusion and misalignment of teeth due to thumb sucking in early childhood are reversible if the habit is substantially arrested by age 6 or 7 years.

When examining for maxillary protrusion (*overbite*) or mandibular protrusion (*underbite*), one should *not* ask the child to "show your teeth," because the upper and lower teeth are aligned reflexly when they are presented for inspection. Rather, ask the child to bite down

Transillumination is absent or diminished when sinusitis is present.

The appearance of the *tongue* may indicate disease. The *coated* tongue is nonspecific, the *smooth* tongue is found in avitaminosis, and the *strawberry* and *raspberry* tongues are seen at specific stages of scarlet fever. The *scrotal* and *fissured* tongues have no significance (see Table 7-20, p. 227).

Dental caries are caused by bacterial activity and reflect poor nutrition and oral hygiene. Extensive decay of the primary teeth may be associated with prolonged bottle feeding ("nursing-bottle caries"), especially in children who take their bottles to bed at night and during naps.

Green coloration of the teeth is seen following severe *erythroblastosis fetalis*; grayish mottling of the enamel may result from the administration of tetracycline to infants and children under 8 years of age; and black lines along the gingival margins signal the ingestion of heavy metals.

Malocclusion is most often due to hereditary predisposition, but may be due to chronic mouth breathing secondary to

as hard as possible. Upon parting the lips you will observe the *true* bite. In normal children the upper teeth slightly override the lower teeth.

The *primary teeth* erupt more predictably than do the secondary teeth. At age 7 months most infants have two upper and two lower central incisors. From that point on, four teeth are added every 4 months, so that there are eight at 11 months, 12 at 15 months, 16 at 19 months, and a full complement of 20 at 23 months. Normally the shedding of primary teeth begins at about age 5 years; it precedes the eruption of corresponding *secondary teeth*, which begins at the beginning of late childhood between 6 and 7 years of age and ends in early adulthood at age 17 to 22 years.

When the *throat* is examined, the size and appearance of the *tonsils* should be noted. In both early and late childhood the tonsils are relatively larger than in infancy and adolescence, as demonstrated by the abundance of lymphoid tissue at this time of life (see figure on p. 561). They appear even larger as they move out of their fossae toward the midline and forward when the gag reflex is elicited or when the tongue is voluntarily protruded and the traditional "ahhh!" is sounded. The tonsils usually have deep crypts on their surfaces, which often have white concretions or food particles protruding from their depths. This does not indicate disease, current or past.

The *adenoids* are not ordinarily visible unless extremely enlarged or unless the soft palate is elevated with the tongue blade to expose them in the nasopharynx. Adenoidal size can be determined indirectly by noting the degree of posterior nasal obstruction present when the patient sniffs through each nostril and the nasal quality they produce in the voice. Their size may also be determined directly by palpation. Adenoidal palpation should be carried out when there is a history of recurrent fever, headaches, and cough and thus the diagnoses of *chronic adenoiditis* and *adenoidal abscess* are entertained.

During this examination, position and restrain the child as for examining the throat (see p. 601). Tape three tongue blades together and, with your left hand, place them between the molars and turn them on edge to ensure wide exposure. Place your plastic-gloved right index finger through the mouth into the nasopharynx behind the soft palate, and very rapidly palpate and thoroughly massage the adenoidal and surrounding lymphoid tissue. The procedure is accomplished with three or four quick strokes of the finger.

obstruction of the nasal airway. Maxillary overgrowth is associated with *chronic hemolytic anemia*. Mandibular overgrowth occurs rarely in the initial stages of *juvenile rheumatoid arthritis*, affecting the temporomandibular joint; micrognathia eventually ensues, however, in chronic cases.

A white exudate over the surface of the tonsils suggests *streptococcal tonsillitis*; a thick, gray, adherent exudate suggests *diphtheritic tonsillitis*; and necrosis (a grayish discoloration of the tonsillar tissue itself, rather than an exudate or a membrane overlying it) suggests *infectious mononucleosis*. All three conditions produce a fetid odor, but no one odor is distinguishable from the others. When one tonsil appears inflamed and unilaterally protrudes toward the midline and forward, a *peritonsillar abscess* is almost certainly present.

In cases of chronic adenoiditis and adenoidal abscess, palpation will reveal enlarged and boggy adenoidal tissue and massage will produce copious amounts of bloody mucus and purulent material.

The child and parents should be warned that this procedure is uncomfortable and is likely to produce vomiting.

The same method may be used to palpate (1) a peritonsillar abscess to determine the presence of fluctuation, and (2) the posterior pharyngeal wall to determine the presence of a retropharyngeal abscess.

Absence or asymmetrical movement of the soft palate in response to gagging and phonation, which indicates paralysis or weakness, should be noted. Asymmetry and corresponding voice change are often observed for varying periods after tonsillectomy.

Often overlooked in the examination of the throat is the presence of a submucosal cleft palate in which the muscles of the medial portion of the soft palate are missing. The mucosa is intact, however, and the underlying defect is easily missed. This condition is usually associated with notching of the posterior margin of the hard palate and a bifid uvula. Children with this anatomic variation may have hypernasal speech, but many have no voice changes. Adenoidectomy should be avoided, since regurgitation of liquids and food into the nasal passages and nasality of speech will surely present difficulties.

The child who has a high fever, croupy cough, hoarseness, drooling, difficulty in swallowing, and signs of upper respiratory tract obstruction may have acute *epiglottitis*. In such a case, the epiglottis is markedly swollen and cherry red. Invoking the gag reflex in this instance could produce complete laryngeal obstruction and a fatal outcome. Therefore, *great care* must be taken in examining the throat. It should be done only once, if at all, and then deftly and gently with the child upright, and with a tracheostomy set at hand to use in case of complete upper airway obstruction resulting from the examination. The danger of such obstruction is sufficiently great that many clinicians prefer to omit direct examination of the throat in suspected cases of acute epiglottitis and to rely on lateral x-rays of the neck to establish the diagnosis.

THE THORAX, BREASTS, AND LUNGS

Infancy

The infant's *thorax* is rounded, with the anteroposterior diameter being equal to the transverse diameter. The *thoracic index*, which is the ratio of the transverse diameter to the anteroposterior diameter, is 1 at birth. At 1 year of age it is 1.25, and it reaches 1.35 at 6 years without much change thereafter.

The chest wall in infancy is thin with little musculature, and the bony and cartilaginous rib cage is very soft and pliant. The tip of the xiphoid process is often seen protruding anteriorly immediately beneath the skin at the apex of the costal angle.

Pectus excavatum may manifest in early infancy by marked midline sternal retractions with normal inspiration; however, it

The *breasts* of the newborn in both male and female are often enlarged and engorged with a white liquid called "witch's milk." This is due to maternal estrogen effect and usually lasts only a week or two. Supernumerary nipples occasionally are found on the thorax or the abdomen along a vertical line below the true nipple(s). They appear as small, round, flat or slightly raised, pigmented lesions and are not clinically significant.

and other thoracic deformities, such as *pectus carinatum* ("chicken breast" deformity), do not ordinarily become evident until early childhood (see p. 257).

The respiratory rate and patterns in infancy and early childhood are discussed on page 578. Breathing is predominantly effected by movement of the diaphragm, with little assistance from the thoracic muscles. This results in protrusion of the abdomen on inspiration and the reverse on expiration—so-called abdominal breathing.

When the pattern of breathing becomes predominantly thoracic, intra-abdominal or intrathoracic pathology, which restricts the use of the diaphragm, should be suspected. On the other hand, an *increase* in abdominal breathing suggests pulmonary disease.

Newborn infants, especially those born prematurely, exhibit irregular breathing characterized by periods of breathing at normal rates (30 to 40 per minute) alternating with "periodic breathing" during which the respiratory rate slows markedly and may even cease three or more times for 3 seconds or longer. These alternating respiratory patterns have been observed in 30% to 95% of premature babies during sleep, but less frequently in full-term infants. The short apneic periods are not accompanied by bradycardia.

Periods of apnea lasting longer than 20 seconds and accompanied by bradycardia may indicate the presence of cardiopulmonary or central nervous system disease or a high risk for *Sudden Infant Death Syndrome* (*SIDS*).

Feel for tactile fremitus in infants by placing your hand on the chest when the baby cries. Place your whole hand, palm and fingertips, over the anterior, lateral, or posterior thorax to detect gross changes in sound transmission through the parenchyma of the lung, pleura, and chest wall. Percuss the infant's chest directly by tapping the thoracic wall with one finger or indirectly by using the finger-on-finger method.

The percussion note is normally hyperresonant throughout. Any decrease in hyperresonance detected over the lung fields has the same significance as dullness in the adult.

Dullness to percussion may be elicited in infants when consolidation of the lung, an intrathoracic mass, or pleural fluid is present.

Use the bell or small diaphragm of the stethoscope when auscultating the infant's chest, to pinpoint findings.

The breath sounds are louder and harsher than in adults because the stethoscope is closer to the origin of the sounds. Breathing in newborns is usually intermittently slow and shallow, then rapid and deep. Breath sounds will often be diminished on the side of the chest opposite the direction in which the head is turned. Fine crackles at the end of deep inspiration may be heard in normal newborns and older infants. Crying, fortunately, will produce all of the deep breaths one could want and

Extension or other movement of the head with inspiration indicates use of accessory muscles of respiration, and usually accompanies severe respiratory disease.

actually enhances auscultation, except in the unusual baby who cries on inspiration as well as expiration.

Because of the smallness of the thoracic cage and the ease of sound transmission within it, breath sounds are rarely absent entirely. Even with atelectasis, effusion, empyema, and pneumothorax, breath sounds are diminished rather than absent. In infants, pure bronchial breathing is rarely heard, even when consolidation is present. *Wheezes,* which are palpable and audible vibrations caused by air rushing through a narrowed segment of the lumen, occur more frequently in infancy and early childhood than in older children and adults because the small lumen of the tracheobronchial tree is easily narrowed by slight swelling of the mucous membrane or by small amounts of mucus.

An inspiratory wheeze indicates narrowing high in the tracheobronchial tree; an expiratory wheeze indicates narrowing lower down.

Where respiratory distress or abnormal findings are manifest on percussion or auscultation of the chest in the newborn, transillumination of the thorax with a high-intensity, fiberoptic light can help to localize and define pathology, such as pleural effusion and pneumothorax.

Early and Late Childhood

Breast development for girls may begin normally as early as 8 years of age. Asymmetrical growth with resulting differences in breast size during preadolescence is the rule, symmetrical breast growth the exception. Completion of growth through adolescence usually corrects these inequalities. It is often helpful to explain this to parents and the young person herself, even if neither mentions the subject.

The breath sounds on auscultation of the lungs are louder and harsher in early and late childhood, as in infancy, than in adulthood because of the continued relative lack of musculature and subcutaneous tissue overlying the thorax. Respiratory patterns are more regular than in infancy, and cooperation in taking deep breaths and conducting other breathing maneuvers during auscultation of the lungs increases with age.

The stethoscope may be threatening to the very young child; therefore, your success in placing it on the chest will be enhanced if you say what it is and if you allow the child to manipulate it or even listen through it.

Generate tactile fremitus by feeling the chest wall while carrying on a conversation with the child. A surprising number say "99" or "1, 2, 3" when asked to. Gain the child's cooperation in deep breathing and breath holding by demonstrating each maneuver. If this is not successful, ask the child to blow out the light in your flashlight. This almost always produces full inspiration.

THE HEART

The examination of the heart in infants and children is, with few exceptions, conducted like that in the adult. The femoral pulses assume greater importance because their diminution (as compared with the radial pulse) or absence may be the only finding to suggest *coarctation of the aorta* in infancy and early childhood.

Feel along the inguinal ligament midway between the iliac crest and the symphysis pubis for the femoral pulse.

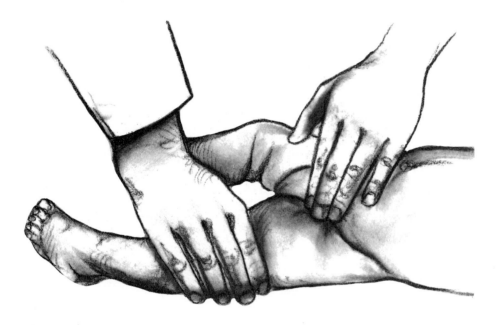

Because the respiratory rate may approximate the heart rate in infancy, breath sounds may be mistaken for murmurs.

Occlude the nares momentarily to interrupt the respirations long enough to clarify this issue.

During the first 48 hours of life, heart murmurs caused by the transition from intrauterine to extrauterine circulation are heard frequently. These are systolic in timing, less than grade II in intensity, and disappear spontaneously upon closure of the ductus arteriosus and the foramen ovale.

There are some distinct cardiac characteristics in normal infants and children that are not found in adults. The apical impulse (PMI), which is often visible, is at the level of the 4th interspace until age 7 years, when it drops to the level of the 5th interspace. It is to the left of the midclavicular line until age 4 years, at the midclavicular line between ages 4 and 6, and to the right of it at age 7. On percussion the heart appears larger than it is because of its more horizontal position and the overlying thymus gland at its base. *Sinus arrhythmia* (heart rate faster on inspiration and slower on expiration) is almost always present, and *premature ventricular*

The physical indications of severe heart disease include those not found with the stethoscope: poor weight gain; delayed development; tachypnea; tachycardia; a prominent, active, heaving or thrusting precordium; cyanosis; and clubbing of the fingers and toes. Heart failure is marked by tachycardia, tachypnea, venous engorgement, pulsus alternans, gallop rhythm, and hepatic enlargement. Pulmonary and peripheral edema appear late in the course of heart failure. (Peripheral edema, when it occurs in children, is more likely to be caused by renal failure.)

When S_2 is equal to or greater than S_1 at the apex, first-degree heart block should be suspected.

contractions are quite common. The heart sounds are louder than those in adults because the chest wall is thinner, and they are of higher pitch and shorter duration. S_1 is louder than S_2 at the apex. Splitting of S_2 at the apex is found in 25% to 33% of infants and children. S_2 is louder than S_1 in the pulmonic area.

In the pediatric cardiac examination the *murmur* assumes great significance in differential diagnosis, because more than 50% of all children (indeed, some say all) develop an innocent murmur at some time during childhood and because significant heart disease in the pediatric age group is infrequent in the absence of a murmur. The examiner must therefore distinguish between the innocent and the organic murmur. The intensity of murmurs is graded on a scale of 1 to 6, as shown on pages 300–301.

The *innocent murmur* has received more than 120 labels, indicative of its benign or functional nature, its origin, or its auscultatory characteristics. It is systolic, is usually of short duration and of grade 3 or less in intensity, and has an empty, low-pitched, vibratory, musical groaning quality. It is usually loudest along the left sternal border, either in the 2nd or 3rd intercostal spaces or in the 4th or 5th intercostal spaces medial to the apex. It is poorly transmitted and is heard best with the patient supine. Its intensity may vary with change in position, with the phase of respiration, with exercise, and from day to day. The most important characteristic of the innocent murmur is that it is heard in the absence of any other demonstrable evidence of cardiovascular disease.

A *venous hum* (see Table 9-15, p. 320) is heard commonly during childhood.

Hemic murmurs are caused by increased blood flow through the heart. This occurs when the body's tissues require more oxygen than usual (increased metabolism or muscular activity) or when hemoglobin-depleted red blood cells are not delivering ordinary amounts of oxygen to the tissues (anemia). These murmurs are located at the base of the heart, are soft (less than grade 3), occur during systole, and are accompanied by tachycardia.

The noninnocent or *organic murmurs* are caused by congenital or acquired heart disease. Almost all acquired heart disease productive of murmurs in childhood is caused by acute rheumatic fever. An organic murmur first appearing before 3 years of age is almost always caused by a congenital cardiac defect; one first appearing after that age is usually caused by rheumatic valvulitis.

The murmurs of congenital cardiac defects are caused either by abnormal communications between the arterial and venous circuits of the heart and great vessels or by valvular deformities. They are usually coarse in character, systolic in timing, and heard best at the base of the heart. The

Murmurs of grade 3 or higher usually indicate heart disease.

In *atrial septal defect* a grade 1 to 3 coarse systolic murmur is heard at the 2nd and 3rd left interspaces. It is less coarse than the murmur of a ventricular septal defect, is rarely accompanied by a thrill, and is not widely distributed. The murmur of *coarctation of the aorta* (adult type) is heard in the same area, is louder, is transmitted to the back medial to the scapula, and may be accompanied by a visible pulsation and palpable thrill at the suprasternal notch. It is also associated with decreased to absent femoral pulses and elevated blood pressure in the upper extremities. The murmurs associated with *tetralogy of Fallot, pure pulmonic stenosis, tricuspid atresia, transposition of the great vessels*, and *Eisenmenger's syndrome* are grades 3 to 5 in intensity, are systolic in timing, may be heard best at the left 2nd and 3rd interspaces, are not well transmitted, may or may not be accompanied by a thrill, and have no

murmurs of *ventricular septal defect* and of *patent ductus arteriosus* have been described on pages 318 and 320, respectively. Those of *aortic stenosis* and *pulmonic stenosis* are described on page 317.

The presence or absence of cyanosis may be helpful to the examiner in differentiating the various types of congenital heart disease that have similar murmurs (see Table 19-5).

Usually the final diagnostic impression must await the results of electrocardiograms, chest x-rays, cardiac catheterization, echocardiograms, and more sophisticated studies.

The murmurs associated with acquired rheumatic heart disease include those of mitral stenosis (see p. 319), mitral regurgitation (see p. 318), aortic stenosis (see p. 317), and aortic regurgitation (see p. 319). Stenosis and regurgitation usually occur concomitantly when either the mitral or aortic valve is affected from rheumatic carditis. Mitral valvular disease occurs in 90% of children who develop heart disease following acute rheumatic carditis, either alone or in combination with aortic valvular disease. Aortic valve involvement occurs in approximately 25% of cases. The tricuspid and pulmonic valves are rarely involved in the rheumatic process.

The examiner should be able to differentiate normal from abnormal findings. Final decisions regarding specific abnormalities, however, must often be left to the pediatric cardiologist, whose experience and access to special diagnostic tools will be more likely to produce accurate diagnoses and appropriate management. Therefore, the infant or child with evidence of congenital or acquired heart disease should be referred to a pediatric cardiologist early on.

distinguishing characteristics. These murmurs may be absent in infancy. In addition, palpable liver pulsations may be present with tricuspid atresia and pure pulmonic stenosis.

Table 19-5 Cyanosis and Congenital Heart Disease

NO CYANOSIS	Septal defects—small Patent ductus arteriosus Pure pulmonic stenosis—mild Coarctation of the aorta *Anomalous origin of left coronary artery *Subendocardial fibroelastosis *Glycogen storage disease
EARLY CYANOSIS	Tetralogy of Fallot—severe Tricuspid atresia Transposition of the great vessels Two- and three-chambered hearts Severe pulmonic stenosis with intact ventricular septum
LATE CYANOSIS	Eisenmenger's complex Pure pulmonic stenosis—mild Tetralogy of Fallot Septal defects—large

* Present with cardiac enlargement, tachycardia, and tachypnea, but without a heart murmur.

THE ABDOMEN

Infancy

The abdomen in infants is protuberant, due to poorly developed abdominal musculature.

A newborn with a concave abdomen should immediately be investigated for *diaphragmatic hernia* with displacement of some of the abdominal organs into the thoracic cavity.

The *umbilical cord* should be checked routinely at birth for the number of vessels present—normally two thick-walled umbilical arteries and one thin-walled umbilical vein. The diameter of the arteries is smaller than that of the vein, and the vein is usually found at the 12 o'clock position at the level of the abdominal wall.

A high correlation exists between the presence of only a *single umbilical artery* and a variety of congenital anomalies.

The umbilicus in the newborn may have a relatively long cutaneous portion (*umbilicus cutis*), which is covered with skin, or a relatively long amniotic portion (*umbilicus amnioticus*), which is of firm gelatinous substance. The amniotic portion dries up within 1 week and falls off within 2, while the cutaneous portion retracts to become flush with the abdominal wall.

Failure of the *navel* to heal, with granulomatous tissue formation at its base, occurs frequently.

Infants are prone to *umbilical hernias* (see p. 362), *ventral hernias*, and *diastasis recti*. However, these are not usually discernible until 2 or 3 weeks of age. All are easily detected with crying.

The presence of diastasis recti may reflect a congenital weakness of the abdominal musculature (rare) or result from a chronically distended abdomen. Most, however, are normal variants and disappear in early childhood.

The defect in the abdominal wall at the umbilicus may be as large as 1½ inches in diameter, and the hernia itself may protrude 3 to 4 inches from the abdominal wall when intra-abdominal pressure is increased. Most umbilical hernias disappear by 1 year of age.

A superficial abdominal venous pattern is observable until puberty. Abdominal reflexes are usually absent until after the first year of life.

Dilated veins may indicate portal vein obstruction. The direction of venous flow in *portal hypertension* is downward in veins below the umbilicus.

Palpation of the infant's abdomen is relatively easy.

Relax the infant by holding the legs flexed at the knees and hips with one hand; palpate with the other.

The *liver edge* and *spleen tip* are more often palpable than not, and frequently both *kidneys* can be felt by using the technique described for adults. The *bladder* is often felt and normally percussed to the level of the umbilicus. The *descending colon* is easily felt and may appear as a sausage-like mass in the left lower quadrant. Any abdominal masses of other origin are easily outlined.

In *Hirschsprung's disease* (congenital megacolon) a midline suprapubic mass representing a feces-filled rectosigmoid is often found.

Differentiate *cysts*, which occur rarely, from solid *tumors* by transillumination.

Avoid the spasm and rigidity encountered in palpating the abdomen of a crying infant by giving a bottle or a sugar nipple.

The infant's abdomen is percussed like that of the adult, but the examiner must allow for a greater amount of air within the stomach and the intestinal lumen because infants frequently swallow air when feeding and crying.

The abdomen should be auscultated before palpation. During auscultation, metallic tinkling every 10 to 30 seconds is heard normally.

The abdominal examination technique is altered when *pyloric stenosis* is suspected.

Place the unclothed infant supine and stand at the foot of the table. Direct a bright light at table height across the abdomen from the patient's right side. Feed the infant a bottle of sugar water or milk and observe the abdomen closely. When pyloric stenosis is present, peristaltic waves are seen to go across the upper abdomen from left to right. These become increasingly large and frequent as the feeding progresses, as shown in the figure below on the right.

An increase in pitch or frequency of bowel sounds, or a marked diminution, indicates *intestinal obstruction* and *ileus*, respectively. A venous hum is a sign of *portal hypertension*.

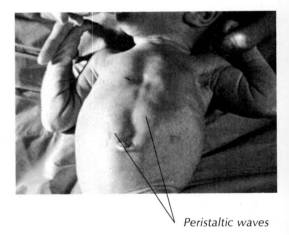

Peristaltic waves

Inevitably, the baby will vomit with projectile force. At this point, palpate deeply in the right upper quadrant with your extended middle finger. This will most likely reveal the presence of an olive-size pyloric mass. Similar palpation with the baby prone may prove more successful.

Early and Late Childhood

A protuberant abdomen, apparent when the child is upright and disappearing when the child is supine, is typical in most children until adolescence.

Children are almost universally ticklish when you first place your hand on their abdominal wall. This reaction disappears in most cases, particularly if you distract the child by conversation and place your whole hand flush on the surface for a few moments without probing with your fingers. With children whose sensitivity persists, place the

child's hand under yours, as shown in the illustration below, to reduce apprehension and increase relaxation of the abdominal musculature. Palpate lightly and then deeply in all quadrants. Examine last the area that the history suggests as the site of pathology.

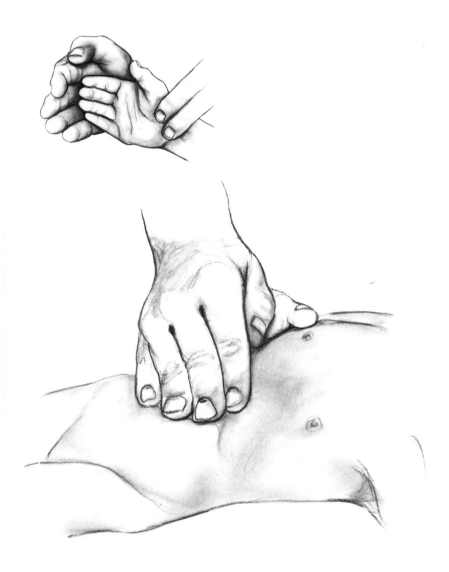

Tenderness may be detected by the child's telling you, by a change in the child's facial expression, or in the pitch of the child's cry.

The *liver* is easily palpated in most children. The edge of the liver is normally felt 1 cm to 2 cm below the right costal margin. It is sharp and soft and moves easily when pushed from below upward during deep inspiration. The size of the liver is better determined by percussion than by palpation. Table 19-6 shows the expected liver span by percussion in the right midclavicular line for male and female patients by age.

A pathologically enlarged liver is usually palpable at more than 2 cm below the costal margin and has a round, firm edge.

The lower border of the liver can be determined with a *scratch test*. Place the diaphragm of your stethoscope just above the right costal margin at the midclavicular line. With your fingernail, lightly scratch the skin of the abdomen along the midclavicular line moving from below the umbilicus towards the costal margin. When your scratching finger reaches the liver's edge, you will hear the scratching sound as it passes through the liver to your stethoscope.

Table 19-6   Expected Liver Span of Infants, Children, and Adolescents by Percussion

AGE IN YEARS	MEAN ESTIMATED LIVER SPAN (cm)		AGE IN YEARS	MEAN ESTIMATED LIVER SPAN (cm)	
	MALES	FEMALES		MALES	FEMALES
.5 (6 mo)	2.4	2.8	8	5.6	5.1
1	2.8	3.1	10	6.1	5.4
2	3.5	3.6	12	6.5	5.6
3	4.0	4.0	14	6.8	5.8
4	4.4	4.3	16	7.1	6.0
5	4.8	4.5	18	7.4	6.1
6	5.1	4.8	20	7.7	6.3

As a rule the *spleen,* like the liver, is felt easily in most children. It too is soft with a sharp edge, and it appears as a downward, tonguelike projection at the left costal margin.

You can often palpate the spleen between the thumb and forefinger of your right hand, and find it to be moveable.

Pulsations in the epigastrium caused by the aorta are seen normally.

The pulsations of an enlarged right ventricle may be transmitted through the diaphragm and be visible in the epigastrium.

Deeply palpate the abdomen to the left of the midline to feel the *aorta* and its pulsations.

Because the omentum is poorly developed in early childhood, localization of intra-abdominal infection or other inflammatory reaction is less apt to occur than in late childhood and adolescence.

Tenderness and spasm of the abdominal musculature are usually diffuse whenever serious pathology occurs within the abdomen; *generalized peritonitis* should be suspected.

Ask the child to sit up from a supine position while you push down against the forehead with your hand.

This maneuver will elicit pain in the right lower quadrant in *acute appendicitis* when the appendix is lying anteriorly. When the appendix lies retrocecally over the psoas and obturator muscles, *psoas* and *obturator signs* are present (see p. 361).

THE GENITALIA AND RECTUM

Infancy

Examining the genitalia in the male infant presents no difficulties. The *foreskin* adheres to the *glans penis*, covers it, and has a tiny orifice at its distal end. It does not retract over the glans until the infant is several months old, and then only if it has been stretched regularly.

Circumcision is still carried out on many male infants in our society in the immediate neonatal period, exposing the glans penis to its base. The number circumcised has diminished in recent years.

The *testes* are normally found in the scrotum, or in the inguinal canal from which they can easily be milked down into the scrotum.

In the newborn female the *labia minora* are prominent; they quickly atrophy and become almost nonexistent until puberty. More often than not there is a bloody, mucoid vaginal discharge during the first week of life, due to the maternal estrogen influence on the cervix and vaginal mucosa. A serosanguinous vaginal discharge may supplant this for a week or two more.

Inspect the perineal structures, the urethral orifice, the hymen, and the vaginal mucosa by separating the labia with the thumb and forefinger of one hand while you press forward and downward from within the rectum with the index finger of your other hand. The rectoperineal portion of this examination should be done only when intravaginal pathology such as a rectovaginal fistula is suspected.

The genitalia of both male and female breech babies may be markedly edematous and bruised for several days following delivery.

The *rectal examination* of infants (and of patients in early and late childhood) should be performed whenever intra-abdominal, pelvic, or perirectal disease is suspected. It should be performed with the patient supine. This allows for deeper penetration of the examining finger and for combined abdominal and rectal examination.

Hold the feet together and flex the knees and hips on the abdomen with one of your hands while introducing the index finger of your other hand into the rectum. Then place your first hand on the abdomen to conduct a bimanual examination. The index finger is preferred for the rectal examination, even for infants, because of its greater tactile sensitivity. Regardless of the size of your examining

Hypospadias is present when the urethral orifice appears at some point along the ventral surface of the glans or the shaft of the penis. The foreskin in these instances is incompletely formed ventrally.

Hydroceles of the testes and the spermatic cord are common in infancy and often associated with actual or potential *inguinal hernias*. Hydroceles may be differentiated easily from hernias in that the former transilluminate and are not reducible.

finger, slight bleeding and protrusion of the rectal mucosa will usually occur upon its removal.

Early and Late Childhood

The size of the *penis* in early childhood and prepubescence is of little significance unless it is very large. In obese boys the fat pad over the symphysis pubis may envelop the penis, obscuring it completely. The testes in young boys are quite retractile and are often found in the inguinal canal rather than in the scrotum.

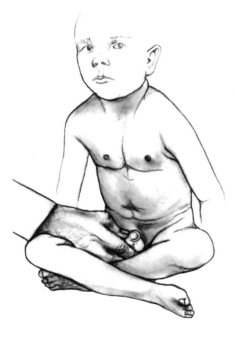

Enlargement of the penis to adolescent or adult size occurs in *precocious puberty*, due to an excess in circulating androgens of adrenal or testicular origin. This occurs with tumors of these organs or of the pituitary gland. Other signs of virilization —pubic and axillary hair, increased testicular size, increased somatic growth and muscle mass, hirsutism, and a deepening voice—usually accompany the penile enlargement.

You can overcome testicular retractibility by having the child sit crosslegged on the examining table, as illustrated here. Undescended testicle should not be diagnosed until you have palpated the inguinal canal and scrotum with the patient in this position.

Cryptorchidism, or undescended testicle, may occur unilaterally or bilaterally, with the testicle remaining in the abdomen or within the inguinal canal.

The examination for *inguinal hernia* in this age group is similar to that performed on the adult and should be done with the patient standing.

The child's cough may not be strong enough to demonstrate a reduced hernia. The hernia can sometimes be made evident if the child attempts to lift a heavy object, such as the end of the examining table or the chair in which you are sitting.

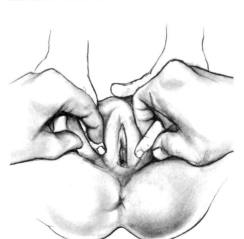

You can often make the examination of the female genitalia in this age group easier for yourself and more comfortable for the child by using the child's own hands to distract and reassure her, as shown here.

Fusion of the labia minora is seen commonly. It may be partial, with only the posterior portion of the labia fused, or it may be complete. A thin membrane that joins the labial edges is easily lysed with a cotton swab or a probe. The labia will also separate if an estrogen-containing cream is applied to the labia once or twice daily for several days.

You can obtain greater relaxation and cooperation during the rectal examination in this age group if you first demonstrate and then ask the child to try breathing in and out rapidly "like a puppy dog."

Perianal skin tabs are common and have no significance. Bimanual rectoabdominal palpation in females reveals a small midline mass, which is the *cervix.* Any other mass that is palpable on this examination should be considered abnormal, since none of the other anatomical structures are normally palpable until adolescence. Vaginoabdominal palpation as a method of examining the pelvic structures and direct visualization of the vagina and cervix are not considered part of the ordinary physical examination in childhood. When visualization of the vagina and cervix is indicated it is done best with an otoscope equipped with a vaginal speculum.

Foreign bodies are often inserted by the child into the vagina and cause irritation and infection, which lead to a purulent vaginal discharge.

Examination of the vagina and cervix is indicated when sexual abuse is suspected.

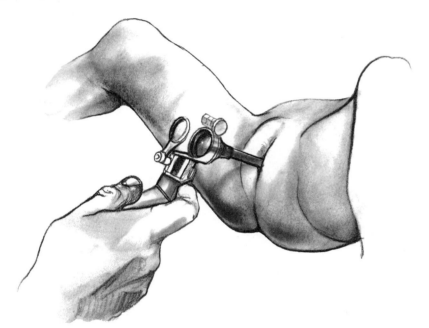

Secondary sexual *hair growth* parallels the development of other secondary sexual characteristics. Pubic hair may appear sparsely as early as the eighth year. Axillary, facial, body, arm, and leg hair proliferate in sequence before and during puberty.

THE MUSCULOSKELETAL SYSTEM

Infancy

The *range of motion* at all joints is greatest in infancy and gradually lessens throughout childhood to adult levels.

At birth, the *feet* may appear deformed if they retain their intrauterine positioning. Such positional deformities can be distinguished by the ease with which the affected foot can be manipulated to neutral and over-

True deformities do not return to the neutral position even through manipulation.

corrected positions. Scratching or stroking along the outer edge of the positionally deformed foot will cause it to assume a normal position.

Look for inversion of the feet. Note the relationship of the forefoot to the hindfoot. Is the forefoot adducted at the metatarsal–tarsal line (a line across the junctions of the tarsal and metatarsal bones)?

When the forefoot is twisted inward on its longitudinal axis (inverted) in addition to being adducted, *metatarsus varus* exists, as shown in the figure below.

Adduction of the forefoot distal to the metatarsal-tarsal line (*metatarsus adductus deformity*) is common; spontaneous correction occurs within the first 2 years of life.

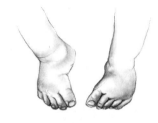

During infancy there is a distinct *bowlegged growth pattern*. This begins to disappear at 18 months of age, when a transition from bowlegs to knock-knees occurs. The *knock-knee pattern* usually persists from 2 until 6 to 10 years of age, when a balancing takes place and, for most, the legs straighten. Some babies exhibit a twisting or torsion of the tibia inwardly or outwardly on its longitudinal axis. This invariably corrects itself during the second year of life.

Talipes varus is present when the forefoot is adducted and the entire foot is inverted.

Talipes equinovarus (clubfoot) is characterized by forefoot adduction and inversion and plantar flexion (equinus position) of the entire foot, as shown below.

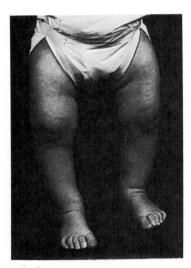   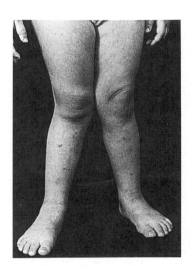

**GENU VARUM
(BOW LEGS)**   **GENU VALGUM
(KNOCK-KNEES)**

(Black-and-white prints of color photographs from Zitelli BJ, Davis HW: Atlas of Pediatric Physical Diagnosis, p. 19.30. St Louis, CV Mosby, 1987. Reproduced with permission.)

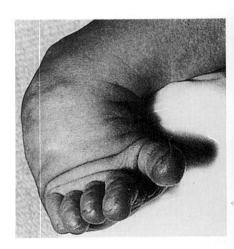

(Reproduced with permission from Prechtl HFR: The Neurological Examination of the Full-Term Newborn Infant, 2nd ed. Philadelphia, JB Lippincott, 1977)

When infants stand, their legs are set wide apart and the weight is borne on the inside of the feet. When they walk, a wide-based gait is used for the first year or two. This causes a certain degree of *pronation of the feet* and incurving of the Achilles tendons (viewed from behind).

The longitudinal arch in infancy is obscured by adipose tissue, giving the foot a flat appearance. This is accentuated by pronation of the foot, so the infant is often misdiagnosed as being flatfooted.

The *hips* of all infants should be examined for signs of dislocation.

Place the baby supine with the legs pointing toward you. Flex the legs to right angles at the hips and knees, placing your index finger over the greater trochanter of each femur and your thumb over the lesser trochanter, as shown in the figures below. Abduct both hips simultaneously until the lateral aspect of each knee touches the examining table. This maneuver is known as the *Ortolani test*.

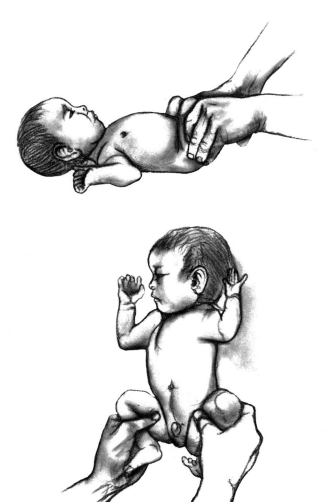

When a *congenitally dislocated hip* is present, you will see, feel, and sometimes hear a "click" as the femoral head, which in this condition lies posterior to the acetabulum, enters the acetabulum at some point in the 90° abduction arc. This finding is known as *Ortolani's sign*.

Beyond the newborn period, as the muscles surrounding the hip increase in strength, the click of the Ortolani sign is less obtainable; then decreased abduction of the flexed legs (at the hip on one or both sides) becomes the significant finding in detecting unilateral or bilateral congenital dislocation of the hip.

Detect an unstable (nondislocated but potentially dislocatable) hip by placing your thumb medially over the lesser trochanter and your index finger laterally over the greater trochanter, as shown in the figure on page 624; press your thumb backward and outward. Feel for movement of the head of the femur laterally against some resistance

as it slips out onto the posterior lip of the acetabulum. Normally no movement is felt. Then, with your index finger, press the greater trochanter forward and inward. Feel for a sudden movement of the femoral head inward as it returns to the hip socket. Again, movement is not normally felt. Movement in both directions constitutes *Barlow's sign.*

Barlow's sign is not diagnostic of a congenital dislocated hip, but it indicates the need to observe the baby very carefully for this possibility.

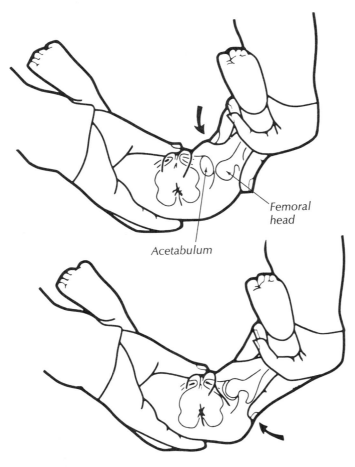

Femoral
head

Acetabulum

(Reproduced with permission from Burnside JW: Physical Diagnosis: An Introduction to Clinical Medicine, 16th ed, p 246. Baltimore, Williams & Wilkins, 1981)

Massive defects in the spine, such as meningomyelocele, are quite obvious at birth, but others that may lead to serious consequences present more subtly.

Palpate the spine carefully, particularly in the lumbosacral region, to determine if there are any deformities of the vertebra or any abnormalities of the overlying skin, pigmented spots, hairy patches, or deep pits that might overlie external openings of sinus tracts that extend to the spinal canal.

Spina bifida occulta (a defect of the vertebral bodies) may be associated with defects of the underlying spinal cord (*diastematomyelia*) that can cause malfunctioning of the bladder and rectum and weakness or paralyses of the lower extremities. A sinus tract provides potential entry to the spinal canal of organisms that can cause meningitis.

Early and Late Childhood

From both in front and behind, watch the child standing upright. You can often detect the presence of musculoskeletal difficulties in this age group by closely observing the child in various postures from the front and the rear (*e.g.,* **while the child is standing upright with the feet together, walking, stooping to obtain an object from the floor, rising from the supine position, and touching the toes or the shins while standing).**

In childhood the thoracic convexity is decreased and the lumbar concavity increased. Lordosis is common and rarely causes symptoms.

Test for severe hip disease with its associated weakness of the gluteus medius muscle by observing the child from behind as the weight is shifted from one leg to the other. The pelvis remains level when the weight is borne on the unaffected side (negative Trendelenburg sign).

The pelvis tilts toward the unaffected hip when weight is borne on the affected side (positive Trendelenburg sign).

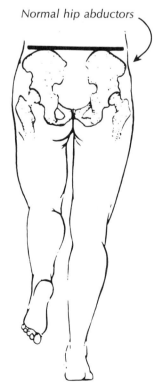

Normal hip abductors

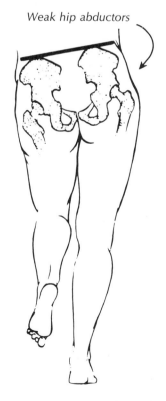

Weak hip abductors

(Reproduced with permission from Chung SMR: Hip Disorders in Infants and Children, p. 65. Philadelphia, Lea & Febiger, 1981)

Determine any *leg shortening* in hip disease by comparing the distance from the anterior superior spine of the ilium to the medial malleolus on each side (see p. 490).

When you suspect *scoliosis* (see p. 500), ask the child to bend forward. Mark the spinous processes with a felt-tip pen. After the child stands erect, look for a curve in the line of ink dots.

THE NERVOUS SYSTEM

Infancy

Neurologic screening includes assessment of positioning, spontaneous and induced movements, cry, and knee and ankle jerk responses, and elicitation of the rooting, grasp, tonic neck, and Moro automatisms. It should be performed on all newborns. Babies showing abnormalities in these areas and those at risk for central nervous system disease should be completely assessed neurologically at frequent intervals.

The findings during the neurologic examination in infancy, especially in the newborn period, differ markedly from those present in children and adults.

The central nervous system at birth is underdeveloped and functions at subcortical levels. Cortical function develops slowly after birth and cannot be tested entirely until early childhood. Thus, in the newborn period and early infancy, findings of normal brainstem and spinal functioning do not ensure an intact cortical system, and abnormalities of the brainstem and spinal cord may exist without concomitant cortical abnormalities. A number of specific reflex activities (*infantile automatisms*) are found in the normal newborn that disappear in early infancy.

The absence of infantile automatisms in the neonate or the persistence of some beyond their expected time of disappearance may indicate severe central nervous system dysfunction.

The neurologic examination in infancy will enable the clinician to detect extensive disease of the central nervous system, but will be of little use in pinpointing minute lesions and specific functional deficits.

The general appearance, positioning, activity, cry, and alertness of the newborn baby should be noted, because these observations are important in the neurologic assessment of this age group.

Test for *motor function* by putting each major joint through its range of motion to determine whether normal muscle tone, spasticity, or flaccidity is present.

Postural indications of severe intracranial disease include persistent asymmetries, predominant extension of the extremities, and constant turning of the head to one side. Marked extension of the head, stiffness of the neck, and extension of the arms and legs (*opisthotonus*) indicate severe meningeal or brainstem irritation, seen in in-

Beyond the newborn period, throughout infancy, specific *gross and fine motor coordination testing* can be done using an age-appropriate protocol, such as the *Denver Developmental Screening Test* (see pp. 571–572). This test also assesses social and language development. Discrepancies in achievement in the motor and communication areas may suggest whether the deficit is in the motor, sensory, or intellectual spheres. Knowledge of when developmental landmarks are normally achieved is essential in assessing the function of the infant's nervous system.

tracranial infection or hemorrhage (see figure below).

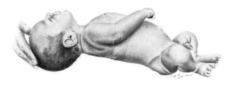

(Redrawn from Paine RS: Neurological examination of infants and children. Pediatr Clin North Am 7:477, 1960)

The *sensory examination* for infants is rather limited in terms of defining neurologic disease. Thresholds of touch, pain, and temperature are higher in older children, and reactions to these stimuli are relatively slow.

Gently touch the baby's arms and legs with a pin, and observe movement of the stimulated extremity or change in the facial expression. If the pin is used vigorously enough, crying will result. Discard the pin after each examination!

The *cranial nerves* are tested in infancy as in the adult. The difficulties encountered in assessing the function of the 2nd and 8th nerves have already been mentioned.

The 12th nerve is easily tested. Pinch the nostrils of the infant. This produces a reflex opening of the mouth and raising of the tip of the tongue.

Because the corticospinal pathways are not fully developed in infants, the *spinal reflex mechanisms* (deep tendon reflexes and plantar response) during infancy are variable. Their exaggerated presence, or their absence, has very little diagnostic significance unless this response is different from that in a previous testing.

The technique for eliciting these reflexes is similar to that used with adults, except that your semiflexed index or middle finger can substitute for the neurologic hammer, its tip acting as the striking point. Your thumbnail may be used to elicit the plantar response.

The *Babinski response* to plantar stimulation can be elicited in some normal infants, and sometimes until 2 years of age. However, a flexion response to plantar stimulation is elicited in more than 90% of normal newborns. The *triceps reflex* is usually not present until after 6 months of age. Rapid, rhythmic plantar flexion of the foot in response to eliciting of the ankle reflex (*ankle clonus*) is common in newborns; as many as eight to ten such contractions in response to one stimulus may occur normally (*unsustained ankle clonus*).

Absence of withdrawal when a painful stimulus is applied to an extremity indicates anesthesia or paralysis. If a facial expression or a cry changes in the absence of withdrawal, paralysis rather than anesthesia is indicated. With spinal cord lesions the extremity withdraws reflexly in response to pain but the baby's facial expression or cry will not change.

If *12th nerve paresis* is present, the tongue tip will deviate toward the affected side.

When the contractions are continuous (*sustained ankle clonus*), severe central nervous system disease should be suspected.

You can also elicit ankle clonus by pressing your thumb over the ball of the infant's foot and abruptly dorsiflexing the foot.

The *abdominal reflexes* are absent in the newborn but appear within the first 6 months of life. The *anal reflex*, however, is normally present in newborns and is important to elicit when spinal cord lesions are present or suspected.

With the baby supine, straighten and raise the lower legs, stroke the perianal region with a paper clip, and observe the external anal sphincter contract.

An absent anal reflex strongly suggests loss of innervation of the external sphincter muscle due to a spinal cord lesion at the level of the lower sacral segments (or higher), such as a congenital anomaly (*spina bifida*), a tumor, or an injury.

INFANTILE AUTOMATISMS

The infantile automatisms are reflex phenomena present at birth or appearing shortly thereafter. Some remain only a few weeks while others persist well into the second year of life. Automatisms have prognostic value for central nervous system integrity. Eliciting any of them (except the rooting, grasp, tonic neck, and Moro responses) should be attempted only when central nervous system function is questionable. Each automatism is listed here with the method of elicitation and the prognostic significance of its presence or absence. All are present at birth unless otherwise indicated. The time of disappearance is also listed.

Blinking (Dazzle) Reflex. Disappears after first year. The eyelids close in response to bright light.

Absence may indicate blindness.

Acoustic Blink (Cochleopalpebral) Reflex. Disappearance time is variable. Both eyes blink in response to a sharp loud noise.

Absence may indicate decreased hearing.

Palmar Grasp Reflex. Disappears at 3 or 4 months

With the baby's head positioned in the midline and the arms semiflexed, place your index fingers from the ulnar side into the baby's hands and press against the palmar surfaces. The baby responds by flexing all of its fingers to grasp your fingers. This method allows for comparison of both hands. If the reflex is absent or weak, you can enhance it by offering the baby a bottle, since sucking facilitates grasping.

Persistence of the grasp reflex beyond 4 months suggests cerebral dysfunction. It should be noted that babies normally clench their hands during the first month of life. Persistence of the clenched hand beyond 2 months also suggests central nervous system damage.

Stroke the ulnar surface of the hand and fifth finger lightly to produce extension of the thumb and other fingers (*digital response reflex*). This is not classified as an infantile automatism. It disappears at 3 or 4 months

Rooting Reflex. Disappears at 3 or 4 months; may be present longer during sleep

Absence of this reflex indicates severe generalized or central nervous system disease.

With the baby's head positioned in the midline and the hands held against the anterior chest, stroke with your forefinger the perioral skin at the corners of the baby's mouth and at the midline of the upper and lower lips.

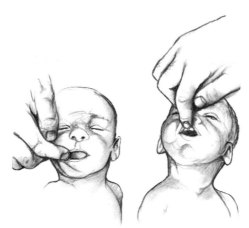

In response, the mouth will open and turn to the stimulated side. When the upper lip is stimulated, the head will extend; when the lower lip is stimulated, the jaw will drop. This response will also occur when the infant's cheek is stimulated at some distance from the corners of the mouth.

Trunk Incurvation (Galant's) Reflex. Disappears at 2 months

Transverse spinal cord lesions may be detected by testing for the presence of this reflex. It is absent in transverse spinal cord lesions or injuries.

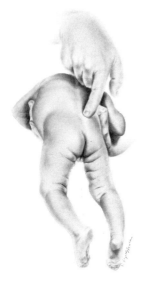

Hold the baby horizontally and prone in one of your hands. Stimulate one side of the baby's back approximately 1 cm from the midline along a paravertebral line extending from the shoulder to the buttocks. This produces a curving of the trunk toward the stimulated side, with shoulders and pelvis moving in that direction.

(Redrawn from Paine RS: Neurological examination of infants and children. Pediatr Clin North Am 7:490, 1960)

Vertical Suspension Positioning. Disappears after 4 months

While you support the baby upright with your hands under the axillae, the head is normally maintained in the midline and the legs are flexed at the hips and knees.

Fixed extension and adduction of the legs (scissoring) indicates *spastic paraplegia* or *diplegia,* as shown on p. 630.

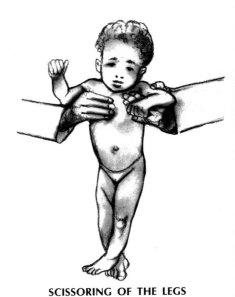

SCISSORING OF THE LEGS

Placing Response. Best elicited after the first 4 days. Disappearance time is variable.

Hold the baby upright from behind by placing your hands under the baby's arms with your thumbs supporting the back of the head, and allow the dorsal surface of one foot to touch the undersurface of a table top. This procedure is demonstrated below.

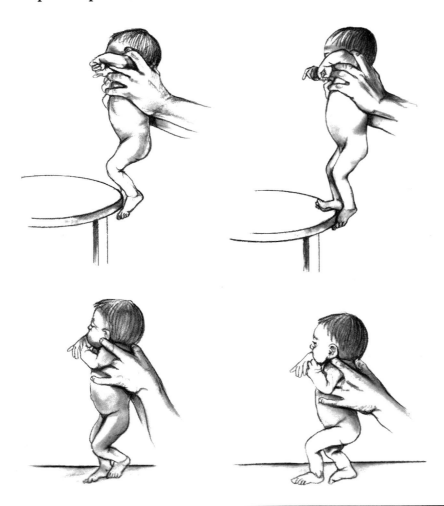

Take care not to plantar flex the foot. The baby responds by flexing the hip and knee and placing the stimulated foot on the table top. Repeat the process, stimulating the other foot. With one foot placed on the table, the opposite leg steps forward and a series of alternate stepping movements occurs as you move the baby gently forward.

These responses are absent when paresis is present and in babies born by breech delivery.

Rotation Test. Disappearance time is variable.

Hold the baby under the axillae, at arm's length facing you, and turn him or her in one direction and then the other. The head turns in the direction in which you turn the baby. If you restrain the head with your thumbs, the baby's eyes will turn in the direction in which you turned (see figure on p. 595).

The head and eyes do not move in the presence of vestibular dysfunction. *Strabismus* may be detected early with this maneuver.

Tonic Neck Reflex. May be present at birth but usually appears at 2 months and disappears at 6 months

With the baby supine, as shown below, turn the head to one side, holding the jaw over the baby's shoulder. The arm and the leg on the side to which the head is turned extend, while the opposite arm and leg flex. This response does not normally occur each time this maneuver is performed.

When this reflex is elicited every time it is evoked, it should be considered abnormal, at any age. It will persist beyond the time of expected disappearance in major cerebral damage.

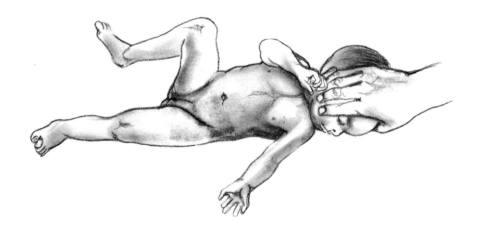

Two mass reflexes occur in the presence of normal subcortical mechanisms that are not yet under significant inhibitory control from higher cerebral centers. They are present at birth and disappear by the third month.

Perez Reflex. Suspend the baby prone in one of your hands. Place the thumb of your other hand on the baby's sacrum and move it firmly

Absence of either reflex during the first 3 months of life indicates severe cerebral insult, injury to the upper cervical cord, advanced anterior horn cell disease, or severe myopathy.

toward the head along the entire length of the spine. Extension of the head and spine, flexion of the knees on the abdomen, a cry, and emptying of the bladder are the usual responses.

The last part of the response occurs with sufficient frequency to be useful in the collection of urine specimens from neonates.

Moro Response (Startle Reflex). **You can produce the Moro response in several ways:**

- **Hold the baby in the supine position, supporting the head, back, and legs. Then suddenly lower the entire body about 2 feet and stop abruptly, as shown below.**

Persistence of the Moro response beyond 4 months may indicate neurologic disease; persistence beyond 6 months is almost conclusive evidence of such. An asymmetrical response in the upper extremities suggests hemiparesis, injury to the brachial plexus, or fracture of the clavicle or humerus. Low spinal injury and congenital dislocation of the hip may produce absence of the response in one or both legs.

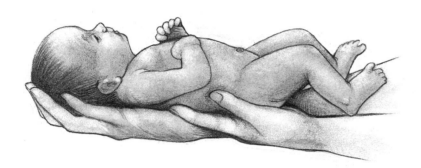

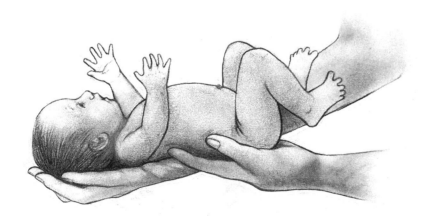

- **Lift the supine baby's head to an angle approximately 30° from the examining table. Suddenly release your grip and allow the head to fall backward, catching it before it hits the table.**
- **Hold the baby supine, supporting the back and pelvis with one hand and arm and the head with the other hand. Then allow the head to drop several centimeters with a sudden, rapid movement.**
- **Produce a loud noise (*e.g.,* strike the examining table with the palms of your hands on both sides of the baby's head).**

The response itself is one in which the arms briskly abduct and extend with the hands open and fingers extended, and the legs flex slightly and abduct (but less so than the arms). The arms then return forward over the body in a clasping maneuver and the baby cries simultaneously.

GENERAL INDICATORS OF CENTRAL NERVOUS SYSTEM DISEASE

The following *general findings in infancy* should suggest to the clinician the presence of central nervous system disease:

1. Abnormal localized neurologic findings
2. Failure to elicit expected responses
3. Asymmetry of normal responses
4. Late persistence of normal responses
5. Reemergence of vanished responses
6. Developmental delays

Certain combinations of findings in infancy suggest specific diagnoses. In a baby with a history of jaundice in the neonatal period, the presence of the setting sun sign, opisthotonos, and a disappearing or absent Moro response suggest *kernicterus.*

In *congenital hemiplegia,* unilaterally absent or diminished movement of an extremity, along with abnormal posturing, is seen. Reflexes and muscle tone may be normal.

Bilateral cerebral injury produces hypotonia with normal or brisk deep tendon reflexes, delay in reaching motor milestones, and persistence of the tonic neck reflex.

Early and Late Childhood

Beyond infancy when the infantile automatisms have disappeared, the neurologic examination is conducted much like the adult examination. Samples of handwriting and figure drawing with both hands help to detect fine motor defects. Capacities for stereognosis, vibration, position, two-point discrimination, number identification, and extinction are not usually testable in the child under 3 years of age and in many under 5 years. The gait should be observed with the child both walking and running. Asymmetric arm movements in walking or running may indicate a hemiparesis, as may unequal wear of the soles and heels on the child's shoes. There are also localized neurologic and orthopedic conditions that may produce unequal shoe wear.

Observe the child rising from the floor from a supine position so that you can note the manner in which the muscles of the neck, trunk,

The *spastic diplegias* produce variable dystonic spasms, followed by hypertonia early in infancy and persistent clenched fists coupled with scissoring after the first few months.

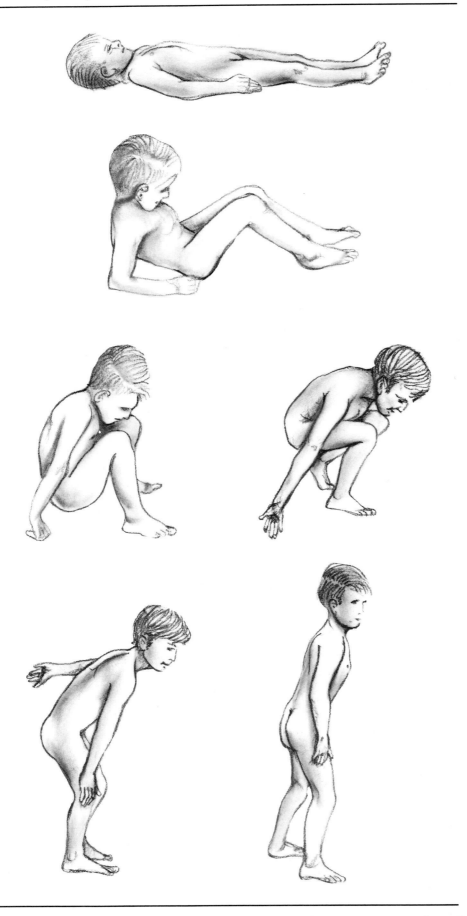

In certain forms of *muscular dystrophy* with pelvic girdle weaknesses, rising from a supine to a standing position is accomplished as shown below (*Gowers's sign*).

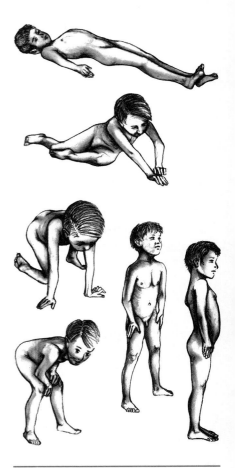

arms, and legs are used to assume first the sitting position and then the standing position (see figures on facing page).

Evidence of neurologic deficits, muscular weaknesses, and orthopedic defects may be detected here that would not otherwise be noted.

When there is nystagmus, unsteady gait, or history of streptomycin therapy, *vestibular function* should be tested. This is accomplished with the *cold caloric test*.

The absence of nystagmus occurs with 8th nerve damage from *drug toxicity, meningitis* or *brain tumor,* or *labyrinthitis.*

Inject ice water into the external auditory canal with an ear syringe. Observe for nystagmus, which should occur within 30 seconds.

At All Ages

In essence, the complete neurologic examination in infancy and childhood includes elements of all parts of the general physical examination as well as the specific components of the neurologic examination outlined here. The clinician is constantly assessing neurologic functioning throughout the course of every patient encounter. All the observations made and impressions gained are used to determine the integrity of the central and peripheral nervous systems. This is equally true in the examination of adults.

Chapter 20
Clinical Thinking: From Data to Plan

Like colors on an artist's palette, clinical data lack form and meaning. The clinician must not only gather data through interviewing and examination; he or she must also analyze them, identify the patient's problems, evaluate the patient's responses to the illness, and, together with the patient, formulate a plan to deal with the situation. This chapter describes this sequence of activities and focuses on the clinical thinking that underlies it.

FROM DATA BASE TO PLAN

Since the introduction of the problem-oriented system of recordkeeping, certain terms have gained wide acceptance. Information given by the patient, or possibly by family members or significant others, is called *subjective data*. *Objective data* include two kinds of information: physical findings and laboratory reports. Since both physical examination and laboratory work are human activities, they too, admittedly, involve subjective elements, and, as we shall see later, all kinds of data are subject to error. A comprehensive set of subjective and objective data, such as you might gather in evaluating a new patient, makes up a *data base* for that patient.

In recording the data base you should describe your findings as accurately as possible, whether they relate to what the patient tells you or to what you observe. Although inference and interpretation inevitably affect the organization of your materials, statements in the data base should describe, not interpret. Thus, "late inspiratory crackles at the bases of both lungs" is appropriate, while "signs of congestive heart failure" is not.

In the *assessment* process, however, you go beyond perception and description to analysis and interpretation. Here you select and cluster relevant pieces of data, think about their possible meanings, and try to explain them logically. For example, a patient's complaint of a "scratchy throat" and "stuffy nose," together with your observations of a swollen nasal mucosa and slight redness of the pharynx, give you the subjective and objective data on which to base a presumptive diagnosis of viral nasopharyngitis.

Assessment also includes the patient's responses to the illness and to your diagnostic and therapeutic ideas. What are the patient's feelings, concerns, questions, and goals?

Once you have made these assessments, you are ready to work out a *plan* with the patient. In the problem-oriented record system, this plan has three parts: diagnostic, therapeutic, and educational. For example, you might decide on a throat culture, a decongestant for the patient's stuffy nose, cautionary advice against overfatigue, and a brief review of upper respiratory infections, their causes, and their modes of transmission.

Defining part of the plan as "educational" has one misleading connotation—that the process of communication is unidirectional. It should not be. The patient should participate in making the plan. Appropriate "education" depends on what the patient already knows and wants to know. Give the patient an opportunity to tell you. Other parts of the plan may well be influenced by the patient's goals, economic means, and competing responsibilities, and the opinions of family or friends—to name just a few variables. Establishing a successful plan requires interviewing skills and interpersonal sensitivity, not just knowledge of diagnostic and therapeutic techniques.

The diagram below summarizes the sequence from data base to plan. The effects of the assessment process on the data base, as implied by the bidirectional arrows between them, are discussed later in the chapter.

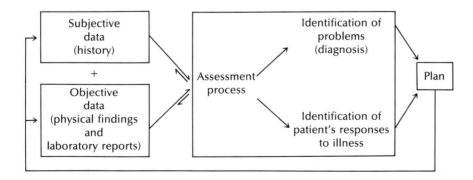

After a plan has been implemented, the process recycles. The clinician gathers more data, assesses the patient's progress, modifies the problem list if indicated, and adjusts the plan appropriately.

ASSESSMENT: THE PROCESS OF CLINICAL THINKING

Because assessment takes place in the clinician's mind, its processes often seem inaccessible, even mysterious, to the beginning student. Experienced clinicians, moreover, think so quickly, with little overt or conscious effort, that they sometimes have difficulty in explaining their own logic. They also think in different ways, with different, individualistic personal styles. Some general principles underlie this analytic process, however, and certain explicit steps may help you to think constructively and purposefully about your data. The thinking process starts at the beginning of your patient encounter, not at the end, but assume for the moment that you already have a data base to consider. You must answer the questions, "What is wrong with the patient? What are the problems?" To do so, try the following steps:

- *Identify the abnormal findings* in the patient's data base. Make a list of the *symptoms* noted by the patient, the *signs* that you observed on physical examination, and any *laboratory reports* that are available to you.

- *Localize these findings anatomically.* This step may be easy. The symptom of scratchy throat and the sign of a reddened pharynx, for example, clearly localize a problem in the pharynx. Other data, however, present greater difficulty. Chest pain, for example, might originate in the heart, the pleural surfaces, the esophagus, or the musculoskeletal system. If the pain consistently occurs with exercise and disappears with rest, either the heart or the musculoskeletal system is probably involved. If the patient notes pain only when carrying groceries with the left arm, the musculoskeletal system becomes the likely culprit. Be as explicit in your localization as your data allow, but no more so. You may have to settle for a body region (*e.g.,* the chest) or a body system (*e.g.,* the musculoskeletal system), or you may be able to define the exact structure involved (*e.g.,* left pectoral muscle). Some symptoms and signs, such as fatigue or fever, have no localizing value but may be useful in the next step, interpreting probable process.

- *Interpret the findings in terms of the probable process.* A patient's problem may stem from a *pathological* process involving a bodily structure. There are a number of such processes, variably classified, including congenital, inflammatory, immunologic, neoplastic, metabolic, nutritional, degenerative, vascular, traumatic, and toxic. Other problems are *pathophysiological,* such as increased gastrointestinal motility or congestive heart failure, while others still are *psychopathological,* such as a disorder of mood or of thought processes. Redness and pain are two of the four classic signs of inflammation, and a red, painful throat, even without the other two signs—heat and swelling—strongly suggests an inflammatory process in the pharynx.

- *Make one or more hypotheses about the nature of the patient's problem.* Here you will have to draw on all the knowledge and experience you can muster, and it is here that reading will be most helpful in learning about abnormalities and diseases. Until your experience and knowledge broaden you may not be able to reach highly explicit hypotheses, but proceed as far as you can with the data and knowledge you have. The following steps should help:

1. *Select the most specific and central findings* around which to construct your hypothesis. If a patient reports loss of appetite, nausea, vomiting, fatigue, and fever, for example, and if you find a tender, somewhat enlarged liver and mild jaundice, build your hypothesis around jaundice and hepatomegaly rather than fatigue and fever. Although the other symptoms are useful diagnostically, they are much less specific.

2. Using your inferences about the structures and processes involved, *match your findings against all the conditions you know that can produce them.* For example, you can match your patient's red throat with a list of inflammatory conditions affecting the pharynx; or you can compare the symptoms and signs of the jaundiced patient with the various inflammatory, toxic, and neoplastic conditions that might produce this kind of clinical picture.

3. *Eliminate the diagnostic possibilities that fail to explain the findings.* You might consider conjunctivitis as a cause of the patient's red eye, for example, but eliminate this possibility because it does not explain the dilated pupil or decreased visual acuity. Acute glaucoma would explain all these findings.

4. *Weigh the competing possibilities* and *select the most likely diagnosis* from among the conditions that might be responsible for the patient's findings. You are looking, of course, for a *close match* between the patient's clinical presentation and a typical case of a given condition. Other clues help in this selection too. The *statistical probability* of a given disease in a patient of this age, sex, race, habits, lifestyle, and locality should have major impact on your selection. You should consider the possibilities of osteoarthritis and metastatic prostatic cancer in a 70-year-old man with back pain, for example, but not in a 25-year-old woman with the same complaint. The *timing of the patient's illness* also makes a difference. Productive cough, purulent sputum, fever, and chest pain that develop acutely over 24 hours suggest quite a different problem than do identical symptoms that develop over 3 or 4 months. In making a tentative diagnosis, you can seldom reach certainty but must often settle for the most probable explanation. Such is the real world of applied science.

5. Finally, in considering possible explanations for a patient's problem, give special attention to *potentially life-threatening and treatable* conditions such as meningococcal meningitis, bacterial endocarditis, or subdural hematoma. Here you are trying to minimize the risk of missing conditions that may occur less frequently or be less probable but that, if present, would be particularly important.

- Once you have made a hypothesis about a patient's problem, you will usually want to *test that hypothesis.* You may need further history, additional maneuvers on physical examination, or laboratory studies to confirm or rule out your tentative diagnosis. When the diagnosis seems clear-cut—a simple upper respiratory infection, for example, or a case of hives—this step may not be necessary.

- You should then be ready to *establish a working definition of the problem.* Make this at the highest level of explicitness and certainty that the data allow. You may be limited here to a symptom, such as "pleuritic chest pain, cause unknown." At other times you can define a problem explicitly in terms of structure, process, and cause. Examples include "pneumococcal pneumonia, right lower lobe," and "hypertensive cardiovascular disease with left ventricular enlargement, congestive heart failure, and sinus tachycardia."

DIFFICULTIES AND VARIATIONS

LIMITATIONS OF THE MEDICAL MODEL. Although medical diagnosis is based primarily on identifying abnormal structures, disturbed processes, and specific causes, you will frequently see patients whose complaints do not fall neatly into these categories. Some symptoms defy analysis, and you may never be able to move beyond simple descriptive categories such as "fatigue" or "anorexia." Other problems relate to the patient's life rather than to the body. Loss of a job or loved one threatens a person, for example, and may increase the risk of subsequent illness. Identifying such life events, evaluating a person's responses to them, and working out a plan to help the person cope with them are just as appropriate as dealing with the pharyngitis or duodenal ulcer. Some people, moreover, seek health care to maintain their health, not to detect and correct a disease. For them, and most others, in fact, "health maintenance" becomes a legitimate item on a list of "problems," and plans may include, for example, updating immunizations, advice on nutrition, exploring feelings about an important life event, and recommendations for seat belts or exercise.

SINGLE VERSUS MULTIPLE PROBLEMS. One of the greatest difficulties faced by the student is deciding whether to cluster the patient's symptoms and signs into one or into several problems. The patient's *age* may help, since young people are more likely to have single diseases while older people tend to have multiple ones. The *timing* of symptoms is frequently useful. An episode of pharyngitis 6 weeks ago is probably unrelated to fever, chills, chest pain, and cough today. To use timing effectively, you need to know the natural history of various diseases. A yellowish discharge from the penis followed in 3 weeks by a painless penile ulcer, for example, suggests two problems, gonorrhea and primary syphilis. A penile ulcer followed in 6 weeks by a maculopapular skin rash and generalized lymphadenopathy, on the other hand, suggests two stages of the same problem: primary and secondary syphilis.

Involvement of *different body systems* may help you to cluster the items of data. While symptoms and signs within a single system can often be explained by one disease, manifestations in different, apparently unrelated systems frequently require more than one explanation. Again, a knowledge of disease patterns is necessary. You might decide, for example, to group a patient's high blood pressure and sustained thrusting apical impulse together with the flame-shaped retinal hemorrhages, place them in the cardiovascular system, and label the constellation "hypertensive cardiovascular disease with hypertensive retinopathy." You will probably develop another explanation for the diarrhea and left lower quadrant tenderness.

Some diseases affect more than one body system. As you gain in knowledge and experience, you will become increasingly adept at recognizing such *multisystem conditions* and at building plausible explanations that link together their seemingly unrelated manifestations. In trying to explain the productive cough, hemoptysis, and weight loss reported by a 60-year-old man who has smoked cigarettes for 40 years, you probably even now would postulate lung cancer as a likely cause. You might even support this hypothesis by your observation of clubbed fingernails. With time you will also recognize that his other symptoms and signs can be linked to the same diagnosis. The dysphagia is caused by extension of the cancer to his esophagus; the pupillary inequality is a Horner's syndrome caused by pressure on the cervical sympathetic chain; and the jaundice results from metastases to the liver.

In another case of multisystem disease, a man's fever, weight loss, chronic diarrhea, dysphagia, white-coated tongue, generalized lymphadenopathy, and purplish skin nodules can all be explained by AIDS. The clinician who has not already explored his risk factors for this disease should do so.

AN UNMANAGEABLE ARRAY OF DATA. In trying to understand a patient's problems, the clinician often is confronted with a relatively long list of symptoms and signs and an equally long list of potential explanations or labels. As already suggested, you can tease out separate clusters of observations and deal with them one cluster at a time.

You can also analyze a given group of observations by asking key questions, the answers to which steer your thinking in one direction and allow you to ignore others temporarily. For example, you may ask what produces and relieves a person's chest pain. If the answer is exercise and rest respectively, you can concentrate on the cardiovascular system (and possibly the musculoskeletal system as well) and put aside the gastrointestinal tract. If the pain results from eating quickly and is relieved by regurgitating the food, you logically concentrate on the upper gastrointestinal tract. A series of such discriminating questions forms a branching logic tree or algorithm and is helpful in collecting data, analyzing them, and reaching conclusions that probably explain them.

QUALITY OF THE DATA. Virtually all the information with which the clinician works is subject to error. Patients forget symptoms, misremember the sequence in which they occurred, hide important but embarrassing facts, and shape their stories toward what interviewers seem to want to hear. Clinicians misunderstand their patients, overlook some relevant information, fail to ask the one key question, jump to premature diagnostic conclusions, or forget to examine the genitals of a patient with asymptomatic testicular carcinoma. You can avoid some of these errors by being thorough, by keeping an open mind as you gather data, and by analyzing any mistakes that you might make. Clinical data, however, including laboratory work, are inherently imperfect. The quality of information may be judged by its accuracy, precision, sensitivity, specificity, and predictive value.

Accuracy refers to the closeness with which a measurement reflects the true value of an object. *Precision,* on the other hand, refers to the reproducibility of a measurement.* These terms are illustrated below by four attempts to hit a target, at the center of which lies "truth."

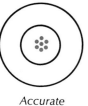

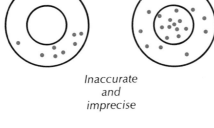

Accurate and precise	Inaccurate but precise	Inaccurate and imprecise

Note that a measurement may be quite precise and inaccurate at the same time, as shown in the second example. In the example on the far right the average of a large number of measurements would be accurate, but because of the imprecision an individual measurement cannot be so considered. In the usual clinical setting both of the imprecise examples, therefore, would have to be considered inaccurate.

Estimates of liver size by percussion illustrate these principles. The fact that such estimates vary between 2 cm and 3 cm depending on the force of percussion demonstrates that liver percussion is not an especially precise technique. The fact that percussion leads to smaller estimates of liver size than do radioisotope liver scans suggests that it is not very accurate either. Even so, percussion provides a better estimate than palpation alone.

Sensitivity of an observation or a test refers to its ability to identify persons with a certain disease or condition among a group of people all

---

* Definitions of these and similar terms vary with the discipline in which they are used. Accuracy, as used here, might also be considered as validity, precision as reliability.

of whom have that particular condition. When an observation fails to identify the abnormality in a person who has it, the result is called falsely negative. A highly sensitive test or observation detects most of the people with a given condition (the true positives) and has few false negatives.

Specificity of an observation or test refers to its ability to identify correctly those people who do *not* have the condition. A test that is 95% specific correctly identifies 95 out of 100 normal people. The other 5 are false positives.

Heart murmurs provide good examples of sensitivity and specificity. The vast majority of patients with significant valvular aortic stenosis have systolic murmurs audible in the aortic area. A systolic murmur is, therefore, quite a sensitive criterion for valvular aortic stenosis. When auscultation for an aortic systolic murmur is used to detect this condition, it finds most of the cases and misses only a few. The false negative rate is low. Such a murmur, however, sorely lacks specificity. Many other conditions, such as increased blood flow across a normal valve or the sclerotic changes associated with aging, may also produce this kind of murmur. If you were to use an aortic systolic murmur as your sole criterion for aortic stenosis, you would falsely label many patients as having it, thus producing many false positives. In contrast, the high-pitched decrescendo diastolic murmur heard best along the left sternal border is a murmur quite specific for aortic regurgitation. Normal people virtually never have such a murmur, and other conditions that might cause a similar sound are uncommon. The specificity of this murmur is very high.

Both sensitivity and specificity of an observation are determined in very atypical situations; either all or none of the people observed or tested have the disease in question. In the usual clinical setting, in contrast, a few of the patients may have this disease and probably most do not. The clinician who has made an observation—either positive or negative—wants to know how well this finding predicts the true condition of the patient. Predictive values give this information.

The *positive predictive value* of an observation or a test is the characteristic that is most relevant to the clinical setting. It refers to the proportion of positive observations that accurately predict the presence of a condition in a given population. In a group of women found to have suspicious breast nodules in a cancer screening program, for example, the proportion later determined to have breast cancer would constitute the positive predictive value of "suspicious nodules."

The *negative predictive value* of an observation or a test refers to the proportion of negative observations that accurately predict the absence of a condition in a population. In a screening program for breast cancer, the proportion of women without suspicious nodules who really have no breast cancer constitutes the negative predictive value of the observation.

Predictive values depend in part on sensitivity and specificity but, unlike them, depend heavily on the prevalence of the condition within the population. Despite unchanging sensitivity and specificity, the positive predictive value of an observation rises with prevalence while the negative predictive value falls.

All these terms can be illustrated with the help of a 2 × 2 table that shows the results of an observation, either positive or negative, in a group of people some of whom have a disease and some of whom do not. In the case below, an observation with a sensitivity of 95% and a specificity of 90% is used in a group of 200 people, half of whom have the disease.

Note that the numbers related to sensitivity and specificity are traditionally located in the left and right columns respectively and are indicated here by vertical red bars. Numbers related to positive and negative predictive values are found in the upper and lower rows respectively and are indicated by horizontal bars.

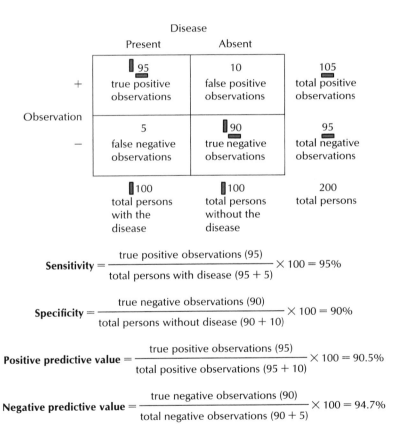

$$\text{Sensitivity} = \frac{\text{true positive observations (95)}}{\text{total persons with disease (95 + 5)}} \times 100 = 95\%$$

$$\text{Specificity} = \frac{\text{true negative observations (90)}}{\text{total persons without disease (90 + 10)}} \times 100 = 90\%$$

$$\text{Positive predictive value} = \frac{\text{true positive observations (95)}}{\text{total positive observations (95 + 10)}} \times 100 = 90.5\%$$

$$\text{Negative predictive value} = \frac{\text{true negative observations (90)}}{\text{total negative observations (90 + 5)}} \times 100 = 94.7\%$$

Two examples further illustrate these principles and show how predictive values vary with prevalence. Consider first an imaginary population *A* with 1000 people. The prevalence of disease X in this population is high—40%. You can quickly calculate that 400 of these people have X. You then set out to detect these cases with an observation that is 90% sensitive and 80% specific. Of the 400 people with X, the observation detects .90 × 400, or 360 (the true positives). It misses the other 40 (400 − 360, the false negatives). Out of the 600 people without X, the observation proves negative in .80 × 600, or 480. These people are truly free of X, as the observation suggests (the true negatives). But the observation misleads you in the remaining 120 (600 − 480). These people are falsely labeled as having X when they are really free of it (the false positives). These figures are summarized below:

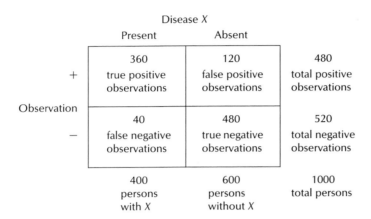

As a clinician who does not have perfect knowledge of who really does or does not have disease X, you are faced with a total of 480 people with positive observations. You must try to distinguish between the true and the false positives, and will undoubtedly use additional kinds of data to help you in this task. Given only the sensitivity and specificity of your observation, however, you can determine the probability that a positive observation is a true positive, and you may wish to explain it to the concerned patient. This probability is calculated as follows:

$$\text{Positive predictive value} = \frac{\text{true positives (360)}}{\text{total positives (360 + 120)}} \times 100 = 75\%$$

Thus 3 out of 4 of the persons with positive observations really have the disease and 1 out of 4 does not.

By a similar calculation, you can determine the probability that a negative observation is a true negative. The results here are reasonably reassuring to the involved patient:

$$\text{Negative predictive value} = \frac{\text{true negatives (480)}}{\text{total negatives (480 + 40)}} \times 100 = 92\%$$

As prevalence of the disease in a population diminishes, however, the predictive value of a positive observation diminishes remarkably while the predictive value of a negative observation, already fairly good in population A, rises further. Consider a second population, B, of 1000 people, only 1% of whom have disease X. Now there are only 10 cases of

X and 990 people without X. If this population is screened with the same observation, which has a 90% sensitivity and an 80% specificity, here are the results:

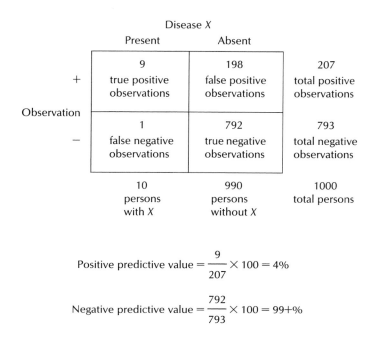

$$\text{Positive predictive value} = \frac{9}{207} \times 100 = 4\%$$

$$\text{Negative predictive value} = \frac{792}{793} \times 100 = 99+\%$$

You are now confronted with possibly upsetting 207 people (all those with positive observations) in order to detect 9 out of the 10 real cases. The predictive value of a positive observation is only 4%. Improving the specificity of your observation without diminishing its sensitivity would be very helpful, if it were possible. For example, if you could increase the specificity of the observation from 80% to 98% (given the same prevalence of 1% and sensitivity of 90%), the positive predictive value of the observation would improve from 4% to 31%—scarcely ideal but certainly better.

THE INTERPLAY OF ASSESSMENT AND DATA COLLECTION

The concepts of sensitivity and specificity help in both the collection and the analysis of data. They even underlie some of the basic strategies of interviewing. A question that is characterized by high sensitivity, if answered in the affirmative, may be particularly useful for screening and for gathering evidence to support a hypothesis. For example, "Have you had any discomfort or unpleasant feelings in your chest?" is a highly sensitive question for angina pectoris, and in patients with this condition would yield few falsely negative responses. It is a good first screening question, but because there are many other causes of chest discomfort it is not at all specific. With additional directed questions about location, quality, and duration of the discomfort, you can test further your hypothesis of angina pectoris. A pain that is retrosternal, pressing, and less than 10 minutes in duration—each a reasonably sensitive attribute of angina pectoris but not by itself specific—would add importantly to your growing evidence for the diagnosis. To confirm a hypothesis, a more specific question, if answered in the affirmative, is especially helpful. Precipitation of the pain by exercise and its prompt relief by rest are answers that serve this purpose.

Data with which to test a hypothesis come from the physical examination as well as from the history, and from both you can often screen, build your case, and clinch a diagnosis even before obtaining further diagnostic tests. Consider the following list of evidence: cough, fever, a shaking chill, left-sided chest pain that is aggravated by breathing, and dullness throughout the left lower posterior lung field with crackles, bronchial breathing, and increased voice sounds. Cough and fever are good screening items for pneumonia, the next items support the hypothesis, and bronchial breathing with increased voice sounds in this distribution is very specific for lobar pneumonia. A chest x-ray would confirm the diagnosis.

A negative response to a question or the absence of physical signs is also diagnostically useful, especially when the symptoms or signs are usually positive in a certain condition, *i.e.*, when they have a high sensitivity. For example, if a patient with cough and left-sided pleuritic chest pain does not have fever, bacterial pneumonia becomes much less likely (except possibly in infancy and old age). Likewise, in a patient with severe dyspnea, the absence of orthopnea makes left ventricular failure a less probable explanation for the shortness of breath.

Skilled clinicians use this kind of logic in making assessments whether or not they are conscious of its statistical underpinnings. They often start to generate tentative hypotheses from the patient's identifying data and the chief complaint, and then build evidence for one or more of these hypotheses and discard others as they ask questions and look for physical signs. In developing a present illness they borrow items from other parts of the history, such as the family history, the past history, and the review of systems. If a middle-aged patient complains of chest pain, the skilled clinician does not stop after determining the attributes of the pain. If the pain suggests coronary artery disease, further questions probe the risk factors for this condition such as smoking, high blood pressure, diabetes mellitus, and a family history of the disease. In both history and physical examination, the clinician also focuses explicitly on other possible manifestations of coronary artery disease, such as congestive heart failure, and on evidence of atherosclerosis elsewhere in the body, such as intermittent claudication and diminished or absent pulses in the legs. By generating hypotheses early and by testing them sequentially, experienced clinicians improve their efficiency and enhance the relevance and value of the data they collect. They dig and collect less ore but they find more gold.

Because prevalence strongly affects the predictive value of an observation, prevalence too influences the assessment process. Because coronary artery disease is much more common in middle-aged men than in young women, you should pursue angina as a cause of chest pain more actively in the former group. The effect of prevalence on predictive value explains why your odds of making a correct assessment are better when you hypothesize a common condition as opposed to a rare one. The combination of fever, headache, myalgias, and cough probably has the same sensitivity and specificity for influenza throughout the year, but your chance of making this diagnosis correctly by using this cluster of symptoms is much greater during a winter flu epidemic than it is during a quiet August.

Prevalence varies importantly with clinical setting as well as with season. Chronic bronchitis is probably the most common cause of hemoptysis among patients seen in a general medical clinic. In the oncology clinic of a tertiary medical center, however, lung cancer might head the list, while in a group of postoperative patients on a general surgical service irritation from an endotracheal tube or pulmonary infarction might be most likely. In certain parts of Asia, in contrast, one should think first of a worm called a lung fluke. When you hear hoofbeats in the distance, according to the familiar saying, bet on horses, not on zebras, unless of course you're visiting the zoo.

While there are enormous values in structuring your data collection so as to test hypotheses, there are also risks. First, initial judgments are often wrong. They allow you to overlook important data and may prevent you from entertaining other, possibly sounder hypotheses. Second, premature formulation of hypotheses may lead you to the premature asking of direct questions, and thus you may miss important parts of the patient's story. Third, focusing in on a single problem may lead you to incomplete assessment. Not every patient needs a complete evaluation, of course, but some have hypertension, some are seriously depressed, and some have cervical cancer. You cannot detect these problems unless you make the proper observations; to do so you have to be reasonably complete.

DEVELOPING A PROBLEM LIST AND PLAN

Turn now to the history and physical examination recorded for Mrs. N. in Chapter 21. Make a list of her symptoms and signs. Group these items together in a clinically rational way. Note that much of this clustering has already been done in constructing Mrs. N.'s present illness, since headache, nausea, vomiting, and psychological stress have all been placed together. You may or may not agree with this organization. Identify the problems to the degree that you can, and assess the patient's response to her illness.

Make a tentative problem list. In the problem-oriented record system, two parallel columns are used: active problems go on the left, inactive ones on the right. The problem list is placed at the front of the patient's clinical record, and all notes refer to these problems by name and number.

Date problem entered	No.	Active problems	Inactive problems
	1		

For each active problem, develop an initial plan insofar as you can. Some problems, of course, may need no immediate attention. Undoubtedly you will want more information in some areas. Make getting it part of your plan.

Chapter 21
The Patient's Record

The clinical record documents the patient's history and physical findings. It shows how clinicians assessed the problems, what plans they made on the patient's behalf, what actions they took, and how the patient responded to their efforts. An accurate, clear, well organized record reflects and facilitates sound clinical thinking. It leads to good communication among the many professionals who participate in caring for the patient, and helps to coordinate their activities. It also serves to document the patient's problems and health care for medicolegal purposes.

When creating a record, you do more than simply make a list of what the patient has told you and what you have found on examination. You must review your data, organize them, evaluate the importance and relevance of each item, and construct a clear, concise, yet comprehensive report. If you are a beginner, organizing the present illness will probably constitute one of the most difficult problems because considerable knowledge is needed to recognize which symptoms and signs are related to each other. That muscular weakness, heat intolerance, excessive sweating, diarrhea, and weight loss all constitute a present illness, for example, may not be apparent to either the patient or the student who is unfamiliar with hyperthyroidism. Until your knowledge and judgment grow, the patient's story itself and the seven key attributes of symptoms listed on page 17 are helpful guides.

Regardless of your experience, certain principles will help you to organize a good record. Order is imperative. Use it consistently and obviously so that future readers, including yourself, can easily find specific points of information. Keep items of history in the history, for example, and do not let them stray into the physical examination. Make your headings clear, use indentations and spacing to accentuate your organization, and asterisk or underline important points. Arrange the present illness in chronological order, starting with the current episode and then filling in the relevant background information. If a patient with long-standing diabetes is hospitalized in coma, for example, start with the events leading up to the coma and then summarize the past history of the diabetes.

The amount of detail to record often poses a vexing problem. As a student, you may wish (or you may be required) to be quite detailed, since doing so is one way to build your descriptive skills, vocabulary, and speed—admittedly a painful, tedious process. Pressures of time, however, will ultimately force some compromises. The following guidelines may be useful in choosing what to record and what to omit:

- *Record all the data—both positive and negative—that contribute directly to your assessment.* No diagnosis should be made, no problem identified, unless you have clearly spelled out the data upon which your assessment is based.

- *Describe specifically any pertinent negative information (i.e.,* the absence of a symptom or a sign) when other portions of the history or physical examination suggest that an abnormality might exist or develop in that area. For example, if the patient has large and unexplained bruises, you should specifically note the negative history for other kinds of bleeding, for injury and physical violence, for medications and nutritional deficits that might lead to bruising, and for familial bleeding disorders. If a patient feels depressed but not suicidal, state both facts. If the patient has no emotional problems, on the other hand, a comment on suicide is clearly unnecessary.

- *Data not recorded are data lost.* No matter how vividly you can recall a detail today, you will probably not remember it in a few months. The phrase "neurologic exam negative," even in your own handwriting, may leave you wondering a few months hence: "Did I really do a sensory exam?"

- On the other hand, information can be buried in a mass of excessive detail, to be discovered by only the most persistent reader. *Omit most of your negative findings* unless they relate directly to the patient's complaints or to specific exclusions in your diagnostic assessment. Do not try to list all the abnormalities that you did *not* observe. Instead, concentrate on a few major ones (such as "no heart murmurs") and try to describe structures in a concise, positive way. "Cervix pink and smooth" indicates that you saw no redness, ulcers, nodules, masses, cysts, or other suspicious lesions, but the description is shorter and much more readable. You can even omit certain bodily structures despite the fact that you examined them. You may thus leave out normal eyebrows and eyelashes even though you looked at them.

- Save valuable time and space by omitting superfluous words. *Avoid redundancies* such as those in parentheses in the following examples: pink (in color), resonant (by percussion), tender (to palpation), both (right and left) ears, (audible) murmur, and (bilaterally) symmetrical thorax. Repetitive introductory phrases such as "The patient reports no . . ." are also redundant and may be omitted. Unless you have indicated otherwise, readers will assume that the patient gave you the history. *Use short words* instead of long and probably fancier ones when they mean the same thing: "seen" for "visualized," and "heard" for "auscultated." Try to *describe what you observed, not what you did.* "Optic discs seen" may mark an exciting moment in your career when you first glimpsed them, and it may be all you can claim during your first few tries at an ophthalmoscopic examination. "Disc margins sharp," however, adds important information with only two additional letters.

- *Be as objective as possible.* Hostility, moralizing comments, disgust, and disapproval have no place in the patient's record, whether conveyed in words, penmanship, or punctuation. Notes such as "PATIENT DRUNK AND LATE TO CLINIC AGAIN!!" tell more about the writer than about the patient and, furthermore, might prove embarrassing in court.

Because records are scientific and legal documents, they should be understandable. Employ abbreviations and symbols only if they are commonly used and understood. Some clinicians may wish to develop an elegant style and should certainly be encouraged to do so. Time is usually scarce, however, and style may be sacrificed in favor of concise completeness. In the sample record that follows, for example, words and brief phrases substitute for whole sentences. Legibility, of course, is always essential. Otherwise, all that you have done is worthless to potential readers.

Diagrams add greatly to the speed and ease with which a record communicates its message. Two examples follow:

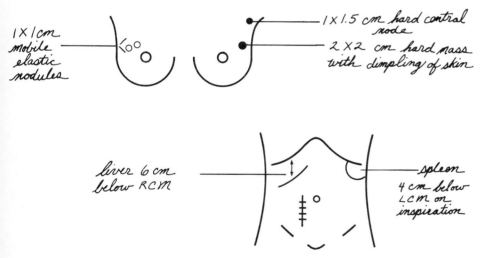

Make measurements in centimeters, not in fruits, vegetables, or nuts. "Pea-sized," "lemon-sized," and "walnut-sized" lesions vaguely convey an idea but make accurate evaluations and future comparisons impossible. How big were the lemons or peas? Did the walnut have a shell?

You should write the record as soon as possible, before the data fade from your memory. In your initial attempts at interviewing, you will probably prefer just to take notes when talking with a patient. As you gain experience, however, work toward recording in final form the past medical history, family history, and review of systems as you take them. Leave spaces for filling in later the present illness, the psychosocial history, and any other complex areas. During a physical examination it is wise to record immediately such specific measurements as the blood pressures in three positions. Recording a large number of items and descriptions interrupts the flow of the examination, however, and you will soon learn to remember your findings until you have finished.

Recording the history and physical examination is simplified, of course, by printed forms. If your institution or agency provides them, you may be expected to use them. You should also, however, be able to create a record without using a form. The example that follows offers one moderately complete guide. Although it is longer than most you may see in patients' charts, it still does not reflect every question and technique that you have learned to use. Note the difference in the statements that introduce the history and the physical examination. The basic identifying data start the history, while a descriptive paragraph that summarizes your general survey begins the physical examination.

Unless forms are used and carefully followed, records are not exactly alike in detail. Detail varies appropriately with the patient's symptoms and signs and with the clinician's diagnostic thoughts about them. In this record, additional pertinent negatives are sometimes listed when an abnormality is described. Because of the edema and varicose veins, for example, the clinician also reported "No stasis pigmentation or ulcers." If there had been neither edema nor varicose veins, these comments would not have been necessary.

Mrs. Audrey N., 1463 Maple Blvd., Capital City
11/13/90
Mrs. N. is a 54-year-old, widowed, white saleswoman, born in the U.S.

REFERRAL. None.

SOURCE. Self, seems reliable.

CHIEF COMPLAINT. Headaches.

PRESENT ILLNESS. For about 3 mo Mrs. N. has been increasingly troubled by headaches: bifrontal, usually aching, occasionally throbbing, mild to moderately severe. She has missed work only once because of headaches, when she felt nauseated and miserable and vomited several times. Otherwise, nausea is associated only occasionally. Headaches now average once a wk, usually are there when she wakes up, and last all day. Little relief from aspirin. It helps to lie down, be quiet, use cold wet towel on head. No other related symptoms, no local weakness, no numbness or visual symptoms.

Mrs. N. first began to have headaches at age 15. "Sick headaches" recurred through her mid-20s, then diminished to one every 2 or 3 mo and finally almost disappeared.

Has recently had increased pressure at work from a new and demanding boss, and is also worried about her daughter (see psychosocial). Thinks her headaches may be like those in the past, but wants to be sure because her mother died of a stroke. Is concerned that they make her irritable with her family.

PAST HISTORY

General Health. Good.

Childhood Illnesses. Only measles and chickenpox.

Adult Illnesses. None serious.

Psychiatric Illness. None.

Injuries. Stepped on glass at beach, 1987, laceration, sutured, healed.

Operations. Tonsillectomy, age 6; appendectomy, age 13.

Hospitalizations. St. Mary's, acute kidney infection, 1978.

CURRENT HEALTH STATUS

*Allergies. Ampicillin (see R.O.S., urinary).

Immunizations. Oral polio vaccine, yr uncertain; tetanus shots × 2 in 1987, followed by a booster 1 yr later; flu vaccine, 11/89, no reaction.

Screening Tests. Pap smear 1987, "normal." No mammograms.

*Environmental Hazards. Medicines kept in unlocked medicine cabinet. Cleaning solutions, furniture polish, and Drano kept in unlocked cabinet below sink. Mr. N.'s shotgun, with a box of shells, is in upstairs closet.

Safety Measures. Seat belt regularly.

Exercise/Leisure. "No time."

Sleep. Generally good, average 7 hr, sometimes has trouble falling asleep, is wakened by alarm.

Diet. Breakfast—orange juice, 2 sweet rolls, black coffee
   Mid-morning—doughnut, coffee
   Lunch—hamburger and bun or fish sandwich, coffee

---

* Asterisk or underline important points.

Dinner—meat or fish, vegetable, potato, sometimes fruit, sometimes cookies

Snacks in evening (*e.g.*, chips, cola)

Has almost no milk or cheese.

Current Medications. Aspirin for headaches, multivitamins. Has taken "water pill" for ankle swelling, but none in past several mo.

Tobacco. About 1 pack cigs per day from age 18 (36 pack yr).†

Alcohol/Drugs. Rare drink (wine) only, doesn't like it. No drugs.

FAMILY HISTORY

(There are two methods of recording the family history. The diagrammatic format is more helpful than the narrative in tracing genetic disorders. The negative family information follows either format.)

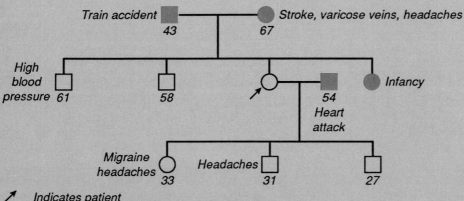

↗ *Indicates patient*

◼ *Deceased male*

● *Deceased female*

□ *Living male*

○ *Living female*

Outline

Father died, 43, train accident
Mother died, 67, stroke, had had varicose veins, headaches
One brother, 61, has high blood pressure, otherwise well
One brother, 58, apparently well but for mild arthritis
One sister, died in infancy, ? cause
Husband died, 54, heart attack
One daughter, age 33, "migraine headaches," otherwise well
One son, 31, headaches
One son, 27, well

† (Age 54 yr − 18 yr) × (1 pack) = 36 pack yr.

No family history of diabetes, tuberculosis, heart or kidney disease, cancer, anemia, epilepsy, or mental illness

*PSYCHOSOCIAL. Born and raised in Lake City, finished high school, married at age 19. Worked as a clerk in store for 2 yr, then moved with husband to Capital City, had 3 children. Mr. N. had a fairly steady factory job, but to help with the family income Mrs. N. went back to work 15 yr ago. Children have all married. 4 yr ago Mr. N. died suddenly of a heart attack, leaving little savings and no insurance. Finances now tight. Has moved to small apartment to be near daughter, Dorothy. Dorothy's husband, Arthur, has a drinking problem and is verbally though not physically abusive. Mrs. N.'s apartment serves as a haven for Dorothy and her 2 children, Kevin, 6 yr, and Linda, 3 yr. Mrs. N. feels responsible for helping them, is tense and nervous, but denies depression. She has a few good friends but doesn't like to bother them with her family's trouble. "I'd rather keep it to myself. I don't like gossip." No church or other organizational support.

Typically up at 7:00 a.m., works 9:00 to 5:30, eats dinner alone. Dorothy or the children visit most evenings and weekends. Moderate number of squabbles and considerable strain.

REVIEW OF SYSTEMS

*General. Has <u>gained</u> about <u>10 lb</u> in the past 4 yr.

Skin. No rashes or other changes.

Head. See present illness. No head injury.

Eyes. Reading glasses for 5 yr, last checked 1 yr ago. No other symptoms.

Ears. Hearing good. No tinnitus, vertigo, infections.

Nose, Sinuses. Occasional mild cold. No hay fever, sinus trouble.

*Mouth and Throat. Some <u>bleeding of gums</u> recently. Last to dentist 2 yr ago. Occasional canker sore, has had one for 4 days.

Neck. No lumps, goiter, pain.

Breasts. No lumps, pain, discharge. Does breast self exams sporadically.

Respiratory. No cough, wheezing, pneumonia, tuberculosis. Last chest x-ray 1978, St. Mary's Hospital, normal.

Cardiac. No known heart disease or high blood pressure; last blood pressure taken in 1983. No dyspnea, orthopnea, chest pain, palpitations. No ECG.

GI. Appetite good; no nausea, vomiting, indigestion. Bowel movement about once daily though sometimes has <u>hard stools, q 2–3 d, when especially tense;</u> no diarrhea or bleeding. No pain, jaundice, gallbladder or liver trouble.

Urinary. <u>Acute kidney infection,</u> 1978, with fever and right flank pain; treated with ampicillin. A generalized rash with itching developed several days later. Kidney x-rays said to be normal, and infection has not recurred. No frequency, dysuria, hematuria; nocturia × 1, large volume; <u>Occasionally loses some urine</u> when coughs hard.

Genital. Menarche at 13, regular periods, tapered off in late 40s and stopped at 49; no bleeding since; mild hot flashes and sweats then, none now.

Gravida 3, para 3, living children 3. Prolonged labor during first pregnancy, otherwise normal. Little sexual interest now, not sexually active.

Musculoskeletal. Mild <u>aching low back pain</u> often after a long day's work; no radiation down legs; used to do back exercises, but not now. No other joint pain.

Peripheral Vascular. <u>Varicose veins</u> appeared in both legs during first pregnancy. Has had swollen ankles after prolonged standing for 10 yr; wears light elastic pantyhose; tried "water pill" 5 mo ago but it didn't help much; no history of phlebitis or leg pain.

Neurologic. No faints, seizures, motor or sensory loss. Memory good.

Hematologic. Except for bleeding gums, no easy bleeding. No anemia.

Endocrine. No known thyroid trouble, temperature intolerance. Sweating average. No symptoms or history of diabetes.

Psychiatric. See present illness and psychosocial.

PHYSICAL EXAMINATION

Mrs. N. is a short, moderately obese, middle-aged woman who walks and moves easily and responds quickly to questions. She wears no makeup but her hair is fixed neatly and her clothes are immaculate. Although her ankles are swollen, her color is good and she lies flat without discomfort. She talks freely but is somewhat tense, with moist, cold hands.

        P 94, regular   R 18   Temp 37.1°C (oral)
        BP 164/98 right arm, lying
            160/96 left arm, lying
            152/88 right arm, lying (wide cuff)

Ht (without shoes) 157 cm (5'2")
Wt (dressed) 65 kg (143 lb)

Skin. Palms cold and moist, but color good. Scattered cherry angiomas over the upper trunk.

Head. Hair of average texture. Scalp and skull normal.

Eyes. Vision 20/30 in each eye. Fields full by confrontation. Conjunctiva pink. Sclera clear. Pupils round, regular, equal, react to light. Extraocular movements intact. Disc margins sharp. No arteriolar narrowing, A–V nicking, hemorrhages, or exudates.

Ears. Wax partially obscures right drum. Left canal clear and drum negative. Acuity good (to whispered voice). Weber midline. AC > BC.

Nose. Mucosa pink, septum midline. No sinus tenderness.

*Mouth. Mucosa pink. Several interdental papillae red and slightly swollen. Teeth in good repair. Tongue midline, negative but for a small (3 × 4 mm), shallow, white <u>ulcer</u> on an erythematous base, located on the undersurface near the tip; it is slightly tender but not indurated. Tonsils absent. Pharynx negative.

Neck. Trachea midline. Thyroid isthmus barely palpable, lobes not felt.

Lymph Nodes. Small (less than 1 cm), soft, nontender, and mobile tonsillar and posterior cervical nodes bilaterally. No axillary or epitrochlear nodes. Several small inguinal nodes bilaterally—soft and nontender.

Thorax and Lungs. Thorax symmetrical. Good expansion. Lungs resonant. Breath sounds normal with no added sounds.

*Cardiovascular. Jugular venous pressure 1 cm above the sternal angle, with head of bed raised to 30°. Carotid pulses normal and symmetrical. Apical impulse barely palpable in the 5th left interspace 8 cm from the midsternal line. Physiologic splitting of S_2. No S_3 or S_4. A grade 2/6 medium-pitched midsystolic <u>murmur</u> heard at the aortic area; does not radiate to the neck. Diastole clear.

Breasts. Large, pendulous, symmetrical. No masses. Nipples erect and without discharge.

Abdomen. Obese, but symmetrical. Well-healed right lower quadrant scar. Bowel sounds normal. Except for a slightly tender sigmoid colon, no masses or tenderness. Liver, spleen, and kidneys not felt. Liver span 7 cm in right midclavicular line. No CVA tenderness.

*Genitalia. Vulva normal. On straining, a mild <u>cystocele</u> appears. Vagina negative. Smooth, pink cervix, nontender. Uterus anterior, midline, smooth, not enlarged. Adnexa difficult to delineate because of obesity

and poor relaxation, but there is no tenderness. Pap smears taken. Rectovaginal examination confirms above.

Rectal. Negative. Brown stool, negative for occult blood.

*Peripheral Vascular

Pulses: 2+ <u>edema</u> of feet and ankles with 1+ edema extending up to just below knees. Moderate <u>varicosities</u> of saphenous veins bilaterally from midthigh to ankles, with venous stars on both lower legs. No stasis pigmentation or ulcers. No calf tenderness.

	RADIAL	FEMORAL	POPLITEAL	DORSALIS PEDIS	POSTERIOR TIBIAL
RT	N	N	N	↓	N
LT	N	N	N	0	N

Musculoskeletal. No joint deformities. Range of motion, including hands, wrists, elbows, shoulders, spine, hips, knees, ankles, is normal.

Neurologic

Cranial Nerves. See head and neck. Also—

N5—Sensation intact, strength good
N7—Facial movement good
N11—Sternomastoids and trapezii strong

Screening. Gait, heel-to-toe, heel and toe walking, knee bends, hops well done. Romberg negative. No pronator drift or winging. Grip and arms strong.

Motor. No involuntary movements or atrophy. Muscle tone normal, Rapid alternating movements of the hands quick and accurate.

Sensory. Pain, vibration, light touch, and stereognosis screened and intact.

Reflexes. (Two methods of recording may be used, depending upon personal preference: a tabular form or a stick figure diagram, as shown below and at right.)

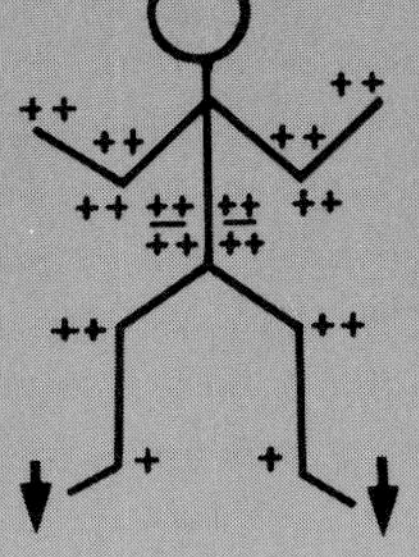

	BICEPS	TRICEPS	SUP	ABD	KNEE	ANKLE	PL
RT	2+	2+	2+	2+/2+	2+	1+	↓
LT	2+	2+	2+	2+/2+	2+	1+	↓

Mental Status. Tense but alert and cooperative. Thought coherent. Oriented. Cognitive testing not done in detail.

Before reading farther, assess Mrs. N.'s symptoms and physical findings. Then construct your own problem list for Mrs. N., as suggested in Chapter 20. You may choose to list the problems in order of their relative importance. In the problem-oriented system, however, problems retain their same numbers over time while their relative importance often changes.

One way to organize Mrs. N.'s problem list is shown below. The clinician constructed the following problem list for Mrs. N. and placed it at the front of the chart. When a new assessment indicates changing the name of a problem, the original name is crossed out and a new name is given to the old number.

DATE PROBLEM ENTERED	NO.	ACTIVE PROBLEMS	INACTIVE PROBLEMS
11/13/90	1	Migraine headaches	
11/13/90	2		Acute kidney infection
11/13/90	3	Allergy to ampicillin	
11/13/90	4	Tensions secondary to family situation, finances, and stress at work	
11/13/90	5	Gingivitis	
11/13/90	6	Low back pain	
11/13/90	7	Varicose veins with venous insufficiency	
11/13/90	8	Cystocele with occasional stress incontinence	
11/13/90	9	Possible high blood pressure	
11/13/90	10	Diet high in calories, fat, and carbohydrates, low in calcium	
11/13/90	11	Home hazards: kitchen supplies, medicines, gun	

Different clinicians often organize somewhat different problem lists for the same patient, and yours probably does not agree exactly with this one. Good lists vary in their emphases, length, and detail according to many factors, including clinicians' philosophies, specialties, and perceptions of their appropriate roles in the care of the patient. The list illustrated here includes problems that need some attention now (such as the headaches) or may need further observation or possible future attention (such as the blood pressure and cystocele). The allergy is listed as an active problem to warn against inadvertent future prescriptions of penicillins.

A few items noted in the history and physical examination, such as canker sores and constipation, do not appear in this problem list because they are relatively common phenomena that do not seem to demand attention. Such judgments are occasionally wrong, of course. Problem lists that are cluttered with relatively insignificant items, however, diminish in value. Some clinicians would undoubtedly judge this list too long; others would bring greater explicitness to problems such as "tensions," "diet," and "gingivitis." No one can specialize in everything.

The patient's record included notes on two of Mrs. N.'s problems:

1. Migraine headaches

   Assessment. Supporting this diagnosis are "sick headaches" in earlier life, recurrent course of headaches, their duration, their relief by cold and quiet, associated nausea and vomiting (once at least), and positive family history. Further, no related neurologic symptoms or signs. Headaches may be somewhat more frequent than typical migraine headaches, pain is usually aching rather than throbbing, and there are obvious tensions at work and at home. Tension headaches should also be considered, therefore, but the headaches fit this pattern less well.

   Plan
   Diagnostic. Observation only. Mrs. N. to look for possible precipitating factors.
   Therapeutic. Continue aspirin as needed.
   Education. Nature of migraine discussed. Patient pleased and relieved

9. Possible high blood pressure.

   Assessment. Some of apparent elevation clearly related to obese arms, and some may be related to anxiety of a first visit. No evidence of target organ damage.

   Plan
   Diagnostic. Repeat BP in one month. Use wide cuff. Urinalysis.
   Therapeutic. None now. Consider diet change on next visit.
   Education. Need for BP checks explained.

A month later Mrs. N. returned for a second visit. Part of the progress notes read as follows:

1. Migraine headaches

   Subjective (S). Has had only 2 headaches, both mild, without associated symptoms. No longer worried about them. Cannot detect any precipitating factors.
   Objective (O). Not reexamined.
   Assessment (A). Improved.
   Plan (P). Return as needed.

4. Tensions

   S. Dorothy is now attending Al-Anon meetings and tensions at home seem somewhat better.
   O. Mrs. N. is more relaxed today.
   A. Somewhat improved.
   P. Encouraged to discuss situation with me as needed.

9. Possible high blood pressure

   S. None.
   O. BP 146/84 right arm, lying (wide cuff). Urinalysis normal.
   A. If the systolic pressure is found high next time, it will indicate borderline isolated systolic hypertension.
   P. Repeat BP in 6 months.

Although you have insufficient information about most of Mrs. N.'s other problems, including her own priorities, try to develop an approach to them. What further data do you need?

What information do you need and how do you obtain it? These questions appear implicitly in Chapter 1 and continue throughout the book —and long afterward. The process of learning about a patient continues far beyond the first encounter, and understanding grows in depth, complexity, and fascination. Although your knowledge of Mrs. N. is incomplete, you know a great deal about her and have the tools with which to expand your knowledge further. Needed now is repetitive practice, with supervision, in using your newly acquired tools.

Bibliography

GENERAL REFERENCES

Anatomy and Physiology

Anderson JE: Grant's Atlas of Anatomy, 8th ed. Baltimore, Williams & Wilkins, 1983.

Basmajian JV, Slonecker CE: Grant's Method of Anatomy, 11th ed. Baltimore, Williams & Wilkins, 1989.

Berne RM, Levy MN: Physiology, 2nd ed. St Louis, CV Mosby, 1988.

Guyton AC: Textbook of Medical Physiology, 7th ed. Philadelphia, WB Saunders, 1986.

Moore KL: Clinically Oriented Anatomy, 2nd ed. Baltimore, Williams & Wilkins, 1985.

Physical Examination

Burnside JW, McGlynn TJ: Physical Diagnosis, 17th ed. Baltimore, Williams & Wilkins, 1987.

Clain A (ed): Hamilton Bailey's Demonstrations of Physical Signs in Clinical Surgery, 17th ed. Bristol, Wright, 1986.

DeGowin & DeGowin's Bedside Diagnostic Examination, 5th ed; DeGowin RL (rev). New York, Macmillan, 1987.

Judge RD, Zuidema GD, Fitzgerald FT (eds): Clinical Diagnosis: A Physiologic Approach, 5th ed. Boston, Little, Brown & Co, 1989.

Lumsden CJ, Whiteside CI: Clinical Methods. New York, Alan R Liss, 1987.

Pappworth MH: A Primer of Medicine, 5th ed. London, Butterworths, 1984.

Sapira JD: The Art and Science of Bedside Diagnosis. Baltimore, Urban & Schwarzenberg, 1990.

Walker HK, Hall WD, Hurst JW: Clinical Methods: The History, Physical, and Laboratory Examinations, 3rd ed. Boston, Butterworths, 1990.

Changes With Age

ADOLESCENTS

American College of Physicians: Health care needs of the adolescent. Ann Intern Med 110:930, 1989.

Hofmann AD, Greydanus DE (eds): Adolescent Medicine, 2nd ed. Norwalk, CT, Appleton & Lange, 1989.

Sanford ND: Providing sensitive health care to gay and lesbian youth. Nurse Pract 14(5):30, 1989.

OLDER PERSONS

Hazzard WR, Andres R, Bierman EL, et al: Principles of Geriatric Medicine and Gerontology, 2nd ed. New York, McGraw-Hill, 1990.

Kane RL, Ouslander JG, Abrass IB: Essentials of Clinical Geriatrics, 2nd ed. New York, McGraw-Hill, 1989.

Lachs MS, Feinstein AR, Cooney LM Jr, et al: A simple procedure for general screening for functional disability in elderly patients. Ann Intern Med 112:699, 1990.

Mezey MD, Rauckhorst LH, Stokes SA: Health Assessment of the Older Individual. New York, Springer-Verlag, 1980.

Rowe JW, Besdine RW: Geriatric Medicine, 2nd ed. Boston, Little, Brown & Co, 1988.

Medicine and Surgery

Branch WT Jr: Office Practice of Medicine, 2nd ed. Philadelphia, WB Saunders, 1987.

Braunwald E, Isselbacher KJ, Petersdorf RG, et al (eds): Harrison's Principles of Internal Medicine, 11th ed. New York, McGraw-Hill, 1987.

Goroll AH, May LA, Mulley AG Jr: Primary Care Medicine: Office Evaluation and Management of the Adult Patient, 2nd ed. Philadelphia, JB Lippincott, 1987.

Harvey AM, Johns RJ, McKusick VA, et al (eds): The Principles and Practice of Medicine, 22nd ed. Norwalk, CT, Appleton & Lange, 1988.

Hurst JW: Medicine for the Practicing Physician, 2nd ed. Stoneham, MA, Butterworths, 1988.

Kelley WN (ed): Textbook of Internal Medicine. Philadelphia, JB Lippincott, 1989.

Sabiston DC Jr (ed): Textbook of Surgery: The Biological Basis of Modern Surgical Practice, 13th ed. Philadelphia, WB Saunders, 1986.

Schwartz SI (ed): Principles of Surgery, 5th ed. New York, McGraw-Hill, 1989.

Wyngaarden JB, Smith LH Jr (eds): Cecil Textbook of Medicine, 18th ed. Philadelphia, WB Saunders, 1988.

CHAPTER 1. INTERVIEWING AND THE HEALTH HISTORY

Beckman HB, Frankel RM: The effect of physician behavior on the collection of data. Ann Intern Med 101:692, 1984.

Billings JA, Stoeckle JD: The Clinical Encounter: A Guide to the Medical Interview and Case Presentation. Chicago, Year Book Medical Publishers, 1989.

Braham R, Furniss K, Holtz H, et al: Hospital Protocol on Domestic Violence. Morristown, NJ, Jersey Battered Women's Service, Inc, 1986.

Cassell EJ: Talking With Patients. Vol. 1: The Theory of Doctor–Patient Communication. Vol. 2: Clinical Technique. Cambridge, MA, MIT Press, 1985.

Coulehan JL, Block MR: The Medical Interview: A Primer for Students of the Art. Philadelphia, FA Davis, 1987.

Enelow AJ, Swisher SN: Interviewing and Patient Care, 3rd ed. New York, Oxford University Press, 1986.

Engel GL, Morgan WL Jr: Interviewing the Patient. Philadelphia, WB Saunders, 1973.

Gjerdingen DK, Simpson DE, Titus SL: Patients' and Physicians' Attitudes Regarding the Physician's Professional Appearance. Arch Intern Med 147:1209, 1987.

Havens LL: Taking a history from the difficult patient. Lancet 1:138, 1978.

King MC, Ryan J: Abused women: Dispelling myths and encouraging intervention. Nurse Pract 14(5):47, 1989.

Levinson D: A Guide to Clinical Interviewing. Philadelphia, WB Saunders, 1987.

Mishler EG, Clark JA, Ingelfinger J, et al: The language of attentive patient care: A comparison of two medical interviews. J Gen Intern Med 4:325, 1989.

The Occupational and Environmental Health Committee of the American Lung Association of San Diego and Imperial Counties: Taking the occupational history. Ann Intern Med 99:641, 1983.

Pomeroy WB, Flax CC, Wheeler CC: Taking a Sex History: Interviewing and Recording. New York, Free Press, 1982. [*The techniques of the Kinsey Institute*]

Suchman AL, Matthews DA: What makes the patient–doctor relation therapeutic? Exploring the connexional dimension of medical care. Ann Intern Med 108:125, 1988.

Three Contrasting Views on Using First Names

Angelou M: I Know Why the Caged Bird Sings. New York, Bantam Books, 1971:21–27. [*The memories of a black woman*]

Conant EB: Addressing patients by their first names. N Engl J Med 308:226, 1983. [*A patient's view*]

Heller ME: Addressing patients by their first names. N Engl J Med 308:1107, 1987. [*Short report of a survey of obstetrical outpatients*]

Understanding Illness

Benner P, Wrubel J: The Primacy of Caring: Stress and Coping in Health and Illness. Menlo Park, CA, Addison-Wesley, 1989.

Kleinman A: The Illness Narratives: Suffering, Healing, and the Human Condition. New York, Basic Books, 1988.

Screening Questions for Alcoholism

Cyr MG, Wartman SA: The effectiveness of routine screening questions in the detection of alcoholism. JAMA 259:51, 1988.

Ewing JA: Detecting alcoholism: The CAGE Questionnaire. JAMA 252:1905, 1984.

Hurt RD, Morse RM, Swenson WM: Diagnosis of alcoholism with a self-administered alcoholism screening test: Results with 1,002 consecutive patients receiving general examinations. Mayo Clin Proc 55:365, 1980.

Mayfield D, McLeod G, Hall P: The CAGE Questionnaire: Validation of a new alcoholism screening instrument. Am J Psychiatry 131:1121, 1974.

Pokorny AD, Miller BA, Kaplan HB: The brief MAST: A shortened version of the Michigan Alcoholism Screening Test. Am J Psychiatry 129:342, 1972.

Woodruff RA Jr, Clayton PJ, Cloninger CR, et al: A brief method of screening for alcoholism. Dis Nerv Sys 37:434, 1976.

See Also

Barnes HN, Aronson MD, Delbanco TL (eds): Alcoholism: A Guide for the Primary Care Physician. New York, Springer-Verlag, 1987.

Gallant DM: Alcoholism: A Guide to Diagnosis, Intervention, and Treatment. New York, WW Norton, 1987.

CHAPTER 2. AN APPROACH TO SYMPTOMS

For most symptoms in this chapter, see the relevant references in later chapters and the texts listed under *Medicine* and *Surgery*.

Duthie EH Jr: Falls. Med Clin North Am 73:1321, 1989.

Fox GN: Restless legs syndrome. Am Fam Physician 33:147, 1986.

Frymoyer JW: Back pain and sciatica. N Engl J Med 318:291, 1988.

Gillin JC, Byerley WF: The diagnosis and management of insomnia. N Engl J Med 322:239, 1990.

Johnson JR, Stamm WE: Urinary tract infections in women. Ann Intern Med 111:906, 1989.

Johnston H, Reisz G: Changing spectrum of hemoptysis: Underlying causes in 148 patients undergoing diagnostic flexible fiberoptic bronchoscopy. Arch Intern Med 149:1666, 1989.

Kales A, Soldatos CR, Kales JD: Sleep disorders: Insomnia, sleepwalking, night terrors, nightmares, and enuresis. Ann Intern Med 106:582, 1987.

Kales A, Vela-Bueno A, Kales JD: Sleep disorders: Sleep apnea and narcolepsy. Ann Intern Med 106:434, 1987.

Krane RJ, Goldstein I, Saenz de Tejada I: Impotence. N Engl J Med 321:1648, 1989.

Lipsky BA: Urinary tract infections in men: Epidemiology, pathophysiology, diagnosis, and treatment. Ann Intern Med 110:138, 1989.

Manolis AS, Linzer M, Salem D, et al: Syncope: Current diagnostic evaluation and management. Ann Intern Med 112:850, 1990.

Mitchell JE, Seim HC, Colon E, et al: Medical complications and medical management of bulimia. Ann Intern Med 107:71, 1987.

Mulligan T, Katz PG: Why aged men become impotent. Arch Intern Med 149:1365, 1989.

Pannill FC III: Practical management of urinary incontinence. Med Clin North Am 73:1423, 1989.

Pincus T, Callahan LF, Brooks RH, et al: Self-report questionnaire scores in rheumatoid arthritis compared with traditional physical, radiographic, and laboratory measures. Ann Intern Med 110:259, 1989.

Resnick NM, Subbarao VY, Laurino E: The pathophysiology of urinary incontinence among institutionalized elderly persons. N Engl J Med 320:1, 1989.

Wrenn K: Fecal impaction. N Engl J Med 321:658, 1989.

CHAPTER 3. MENTAL STATUS

American Psychiatric Association: Diagnostic and Statistical Manual of Mental Disorders, 3rd ed, rev. Washington, DC, American Psychiatric Association, 1987.

Blazer D: Depression in the elderly. N Engl J Med 320:164, 1989.

Drugs that cause psychiatric symptoms. Med Lett Drugs Ther 31:113, 1989.

Evans DA, Funkenstein HH, Albert MS, et al: Prevalence of Alzheimer's disease in a community population of older persons. JAMA 262:2551, 1989.

Kaplan HI, Sadock BJ (eds): Modern Synopsis of Comprehensive Textbook of Psychiatry/V, 5th ed. Baltimore, Williams & Wilkins, 1989.

Kermis MD: Mental Health in Late Life: The Adaptive Process. Boston, Jones & Bartlett, 1986.

Koenig HG, Meador KG, Cohen HJ, et al: Depression in elderly hospitalized patients with medical illness. Arch Intern Med 148:1929, 1988.

Lipowski ZJ. Delirium in the elderly patient. N Engl J Med 320:578, 1989.

Nicholi AM Jr (ed): The New Harvard Guide to Psychiatry, 2nd ed. Cambridge, Belknap Press of Harvard University Press, 1988.

Reich P: Panic attacks and the risk of suicide. N Engl J Med 321:1260, 1989.

Strub RL, Black FW: The Mental Status Examination in Neurology, 2nd ed. Philadelphia, FA Davis, 1985.

Talbott JA, Hales RE, Yudofsky SC (eds): American Psychiatric Press Textbook of Psychiatry. Washington, DC, American Psychiatric Press, 1988.

Teasdale G, Jennett B: Assessment of coma and impaired consciousness: A practical scale. Lancet 2:81, 1974. [*The Glasgow coma scale*]

Weissman MM, Klerman GL, Markowitz JS et al: Suicidal ideation and suicide attempts in panic disorder and attacks. N Engl J Med 321:1209, 1989.

CHAPTER 4. PHYSICAL EXAMINATION: APPROACH AND OVERVIEW

Oboler SK, LaForce FM: The periodic physical examination in asymptomatic adults. Ann Intern Med 110:214, 1989.

Report of the U.S. Preventive Services Task Force: Guide to Clinical Preventive Services. Baltimore, Williams & Wilkins, 1989.

CHAPTER 5. THE GENERAL SURVEY

Tanner JM: Growing up. Sci Am 229(3):34, 1973.

CHAPTER 6. THE SKIN

Baran R, Dawber RPR: Diseases of the Nails and Their Management. Oxford, Blackwell Scientific Publications, 1984.

Beaven DW, Brooks SE: Color Atlas of the Nail in Clinical Diagnosis. Chicago, Year Book Medical Publishers, 1984.

Chanda JJ: The clinical recognition and prognostic factors of primary cutaneous malignant melanoma. Med Clin North Am 70:39, 1986.

Fitzpatrick TB, Polano MK, Suurmond D: Color Atlas and Synopsis of Clinical Dermatology. New York, McGraw-Hill, 1983.

Friedman-Kien AE (ed): Color Atlas of AIDS. Philadelphia, WB Saunders, 1989.

Jeghers H, Edelstein LM: Skin color in health and disease. In Blacklow RS (ed): MacBryde's Signs and Symptoms: Applied Pathologic Physiology and Clinical Interpretation, 6th ed. Philadelphia, JB Lippincott, 1983.

Lampe RM, Kagan A: Detection of clubbing—Schamroth's sign: Closing the window and opening the angle. Clin Pediatr 22:125, 1983.

Marks R: Skin Disease in Old Age. Philadelphia, JB Lippincott, 1987.

McLaury P: Head lice: Pediatric social disease. Am J Nurs 83:1300, 1983.

Rosen T, Martin S: Atlas of Black Dermatology. Boston, Little, Brown & Co, 1981.

Sauer GC: Manual of Skin Diseases, 5th ed. Philadelphia, JB Lippincott, 1985.

CHAPTER 7. THE HEAD AND NECK

Eyes

Michaelson IC: Textbook of the Fundus of the Eye, 3rd ed. Edinburgh, Churchill Livingstone, 1980.

Newell FW: Ophthalmology: Principles and Concepts, 6th ed. St Louis, CV Mosby, 1986.

Vaughan D, Asbury T, Tabbara KF: General Ophthalmology, 12th ed. Norwalk, CT, Appleton & Lange, 1989.

Ears, Nose, and Throat

Bull TR: A Colour Atlas of E.N.T. Diagnosis, 2nd ed. London, Wolfe Medical Publications, 1987.

De Weese DD, Saunders WH, Schuller DE, et al: Otolaryngology—Head and Neck Surgery, 7th ed. St Louis, CV Mosby, 1988.

Harnisch JP, Tronca E, Nolan CM, et al: Diphtheria among alcoholic urban adults: A decade of experience in Seattle. Ann Intern Med 111:71, 1989.

Hawke M, Keene M, Alberti PW: Clinical Otoscopy: A Text and Colour Atlas. Edinburgh, Churchill Livingstone, 1984.

Huovinen P, Lahtonen R, Ziegler T, et al: Pharyngitis in adults: The presence and coexistence of viruses and bacterial organisms. Ann Intern Med 110:612, 1989.

Komaroff AL, Pass TM, Aronson MD, et al: The prediction of streptococcal pharyngitis in adults. J Gen Intern Med 1(1):1, 1986.

Stafford ND, Youngs R: ENT. Edinburgh, Churchill Livingstone, 1988.

Mouth

Cawson RA, Eveson JW: Oral Pathology and Diagnosis: Color Atlas with Integrated Text. Philadelphia, WB Saunders, 1987.

Connolly GN, Winn DM, Hecht SS, et al: The reemergence of smokeless tobacco. N Engl J Med 314:1020, 1986.

Lynch MA, Brightman VJ, Greenberg MS (eds): Burket's Oral Medicine: Diagnosis and Treatment, 8th ed. Philadelphia, JB Lippincott, 1984.

Pindborg JJ: Atlas of Diseases of the Oral Mucosa, 4th ed. Philadelphia, WB Saunders, 1985.

Regezi JA, Sciubba JJ: Oral Pathology: Clinical–Pathologic Correlations. Philadelphia, WB Saunders, 1989.

Scully C, Cawson RA: Oral Medicine. Edinburgh, Churchill Livingstone, 1988.

Neck

Ingbar SH: The thyroid gland. In Wilson JD, Foster DW (eds): Williams Textbook of Endocrinology, 7th ed. Philadelphia, WB Saunders, 1985. [*See pp. 742–743 for inspection and palpation.*]

Jeghers H, Clark SL Jr, Templeton AC: Lymphadenopathy and disorders of the lymphatics. In Blacklow RS (ed): MacBryde's Signs and Symptoms: Applied Pathologic Physiology and Clinical Interpretation, 6th ed. Philadelphia, JB Lippincott, 1983.

Nordyke RA, Gilbert FI Jr, Harada ASM: Graves' disease: Influence of age on clinical findings. Arch Intern Med 148:626, 1988.

CHAPTER 8. THE THORAX AND LUNGS

Textbooks

Baum GL, Wolinsky E (eds): Textbook of Pulmonary Diseases, 4th ed. Boston, Little, Brown & Co, 1989.

Murray JF, Nadel JA: Textbook of Respiratory Medicine. Philadelphia, WB Saunders, 1988.

Assessment of the Lungs

Cugell DW: Lung sound nomenclature. Am Rev Respir Dis 136:1016, 1987.

Epler GR, Carrington CB, Gaensler EA: Crackles (rales) in the interstitial pulmonary diseases. Chest 73:333, 1978.

Forgacs P: Lung Sounds. London, Bailliere Tindall, 1978.

Kraman SS: Vesicular (normal) lung sounds: How are they made, where do they come from, and what do they mean? Semin Respir Med 6:183, 1985.

Kraman SS: Lung sounds for the clinician. Arch Intern Med 146:1411, 1986.

Lal S, Ferguson AD, Campbell EJM: Forced expiratory time: A simple test for airways obstruction. Br Med J 1:814, 1964.

Lehrer S: Understanding Lung Sounds. Philadelphia, WB Saunders, 1984. [*With audiocassette.*]

Loudon RG: The lung exam. Clin Chest Med 8:265, 1987.

Murphy RLH Jr: Discontinuous adventitious lung sounds. Semin Respir Med 6:210, 1985.

Nath AR, Capel LH: Inspiratory crackles—early and late. Thorax 29:223, 1974.

Nath AR, Capel LH: Lung crackles in bronchiectasis. Thorax 35:694, 1980.

CHAPTER 9. THE CARDIOVASCULAR SYSTEM

Cardiac Assessment

Abrams J: Essentials of Cardiac Physical Diagnosis. Philadelphia, Lea & Febiger, 1987.

Devereux RB, Kramer-Fox R, Kligfield P: Mitral valve prolapse: Causes, clinical manifestations, and management. Ann Intern Med 111:305, 1989.

Ewy GA: The abdominojugular test: Technique and hemodynamic correlates. Ann Intern Med 109:456, 1988.

Hurst JW, Schlant RC, Rackley CE, et al (eds): The Heart, Arteries, and Veins, 7th ed. New York, McGraw-Hill, 1990.

Lembo NJ, Dell'Italia LJ, Crawford MH, et al: Bedside diagnosis of systolic murmurs. N Engl J Med 318:1572, 1988.

Novey DW, Pencak M, Stang JM: The Guide to Heart Sounds: Normal and Abnormal. Boca Raton, FL, CRC Press, 1988. [*Audiocassette with pamphlet.*]

Perloff JK: Physical Examination of the Heart and Circulation. Philadelphia, WB Saunders, 1982.

Tilkian AG, Conover MB: Understanding Heart Sounds and Murmurs: With an Introduction to Lung Sounds, 2nd ed. Philadelphia, WB Saunders, 1984. [*with audiocassette*]

Wenger NK, O'Rourke RA, Marcus FI: The care of elderly patients with cardio-vascular disease. Ann Intern Med 109:425, 1988.

Blood Pressure

The 1988 Report of the Joint National Committee on Detection, Evaluation, and Treatment of High Blood Pressure, U.S. Department of Health and Human Services, Public Health Service, National Institutes of Health, 1988.

Adams CE, Leverland MB: Environmental and behavioral factors that can affect blood pressure. Nurse Pract 10(11):39, 1985.

Frohlich ED, Grim C, Labarthe DR, et al: Recommendations for human blood pressure determination by sphygmomanometers. Report of a special task force appointed by the Steering Committee, American Heart Association. Circulation 77:501A, 1988.

Lipsitz LA: Orthostatic hypotension in the elderly. N Engl J Med 321:952, 1989.

CHAPTER 10. THE BREASTS AND AXILLAE

Pubertal Changes

Harlan WR, Harlan EA, Grillo GP: Secondary sex characteristics of girls 12 to 17 years of age. The U.S. Health Examination Survey. J Pediatr 96:1074, 1980.

Marshall WA, Tanner JM: Variations in pattern of pubertal changes in girls. Arch Dis Child 44:291, 1969.

Tanner JM: Growth at Adolescence, 2nd ed. Oxford, Blackwell Scientific Publications, 1962.

Examination and Diseases

Cavanaugh J, Niewoehner CB, Nuttall FQ: Gynecomastia and cirrhosis of the liver. Arch Intern Med 150:563, 1990.

Donegan WL, Spratt JS: Cancer of the Breast, 3rd ed. Philadelphia, WB Saunders, 1988.

Haagensen CD: Diseases of the Breast, 3rd ed. Philadelphia, WB Saunders, 1986.

Harris JR, Hellman S, Henderson IC, et al: Breast Diseases. Philadelphia, JB Lippincott, 1987. Within this text, see Love SM, Schnitt SJ, Connolly JL, et al: Benign breast disorders: 15–53, and Miller AB: Early detection of breast cancer: 122–134. [*The latter reviews the biases in evaluation and assesses breast self-examination, physical examination, and mammography.*]

Love SM, Gelman RS, Silen W: Fibrocystic "disease" of the breast—a nondisease? N Engl J Med 307:1010, 1982.

Niewoehner CB, Nuttall FQ: Gynecomastia in a hospitalized male population. Am J Med 77:633, 1984.

CHAPTER 11. THE ABDOMEN

Textbooks

Silen W: Cope's Early Diagnosis of the Acute Abdomen, 17th ed. New York, Oxford University Press, 1987.

Sleisenger MH, Fordtran JS: Gastrointestinal Disease: Pathophysiology, Diagnosis, Management, 4th ed. Philadelphia, WB Saunders, 1989.

Examination of the Liver

Castell DO, O'Brien KD, Muench H, et al: Estimation of liver size by percussion in normal individuals. Ann Intern Med 70:1183, 1969.

Sapira JD, Williamson DL: How big is the normal liver? Arch Intern Med 139:971, 1979.

Castell DO: How big is the normal liver, indeed! Arch Intern Med 139:968, 1979.

Srainka B, Stahlhut J, Fulbeck CL, et al: Measuring liver span: Bedside examination versus ultrasound and scintiscan. J Clin Gastroenterol 8:267, 1986.

Examination of the Spleen

Castell DO: The spleen percussion sign: A useful diagnostic technique. Ann Intern Med 67:1265, 1967.

Sullivan S, Williams R: Reliability of clinical techniques for detecting splenic enlargement. Br Med J 2:1043, 1976.

CHAPTER 12. MALE GENITALIA AND HERNIAS

Pubertal Changes

Harlan WR, Grillo GP, Cornoni-Huntley J, et al: Secondary sex characteristics of boys 12 to 17 years of age. The U.S. Health Examination Survey. J Pediatr 95:293, 1979.

Marshall WA, Tanner JM: Variations in the pattern of pubertal changes in boys. Arch Dis Child 45:12, 1970.

Tanner JM: Growth at Adolescence, 2nd ed. Oxford, Blackwell Scientific Publications, 1962.

Textbooks of Urology

Tanagho EA, McAninch JW: Smith's General Urology, 12th ed. East Norwalk, CT, Appleton & Lange, 1988.

Walsh PC, Gittes RF, Perlmutter AD, et al: Campbell's Urology, 5th ed. Philadelphia, WB Saunders, 1986.

Hernias

Morton JH: Abdominal wall hernias. In Schwartz SI (ed): Principles of Surgery, 5th ed. New York, McGraw-Hill, 1989.

Nyhus LM, Bombeck CT: Hernias. In Sabiston DC Jr (ed): Textbook of Surgery: The Biological Basis of Modern Surgical Practice, 13th ed, Philadelphia, WB Saunders, 1986.

Sexually Transmitted Diseases

DeVita VT Jr, Hellman S, Rosenberg SA (eds): AIDS: Etiology, Diagnosis, Treatment, and Prevention, 2nd ed. Philadelphia, JB Lippincott, 1988.

Holmes KK, Mardh P-A, Sparling PF (eds): Sexually Transmitted Diseases, 2nd ed. New York, McGraw-Hill, 1990.

Nettina SL, Kauffman FH: Diagnosis and management of sexually transmitted genital lesions. Nurse Pract 15(1):20, 1990.

CHAPTER 13. THE FEMALE GENITALIA

Pubertal Changes

See the references listed on this topic in Chapter 10.

Sexually Transmitted Diseases

See the references listed on this topic in Chapter 12.

Textbooks of Gynecology

Greydanus DE, Shearin RB: Adolescent Sexuality and Gynecology. Philadelphia, Lea & Febiger, 1990.

Jones HW III, Wentz AC, Burnet LS: Novak's Textbook of Gynecology, 11th ed. Baltimore, Williams & Wilkins, 1988.

Scott JR, DiSaia PJ, Hammond CB, et al (eds): Danforth's Obstetrics and Gynecology, 6th ed. Philadelphia, JB Lippincott, 1990.

The Pelvic Examination

Brink CA, Sampselle CM, Wells TJ, et al: A digital test for pelvic muscle strength in older women with urinary incontinence. Nurs Res 38:196, 1989.

Hein K: The first pelvic examination and common gynecological problems in adolescent girls. Women Health 9(2/3):47, 1984.

Magee J: The pelvic examination: A view from the other end of the table. Ann Intern Med 83:563, 1975.

Primrose RB: Taking the tension out of pelvic exams. Am J Nurs 84:72, 1984.

Sampselle CM, Brink CA, Wells TJ: Digital measurement of pelvic muscle strength in childbearing women. Nurs Res 38:134, 1989.

Taylor PT Jr, Andersen WI, Barber SR, et al: The screening Papanicolaou smear: Contribution of the endocervical brush. Obstet Gynecol 70:734, 1987.

Vaginitis

Chantigian PDM: Vaginitis: A common malady. Prim Care 15:517, 1988.
McCue JD: Evaluation and management of vaginitis: An update for primary care practitioners. Arch Intern Med 149:565, 1989.

CHAPTER 14. THE PREGNANT WOMAN

Beebe JE, Duperret M (consultants): Programmed instruction: Examination of the female pelvis, Part I. Am J Nurs 78:10, 1978.
Cunningham FG, MacDonald PC, Gant NF: Williams Obstetrics, 18th ed. Norwalk, CT, Appleton & Lange, 1989.
Myles M: Textbook for Midwives, 9th ed. London, E & S Livingstone, 1981.
Oxorn H: Oxorn-Foote Human Labor and Birth, 5th ed. Norwalk, CT, Appleton-Century-Crofts, 1986.
Public Health Service, DHHS: Caring for Our Future: The Content of Prenatal Care. Washington, DC, U.S. Government Printing Office, 1989.
Thompson JE: Primary health care nursing for women. In Mezey MD, McGivern DO: Nurses, Nurse Practitioners. Boston, Little, Brown & Co., 1986.
Varney H: Nurse-Midwifery, 2nd ed. Boston, Blackwell Scientific Publications, 1987.

CHAPTER 15. THE ANUS, RECTUM, AND PROSTATE

Schrock TR: Examination of the anorectum, rigid sigmoidoscopy, flexible sigmoidoscopy, and diseases of the anorectum. In Sleisenger MH, Fordtran JS: Gastrointestinal Disease: Pathophysiology, Diagnosis, Management, 4th ed. Philadelphia, WB Saunders, 1989.

CHAPTER 16. THE PERIPHERAL VASCULAR SYSTEM

Allman RM: Pressure ulcers among the elderly. N Engl J Med 320:850, 1989.
Jeghers H, Clark SL Jr, Templeton AC: Lymphadenopathy and disorders of the lymphatics. In Blacklow RS (ed): MacBryde's Signs and Symptoms: Applied Pathologic Physiology and Clinical Interpretation, 6th ed. Philadelphia, JB Lippincott, 1983.
Spittell JA Jr (ed): Clinical Vascular Disease. Cardiovasc Clin 13(2), 1983.

CHAPTER 17. THE MUSCULOSKELETAL SYSTEM

Deyo RA, Loeser JD, Bigos SJ: Herniated lumbar intervertebral disk. Ann Intern Med 112:598, 1990.
Hoppenfeld S: Physical Examination of the Spine and Extremities. East Norwalk, CT, Appleton-Century-Crofts, 1976.

Katz JN, Larson MG, Sabra A, et al: The carpal tunnel syndrome: Diagnostic utility of the history and physical examination findings. Ann Intern Med 112:321, 1990.

Kelley WN, Harris ED Jr, Ruddy S, et al: Textbook of Rheumatology, 3rd ed. Philadelphia, WB Saunders, 1989.

McCarty DJ (ed): Arthritis and Allied Conditions: A Textbook of Rheumatology, 11th ed. Philadelphia, Lea & Febiger, 1989.

Polley HF, Hunder GG: Rheumatologic Interviewing and Physical Examination of the Joints, 2nd ed. Philadelphia, WB Saunders, 1978.

Schumacher HR, Klippel JH, Robinson DR (eds): Primer on the Rheumatic Diseases, 9th ed. Atlanta, GA, Arthritis Foundation, 1988.

CHAPTER 18. THE NERVOUS SYSTEM

Anatomy and Physiology

De Groot J, Chusid JG: Correlative Neuroanatomy, 20th ed. East Norwalk, CT, Appleton & Lange, 1988.

Gilman SG, Newman SW: Manter and Gatz's Essentials of Clinical Neuroanatomy and Neurophysiology, 7th ed. Philadelphia, FA Davis, 1987.

Neurology

Adams RD, Victor M: Principles of Neurology, 4th ed. New York, McGraw-Hill, 1989.

Rowland LP (ed): Merritt's Textbook of Neurology, 8th ed. Philadelphia, Lea & Febiger, 1989.

Sudarsky L: Geriatrics: Gait disorders in the elderly. N Engl J Med 322:1441, 1990.

The Neurologic Examination

Aids to the Examination of the Peripheral Nervous System: Medical Research Council Memorandum No. 45. London, Her Majesty's Stationery Office, 1976.

Bickerstaff ER: Neurological Examination in Clinical Practice, 5th ed. St. Louis, CV Mosby Yearbook, 1989.

DeJong RN: The Neurological Examination: Incorporating the Fundamentals of Neuroanatomy and Neurophysiology, 4th ed. Hagerstown, Harper & Row, 1979.

Rodnitsky RL: Van Allen's Pictorial Manual of Neurologic Tests, 3rd ed. Chicago, Year Book Medical Publishers, 1988.

CHAPTER 19. THE PHYSICAL EXAMINATION OF INFANTS AND CHILDREN

Battaglia FC, Lubchenco LO: A practical classification of newborn infants by weight and gestational age. J Pediatr 71:159, 1967.

Burnside JW: Physical Diagnosis: An Introduction to Clinical Medicine, 17th ed. Baltimore, Williams & Wilkins, 1987.

Caceres CA, Perry W: The Innocent Murmur: A Problem in Clinical Practice. Boston, Little, Brown & Co, 1967.

Capraro VJ: Gynecological examination in children and adolescents. Pediatr Clin North Am 19:511, 1972.

Chung SM: Hip Disorders in Infants and Children. Philadelphia, Lea & Febiger, 1981.

Dubowitz LV, Dubowitz C, Goldberger C: Clinical assessment of gestational age in the newborn infant. J Pediatr 77:1, 1970.

Frankenburg WK, Camp BW (eds): Pediatric Screening Tests. Springfield, IL, Charles C Thomas, 1975.

Fuller GN, Hargreave MR, King DM: Scratch test in clinical examination of liver. Lancet 1:181, 1988.

Gorman JJ, Cogan DG, Gellis SS: An apparatus for grading the visual acuity of infants on the basis of opticokinetic nystagmus. Pediatrics 19:1088, 1957.

Gundy JH: Assessment of the Child in Primary Health Care. New York, McGraw-Hill, 1981.

Hoekelman RA: An appraisal of the effectiveness of child health supervision. Curr Opin Pediatr 1:146, 1989.

Hoekelman RA, et al (eds): Primary Care Pediatrics. St Louis, CV Mosby, 1987. [1776-page general textbook]

Illingworth RS: An Introduction to Developmental Assessment in the First Year. London, National Spastics Society Medical Education and Information Unit, 1962.

Lawson EE, Grand RJ, Neff RK, Cohen LF: Clinical estimation of liver span in infants and children. Am J Dis Child 132:474, 1978.

Lowrey GH: Growth and Development of Children, 8th ed. Chicago, Year Book Medical Publishers, 1986.

Lubchenco LO, Searls DT, Brazie JV: Neonatal mortality rate: Relationship to birth weight and gestational age. J Pediatr 81:814, 1972.

Nadas AS, Fyler DC: Pediatric Cardiology, 3rd ed. Philadelphia, WB Saunders, 1972.

Newell FW: Ophthalmology: Principles and Concepts, 6th ed. St Louis, CV Mosby, 1986.

Paine RS: Neurological examination of infants and children. Pediatr Clin North Am 7:471, 1960.

Rodnitzky RL: Van Allen's Pictorial Manual of Neurologic Tests. 3rd ed. Chicago, Year Book Medical Publishers, 1988.

Sweet AY: Classification of the low-birth-weight infant. In Klaus MH, Fanaroff AA (eds): Care of the High-Risk Neonate, 3rd ed. Philadelphia, WB Saunders, 1986.

Tachdjian MO: Diagnosis and treatment of congenital deformities of the musculoskeletal system in the newborn and the infant. Pediatr Clin North Am 14:307, 1967.

Thomas A, Chesni Y, Dargassies SS: The Neurological Examination of the Infant. London, National Spastics Society Medical Education and Information Unit, 1960.

CHAPTER 20. CLINICAL THINKING: FROM DATA TO PLAN

Cutler P: Problem Solving in Clinical Medicine: From Data to Diagnosis, 2nd ed. Baltimore, Williams & Wilkins, 1985.

Kassirer JP: Diagnostic reasoning. Ann Intern Med 110:893, 1989.

Kassirer JP: Our stubborn quest for diagnostic certainty: A cause of excessive testing. N Engl J Med 320:1489, 1989.

CHAPTER 21. THE PATIENT'S RECORD

Burnum JF: The misinformation era: The fall of the medical record. Ann Intern Med 110:482, 1989.

Hurst JW, Walker HK (eds): The Problem-Oriented System. New York, Medcom Press, 1972.

Index

NOTE: A *t* following a page number indicates tabular material. Page numbers in **bold face** indicate color plates. Drugs are listed under their generic names. When a drug trade name is listed, the reader is referred to the generic name.

Acoustic (eighth cranial) nerve, function of, 511*t*
  nystagmus and, 635
  testing, 518
Acquired immunodeficiency syndrome (AIDS), Kaposi's sarcoma in, **152**
Acrocyanosis, at birth, 583
Acromegaly, facies in, 197*t*
Acromioclavicular arthritis, 496*t*
Acromion, 463
Actinic keratoses, 141, **152**
Acuity
  auditory, testing, 187–188
  visual
    in aging patients, 171
    testing, 172–173
Acute necrotizing gingivitis, 225*t*
Addison's disease, 65, 70
Adduction, at hip, testing, 527
Adductor tubercle, 467
Adenitis. *See also* Lymphadenitis
  cervical, 592
Adenoiditis, chronic, 608
Adenoids, 608–609
  abscess of, 608
  palpation of, 608–609
Adhesive capsulitis, 496*t*
Adie's pupil, 179, 204*t*
Adjustment disorder, with anxious mood, 116*t*
Adnexa, 387
  on bimanual examination, 397–398
  in pregnancy, 421
Adnexal masses, 398, 408*t*
Adolescents
  acne in, 169
  breast development in
    in females, 323–325
    in males, 326
  comedones in, 169
  genital development in
    in females, 387–389
    in males, 371–373
  growth spurt in, 129, 473
  head and neck changes in, 169
  interviewing, 25
  lymph nodes in, 440
  mental status changes in, 100
  musculoskeletal system in, 473
  pubertal changes in
    in females, 324
    in males, 373
  skin changes in, 140–141
Adrenal cortical hyperfunction, 65
Adult, comprehensive history in, 5–9
Adventitious lung sounds, 250, 255, 259*t*
Aerophagia, 47

Affect. *See also* Mood
  assessment of, 104
  definition of, 100
African Americans
  newborn, skin pigmentation in, 583
  normal ocular fundi in, **213**
  sclera in, 157
  skin and nails in, 140, 143–144
Afterload, 273
AGA. *See* Appropriate for gestational age
Aging patients
  abdominal changes in, 342
  abdominal pain in, 342
  accommodation in, 170
  asteatosis in, 141
  breasts in, 326
  brown macules in, 141
  cataracts in, 170
  colloid bodies of eye in, 170–171
  corneal arcus in, 170
  decreased sense of taste in, 171
  delirium in, 101
  dementia in, 101, 115*t*
    depression differentiated from, 115*t*
  diminished salivary secretions in, 171
  drusen in, 170–171
  dry eyes in, 170
  dry skin in, 141
  ears in, 170
  ectropion in, 170
  entropion in, 170
  extraocular movements in, 170
  eyes in, 170
  female genitalia in, 389
  fundus of eye in, 170–171, **214**
  gait in, 553*t*
  hair in, 142
  head and neck changes in, 169–171
  hearing in, 171
  height/growth/habitus in, 129, 131, 473–474
  interviewing, 25–26
  iris in, 170
  lens of eye in, 170
  lens opacities in, 170
  male genitalia in, 373
  mental status changes and, 101
  motor system in, 513
  mouth in, 170
  musculoskeletal changes in, 473–474
  nails in, 142
  nervous system assessment in, 512–513
  periodontal disease in, 171
  peripheral vascular system in, 440
  prostate gland in, 426
  reflexes in, 513
  resorption of bony ridges of jaw in, 171
  skin changes in, 141–142

  teeth in, 171
  tonsils in, 169–170
  vision in, 40, 171
  vitreous floaters in, 171
Agoraphobia, 116*t*
AIDS (acquired immunodeficiency syndrome), Kaposi's sarcoma in, **152**
Air conduction, 163, 518
Ala nasi, tenderness of, 189
Albinism, 146*t*
Alcoholism, and interviewing inebriated patients, 28–29
Alcohol use, interview questions about, 20–21
Allen test, 449–450
Allergic rhinitis, 42
  nasal mucosa in, 189
  perennial, facies in in children, 591*t*
"Allergic salute", 591*t*
"Allergic shiners", 591*t*
Alternating movements, rapid
  of arms, 530
  of legs, 531
Altitudinal (horizontal) visual field defect, 174, 198*t*
Alzheimer's disease, dementia caused by, 101, 118*t*
Amblyopia, 597
Amenorrhea, 56
  in pregnancy, 412*t*
  primary, 56
  secondary, 56
Amnestic syndrome, 118*t*
Anal canal, 425, 426
Anal fissure, 431*t*
Analgesia, definition of, 540
Anal reflex, in newborns, 628
Anarthria, 114*t*
Anemia, 65
  hemolytic
    jaundice caused by, 51
    maxillary overgrowth in, 608
  of pregnancy, 417
Anesthesia, definition of, 540
Aneurysm
  aortic, dissecting, chest pain in, 72–73*t*
  femoral, 443
  popliteal, 443
"Angel kisses", in newborns, 584
Anger, interviewing techniques and, 28
Angina pectoris, chest pain in, 72–73*t*
Angioedema, of lip, 223*t*
Angioma
  cherry, 141, **151**
  spider, **151**
Angle of Louis (sternal angle,), 231, 232
Angular stomatitis, 171, 222*t*
Anisocoria, pupillary reactions in, 178
Anisometropia, 597

Bile ducts, extrahepatic, jaundice caused by obstruction of, 52
Biliary colic, 78–79t
Bilirubin, in jaundice, 51–52
Bimanual examination, 396–398
  in children, 621
  in pregnant woman, 420–421
Biot's breathing, 256t
Bipolar disorder, 115t
Birth weight, newborn classified by, 566
Bisferiens pulse, 308t
Bismuth line, 226t
Bitemporal hemianopsia, 174, 198t
Black-heads. *See* Comedones
Black persons
  sclera in, 157
  skin and nails in, 140, 143–144
  newborn, skin pigmentation in, 583
  normal ocular fundi in, **213**
Bladder
  in infants, 615
  symptoms related to disorders of, 53
Bleeding
  generalized disorder of, 65
  from gums, 42
  intermenstrual, 57
  from nose (epistaxis), 42
  postcoital, 57
  postmenopausal, 57
  in stools, 50
  in urine, 54
Blepharitis, 176
Blind eye, pupil abnormalities in, 203t
Blindness
  legal, 173
  unilateral, 198t
    pupil abnormalities in, 203t
Blind patients, interviewing techniques and, 31–32
Blind spot, 158–159
Blink reflex
  absence of, 517
  acoustic, in newborns, 600, 628
  in newborns, 628
Blocking, 106t
Blood, coughing, 46
Blood pressure, 274–275
  abnormal, definition of, 284–285
  assessment of, 281–286
    in infants and children, 579–581
    in leg, 285–286
    special problems in, 285–286
  diastolic, 284
    age affecting, 278
    determining, 283
    in infants and children, 580
    normal, 285
  factors affecting, 274–275
  in infants and children, 579–581
    in females, 580
    in males, 580

normal, 285
  in pregnancy, 416
  systolic, 284
    age affecting, 278
    determining, 283
    estimating, 282
    in infants and children, 579, 580
    normal, 285
Blood pressure cuff, size of, 281, 282
  in infants and children, 579
Body frame, 132–133
Body habitus, 129
  aging affecting, 129, 131t, 473–474
  assessment of, 134
Body odors, assessment of, 136
Body temperature
  assessment of, 136–137
    in infants and children, 577
  normal, 137
    in infants and children, 577
Body weight, changes in, 37
Bone conduction, 163, 518
Borborygmi, 346
Bouchard's node, 491t
Boutonniere deformity, 491t
Bowel function, 50
Bowel sounds, 346, 364t
  in infants, 616
Bow legs, in infants and children, 622
Brachial pulse, 435
  assessment of, 281, 441
Brachioradialis reflex
  assessment of, 534
  spinal segments involved in, 504
Bradycardia, sinus, 304t, 306t
Bradykinesia, 506
Bradypnea, 256t
Brain, anatomy and physiology of, 501–502
Brainstem, 501, 502
Brain tumors
  headaches with, 68–69t
  in infants and children, 583
    Macewen's sign in, 587
Breasts
  female
    in adolescents, 323–325
      examination of, 329
    in adults, 325
    age affecting, 323–326
    in aging patients, 326
    anatomy and physiology of, 321–323
    in assessment of tactile fremitus, 252
    cancer of, 328–331, 336t, 337t
      differentiation of from other nodules, 337t
      risk factors and, 328
      visible signs of, 328–331, 336t

in children, 611
    consistency of, 332
    cysts of, 337t
    dimpling of, 329–331, 336t
    examination of, 124, 328–334
      inspection in, 328–331
      palpation in, 331–334
      in pregnancy, 417–418
    fatty tissue of, 322
    fibroadenoma of, 337t
    fibrous tissue of, 322
    glandular tissue of, 322
    in newborns, 610
    nodules in, 332–333
      differentiation of, 337t
    palpation of chest and, 253
    percussion of chest and, 253
    in pregnancy, 410
      examination of, 417–418
      tenderness of, 412t
    retraction of, 329–331, 336t
    in review of systems, 8
    supernumerary, 323
    symptoms related to, 43. *See also specific type*
    tenderness of, 332
    thickening of skin of, 329, 336t
  male, 323
    in adolescents, 326
    cancer of, 334
    examination of, 334
    in newborns, 610
Breathing (respiration), 238–240
  abdominal, in infants, 610
  abnormalities in rate and rhythm of, 256t
  assessment of, 241–242
  ataxic, 256t
  Biot's, 256t
  Cheyne-Stokes, 256t
  in children, 578, 611
  diaphragmatic, in infants and children, 578
  difficulty in, 44–45. *See also* Dyspnea
  in infants, 578, 605, 610
  normal, 256t
  obstructive, 256t
  "periodic", in infants, 610
  rapid deep, 256t
  rapid shallow, 256t
  sighing, 256t
  slow, 256t
  thoracic, in infants, 610
Breath odors, assessment of, 136
Breath sounds (lung sounds), 249–251, 255. *See also specific type*
  adventitious, 250–251, 255, 259t
  in airless lung, 258t
  characteristics of, 249t
  in children, 611

Corneal reflections, asymmetry of, 179
Corneal reflex
  in newborns, 595
  testing, 517
Corona of penis, 369, 370
Corpus luteum, in pregnancy, 413
Corticospinal tract, 505
  damage of, 506
Costal angle, 231
Costal cartilages, 232
Costal margin, 231, 339
Costochondral junctions, 231
Costovertebral angle, tenderness in, 357, 488
Cotton wool patches, 210t
  measurement of, 185
Cough, 45–46, 76t
  abdominal pain and, 350–351
Cough syncope, 94–95t
Cover test, 179, 205t
  in children, 597, 598–599
"Crabs." See Lice
Crackles, 250, 259t
  in infants, 610
Cramps, leg, 60
Cranial bones, in newborn, 586
Cranial nerves. See also specific type
  anatomy of, 502
  functions of, 511–512
    testing, 125, 514–519
      screening, 514
  in infants, 627
  tumor pressing on, vertigo caused by, 71t
Cranial vault, in infants, 586
Craniosynostosis, 587
Craniotabes, 587
Crepitus (crepitation), 475
  of patellofemoral compartment, 483
Crescendo-decrescendo murmurs, 300
Crescendo murmurs, 300
Crescents, around optic disc, 206t
Cretinism (congenital hypothyroidism)
  facies in, 590t
  in newborns
    and quality of cry, 605
    skin in, 583
Cricoid cartilage, 167
Crohn's disease, diarrhea in, 82–83t
Crossed straight leg-raising sign, 490
Cruciate ligaments, of knee, 467
Crude touch, fibers carrying sensation of, 508
Crust, 148t, **154**
Cry, quality of, in infants, 605
Crying, interviewing techniques and, 29
Cryptorchidism, 376, 381t, 620

Cuff, blood pressure, size of, 281, 282
  in infants and children, 579
Cupping of optic disc
  glaucomatous, 207t
  physiologic, 183, 206t
Current health status, 4
  in adults, 6–7
  in children, 11–12
  recording, 655–656
Curved nails, 149t
Cushing's syndrome, 65
  facies in, 197t
Cutaneous hyperesthesia, in appendicitis, 361
Cutis marmorata, 583
Cyanosis, 140, 143, 145t, 241
  in children with heart disease, 614
Cyclopentolate, for mydriasis in infants, 596
Cyclothymia, 115t
Cystitis, painful urination caused by, 53
Cystocele, 393, 402t
  in pregnancy, 420
Cystourethrocele, 402t
Cysts
  abdominal, in infants, 615
  Baker's, 487
  breast, 337t
  of epididymis, 380t
  Nabothian, 403t
  ovarian, 408t
  pilonidal, 431t
  porencephalic, transillumination in, 587
  retention
    cervical, 403t
    mucous, of lip, 223t
  sebaceous
    of ear, 219t
    scrotal, 380t
    of vulva, 321t
  thyroglossal duct, 588
Cytomegalic inclusion disease, and retinal changes in infants, 596

Dacryocystitis, 200t
  in infants, 596
Darwin's tubercle, 219t
Data
  identifying, in health history, 3–4
    in adults, 5
    in children, 9
  obtaining
    in health history interview, 17
    and interplay with assessment, 647–649
  planning and, 637–638
  quality of, 643–647
  unmanageable array of, 642

Date, in health history, 3, 5
Dazzle reflex (blink reflex)
  absence of, 517
  acoustic, in newborns, 600, 628
  in newborns, 628
DDST. See Denver Developmental Screening Test
Deafferented pupil, 203t
Deafness. See also Hearing loss (hearing impairment)
  "selective", 604
Decerebrate rigidity, 560t
Decorticate rigidity, 560t
Decrescendo murmurs, 300
Deep tendon reflexes, 503–504
  assessment of, 531–532
  in infants, 627–628
Deep veins, of legs, 437
Deep venous thrombosis, 446–447
Defervescence, 38
Degenerative joint disease (osteoarthritis). See also Arthritis
  crepitus in, 475
  hands involved in, 491t
  Heberden's nodes in, 478, 491t
  of knee, 483, 484
  pain in, 90–91t
Delayed ejaculation, 59
Delirium, 118t
  in aging patients, 101
  organic causes of, 118t
Delusions, 107t, 117t
  organic causes of, 118t
Demeanor, of clinician, in health history interview, 16
Dementia, 118t
  in aging patients, 101, 115t
    depression differentiated from, 115t
  organic causes of, 118t
Dental caries, 226t
  in children, 607
  "nursing bottle", 607
Dentate line, 425
Dentures, removal of for oral examination, 192
Denture sore mouth, 192
Denver Developmental Screening Test, 570, 571–572
Deoxyhemoglobin, color of skin affected by, 140, 145t
Depersonalization, feelings of, 107t
Depression
  in aging patients, 101, 115t
    dementia differentiated from, 115t
  causes of, 115t
  constipation and, 81t
  interviewing techniques and, 29
Depressive episode, major, 115t
Dermatitis, atopic, **154**

Hearing loss (hearing impairment), 40–41, 518
in aging patients, 171
in children
after otitis media, 604
screening for, 603–604
conduction, 40, 188, 220–221t
in infants, screening for, 600–601
interviewing techniques and, 31
patterns of, 220–221t
sensorineural, 40, 188, 220–221t
Heart. *See also* Cardiovascular system
anatomy of, 263–266
''base of'', 271
chambers of, anatomy of, 265–266
displacement of, 291
examination of, 288–303
auscultation in, 289, 295–301, 302. *See also* Cardiac auscultation
general approach to, 288–289
inspection in, 290
palpation in, 290–295
percussion in, 295
in pregnancy, 417
in infants and children, 612–614
as pump, 273–274
in review of systems, 8
Heart block
complete, 304t, 306t
second-degree, 304t, 306t
Heartburn, 47
in pregnancy, 412t
Heart disease, rheumatic, murmurs associated with, 614
Heart failure
left-sided
cough and hemoptysis in, 76t
dyspnea in, 74–75t
physical signs in, 260t
right-sided, edema caused by, 455t
Heart murmurs (cardiac murmurs), 270
age affecting, 277
aortic systolic, 277–278
attributes of, 298–301
auscultatory areas for detection of, 296
cervical systolic, 278
continuous, 300, 320t
diastolic, 299, 319t
ejection (midsystolic), 299, 316–317t
hemic, 613
holosystolic, 299, 318t
in infants and children, 613–614
innocent, 277, 301
in infants and children, 613
intensity of, 300–301
mechanisms of, 315t
midsystolic, 299, 316–317t
in newborns, 612
organic, 613–614

pansystolic, 299, 318t
pitch of, 301
in pregnancy, 417
quality of, 301
shape of, 300
systolic, 299, 316–317t, 318t
auscultation of, 298
of mitral regurgitation, 278
timing of, 299–300
Heart rate
assessment of, 279
in infants and children, 578
cardiac output affected by, 273
differentiation of, 304t
in infants and children, 518
Heart rhythm. *See also* Arrhythmias
assessment of, 279
differentiation of, 304t
irregular, 307t
regular, 305–306t
quadruple, 313t
Heart sounds, 289
auscultatory areas for detection of, 296
extra. *See also specific type*
in diastole, 313t
in systole, 312t
first, 268
auscultation of, 298
in infants and children, 612, 613
split, 270, 298, 310t
causes of, 314t
variations in, 310t
fourth, 268, 269, 313t
age affecting, 277
auscultation of, 298
palpable, 290, 293
and split S_1, 314t
relative intensity of, 289
second, 268
auscultation of, 298
in infants and children, 612, 613
split, 270, 298, 311t
age affecting, 277
variations in, 311t
splitting of, 269–270
third, 269, 313t
age affecting, 277
auscultation of, 298
palpable, 290, 293
timing of, 289
Heavy metal ingestion, gingival indications of, 607
Heberden's nodes, 478
Heels, walking on, for neurologic screening, 520
Heel-to-toe walking, for neurologic screening, 520
Hegar's sign, 411, 421

Height, 129
aging affecting, 129, 131t, 473
assessment of in infants and children, 581–582
Height spurt
in adolescent females, 389
in adolescent males, 373
Height/weight table for adults, 132t
in girls and boys, 563–564
Helix of ear, nodule in, 219t
Hemangioma, capillary, in newborns, 584
Hematemesis, 50
Hematochezia, 50
Hematologic system
in review of systems, 9
symptoms related to, 64–65. *See also specific type*
Hematoma, subdural
chronic, 68–69t
in infants and children, 583
and retinal hemorrhages in infants, 595
Hematuria, 54
Hemianopsia
bitemporal, 174, 198t
homonymous, 174, 198t
Hemic murmurs, 613
Hemiparesis
definition of, 525
spastic, 552t
Hemiplegia
abnormal postures in, 560t
congenital, nervous system findings in, 633
definition of, 525–526
flaccid, 545–546
and weak dorsiflexion, 526
Hemolytic anemia
jaundice caused by, 51
maxillary overgrowth in, 608
Hemoptysis, 46, 76t
Hemorrhages
pontine, small fixed pupils caused by, 204t
preretinal, 209t
retinal, 209t
in hypertensive retinopathy, **214**
in newborns, 595
scleral, in newborns, 595
splinter, in nail bed, 149t
subarachnoid, and retinal hemorrhages in infants, 595
subconjunctival, 201t
in infants, 595
subhyaloid, 209t
Hemorrhoids
external, 432t
internal, 432t
in pregnancy, 420

Hepatic bruit, 364t
Hepatic friction rub, 364t
Hepatojugular reflux (abdominojugular test), 288
Hepatomegaly, 367–368t
  abdominal pain and tenderness in, 365t
  irregular, 368t
  palpation in assessment of, 351–353
  percussion in assessment of, 346–348
  smooth nontender, 368t
  smooth tender, 268
Hernia
  constipation in, 81t
  diaphragmatic, in infants, 614
  epigastric, 362t
  femoral
    in females, 400
    in males, 371, 383t
      assessment of, 377–378
      course and presentation of, 382
  of groin
    in females, 400
    in males
      course and presentation of, 382
      differentiation of, 383t
      examination of, 377–378
  incarcerated, 378
  incisional, 361, 362t
  inguinal, 371, 383t
    assessment of, 377–378
    in children, 620
    direct, 383t
      course and presentation of, 382
    indirect
      in females, 400
      in males, 376, 383t
      in infants, hydrocele and, 619
  scrotal, 380t
  strangulated, 378
  umbilical, 361, 362t
    in infants, 615
  ventral, 362t
    assessment of, 361
    in infants, 615
Herniated fat, of eyelid, 199t
Herpes simplex infection
  genital
    penis involved in, 379t
    vulva involved in, 401t
  of lip, 222t
Heterochromia, in Horner's syndrome, 204t
"Hip pain", 60
Hips, 469–470
  abduction of, testing, 527
  in children, 625
  congenitally dislocated, 623–624
  flexion at, testing, 527

in infants, 623–624
  movements of, 470
    assessment of, 485–486
Hirschberg test, 597–598
Hirschsprung's disease, in infants, 615
Hirsutism, 172
History, 3–12. See also Interview
  in adults, 5–9
  in children, 9–12
  confusing, 29–30
  content of, 4–14
  family, 4
    in adults, 7
    in children, 12
    recording, 656–657
  past, 4
    in adults, 6
    in children, 10–11
    recording, 655
  pregnancy, 413–414
  psychosocial, 4
    in adults, 7
    recording, 657
  recording, 654–657
  sexual, 21–22
  structure of, 3–4
Hoarseness, 42–43, 518
Hodgkin's disease, lymphadenopathy in children caused by, 593
Holosystolic murmurs, 299, 318t
Homonymous hemianopsia, 174, 198t
Homonymous quadrantic defect, 174, 198t
"Hooking technique", 353
Hopping, for neurologic screening, 520
Hordeolum, acute, 200t
Horizontal visual field defect, 174, 198t
Horner's syndrome
  ptosis in, 199t, 204t
  pupillary abnormalities in, 204t
Hostility, interviewing techniques and, 28
Hot flushes (hot flashes), 57
Housemaid's knee, 482
Houston, valves of, 425, 426
Hum, jugular venous, 278
Humerus, greater tubercle of, 463
Huntington's disease, 555t
Hutchinson's teeth, 226t, 590t
Hydrocele, 376, 380t
  in infants, 619
  transillumination of, 377
Hydrocephalus, 583
Hydrocephaly, 587, 589t
Hygiene, personal, assessment of, 103–104, 135–136
Hymen
  imperforate, 399
  in infants, 619

Hyoid bone, 167
Hypalgesia, definition of, 540
Hyperalgesia, definition of, 540
Hyperemesis, and weight loss in pregnancy, 416
Hyperesthesia
  cutaneous, in appendicitis, 361
  definition of, 540
Hyperkinetic impulse, 293, 309t
Hyperopia (farsightedness), 40
  headaches with, 66–67t
  ophthalmoscopic examination in, 182, 183
Hyperperistalsis, 346
Hyperpnea, 256t
Hyperpyrexia, 136
Hyperreactive reflexes, 532, 538
Hyperresonance, 247, 253
  characteristics of, 247t
Hypertension
  in aging patients, 278
  definition of, 284–285
  in infants and children, 579, 580–581
  portal, in infants, 615, 616
  pregnancy-induced, 416, 422
  pulmonary, pulsations in, 295
  retinal arterioles in, 208t
Hypertensive retinopathy
  with macular star, **215**
  ocular fundus in, **214**
Hyperthyroidism
  bruits in, 196
  in children, facies in, 591t
  convergence in, 180
  exophthalmos and, 199t
  hair in, 172
  lid lag in, 180
  signs of, 229t
  symptoms of, 229t
Hypertrophic cardiomyopathy, murmurs in, 317t
Hypertrophy, definition of, 524
Hyperventilation, 256t
  and anxiety, dyspnea in, 74–75t
  hypocapnia caused by, 94–95t
Hypesthesia, definition of, 540
Hypoactive sexual desire disorder
  in females, 58
  in males, 59
Hypoalbuminemia, edema caused by, 455t
Hypocalcemic tetany, in infants and children, 587
Hypocapnia, 94–95t
Hypogastric pain, 48
Hypogastric area, 340
Hypoglossal (twelfth cranial) nerve
  function of, 512t
    in infants, 627
    testing, 519

Interview. *See also* History
  age of patient affecting style of, 23–26
  and approach to present illness, 14–16
  of children, 24–25, 570–573
  clinician's demeanor during, 16
  closing, 22–23
  environment for, 12–13
  note taking during, 13–14
  obtaining data for, 17
  reviewing chart before, 12
  review of systems and, 18–19
  sensitive topics in, 19–22
  setting stage for, 12–14
  special problems in, 26–33
  transitions in, 18
Intestinal obstruction
  in infants, 616
  mechanical, 81*t*
Intoxicated patients, interviewing, 28–29
Intracranial pressure, increased, in
      infants, 586
Intraductal papilloma, 334
Introitus
  examination of, 392
  parous relaxation of, 420
  small, 399
Intussusception, constipation in, 81*t*
Involuntary movements, 64, 554–556.
      See also specific type
  assessment of, 523
Iridectomy, pupillary irregularity caused
      by, 203*t*
Iris, 157
  in aging patients, 170
  examination of, 178
    in newborns, 596
  innervation of, 160
Iris lesion, **153**
Iritis, acute, 201*t*
Irritable bowel syndrome
  constipation in, 81*t*
  diarrhea in, 82–83*t*
Irritants, cough and hemoptysis caused
      by, 76*t*
Itching, 39
  in eyes/nose/throat, 42
  in jaundiced patients, 52
  vulvovaginal, 57

Jacksonian seizures, 96*t*
Jaundice, 51–52
  assessment of, 143, 146*t*
  in newborns, 584
  physiologic, in newborns, 584
Jaw, 166
  resorption of bony ridges of in aging
      patients, 171

Joints. *See also specific type*
  crepitus and, 475
  deformities of, 476
  degenerative disease of (osteoarthritis).
      See also Arthritis
    crepitus in, 475
    hands involved in, 491*t*
    Heberden's nodes in, 478, 491*t*
    of knee, 483, 484
    pain in, 90–91*t*
  examination of, 475–490
  increase in mobility of, 475
  inflammation of, 475
  limitation of motion of, 61, 475
    describing, 490
  pain in, 60–61, 90–91*t*
  stiffness of, 61
  structure and function of, 459
  tenderness/warmth/redness of, 62
Judgment
  assessment of, 108
  definition of, 99–100
Jugular veins, 168
  examination of, 196, 275–277, 286–
      288
Jugular venous hum, 278
Jugular venous pressure, 275–277, 286–
      288
Jugular venous pulsations, 275–277, 288
  carotid pulsations differentiated from,
      287*t*
JVP. *See* Jugular venous pressure

Kaposi's sarcoma, in AIDS, **152**
Kawasaki's disease, lymphadenopathy in
      children caused by, 593
Keloid, 148*t*
  of ear, 219*t*
Keratoses
  actinic (senile), 141, **152**
  seborrheic, 141, **152**
Kernicterus, nervous system findings in,
      633
Kernig's sign, 542, 593
Kidney pain, 53
Kidneys, 340, 341
  enlargement of, 356
  left
    enlargement of, versus enlarged
        spleen, 355–356, 356–357
    palpation of, 356–357
  palpation of, 356–357
  right, palpation of, 356
  tenderness of, 357
Klinefelter's syndrome, small testes in,
      381*t*
Knee bend, for neurologic screening, 520
Kneecap. *See* Patella

Knee reflex
  in aging patients, 513
  assessment of, 534–535
  in pregnancy, 422
  spinal segments involved in, 504
Knees, 467–469
  examination of, 481–485
    inspection in, 481
  extension at, testing, 528
  flexion at, testing, 528
  fluid in, 482–483
  housemaid's, 482
  knock, in infants and children, 622
  movements of, 469
    assessment of, 485
  swelling of, 482
Knock-knees, in infants and children,
      622
Koilonychia, 149*t*
Koplik's spots, 605–606
Korotkoff sounds, 283
  weak or inaudible, 286
Kyphoscoliosis, thoracic, 257*t*
Kyphosis, 240, 499*t*
  of aging, 473

Labia
  in aging patients, 389
  enlargement of, in pregnancy, 420
  majora, 385
  minora, 385
    examination of, 392
    fusion of, 620
    in infants, 619
  varicosities of in pregnancy, 420
Labyrinthitis, acute, 71*t*
Lacrimal apparatus, examination of, 176
      Lacrimal gland, 157
  enlargement of, 200*t*
Lacrimal puncta, 157
Lacrimal sac, 157
  inflammation of, 200*t*
Lactation
  mammary souffle and, 277
  milky discharge after, 333
Lactose intolerance, diarrhea in, 82–83*t*
Language
  assessment of, 104–105
  definition of, 100
Language barriers, in interviewing, 31
Lanugo, 583
Large for gestational age
  definition of, 567
  mortality rate and, 567
Laryngitis, cough and hemoptysis in, 76*t*
Last menstrual period, 414
Lateral collateral ligament, of knee, 467

Lung sounds (breath sounds) (*continued*)
  in infants, 610–611
  intensity of, 250
  listening to, 250
  normal, 258*t*
Lymphadenitis. *See also* Adenitis
  acute anterior cervical, 592
  acute posterior cervical, 592
Lymphadenopathy, 442
  cervical
    in children, 592–593
    in infants, 588
  occipital, in children, 593
Lymphangitis, acute, 88–89*t*
Lymphatics, 438–439
  of breast, 326–327
  of female genitalia, 387
  of male genitalia, 370
Lymphatic stasis, edema and, 456*t*, 457*t*
Lymphedema, 456*t*, 457*t*
  of arm, 441
Lymph nodes, 438–439
  of arm, 438
  auricular, posterior, examination of, 194
  axillary, 326–327, 438, 439
    breast nodules differentiated from, 332
    enlarged, 335
    examination of, 124, 335
  cervical, 168–169
    in children, 592–593
    examination of, 193–195
    in infants, 588
  in children, 592–593
  by ears, 219*t*
  epitrochlear, 438, 439
    enlargement of, 442
    examination of, 124, 442
  female genitalia draining to, 387
  hard or fixed, 194
  of head and neck, 168–169
    examination of, 193–195
  infraclavicular, 438
  inguinal, 438, 439
    female genitalia draining to, 387
    male genitalia draining to, 370
    palpation of, 442
  lateral, examination of, 335
  occipital, examination of, 194
  pectoral, 326
    examination of, 335
  preauricular, 438
    examination of, 194
  submaxillary, 168, 169
    examination of, 194
  submental, 169
    examination of, 194

subscapular, 326
supraclavicular, 168
  enlargement of, 194
  examination of, 194
tender, 194
tonsillar, 168, 169
  carotid artery mistaken for, 194
  examination of, 194
Lymphoma, non-Hodgkin's, lymphadenopathy in children caused by, 593

Macewen's sign, 587
Macula, 157–158
  examination of, 184
  microaneurysms of, 209*t*
  senile degeneration of, 184
Macular star, **215**
Macule, 147*t*, **153**
  brown, in aging patients, 141
Major depressive episode, 115*t*
Malabsorption syndromes, diarrhea in, 82–83*t*
Male genitalia, 369–383. *See also specific structure*
  in adolescents, 371–373
  age affecting, 371–373
  in aging patients, 373
  anatomy and physiology of, 369, 370–371
  in children, 620
  examination of, 125, 374–378
    sexual development assessment, 374
  in infants, 619
  in review of systems, 8
  symptoms related to, 58–60. *See also specific type*
Malignant melanoma, of skin, **152**
Malleolus
  lateral, 466
  medial, 466
Malleus, 161, 162
  examination of, 187
Malnutrition, 38
  in infants, 570
Malocclusion, 607–608
Mammary duct ectasia, 332
Mammary souffle, 277
Mandible, 167
Mandibular protrusion, 607–608
Mania, causes of, 115*t*
Manic episode, 115*t*
Manual compression test, 448
Manubrium, 231
Marcus Gunn pupil, 203*t*
Mask of pregnancy, 145, 417
Masseter muscles, palpating, 516
Mastoiditis, in children, 603–604

Mastoid process, 161, 162
  lymph nodes near, 219*t*
Maxillary protrusion, 607–608
Maxillary sinuses, 165
  tenderness of, 190
  transillumination of, 191
    in children, 607
Maximal rate of expiration, age affecting, 240
MCP. *See* Metacarpophalangeal joint
Meatus, urethral (urethral orifice)
  in females, 385
    examination of, 392
    in infants, 619
  in males, 369, 370
    examination of, 375
Medial collateral ligament, of knee, 467
Medial epicondylitis, 494*t*
Median nerve
  distribution of, 509, 510
  weak opposition of thumb in disorders of, 527
Mediastinal crunch, 259*t*
Medical model, limitations of, 641
Medulla, 502
Medullated nerve fibers, of optic disc, 206*t*
Megacephaly, 587
Megacolon, congenital, 615
Meibomian glands, 157
  inflammatory lesions of (chalazion), 200*t*
Melanin, color of skin affected by, 140, 145*t*, 146*t*
Melanin pigmentation, of gums, 226*t*
Melanoma, malignant, of skin, **152**
Melasma, 145, 417
Melena, 50, 80*t*
Memory
  assessment of, 70, 108–110
  and "benign forgetfulness", 101
  definition of, 99
Menarche, 56, 325, 388–389
  imperforate hymen delaying, 399
Meniere's disease, 71*t*
Meningeal irritation, 68–69*t*
  in children, 593–594
Meningeal signs, 542–543
Menopause, 57
Menorrhagia, 56
Menstrual period, last, 414
Menstruation, 56–57
  absence of, 56
  cessation of, 389
  pain related to, 57
Mental retardation
  in Down's syndrome, 591*t*
  interviewing techniques and, 30–31

Muscles
    atrophy of, 523–525
    bulk of, assessment of, 523–525
    hypotonic (flaccid), 525
    skeletal, in aging patients, 474
    strength of
        assessment of, 525–529
        in trunk, 527
    tone of, assessment of, 525
    weakness of, 38, 64
Muscle stretch reflexes, 503
Muscle wasting. *See also* Atrophy
    in aging patients, 512–513
Muscular dystrophy, 634
Muscular guarding, 350
    in aging patients, 342
Musculoskeletal system, 459–500. *See also specific structure*
    in adolescents, 473
    age affecting, 473–474
    in aging patients, 473–474
    anatomy and physiology of, 459–474
    in children, 625–626
    examination of, 475–490
        approach to, 125, 475–476
        in patient lying down, 480–487
        in sitting patient, 476–479
        special maneuvers for, 488–490
        in standing patient, 487–488
    in infants, 621–625
    in review of systems, 9
    symptoms related to, 60–63, 90–93t. *See also specific type*
Mushrooms, anticholinergic, dilated fixed pupils caused by, 204t
Myalgias, 61
Mycoplasma pneumonia, cough and hemoptysis in, 76t
Mydriacyl. *See* Tropicamide
Mydriasis, 178
    contraindications to, 180
    for ophthalmoscopic examination, 180
    in infants, 596
Myocardial contractility, 273
Myocardial infarction
    chest pain in, 72–73t
    syncope in, 94–95t
Myoclonus, 97t, 556t
Myomata, uterine, in pregnancy, 421
Myopathy, proximal weakness and, 527
Myopia (nearsightedness), 40, 172
    ophthalmoscopic examination in, 182, 183
Myringitis, bullous, **217**
Myxedema, facies in, 197t

Nabothian cysts, 403t
Nails, 139
    abnormalities and variations of, 149t

in aging patients, 142
    assessment of, 144
Nares, 164
Narrow-angle glaucoma, 170, 178
Nasal atresia, posterior, 568
Nasal breathers, obligate, 604
Nasal cavity. *See also* Nose
    anatomy of, 164
    functions of, 164
    inspection of, 164–165
Nasal mucosa, examination of, 189
Nasal obstruction, 189
    in infants, 604
Nasal polyps, 190
Nasal septum, 164
    deviation of, 189
    examination of, 189–190
    perforation of, 190
Nasal speculum, 189
Nasal stuffiness, 42
Nasal ulcers, 190
Nasolabial fold, flattening of, 517
Nasolacrimal duct obstruction
    assessment of, 176
    in infants, 596
Nausea, 49
    in pregnancy, 412t
Navel, failure of to heal, 615
Near gaze, pupillary constriction with, 160
Near reaction, 160, 179, 515
Nearsightedness (myopia), 40, 172
    ophthalmoscopic examination in, 182, 183
Near syncope, 63
Near vision, testing, 173
Neck, 155–229. *See also* Head
    in adolescents, 169
    age affecting, 169–171
    in aging patients, 169–171
    anatomy and physiology of, 167–169
    examination of, 123, 193–196
        of cervical spine, 477
        in pregnancy, 417
    great vessels of, 168
    in infants, 588
    lymph nodes of, 168–169
        in children, 592–593
        examination of, 193–195
    mobility of, in infants and children, 593–594
    movement at, 471–472
    pain in, 63, 93t
    in review of systems, 8
    survey of, 193
    symptoms related to, 42–43. *See also specific type*
Negative predictive value, of observation or test, 644–647

Neisseria gonorrhoeae. See also under Gonococcal *and* Gonorrhea
    cervicitis caused by, 404t
    pelvic inflammatory disease caused by, 408t
Neologisms, 106t
Neovascularization, in retina, 209t
Nephrotic syndrome, facies in, 197t
Nerve fibers, medullated, of optic disc, 206t
Nerve roots
    peripheral, position sense affected by lesions of, 541
    posterior, 503
Nervousness, assessment of, 70
Nervous system (neurologic system), 501–560. *See also specific structure*
    age affecting, 512–513
    anatomy and physiology of, 501–513
    disease indicators and, in infants and children, 633–635
    examination of, 125–126, 514–547
        screening, 125, 520–523
            in infants, 626
        special maneuvers for, 542–547
    in infants, 626–633
    in review of systems, 9
    symptoms related to, 63–64, 94–97t. *See also specific type*
Neuralgia, trigeminal, 68–69t
Neurofibromatosis, **154**
Neurologic disorders, constipation in, 81t
Neurologic screening examination, 125, 520–523
    in infants, 626
Neuronitis, vestibular, 71t
Neuropathy, peripheral, vibration sense affected in, 540
Neurotrophic ulcer, on foot, 498t
Nevus, 148t
    flammeus, 584
    telangiectatic, 584
    vasculosus, 584
Newborns. *See also* Infants
    classification of, 566–567
    definition of, 566
    examination of, 566–569
    eyes in, 594–597
    skin in, 583–584
New learning ability, assessment of, 110
Night sweats, 38
Nipples
    in females, 321, 323
        in aging patients, 326
        discharge from, 43, 329, 333–334
        inspection of, 329–331
        in pregnancy, 417
        Paget's disease of, 336t

Otitis
externa, 603
ear canal in, 187
pain in, 186, 603
media, 603
eardrum in, 187
hearing loss after, 604
mobility of eardrum in, 187, 603
pain in, 186, 603
with purulent effusion, **217**
serous, **217**, 603
Otoscope
for children, 603
nasal examination with, 189
pneumatic
for children, 603
mobility of eardrum evaluated with, 187
Ovaries, 387
in aging patients, 389, 397–398
on bimanual examination, 397–398
cysts of, 408*t*
function of, in aging patients, 389
infection of, 408*t*
in pregnancy, 413
tumors of, 408*t*
Overanxious disorder, 116*t*
Overbite, 607–608
Overflow incontinence, 86–87*t*
Overtalkative patients, interviewing techniques for, 27
Overweight patients, 37
Oxyhemoglobin, color of skin affected by, 140, 143, 145*t*, 146*t*

P$_2$ component of second heart sound, 270
abnormalities of, 311*t*
auscultation of, 298
Paget's disease, of nipple, 336*t*
Pain
abdominal, 48–49
back, 62, 92*t*
chest, 43–44, 72–73*t*
chest wall, 72–73*t*
in ear, 41
epigastric, 48
facial, testing for, 516
hypogastric, 48
neck, 63, 93*t*
parietal, 48
periumbilical, 48
pleural, 72–73*t*
referred, 48–49
rest, 88–89*t*
sacral, 48

sensation of
assessment of, 540
in infants, 627
fibers carrying, 507
suprapubic, 48
visceral, 48
Palate
cleft, 609
hard, 166
abnormalities of, 224*t*
examination of, 192
in newborns, 604–605
paralysis of, 518
soft, 166
in newborns, 604
weakness of, 518
Pallor
in chronic arterial insufficiency, 450
in newborns, 583
in ulnar arterial occlusion, 450
Palmar grasp reflex, 628
Palmar space infections, 492*t*
Palpation. *See specific system or structure*
Palpebral conjunctiva, 156
examination of, 176–177
upper, examination of, 177
Palpebral fissure, 156
Palpitations, 44
Palsy. *See also* Paralysis
Bell's, 518, 550*t*
facial nerve, in children, 590*t*
Pancreas, 341
cancer of, abdominal pain in, 78–79*t*
Pancreatitis
acute, abdominal pain and tenderness in, 78–79*t*, 366*t*
chronic, abdominal pain and tenderness in, 78–79*t*
Panic disorder, 116*t*
Pansystolic murmurs, 299, 318*t*
Papanicolaou smears, obtaining specimens for, 395–396
in pregnant woman, 416, 420
Papilledema, 207*t*
in infants, 596
and measurement of elevated optic disc, 185
Papilloma, intraductal, 334
Papule, 147*t*, **153**
Paradoxical pulse, 303, 308*t*
Paralysis, 64. *See also* Palsy
definition of, 525
facial, 518
in children, 590*t*
types of, 550–551*t*
flaccid, in coma, 545–546
of palate, 518
Paralytic strabismus, 205*t*

Paranasal sinuses. *See also specific type*
anatomy of, 165
examination of, 123, 190–191
in review of systems, 8
symptoms related to, 42. *See also specific type*
transillumination of, 190–191
Paranoid disorder, 117*t*
Paraphasias, 104
Paraphimosis, 375
Paraplegia
definition of, 526
spastic, scissoring in, 629, 630
Parasternal impulse, palpation of, 290
Parasternal muscles, in breathing, 239
Parasympathetic nervous system, innervation of eye and, 160–161
Paraurethral glands, 385
Paravertebral muscles, examination of, 488
Parental deprivation, 570
Parent-child interaction, assessment of, 573
Parent-infant interaction, assessment of, 569–570
Parents, interviewing, 23–24
Paresis, definition of, 525
Paresthesias, 64
Parietal cortex, lesion of, 515
Parietal pain, 48
Parkinsonism, differentiation of, 557*t*
Parkinson's disease
differentiation of, 557*t*
facies in, 197*t*
gait in, 553*t*
Paronychia, 149*t*
Parotid ducts, 166
Parotid gland, 155
enlargement of in children
assessment of, 592
facies in, 197*t*
Paroxysmal auricular tachycardia, 578
Paroxysmal nocturnal dyspnea, 45
Pars
flaccida, 162, 163
examination of, 187
tensa, 162, 163
examination of, 187
Partial seizures, 96–97*t*
Passive stretch, resistance to, 525
Past history, 4
in adults, 5
in children, 10–11
recording, 655
Past pointing, 531
Patch, 147*t*, **154**
Patella, 467
"floating", ballottement of, 483

Stroke volume
  cardiac output affected by, 273
  definition of, 273
Stupor, 113t. *See also* Coma
  assessment of, 543–547
Sturge-Weber syndrome, 584
Sty, 200t
Subacromial bursa, 465
Subarachnoid hemorrhage, and retinal
    hemorrhages in infants, 595
Subconjunctival hemorrhage, 201t
  in infants, 595
Subcutaneous tissues, 139
Subdural effusion, transillumination in,
    587
Subdural hematoma
  chronic, 68–69t
  in infants and children, 583
  and retinal hemorrhages in infants,
    595
Subhyaloid hemorrhage, 209t
Submandibular gland, 155
Submaxillary gland, 155
  ducts of, 166
Submaxillary lymph nodes, 168, 169
  examination of, 194
Submental lymph nodes, 169
  examination of, 194
Submucosal cleft palate, 609
Subscapular lymph nodes, 326
Subscapularis muscle, 465
Subtalar joint, motions at, 466
  assessment of, 481
Subxiphoid area, palpation of, 294–295
Sudden Infant Death Syndrome, 578,
    610
Summation gallop, 313t
Superficial infrapatellar bursa, 468
Superficial peroneal nerve, distribution
    of, 509, 510
Superficial temporal artery, 155
Superficial veins, of legs, 437
Superior vena cava, anatomy of, 265
Supernumerary breasts, 323
Supernumerary nipples, 323, 610
Supinator reflex
  assessment of, 534
  spinal segments involved in, 504
Supraclavicular, definition of, 235
Supraclavicular lymph nodes, 168
  enlargement of, 194
  examination of, 194
Suprapatellar pouch, 482
  palpation of, 482
Suprapubic pain, 48
Suprapubic area, 340
Supraspinatus muscle, 464
Suprasternal notch, 231

Supraventricular premature contractions,
    304t, 307t
Supraventricular tachycardia, 304t, 305t
Survey, general, 123, 129–137
  anatomy and physiology relevant to,
    129–133
  examination techniques in, 134–137
  in infants and children, 576–583
Sutures (cranial), 585–586
  premature closure of, 582
Swallowing
  difficulty in. *See* Dysphagia
  pain on. *See* Odynophagia
Swan neck deformity, 491t
S wave, of electrocardiogram, 272
Sweat glands, 139–140
Sweating, in thyroid dysfunction, 70
Swelling
  of feet and legs, in peripheral vascular
    disease, 60
  of joints, 61
Swinging flashlight test, for Marcus
    Gunn pupil, 203t
Sydenham's chorea, 555t
Sympathetic nerves, innervation of eye
    and, 161
Symphysis pubis, 339
Symptoms, 35–97. *See also specific type
    and structure affected*
  general, 37–39
    in musculoskeletal disorders, 62
  mental status screening and, 70
  multiple, interviewing techniques and,
    27–28
  related to breasts, 43
  related to chest, 43–46, 72–76t
  related to ears, 40–41, 71t
  related to endocrine system, 65–70
  related to eyes, 39–40
  related to female genital system, 55–58
  related to gastrointestinal tract, 46–52,
    77–83t
  related to head, 39, 66–69t
  related to hematologic system, 64–65
  related to male genital system, 58–60
  related to mouth, 42–43
  related to musculoskeletal system, 60–
    63, 90–93t
  related to neck, 42–43
  related to nervous system, 63–64, 94–
    97t
  related to nose, 42
  related to peripheral vascular system,
    60, 88–89t
  related to sinuses, 42
  related to skin, 39
  related to throat, 42–43
  related to urinary tract, 53–55, 84–87t

Syncope, 63, 94–95t
  in aging patients, 278
Synovial inflammation, 482 Synovial
    membrane, 459
Synovitis, 475
Syphilis
  chancre of
    on lip, 222t
    on penis, 379t
    on vulva, 401t
  congenital
    craniotabes and, 587
    facies in, 590t
  Hutchinson's teeth in, 226t
  neural, Argyll-Robertson pupils in,
    204t
  secondary, vulva affected in, 401t
Syringomyelia
  motor changes associated with, 559t
  sensory deficit and, 559t
Systemic venous pressure, 275–276
Systems, review of, 4, 7–9, 18–19
  recording, 657–658
Systole, 267, 268
  extra heart sounds in, 312t. *See also
    specific type*
  auscultation of, 298
Systolic blood pressure, 284
  age affecting, 278
  determining, 283
  estimating, 282
  in infants and children, 579, 580
  normal, 285
Systolic clicks, 312t
  auscultation of, 298
  early, and split S_1, 314t
Systolic ejection sounds, early, 268, 312t
Systolic hypertension, in aging patients,
    278
Systolic murmurs, 299, 316–317t, 318t
  aortic, 277
  auscultation of, 298
  cervical, 278
  innocent, 277, 301
  of mitral regurgitation, 278

Tabes dorsalis, and Argyll-Robertson
    pupils, 204t
Tachycardias. *See also specific type*
  differentiation of, 304t, 305t
  in infants and children, 578
Tachypnea, 256t
Tactile fremitus
  in airless lung, 258t
  assessment of, 243–244, 252
  in children, 611
  in infants, 610
  normal, 258t

ISBN 0-397-54781-1

9 780397 547814

90000